SLEEP APNEA

LUNG BIOLOGY IN HEALTH AND DISEASE

Executive Editor

Claude Lenfant
Director, National Heart, Lung and Blood Institute
National Institutes of Health
Bethesda, Maryland

ADDITIONAL VOLUMES IN PREPARATION

The opinions expressed in these volumes do not necessarily represent the views of the National Institutes of Health.

SLEEP APNEA
IMPLICATIONS IN CARDIOVASCULAR AND CEREBROVASCULAR DISEASE

Edited by

T. Douglas Bradley

*Toronto General Hospital
of the University Health Network
Toronto Rehabilitation Institute
and Mount Sinai Hospital
University of Toronto
Toronto, Ontario, Canada*

John S. Floras

*Mount Sinai Hospital
and Toronto General Hospital
of the University Health Network
University of Toronto
Toronto, Ontario, Canada*

MARCEL

DEKKER

MARCEL DEKKER, INC.   NEW YORK · BASEL

ISBN: 0-8247-0299-9

This book is printed on acid-free paper.

Headquarters
Marcel Dekker, Inc.
270 Madison Avenue, New York, NY 10016
tel: 212-696-9000; fax: 212-685-4540

Eastern Hemisphere Distribution
Marcel Dekker AG
Hutgasse 4, Postfach 812, CH-4001 Basel, Switzerland
tel: 41-61-261-8482; fax: 41-61-261-8896

World Wide Web
http://www.dekker.com

The publisher offers discounts on this book when ordered in bulk quantities. For more information, write to Special Sales/Professional Marketing at the headquarters address above.

INTRODUCTION

*Interest in sleep and disease has existed since the dawn of history.
Perhaps only love and human conflict have received more attention
from poets and writers.*

William C. Dement (1)

Indeed, one can find comments about sleep in the writings of Aristotle, Galen, and Hippocrates among others. However, closer to our times, much credit must go to William Shakespeare on the one hand and Charles Dickens on the other for having stimulated a new interest in sleep and its disorders.

Shakespeare must have been fascinated by sleep. One of his heroes was Sir John Falstaff, who had an important part in several plays. His behavior in one of them (*Henry IV*) is strongly reminiscent of sleep apnea, but, admittedly, alcohol may also have influenced his irregular sleep. Elsewhere, Shakespeare presents to us another aspect of sleep disorder: parasomnia. In *Macbeth*, Lady Macbeth exhibits much sleepwalking and also sleep-talking.

But it is surely Charles Dickens and his character Samuel Pickwick who brought to public light the problems of sleep disorders. Indeed, it has been reported that Dickens' ''sleep pathology was often better than that of the doctors of his time'' (2).

Today, sleep and its disorders have moved from being the object of literary considerations to being an area of scientific inquiry that attracts basic scientists as well as clinical investigators. Since the publication of the first monograph in

1976, the Lung Biology in Health and Disease series has included three volumes with "sleep" in their title and five others that have significant sections on sleep and its disorders. Such an abundance reflects the huge interest of the biomedical community in this topic and, in particular, the recognition that sleep disorders are a major public health problem that affects all strata of society.

The clinical expressions of sleep disorders are many, but there is one biological system in which they have huge immediate and long-term consequences, that is, the cardiovascular system. Surprisingly, this impact has been recognized only very slowly, and we should not hide the fact that its recognition is far from universal!

Sleep Apnea: Implications in Cardiovascular and Cerebrovascular Disease, edited by T. Douglas Bradley and John S. Floras, is unique because of its focus and the comprehensiveness of its presentation. The editors have assembled a roster of authors who have devoted years of investigation to many aspects of the impact of sleep apnea on the cardiovascular system. Undoubtedly, other researchers will be challenged by this text, but just as important—if not more important—this volume will increase awareness of the problem and thus benefit patients.

As editor of the Lung Biology in Health and Disease series, I am proud to present this volume, and grateful to Drs. Bradley and Floras and their contributors for this opportunity.

Claude Lenfant, M.D.
Bethesda, Maryland

References

1. Dement WC. History of sleep physiology and medicine. In: Kryger M, Roth T, Dement WC, eds. Principles and Practice of Sleep Medicine. 2nd ed. Philadelphia: WB Saunders, 1994:3–15.
2. Johnston AJ. A Pickwick Portrait Galley. London: Chapman and Hall, 1936:188.

PREFACE

I sleep, but my heart waketh.

Song of Solomon, ch 5 v 2

As alluded to in the above passage, the onset of sleep should herald relaxation of the cardiovascular system, and autonomic neural quiescence. When this pacific state is disrupted, the heart and circulation may not enjoy fully the restorative effects of sleep. Apnea, a condition common in patients with cardiovascular and cerebrovascular disease, not only disrupts sleep but places direct mechanical and neurohumoral stresses on the heart and vasculature. In some instances, these can exceed those experienced during active wakefulness. Nevertheless, it is our impression that these pathophysiological effects of sleep apnea on the cardiovascular system are not fully appreciated in the broader medical research and clinical communities.

For these reasons, we accepted with great enthusiasm the invitation from Dr. Claude Lenfant to develop and edit this first comprehensive monograph to specifically address the cardiovascular and cerebrovascular consequences of sleep apnea. Since joining the faculty of the University of Toronto in 1985, as a respirologist and cardiologist, respectively, we have shared the concern that cardiovascular turmoil triggered by sleep-related breathing disorders may be fundamental to the initiation, exacerbation, and perhaps mortality of many patients with common and debilitating conditions such as heart failure, hypertension, and nocturnal angina and conduction disturbances. At the time this concept was not generally appreciated. There was a paucity of scholarly literature on this topic, and the majority of clinicians and investigators in the subspecialties of cardiology, neurology, respirology, and hypertension seemed indifferent to the potential adverse impact of sleep-related breathing disorders on their patients. Indeed, attention was focused on cardiovascular event rates during the first few hours after waking, rather than during sleep.

Over the last decade, the concerted efforts of many integrative physiologists, epidemiologists, and clinical investigators worldwide have transformed our understanding and appreciation of the many mechanisms by which apneas during sleep may contribute to the pathophysiology or complications of cardiovascular and cerebrovascular disease. These are the most common life-threatening and debilitating diseases affecting the adult Western population; as life expectancy in developed and developing countries extends, the number of individuals suffering from one or more of these conditions will increase greatly. These several considerations underscored the compelling need for a comprehensive reference text on this topic.

Our overall objective was to assemble the experimental and clinical literature on this topic into a single authoritative and timely monograph useful to basic and clinical scientists interested in these concepts, and to practicing physicians managing such patients. The text is divided into four parts, addressing, in turn, the influence of normal sleep and respiration on the cardiovascular system, the effects of sleep apnea on blood pressure, the relationship of sleep apnea to coronary and cerebrovascular disease, and the pathophysiological interactions between sleep apnea and congestive heart failure. Our contributors were invited to review critically the current literature in their area of expertise, and encouraged to highlight, whenever possible, those novel observations and important concepts arising from their laboratories with the greatest impact. Any success we have achieved toward this goal must be attributed to these authors, who are to be commended for the quality, comprehensiveness, and timeliness of their contributions.

Excitement in any new and emerging field of scientific endeavour is stimulated by the controversies that inevitably arise whenever investigators from different laboratories attempt to interpret and synthesize observations from a variety of experimental models (each with its own specific limitations) and relate these to human disease. Thus, the astute reader should not be surprised to discover that rigorous experiments by highly talented investigators have often yielded conflicting conclusions as to the mechanisms and impact of specific respiratory events on cardiac function and circulatory regulation. In our view, the intensity and sophistication of such debate render current sleep apnea research all the more interesting. We believe that our role as editors was not to adjudicate the relative merits of the assumptions, methods, or conclusions of individual authors, but rather to allow these experienced investigators to develop their points of view as they saw fit, and allow the critical reader to judge the validity of the arguments presented and their relevance for patients with sleep apnea. Our own experience, as clinician scientists focused on human disease, has enhanced our awareness of the difficulties inherent in application of the integrative approach to the identification of discrete mechanisms triggered by apnea during sleep, and its consequences. However, we have been gratified and stimulated by the positive impact of our research findings on the outcomes of our patients with these co-related conditions. Indeed, we undertook this project with the confidence that transmission of this information to a broader readership would ultimately benefit patients who suffer from sleep apnea and its complications.

We would like to thank Dr. Claude Lenfant of the National Heart, Lung, and Blood Institute and Ms. Sandra Beberman at Marcel Dekker, Inc., for their patience and good humor during the editing and publishing process. We have enjoyed the opportunity to create this volume and trust that our readers will profit from its contents.

T. Douglas Bradley
John S. Floras

CONTRIBUTORS

Amit Anand, M.D.   Research Fellow, Pulmonary and Critical Care Division, Department of Medicine, Beth Israel Deaconess Medical Center, and Harvard Medical School, Boston, Massachusetts

Gang Bao, M.D.   Assistant Professor, Division of Respiratory, Critical Care, and Environmental Medicine, Department of Medicine, University of Louisville School of Medicine, Louisville, Kentucky

Israel Belenkie, M.D.   Professor, Department of Medicine, The University of Calgary, Calgary, Alberta, Canada

T. Douglas Bradley, M.D., F.R.C.P.(C)   Director, Cardiopulmonary Sleep Disorders and Research Centre, Department of Medicine, the Toronto General Hospital of the University Health Network, the Toronto Rehabilitation Institute, and the Mount Sinai Hospital, and Professor, Department of Medicine, University of Toronto, Toronto, Ontario, Canada

Craig A. Chasen, M.D.   Associate Professor, Department of Medicine, University of Kentucky Medical Center, Lexington, Kentucky

Andrew J. S. Coats, M.A., D.M., F.R.A.C.P., F.R.C.P., F.E.S.C., F.A.C.C.   Viscount Royston Professor of Clinical Cardiology, National Heart and Lung Institute, Imperial College of Science, Technology and Medicine, Royal Brompton Hospital, London, England

Mark Eric Dyken, M.D. Associate Professor, Sleep Disorders Center, Department of Neurology, University of Iowa College of Medicine, Iowa City, Iowa

Eugene C. Fletcher, M.D. Professor of Medicine and Director, Division of Respiratory, Critical Care, and Environmental Medicine, Department of Medicine, University of Louisville School of Medicine, Louisville, Kentucky

John S. Floras, M.D., D.Phil. (Oxon.), F.R.C.P.(C) Site Director of Cardiology, Department of Medicine, the Mount Sinai Hospital; Director, Cardiology Research, the Toronto General Hospital of the University Health Network; and Professor, Department of Medicine, University of Toronto, Toronto, Ontario, Canada

Darrel P. Francis, M.A., M.D., M.R.C.P. Clinical Research Fellow, Department of Cardiology, Royal Brompton Hospital, London, England

Patrice G. Guyenet, Ph.D. Professor, Department of Pharmacology, University of Virginia School of Medicine, Charlottesville, Virginia

Patrick J. Hanly, M.D., M.R.C.P.I., F.R.C.P.C., A.B.S.M. Associate Professor, Department of Medicine, University of Toronto, and Director, Sleep Laboratory, St. Michael's Hospital, Toronto, Ontario, Canada

Richard L. Horner, Ph.D. Departments of Medicine and Physiology, University of Toronto, Toronto, Ontario, Canada

Shahrokh Javaheri, M.D. Sleep Disorders Laboratory, Department of Veterans Affairs Medical Center, and Professor, Department of Medicine, University of Cincinnati College of Medicine, Cincinnati, Ohio

Michael C. K. Khoo, Ph.D. Professor, Biomedical Engineering Department, University of Southern California, Los Angeles, California

Sandrine H. Launois, M.D. Instructor, Pulmonary and Critical Care Division, Department of Medicine, Beth Israel Deaconess Medical Center, and Harvard Medical School, Boston, Massachusetts

Barbara J. Morgan, Ph.D. Associate Professor, Department of Surgery, University of Wisconsin–Madison and Middleton Memorial Veterans Hospital, Madison, Wisconsin

James E. Muller, M.D.* Chief, Division of Cardiovascular Medicine, Department of Medicine, University of Kentucky Medical Center, Lexington, Kentucky

Krzysztof Narkiewicz, M.D., Ph.D. Department of Hypertension and Diabetology, Medical University of Gdansk, Gdansk, Poland

C. P. O'Donnell, Ph.D. Division of Pulmonary and Critical Care Medicine, Department of Medicine, Johns Hopkins University, Baltimore, Maryland

Paul E. Peppard, Ph.D. Department of Preventive Medicine, University of Wisconsin–Madison, Madison, Wisconsin

Bradley G. Phillips, Pharm.D. Division of Clinical and Administrative Pharmacy, University of Iowa College of Pharmacy, Iowa City, Iowa

Piotr Ponikowski, M.D., Ph.D. Consultant Cardiologist, Cardiac Department, Military Hospital, Wroclaw, Poland

Steven M. Scharf, M.D., Ph.D. Pulmonary and Critical Care Division, Long Island Jewish Medical Center, and Professor, Department of Medicine, Albert Einstein College of Medicine, New Hyde Park, New York

C. D. Schaub Division of Pulmonary and Critical Care Medicine, Department of Medicine, Johns Hopkins University, Baltimore, Maryland

H. Schneider, M.D. Division of Pulmonary and Critical Care Medicine, Department of Medicine, Johns Hopkins University, Baltimore, Maryland

James B. Skatrud, M.D. Professor, Department of Medicine, University of Wisconsin–Madison and Middleton Memorial Veterans Hospital, Madison, Wisconsin

Virend K. Somers, M.D., Ph.D. Division of Hypertension and Division of Cardiovascular Disease, Department of Internal Medicine, Mayo Clinic and Mayo Foundation, Rochester, Minnesota

Claudette M. St. Croix, Ph.D. Postdoctoral Fellow, Department of Preventive Medicine, University of Wisconsin–Madison and Middleton Memorial Veterans Hospital, Madison, Wisconsin

---

* *Current affiliation*: Associate Director, CIMIT Program, and Director, Clinical Research in Cardiology, Massachusetts General Hospital, Boston, Massachusetts.

Ruzena Tkacova, M.D., Ph.D.   Research Fellow, Department of Medicine, the Toronto General Hospital of the University Health Network, the Toronto Rehabilitation Institute, and University of Toronto, Toronto, Ontario, Canada

John Trinder   Professor, Department of Psychology, University of Melbourne, Parkville, Victoria, Australia

John V. Tyberg, M.D., Ph.D.   Professor, Department of Medicine and Department of Physiology and Biophysics, The University of Calgary, Calgary, Alberta, Canada

Richard L. Verrier, Ph.D., F.A.C.C.   Associate Professor, Department of Medicine, Harvard Medical School, and Director, Institute for Prevention of Cardiovascular Disease, Beth Israel Deaconess Medical Center, Boston, Massachusetts

J. Woodrow Weiss, M.D.   Associate Professor, Pulmonary and Critical Care Division, Department of Medicine, Beth Israel Deaconess Medical Center, and Harvard Medical School, Boston, Massachusetts

Terry Young, Ph.D.   Professor, Department of Preventive Medicine, University of Wisconsin–Madison, Madison, Wisconsin

CONTENTS

SLEEP APNEA

1

Influence of Respiration on Autonomic Control of Heart Rate and Blood Pressure

BARBARA J. MORGAN, CLAUDETTE M. ST. CROIX, and JAMES B. SKATRUD

University of Wisconisin–Madison
and Middleton Memorial Veterans Hospital
Madison, Wisconsin

I. Introduction

Respiration-synchronous oscillations in sympathetic nerve discharge were de-scribed by Adrian and colleagues more than 50 years ago (1); however, despite considerable study by many investigators, the mechanisms responsible for respi-ratory modulation of autonomic activity remain incompletely understood today. One reason for the indecision and controversy surrounding this topic is that sev-eral breathing-related phenomena are clearly capable, *in isolation*, of modulating autonomic outflow to the cardiovascular system (Table 1). In this chapter we propose to show that inconsistencies existing in the literature may be more appar-ent than real, because the wide range of experimental strategies used to investi-gate this topic has led to a variety of conclusions about the relative importance of each mechanism.

At normal breathing frequencies, heart rate rises during inspiration and falls during expiration (2–4). This pattern of breathing-related heart rate fluctuation, which has been termed the respiratory sinus arrhythmia (RSA) (Fig. 1), is pro-duced mainly by oscillations in parasympathetic outflow to the sinoatrial node (5). In contrast, the pattern of respiration-induced blood pressure fluctuation, which is produced mainly by oscillations in sympathetic vasoconstrictor outflow, is much

1

Table 1 Respiratory Modulation of Heart Rate and Blood Pressure: Potential Contributing Factors

Stimulus	Potentially Important Elements	Influence of Inspiration	Effects on Cardiac Vagal Outflow	Effects on Cardiac Sympathetic Outflow	Effects on Sympathetic Vasoconstrictor Outflow
Central mechanisms					
Output of central respiratory oscillator	Respiratory premotor neurons	—	→	↑	↑
Peripheral mechanisms					
Change in lung volume	Pulmonary stretch receptors	+	→	↑ or ←	→ or ↑
Change in intrathoracic pressure	Carotid sinus baroreceptors	+ or −	↑ or ←	→ or ←	→
	Aortic arch baroreceptors	+	←	←	↑
	Atrial receptors with myelinated vagal afferents	+	↑		
	Atrial/ventricular receptors with unmyelinated vagal afferents	+	←	↑	→
Fluctuations in O_2, CO_2	Carotid sinus chemoreceptors	—	→	→	→
Respiratory airflow	Laryngeal receptors	+	←	↑	←
	Nasal/pharyngeal receptors	+	←	↑←	←
Respiratory muscle contraction	Mechano- and metaboreceptors with group III and IV afferents	+	↑	←	←

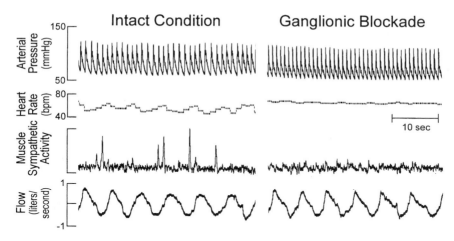

Figure 1 Respiration-related fluctuations in heart rate and blood pressure in the intact human (left) and during ganglionic blockade (right).

harder to discern. This difficulty exists at least in part because vascular smooth muscle cannot respond faithfully to neural signals oscillating with a frequency greater than 3–4 cycles per minute (6). Thus, the relatively long time constant between generation of sympathetic vasoconstrictor impulses in the brainstem and the subsequent vascular response makes it impossible to correlate blood pressure changes with the appropriate portion of the breath cycle. In addition, respiratory modulation of blood pressure is likely to involve a greater number of mechanical and reflex stimuli (some with opposing influences on blood pressure) than does respiratory modulation of heart rate. Consequently, previous investigators have demonstrated that blood pressure can either increase (3) or decrease (4,7,8) during inspiration. Breathing-related swings in blood pressure seem to depend not only on respiratory rate but also on the fullness of the central circulation and the direction and magnitude of intrathoracic pressure change produced during the breath (9,10).

II. Respiratory Modulation of Cardiac Vagal (Parasympathetic) Activity

A predominantly neural basis for RSA has been demonstrated by its elimination or substantial attenuation following cervical vagotomy (2), ganglionic blockade (11), cholinergic blockade (5), and heart transplantation (4,12). Although it is likely that multiple afferent mechanisms contribute to RSA (Table 1), the principal efferent pathway is composed of cardiac vagal motor neurons (5) that discharge during expiration (13,14). In contrast, sympathetic outflow to the heart is not a prominent determinant of RSA because respiratory modulation of heart rate persists after removal of the stellate ganglion (2,15) and β-adrenergic blockade (5,16–17).

A.   Central Neural Influences on Respiratory Sinus Arrhythmia

The role played by central respiratory neurons in causing RSA has been studied in reduced preparations as well as in intact animals and humans. Experimental approaches have included 1) augmentation of respiratory motor activity with hypoxia, hypercapnia, and voluntary efforts while attempting to keep other variables constant and 2) elimination of respiratory motor activity with voluntary, hypocapnia-induced, or mechanical ventilator–induced apnea.

Variation of heart rate in phase with phrenic motor output, even in the absence of lung or chest wall motion (5,18–20), provides evidence for central respiratory modulation of cardiac vagal activity. In experimental animals, RSA persists after cessation of mechanical ventilation (5,18–19). When constant-flow mechanical ventilation was used to eliminate input from pulmonary stretch receptors, baroreceptors, chemoreceptors, and presumably any other phasic inputs related to respiratory excursions, heart rate modulation continued to occur synchronously with phrenic nerve activity at a similar magnitude to that observed during spontaneous breathing (20). In addition, the magnitude of RSA was similar for a given level of phrenic motor output when respiratory drive was enhanced with hypoxia and hypercapnia, suggesting that the influence of both peripheral and central chemoreceptors was mediated by their effect on central respiratory drive. In contrast, evidence against the importance of central respiratory output in generating RSA was provided in patients following bilateral lung transplantation (4). Despite the presence of intact cardiovagal innervation as demonstrated by a tachycardic response to atropine and hypoxia (21), RSA was nearly abolished. The small residual respiratory modulation of heart rate was comparable to that observed in heart transplant recipients whose sinus nodes lacked efferent vagal innervation.

Studies that have used apnea to test the importance of central respiratory activity to RSA have been less definitive because of the inability to control for confounding influences, including those that were introduced by the experimental technique. For example, a voluntary breath-hold in humans eliminated RSA (22); however, attributing an important independent role to central mechanisms is probably not warranted because breath-holds cause perturbations in arterial pressure and blood gases. These stimuli would be expected to increase cardiovagal activity via baroreflex and chemoreflex mechanisms. Posthyperventilation apnea produced in relaxed, awake dogs was associated with persistence of RSA on the first phantom breath following cessation of mechanical ventilation(23). This transient residual modulation of heart rate was attributed to a memory effect of the previous lung inflation caused by the mechanical ventilator, because the investigators were unable to demonstrate evidence of residual central respiratory neural activity. More relevant to the role of central respiratory drive in RSA was the reappearance of heart rate fluctuations consistent with RSA toward the end of the apnea before the reinitiation of spontaneous breathing. These findings suggest that central respiratory drive may have caused oscillations in heart rate despite being at a level that was insufficient to cause rhythmic breathing.

Previous investigators who have used passive positive-pressure mechanical ventilation to decrease inspiratory muscle activity (and, by presumption, central inspiratory neuron discharge) in humans have demonstrated an attenuation of RSA compared to spontaneous breathing at equal volumes and frequencies (4,8,24). Although this finding suggests an important role for central respiratory activity in causing RSA, experiments using passive *negative*-pressure mechanical ventilation point to an alternative explanation. When equivalent tidal volumes and breathing frequencies were achieved with negative-pressure mechanical ventilation, the amplitude of the RSA was *not* reduced relative to spontaneous breathing (24). Taken together, these findings suggest that positive-pressure ventilation suppressed RSA because it altered the influence of inspiration on peripheral reflex mechanisms (*e.g.*, atrial stretch reflex, cardiac or aortic baroreflexes) rather than via an effect on central respiratory drive. On the other hand, it is not possible to document whether inspiratory muscle activity was actually eliminated in these experiments (or at least reduced to a comparable degree by positive- and negative-pressure mechanical ventilation).

Thus, the importance of central respiratory activity in causing RSA remains incompletely understood. On the one hand, there is convincing evidence that central respiratory activity plays a role in causing RSA in experimental animals (5,18–20,23). On the other hand, the presence of central respiratory activity clearly is not sufficient to produce a normal RSA in human lung transplant recipients—individuals in whom vagal feedback from the lung has been surgically interrupted (4).

B. Peripheral Reflex Contributions to Respiratory Sinus Arrhythmia

The demonstration of a central respiratory component to RSA in animals does not rule out potential contributions from a variety of peripheral mechanisms. Many respiration-related neural and mechanical events influence heart rate and thereby contribute to fluctuations in heart rate that occur at the breathing frequency (Table 1).

Influence of Lung Inflation

Lung inflation can modulate heart rate by at least two potential mechanisms. First, passive lung inflation with modest positive pressures causes a reflex increase in heart rate (16,25–27) that is eliminated by interruption of the cervical vagosympathetic nerves (15–17) yet persists following excision of the stellate ganglion (15). The critical importance of vagal afferents from the lung is demonstrated by abolition of this heart rate response after selective section of the pulmonary branches of the vagi (2). It is not clear whether stimulation of pulmonary vagal afferents by lung stretch inhibits vagal outflow to the heart directly or acts via inhibition of central respiratory neurons (2,28). Second, pulmonary stretch receptor activation can modify the effectiveness of other sensory inputs, such as those from baroreceptors and chemoreceptors, as described below (29–33).

An obligatory role for vagal feedback from the lungs in causing RSA was demonstrated in humans following double lung transplantation, an operation that interrupts pulmonary afferent feedback while leaving the cardiovagal efferent pathway intact (4). These individuals were shown (during sleep) to have no inhibition of respiratory motor output in response to held lung inflation up to 80% of total lung capacity (*i.e.*, no Breuer-Hering reflex), even though their airways were shown to be innervated above the carina (34). Furthermore, vagal efferent innervation of the heart was intact and functional, as documented by cardioacceleration in response to atropine and to hypoxia (4,21). It was presumed, then, that the only relevant neural pathway missing in these individuals was that comprising pulmonary vagal afferents. Whether the transplantation procedure may also have interfered with atrial receptors with myelinated vagal afferents was not documented, although there was no specific reason to suspect that these receptors had been affected by the operation (35). Lung transplant recipients showed a marked attenuation of RSA despite the continued presence of central respiratory activity, intrathoracic pressure changes, and cardiac intrinsic mechanisms. Therefore, interruption of vagal afferents from the lung in humans prevented alternative central or peripheral mechanisms from altering cardiovagal tone in a manner that would produce a normal RSA. In addition, the amplitude of RSA was not decreased at faster breathing frequencies or increased at larger tidal volumes in lung or heart transplant recipients as compared with intact subjects. Thus, regulation of RSA in the human at all levels of ventilation is uniquely sensitive to reflexes from the lung. This finding is surprising, given the relative weakness of the Breuer-Hering reflex in humans as compared with other species (36,37).

Influence of Fluctuations in Intrathoracic Pressure

Several sets of mechanoreceptors, each with the ability to reflexly affect heart rate, are influenced by breathing-induced intrathoracic pressure swings (Table 1). Inspiratory decreases in intrathoracic pressure augment venous return (38), thereby causing distention of the right atrium. Atrial distention reflexly increases heart rate; however, the efferent arm of this reflex is thought to be sympathetic outflow to the heart (39), a pathway not critical to RSA. In addition, stretch of the sinoatrial node in isolated hearts causes heart rate speeding (40–42). Because neither of these mechanisms operates via the cardiac vagal efferent pathway, they are unlikely to be major determinants of the RSA in intact animals. However, they may contribute to the small, residual respiratory-related oscillations in heart rate that are observed in patients with denervated hearts (4,12) and after lung transplantation (4).

Previous investigators have used experimental manipulations of intrathoracic pressure to study breathing-related heart rate fluctuations in humans. The effect of negative intrathoracic pressure versus lung stretch on RSA was studied by using resistive breathing and positive- and negative-pressure mechanical ventilation (43). At the same lung volume, greater negative intrathoracic pressure with resistive breathing resulted in a larger amplitude of RSA, implying the importance of additional non–lung-stretch-related influences. The attenuation of RSA with positive-vs. negative-pressure mechanical ventilation also supported the contribution of alternative modulators to RSA. The authors attributed these findings to reflexes arising in the cardiovascular system; however, this study also emphasizes the importance of lung stretch, because a larger tidal volume achieved at the same negative intrathoracic pressure (a resistive load was used with the smaller tidal volume) caused a larger amplitude of RSA.

Pulsed Doppler ultrasound was used to investigate the temporal relationships between within-breath changes in left ventricular stroke volume, arterial pressure, and heart rate (44). When inspiratory and expiratory resistive loads were applied to human subjects breathing at fixed tidal volumes and frequencies, the magnitude of RSA increased. This finding, along with the observation that the phase relationship between stroke volume, arterial pressure, and cardiac interval remained constant during loaded and unloaded breathing, suggests that arterial baroreflexes are an important determinant of RSA. On the other hand, in these same subjects, resistive breathing caused a decrease in the magnitude of the RSA in relation to the magnitude of the within-breath arterial pressure change, suggesting that factors other than within-breath fluctuations in arterial pressure were important in modifying the RSA during resistive breathing.

It is unlikely that carotid sinus baroreceptors are the sole determinants of within-breath heart rate changes because fluctuations in arterial pressure associated with breathing are not consistent either in magnitude or direction, whereas the pattern of RSA is quite stereotypical. At slow respiratory rates, inspiratory increases in heart rate are often associated with increases in arterial pressure that would be expected to slow heart rate if carotid sinus baroreceptors were the primary determinant of RSA. When normal subjects breathed at increased tidal volumes, the amplitude of RSA increased without any lowering of inspiratory arterial pressure (Fig. 2) (4). It is likewise improbable that aortic arch baroreceptors by themselves are responsible for inspiratory speeding of heart rate, because they are activated, not deactivated, during inspiration (via an increase in aortic transmural pressure) (45).

Nevertheless, two aspects of baroreflex function could modulate the magnitude of RSA. First, baroreceptor activity is an important determinant of baseline vagal tone, which, in turn, influences the amplitude of RSA. Second, the effect of baroreceptor activity on cardiovagal efferents is variable throughout the respiratory cycle. During early inspiration, cardiovagal neurons become refractory to incoming baroreceptor impulses (29–33). Therefore, even with a constant level of baroreceptor input throughout the respiratory cycle, the variable accessibility of baroreceptor impulses to the cardiovagal neurons would accentuate the in-

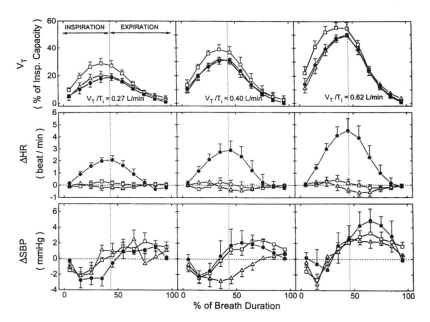

Figure 2   Effect of increasing tidal volume [VT; expressed as a percentage of inspiratory capacity (IC)] and inspiratory flow rate (VT/inspiratory time) on magnitude of within-breath variations in heart rate (HR) and systolic blood pressure (SBP) in normal subjects (healthy subjects, $n = 5$; liver transplant recipients, $n = 2$), lung-denervated subjects (double lung transplant recipients, $n = 5$), and heart-denervated subjects (heart transplant recipients, $n = 3$; double lung transplant recipients, $n = 2$). Breathing frequency was fixed at 10 breaths per minute and inspiratory time/total time was 50% in all subjects at all tidal volumes. (From Ref. 4.)

crease in heart rate during inspiration and contribute to the slowing of heart rate during expiration.

In conclusion, experimental manipulations of the magnitude and/or direction of intrathoracic pressure change during inspiration point to an important role for arterial baroreflexes in causing RSA. This modulatory influence is sometimes difficult to discern because the aortic arch and carotid sinus baroreceptors can be differentially activated during breathing-related changes in intrathoracic pressure (46). The important modulatory role for arterial baroreflexes in causing RSA is likely to be mediated via variable accessibility of medullary vagal neurons to incoming baroreceptor stimuli, a phenomenon that is critically dependent on phasic input from pulmonary stretch receptors (29,31). Atrial and/or sinus node stretch also contributes in a minor way to the generation of RSA (4,12).

Influence of Within-Breath Fluctuations in Blood Gas Composition

The effect of systemic hypoxia or hypercapnia on RSA is obscured by the associated ventilatory stimulation, which increases both tidal volume and breathing frequency and may have other effects on RSA independent of classical chemoreceptor stimulation. For example, even though stimulation of isolated carotid body chemoreceptors in experimental animals produces bradycardia, systemic hypoxia in intact animals is associated with tachycardia (30,47–49). In humans, breath-holds are inconsistently associated with bradycardia, and if the heart rate does slow, the reduction is small and not closely related to the degree of hypoxemia (21,50,51). In carotid body–denervated humans, the normal tachycardic response to systemic hypoxia is exaggerated (52). These findings do not suggest a dominant bradycardic effect of peripheral chemoreceptor stimulation but rather indicate a limiting influence on the tachycardic response to hypoxia. Therefore, if chemoreceptor activation has a causative effect on RSA, it is more likely to be mediated by within-breath fluctuations in chemical stimuli than by the steady-state level of chemoreceptor activity.

Within-breath oscillations in carotid chemoreceptor activity have been identified in relationship to changing blood levels of Pa_{CO_2} (53,54). In anesthetized animals, transient reductions in carotid sinus nerve activity during inspiration have been observed at breathing frequencies up to 30 per minute (54). The magnitude of these fluctuations in chemoreceptor discharge is proportional both to the rate of change of Pa_{CO_2} and to its mean value (53). The reflex effects of such transient changes in chemoreceptor firing on heart rate are not known; however, it is well established that central access of peripheral chemoreceptor discharge to cardiovagal efferents varies throughout the respiratory cycle. Specifically, the bradycardic effect of chemoreceptor stimulation is more pronounced when the stimulus is delivered during expiration versus inspiration (29). Because peak chemoreceptor discharge occurs during expiration, when the cardiovagal neurons are most susceptible, peripheral chemoreceptors may indeed contribute to expiratory slowing of heart rate. In contrast, central chemoreceptors are not likely to contribute to within-breath fluctuations in heart rate because of the relatively long latency between CO_2 accumulation and acidification of the medullary chemoreceptor (55).

Influence of Flow and Pressure Alterations in the Upper Airway

Stimulation of afferents from the upper airway (nasal passages, naso- and oropharynx, and larynx) triggers reflex alterations in breathing pattern and airway patency (56). In experimental animals, stimulation of upper airway receptors also elicits reflex changes in the cardiovascular system, the most striking of which is marked heart rate slowing (in some cases, asystole) (56–59). The finding that within-breath heart rate fluctuations are nearly abolished in lung transplant patients argues against an important role for upper airway reflexes in causing RSA. In these individuals, innervation above the carina is preserved, as evidenced by an intact cough reflex (34).

In conclusion, experiments in human lung transplant recipients demonstrate that normal RSA is critically dependent on afferent feedback from the lung, regardless of the extent of central respiratory drive or the level of negative intrathoracic pressure (4). Given the relative weakness of the Breuer-Hering reflex in humans (60), this obligatory role for lung inflation in causing RSA is indeed surprising. Furthermore, the reduction in RSA caused by passive positive-pressure ventilation in normal subjects demonstrates that in the presence of afferent feedback from the lung, other peripheral and/or central mechanisms are important in generating RSA. Although the lung transplant model has provided valuable information about the causes of RSA, key questions remain unanswered. For example, do the other ''important peripheral mechanisms'' (see above) involve atrial stretch receptors, sinoaortic baroreceptors, chemoreceptors, or mechanical influences on heart rate? Is the obligatory role of lung inflation in generating RSA caused by its ability to limit accessibility of medullary vagal neurons to sensory inputs from baro- and chemoreceptors?

III. Respiratory Modulation of Sympathetic Outflow

The temporal relationship between breathing and the discharge of pre- and postganglionic sympathetic neurons has been studied in several mammalian species, including humans (8,33,61–69). Differences in methodology and species have led to seemingly disparate conclusions about the nature of the relationship between respiration and sympathetic outflow; nevertheless, the following unifying principles have emerged.

First, respiratory modulation is not uniform among functional types of sympathetic neurons. For example, sympathetic vasoconstrictor outflow targeted to skeletal muscle and abdominal viscera exhibits a strong coherence with phrenic discharge, whereas activity in sympathetic sudomotor neurons and in cutaneous vasoconstrictor neurons does not (70). Because this chapter focuses on the influence of respiration on heart rate and blood pressure, we restrict our discussion to sympathetic neurons that innervate the heart and vascular beds with significant contributions to total peripheral vascular resistance (i.e., the renal, skeletal muscle, and splanchnic vascular beds). For a comprehensive discussion of the influence of breathing on a wider range of sympathetic neurons, the reader is directed to a recent review by Häbler and co-workers (70).

Second, respiratory modulation of sympathetic outflow depends on both central neural and peripheral reflex components. In anesthetized, vagotomized animals with sinoaortic denervation, regularly occurring fluctuations in perfusion pressure of the vascularly isolated hindlimb have been observed (71,72). These periodic vasoconstrictions, which occurred with the same frequency as phrenic discharge and inspiration-synchronous bursts of sympathetic activity, disappeared during post-hyperventilation apnea and electrical stimulation of the superior laryngeal nerve, two conditions that elicited phrenic silence (71). In animals *without* sinoaortic denervation, a respiratory rhythmicity in perfusion pressure was also observed; however, these vasoconstrictions occurred in synchrony with ventilation-associated blood pressure fluctuations and were attributed to baroreflex mechanisms (72). Thus, these findings illustrate the concept that both central and peripheral components contribute to respiratory modulation of blood pressure in the intact organism.

A. Central Coupling of Phrenic Discharge and Sympathetic Vasoconstrictor Outflow

The independent influence of the respiratory rhythm generator on the timing of sympathetic outflow has been studied using reduced preparations in which peripheral reflex mechanisms and the mechanical effects of breathing were eliminated. This approach in anesthetized or decerebrate animals involved some or all of the following interventions: 1) vagotomy (to eliminate feedback from pulmonary stretch receptors and cardiopulmonary baroreceptors with vagal afferents), 2) sinoaortic denervation (to eliminate feedback from carotid sinus and aortic arch baroreceptors), and 3) thoracotomy and/or artificial ventilation with neuromuscular blockade (to eliminate breathing-related fluctuations in intrathoracic pressure or to dissociate phrenic motor output from lung inflation and intrathoracic pressure changes).

Experiments in which peripheral feedback is eliminated clearly demonstrate that pre- and postganglionic sympathetic outflow to several different organs and vascular beds occurs with the same frequency as phrenic motor outflow. Nevertheless, there is a lack of consensus among previous studies about the temporal relationship between sympathetic discharge and phrenic discharge. Several investigators have demonstrated on the basis of whole-nerve recordings from cats that sympathetic nerves fire mainly during inspiration (i.e., in synchrony with phrenic discharge), with their minimum activity occurring during expiration (1,61,73). Other investigators have shown, using a rat model, that sympathetic activity in some nerves is suppressed during inspiration and maximal in expiration, whereas in other nerves the pattern is reversed (66,74,75). Still other investigators have found that sympathetic discharge spans inspiration and expiration rather than being locked to a single phase of the respiratory cycle (62).

The lack of consensus regarding the temporal relationship between phrenic discharge and sympathetic outflow is probably due at least in part to the use of whole nerve recordings by many investigators (1,61,62,66,74,75). It has become clear from single-fiber recordings that distinct firing patterns can be exhibited by different fibers within the same nerve (64,76) and that the firing pattern exhibited by a particular neuron depends on the functional subpopulation of sympathetic neurons to which it belongs. In the cat, most visceral and muscle vasoconstrictor neurons fire mainly during inspiration, whereas most cutaneous vasoconstrictor neurons show no respiratory modulation (63). In the rat, most muscle and cutaneous vasoconstrictor neurons fire in expiration (77).

Although it is possible that species differences are responsible for some of the disagreement about the temporal relationship between phrenic discharge and sympathetic outflow, Barman and Gebber found distinct patterns of phrenic-sympathetic coupling within the same species (61). In some cats, the onset of sympathetic activity in the external carotid nerve was coincident with the onset of phrenic discharge, whereas in others, sympathetic activation preceded phrenic activation. In both cases, sympathetic activity reached a peak in inspiration. In still other cats, sympathetic activation began after the start of inspiration and reached a peak in early expiration. These investigators also noted shifts in phrenic-sympathetic coupling that were related to changes in respiratory rate, and they showed examples where the phrenic discharge and sympathetic activity were not locked in a 1:1 ratio. Thus, the time course of respiratory modulation of sympathetic outflow was not fixed, even within the same animal during the same experiment.

The close temporal relationship between the rhythmic discharges in phrenic and sympathetic nerves has prompted the hypothesis that the two neural outputs either arise from the same brainstem neurons or are driven by a common oscillator (78,79). Two lines of evidence support this view. First, phrenic activity and sympathetic activity maintain a 1:1 relationship over a wide range of respiratory frequencies (78). Second, some investigators have found that respiration-related oscillations in sympathetic outflow disappear during phrenic silence elicited by posthyperventilation apnea (62,73,80).

The contrasting view—i.e., that independent brainstem oscillators give rise to phrenic and sympathetic outflows—also has experimental support. As mentioned above, phase relationships between phrenic and sympathetic discharge have been shown to vary as a function of respiratory rate, and the two neural outputs are not always locked in a 1:1 relationship (61). Relationships other than 1:1 would presumably not be possible if a single oscillator were responsible for driving both phrenic and sympathetic outflows. Partial coherence analysis of activity in pairs of sympathetic nerves (cardiac, splenic, or renal) revealed that activity remained correlated after the portion of coherence attributable to phrenic activity was mathematically eliminated, suggesting that both nerves were driven by an oscillator distinct from the one responsible for the central respiratory rhythm (81). In anesthetized cats, a persistent rhythmicity in sympathetic discharge was observed when phrenic activity was silenced during hypocapnia (61,82). During posthyperventilation apnea characterized by disappearance of both phrenic and sympathetic outflows, the return of sympathetic activity preceded the return of phrenic activity, suggesting that the two neural outputs arise from different brainstem neurons with different sensitivities to CO_2 (82).

B. Peripheral Reflex Contributions to Respiratory Rhythm in Sympathetic Outflow

Influence of Lung Inflation

Lung volume is sensed by slowly adapting stretch receptors located in the smooth muscle of the extra- and intrapulmonary airways (83). Afferent information from these receptors is conveyed centrally via the pulmonary branches of the right and left vagi. When stimulated, pulmonary stretch receptors reflexly inhibit inspiratory neurons in the medulla (Breuer-Hering reflex). In addition to their well-known role in the regulation of breathing, these receptors also participate in reflex control of the peripheral circulation. In anesthetized dogs (37,84–86) and rabbits (87), passive lung inflation produces reflex vasodilation in the cutaneous, muscle, and splanchnic vascular beds which is abolished by cutting the cervical vagosympathetic nerves or by interrupting the sympathetic pathways to the blood vessels. Furthermore, tidal volume increases of only 50 mL are sufficient to decrease vascular resistance, suggesting that this lung inflation reflex is operative during eupneic breathing (37,84).

These early findings of a lung inflation-systemic vasodilation reflex have more recently been supported by studies demonstrating a depressant action of lung inflation on directly measured sympathetic nerve activity (88–90). In anesthetized rats, lung inflation invoked reflex decreases in sympathetic activity recorded in the genital femoral nerve that were coincident with increases in the diameter of small arterioles supplying the cremaster muscle and decreases in systemic blood pressure (90).

It is not clear whether pulmonary afferents have a direct influence on sympathetic outflow or whether they act via the central respiratory network. In anesthetized cats, the inhibitory influence of lung inflation on the discharge of sympathetic preganglionic neurons showed a distinctive pattern of distribution, with the neurons whose discharge had an inspiration-synchronous component showing the most sensitivity to activation of the pulmonary afferents (88). This finding suggests that the inhibitory effect of lung inflation is predominantly relayed to the sympathetic pre-ganglionic neuron pool via the respiratory center. This concept is supported by the observation that cervical neurons whose firing was sensitive to the activation of the pulmonary inflation reflex became insensitive to lung inflation when central inspiratory activity was suppressed by hypocapnia (88). Based on these findings, it was proposed that the reflex vasodilation induced by stimulation of pulmonary stretch receptors is caused by a decrease in firing of medullary inspiratory neurons, which secondarily results in sympathoinhibition during inspiration (70,88). In contrast, Daly (91) has argued that there must also be a second independent pathway influencing sympathetic discharge, because when inspiratory activity in sympathetic neurons is suppressed by hypocapnia, lung inflation still causes a reflex systemic vasodilation (37).

Further support for the argument that reflex inhibition of sympathetic discharge in response to lung inflation acts via circuits different from those of the Breuer-Hering reflex comes from recordings of efferent splanchnic and cervical sympathetic nerve discharge in the paralyzed, anesthetized cat with intact vagi (89). When lung inflation was stopped for one inspiratory phase, thereby eliminating the Breuer-Hering reflex, there was inspiratory prolongation but no change in slope of the integral of phrenic activity. However, there was an increase in the slope of the integrated sympathetic discharge. In addition, lung inflation was found to inhibit sympathetic discharge during both the inspiratory and expiratory phases of the phrenic discharge cycle.

The Breuer-Hering reflex is clearly weaker in humans than in experimental animals (36,37); therefore, it is possible that there are also species differences in the role played by pulmonary stretch receptors in reflex control of the circulation. Nevertheless, a distinct pattern of muscle sympathetic nerve activity (MSNA) is evident during eupneic breathing, with the majority of the activity occurring during the low-lung-volume phase of the breath cycle (33,68,69,92). This within-breath pattern of MSNA was shown to be augmented when tidal volume was increased with a voluntary increase in respiratory motor output (68), suggesting that the modulation may be mediated in part by pulmonary stretch reflexes. In addition, the within-breath variation in MSNA was dependent upon both the end-expiratory lung volume and the rate of lung inflation (68).

The main difficulty in determining the role of the pulmonary afferent feedback in affecting sympathetic nerve activity in the human rests in isolating this reflex from the coincident effects of lung inflation on intrathoracic pressure, cardiac filling, and systemic arterial pressure. The most direct information concerning the role played by lung inflation reflexes in respiratory modulation of sympathetic outflow in humans has been obtained in patients following heart-lung transplantation (69). This operation interrupts all afferent connections between the heart and lungs and the central nervous system (it abolishes the Breuer-Hering reflex) while leaving other pathways such as baroreflexes and upper airway reflexes intact. During eupneic breathing, the heart-lung transplant recipients showed similar high- to low-lung-volume differences in MSNA during normal levels of tidal breathing as controls, indicating that stretch-sensitive pulmonary vagal afferents are not required for the lung volume–dependent within-breath variation in MSNA (Figs. 3 and 4). However, when tidal volume was increased to over 50% of inspiratory capacity, respiratory modulation of MSNA became more pronounced in the intact subjects but remained unchanged in the transplant recipients. This finding suggests that potentiation of within-breath variations in MSNA at high lung volumes is critically dependent upon pulmonary vagal feedback, a concept consistent with the demonstration of the Breuer-Hering reflex only at high lung volumes in humans (34). It also suggests that pulmonary vagal afferents do not play a critical role in respiratory modulation of MSNA during eupneic breathing in humans.

Influence of Intrathoracic Pressure Fluctuations

Alterations in intrathoracic pressure are sensed by several sets of mechanoreceptors involved in reflex regulation of the cardiovascular system. The aortic arch baroreceptors and cardiac (low-pressure) baroreceptors, because of their locations within the chest, are directly influenced by changes in intrathoracic pressure. Their receptive fields are deformed by increases in transmural pressure (intravascular pressure minus intrathoracic pressure) across the wall of the chamber or vessel in which they are located. Carotid sinus baroreceptors are influenced indirectly by changes in intrathoracic pressure through respiration-induced fluctuations in intravascular pressure.

Atrial receptors with myelinated vagal afferents are located mainly at the veno-atrial junctions (93). In experimental animals, stimulation of these receptors by atrial distention reflexly increases heart rate and decreases sympathetic outflow to the kidney, whereas sympathetic outflow to other vascular beds remains unaffected (93–95). Atrial receptors with unmyelinated vagal afferents are widely distributed throughout the atria (96). In experimental animals, stimulation of these receptors evokes a generalized depressor response caused by reflex dilation in several vascular beds (97–99). Both types of atrial receptor are known to fire in

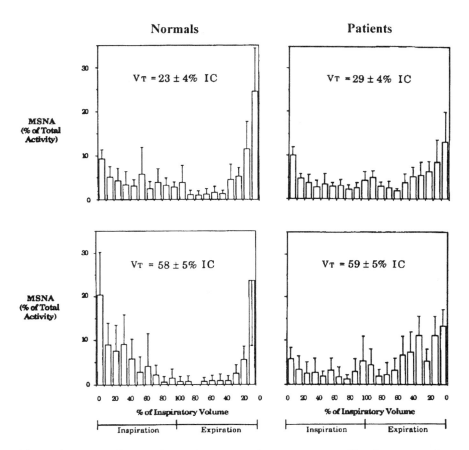

Figure 3 Effect of tidal volume (VT) expressed as a percentage of inspiratory capacity (IC) on within-breath distribution of muscle sympathetic nerve activity (MSNA) in normal subjects (left; $n = 6$) and patients following heart-lung transplantation (right; $n = 4$). Note the presence of within-breath variation in MSNA in the transplant recipients during control VT (upper panel) but, in contrast to normal subjects, the lack of potentiation with elevated VT (lower panel). (Adapted from Ref. 69.)

synchrony with respiration (93,100); however, the reflex effects of such activation on sympathetic outflow have not been determined. Mechanoreceptors subserved by C-fiber afferents are located in both ventricles (96); however, ventricular receptor firing is not influenced by phase of respiration, either during eupneic breathing or when the depth of respiration is increased with CO_2 (93,100). There-

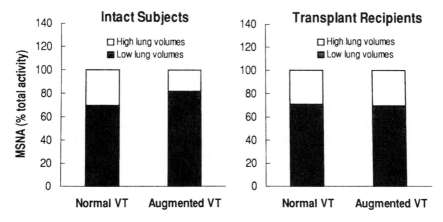

Figure 4 Within-breath partitioning of MSNA in intact subjects and lung-transplant recipients. Note that at normal VT (20–30% of inspiratory capacity), a larger portion of sympathetic bursts occurred in the low (last 50% of expiration + first 50% of inspiration) vs. high (last 50% of inspiration + first 50% of expiration) lung-volume phases of the breath cycle in both intact subjects and transplant recipients. This low- to high-lung-volume MSNA difference widened at augmented VT (50–60% inspiratory capacity) in the normal subjects, but not the transplant recipients. Diastolic blood pressure did not differ in the low- vs. high-lung-volume phases in either group. (Adapted from Ref. 69.)

fore, there is presently no direct evidence to suggest that cardiac (low-pressure) baroreceptors contribute to respiratory modulation of sympathetic outflow.

The carotid sinus and aortic arch (high-pressure) baroreceptors respond to increased transmural pressure by reflexly augmenting parasympathetic outflow to the heart and inhibiting sympathetic outflow to many vascular beds (101). Aortic arch baroreceptors are activated during inspiration because aortic transmural pressure rises as intrathoracic pressure falls (45,46,102). Because systemic arterial pressure can either increase or decrease during inspiration, the effects of breathing on carotid sinus baroreceptor activity are less predictable. In vagotomized animals, respiration-synchronous arterial pressure fluctuations contribute importantly to respiratory modulation of sympathetic discharge, an effect attributed to phasic alterations in baroreflex activity (67,103,104). In contrast, in intact humans, manipulation of the direction and magnitude of intrathoracic pressure change does not affect within-breath modulation of sympathetic outflow to skeletal muscle (68,69). Taken together, these findings from animals and humans suggest that the role of sinoaortic baroreflexes in respiratory modulation of sympathetic outflow, which appears important in reduced preparations, may be masked by other mechanisms in the intact organism. Modulation of sympathetic outflow attributable to breathing-related blood pressure swings is nearly abolished by carotid occlusion in animals with and without vagotomy (63,104). This finding suggests that the high-pressure baroreflexes contribute more importantly than low-pressure baroreflexes in respiratory modulation of sympathetic outflow, at least when intrathoracic pressure is within the physiological range.

The preceding discussion focuses on the autonomic effects of relatively small, physiological fluctuations in intrathoracic pressure; however, in pathological conditions such as sleep apnea syndrome, breathing-related decreases in intrathoracic pressure are much larger in magnitude (*e.g.*, 0 to -60 cmH$_2$O during obstructed inspiratory efforts) (Fig. 5). Large decreases in intrathoracic pressure during inspiration are also seen in chronic obstructive pulmonary disease and in healthy individuals during heavy exercise. Experiments in normal subjects have demonstrated that highly negative inspiratory pressures generated during Mueller maneuvers have transient inhibitory effects on sympathetic outflow to skeletal muscle (11,105) (Fig 6). Obstructed inspiratory efforts during sleep apnea would be expected to activate aortic arch baroreceptors via an increase in aortic transmural pressure while at the same time deactivating carotid sinus baroreceptors via a decrease in systemic arterial pressure (45). In previous experiments that employed simultaneous activation of aortic baroreceptors and deactivation of carotid baroreceptors, sympathetic outflow was inhibited, and this effect was attributed to aortic baroreflex activation (106). Whether this finding indicates a predominant influence of aortic vs. carotid sinus baroreceptors in the control of MSNA is not clear, however, because the converse experiments were not performed (simultaneous carotid sinus *activation* and aortic arch *deactivation*).

The reflex effects of large, abrupt increases in intrathoracic pressure (*i.e.*, Valsalva maneuvers) are well documented. Marked sympathoexcitation and cardioacceleration occur during Valsalva-induced reductions in blood pressure, whereas sympathoinhibition and heart rate slowing accompany the small, transient rise in blood pressure at the onset of the maneuver and the larger, sustained rise in blood pressure that follows release of the expiratory strain (Fig. 7). These reflex responses are elicited by a series of hemodynamic events in which inputs from carotid sinus and aortic arch baroreceptors are at first conflicting and later congruent. At the onset of a sustained Valsalva maneuver, when carotid baroreceptors are activated and aortic baroreceptors are deactivated, sympathetic outflow is inhibited, indicating that carotid baroreceptors predominate in this instance (107). This finding has prompted the hypothesis that when inputs from aortic arch and carotid sinus baroreceptors conflict, the net sympathetic response is determined by input from the set of receptors that are *activated* (107). This concept is consistent with the demonstration that sympathoinhibition also occurs in the initial moments of a Mueller maneuver, when negative intrathoracic

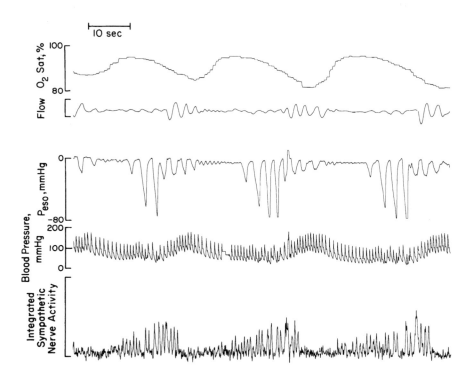

Figure 5   Neurocirculatory consequences of mixed (central and obstructive) sleep apnea. Note that obstructed inspiratory efforts produce transient reductions in muscle sympathetic nerve activity and blood pressure. The primary hemodynamic response to each apnea is a marked increase in blood pressure that occurs after resumption of breathing. Sympathetic activity, which rises more or less progressively (excluding the aforementioned transient reductions) during the apnea, is abruptly inhibited after the resumption of breathing and associated blood pressure rise. (From Ref. 127. © 1996, American Sleep Disorders Association and the Sleep Research Society, Rochester, MN.)

pressure activates aortic and deactivates carotid sinus baroreceptors (11,104) (Fig. 6).

Influence of Within-Breath Fluctuations in Arterial Blood Gas Composition

Although within-breath fluctuations in carotid sinus nerve activity can be detected (52,53), the duration and magnitude of the antecedent O_2 and CO_2 oscillations are quite small relative to level of stimulation required for sympathetic activation

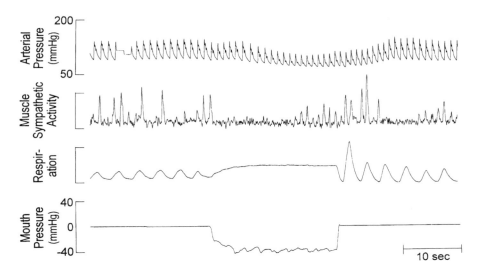

Figure 6 Neurocirculatory responses to a sustained Mueller maneuver. During the initial seconds of the Mueller maneuver, arterial pressure and sympathetic activity decreased; then, arterial pressure returned toward baseline and sympathetic activity increased above baseline. On release of the maneuver, there was a further increase in arterial pressure, followed by a reduction in sympathetic activity.

in humans (108). Thus, it is unlikely that chemoreceptor stimulation is an important determinant of the mean level of MSNA in normoxic, normocapnic conditions. Nevertheless, because the effectiveness of chemoreceptor input, like baroreceptor input, varies throughout the respiratory cycle (109), this mechanism may be in part responsible for the partitioning of MSNA between inspiration and expiration, particularly under hypoxic, hypercapnic conditions.

Influence of Flow and Pressure Alterations in the Upper Airway

Stimulation of nasal and laryngeal receptors causes a reflex increase in lumbar and cervical sympathetic outflow and vasoconstriction in several vascular beds (58,59,110); however, the effects on blood pressure are small and variable. Aside from potential effects of anesthesia on vascular smooth muscle, the most likely explanation for failure of this vasoconstriction to raise blood pressure is the concomitant profound decrease in cardiac output.

Laryngeal receptors with superior laryngeal nerve afferents fire in response to negative pressure in the larynx even at eupneic breathing levels; thus, they may exert some tonic control over breath timing. Whether there is a parallel

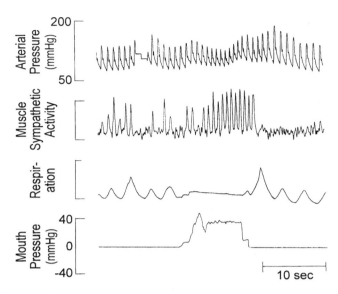

Figure 7 Neurocirculatory responses to a sustained Valsalva maneuver. At the onset of the maneuver, arterial pressure rose transiently, followed by a substantial decrease in systolic and pulse pressure that was accompanied by marked sympathetic activation. On release of the expiratory strain, there was a sustained increase in arterial pressure and sympathetic inhibition.

influence on cardiovascular control is not known; however, it is likely that upper airway reflexes do perturb the cardiovascular system in unusual situations such as suctioning of the respiratory tract, tracheal intubation, and perhaps obstructive sleep apnea syndrome.

Influence of Respiratory Muscle Contraction

During contraction of limb muscles, stimulation of mechano- and metaboreceptors with group III and IV afferents reflexly increases sympathetic outflow and arterial pressure (111,112). Because group III and IV (thinly myelinated and unmyelinated) fibers make up the largest proportion of afferents in the phrenic nerve (113,114), the existence of an analogous sympathoexcitatory reflex arising from diaphragm receptors has been sought by several groups of investigators. In anesthetized cats, electrical stimulation of phrenic afferents elicits reflex increases in sympathetic outflow to the heart and renal vascular bed (115,116). In anesthetized dogs, either electrical or chemical (via capsaicin injection or ischemia) stimulation of phrenic afferents reflexly increases arterial pressure and vascular resistance in several important vascular beds (117,118). Whether physiological activation of these afferents plays an important role in cardiovascular regulation is unknown; however, in humans, augmentation of the amount of respiratory muscle work performed during maximal exercise has been shown to cause vasoconstriction in the leg (119). In these same experiments, leg vascular resistance fell and norepinephrine spillover across the vascular bed of the limb muscle decreased when the work of breathing was reduced. These findings suggest that respiratory muscle contraction exerts some control over perfusion of locomotor muscles, at least during maximal exercise when respiratory muscles must compete with leg muscles for the available cardiac output. The amount of respiratory muscle work required to elicit such reflex vasoconstriction is evidently quite high. Increasing the work of breathing via addition of an inspiratory resistive load or by CO_2 administration in resting humans, while it did increase within-breath modulation of sympathetic outflow, did not increase the mean level of MSNA (68,69).

IV. Summary and Conclusions

A wide variety of experimental approaches have yielded divergent conclusions regarding the importance of central and peripheral mechanisms in modulating autonomic outflow to the cardiovascular system. The conflicting results of these previous investigations illustrate the concept that breathing-related fluctuations in vagal and sympathetic activities are produced by multiple redundant and interrelated mechanisms, each of which can be unmasked in the proper set of experimental circumstances. For example, there is convincing evidence for a role for central respiratory activity in causing RSA in anesthetized animals, yet this mechanism is not sufficient to produce RSA in human lung transplant recipients. Absence of RSA in these individuals demonstrates the critical importance of intact pulmonary vagal innervation to respiratory modulation of heart rate. In contrast, lung denervation does not alter breathing-related oscillations in sympathetic outflow to skeletal muscle during eupneic breathing. This finding underscores the importance of other central or peripheral mechanisms (such as arterial baroreflexes) in respiratory modulation of sympathetic nerve activity in the intact organism.

Another concept that seems clear is that breathing modulates but does not determine the absolute level of autonomic outflow. Mean heart rate is not changed during various combinations of tidal volume or frequency; only the amplitude of RSA is changed (120). This suggests that a change in breathing frequency or tidal volume redistributes the cardiovagal activity between inspiration and expiration but does not change its overall level. A similar within-breath redistribution of MSNA, without a change in mean sympathetic activity, has been observed (68).

As the preceding review of literature indicates, considerable progress has been made toward understanding respiratory-cardiovascular interactions. Nevertheless, several key questions regarding respiratory modulation of autonomic outflow remain unanswered. First, what are the relative contributions of central and peripheral mechanisms (Table 1) to within-breath modulation of parasympathetic and sympathetic outflows in intact animals and humans? Information obtained using reduced preparations can point to potential roles for isolated mechanisms but cannot explain how these complex and sometimes redundant control systems interact in vivo. Second, are breathing-induced fluctuations in autonomic outflow dependent on the level of activity in the central respiratory oscillator? If so, the strength of RSA and breathing-related fluctuation in MSNA should be altered by interventions that increase and decrease respiratory "drive." Third, are the same medullary neurons responsible for driving rhythmic, breathing-related oscillations in vagal and sympathetic discharge? One approach that might prove helpful in answering this question is posthyperventilation apnea, an experimental model that can be applied in human subjects. Although complete absence of rhythmic discharge in medullary respiratory neurons cannot be inferred from disappearance of inspiratory muscle activity (121), this model could be used to determine whether oscillations in autonomic outflows persist during posthyperventilation apnea when phrenic discharge is suppressed. Differential effects of posthyperventilation apnea on RSA and MSNA would suggest that independent oscillators govern vagal and sympathetic outflows. Alternatively, simultaneous suppression of both outflows would suggest that the same medullary neurons are responsible for imposing a respiratory pattern on both vagal and sympathetic outflow. Finally, why is respiratory modulation of heart rate during eupneic breathing critically dependent on input from pulmonary stretch receptors, whereas respiratory modulation of sympathetic outflow is not dependent on intact pulmonary afferent innervation?

It is also unclear whether respiratory modulation of autonomic outflow is of benefit to the organism. What purpose is served by waxing and waning of cardiovascular function in phase with respiration? Previous investigators have theorized that the physiological importance of respiratory modulation of autonomic outflow may be to ensure coordination of the two organ systems responsible for exchange of gases between cells of the body and the environment (70). Recent evidence in support of this concept has been obtained using variable-rate electrical stimulators implanted onto the cardiac branches of the vagus nerves of anesthetized dogs (122). In this model, vagal pacing allowed the heart rate to be increased during inspiration (simulated RSA) or during expiration (reverse RSA) or to be maintained at a constant rate throughout the respiratory cycle. Compared to constant heart rate control, simulated RSA caused a decrease in dead space: tidal volume ratio of 10% and a decrease in physiological shunt of 51%. In contrast, reverse RSA increased both the dead space and shunt. Thus, coupling of heart rate to respiratory rate may have a positive influence on gas exchange at the level of the lung via more effective ventilation perfusion matching. This mechanism may be particularly important during NREM sleep, when high vagal activity and prominent RSA may partially offset the detrimental effects of hypoventilation on gas exchange (123,124). In patients with sleep apnea, inspiratory tachycardia increases over the course of an obstructive apnea and becomes most prominent on the first nonobstructed breath (125). Hypoxia has also been shown to enhance the inspiratory-related tachycardia (126). Thus, the accentuation of the RSA over the course of an apnea or hypopnea, with maximum tachycardia occurring during inspiration on the first unobstructed breath, may serve to match perfusion with ventilation more efficiently and thereby minimize the effect of sleep-disordered breathing events on oxygen delivery. Absence of respiratory-cardiovascular coupling in patients dependent on positive-pressure mechanical ventilators may negatively influence gas exchange in such individuals.

Exercise is another activity of daily living in which respiratory modulation of cardiovascular function may benefit oxygen delivery. It is interesting to speculate whether any portion of the exercise intolerance demonstrated by patients with congestive heart failure, heart-lung transplantation, and diabetic neuropathy could be attributed to the greatly reduced RSA associated with these conditions. The answers to these and other more basic questions regarding the mechanisms of respiratory-cardiovascular coupling await further investigation.

Acknowledgments

The authors would like to thank Mr. Dominic Puleo for assistance in preparing the illustrations and Professor Jerome A. Dempsey for his critical review of the manuscript. This work was supported by the National Heart, Lung, and Blood Institute, the American Heart Association, the Hazel B. Mayer Trust, and the VA Medical Research Service.

References

1. Adrian ED, Bronk DW, Phillips G. Discharges in mammalian sympathetic nerves. J Physiol Lond 1932; 74:115–133.
2. Anrep GV, Pascual W, Rössler R. Respiratory variations in heart rate: I. The reflex mechanism of the respiratory arrhythmia. Proc R Soc Lond B Biol Sci 1936; 119B: 191–217.
3. Eckberg DL. Human sinus arrhythmia as an index of vagal cardiac outflow. J Appl Physiol 1983; 54:961–966.
4. Taha BH, Simon PM, Dempsey JA, Skatrud JB, Iber C. Respiratory sinus arrhyth-

mia in humans: an obligatory role for vagal feedback from the lungs. J Appl Physiol 1995; 78:638–645.

5. Hamlin RL, Smith CR, Smetzer DL. Sinus arrhythmia in the dog. Am J Physiol 1966; 210:321–328.

6. Rosenbaum M, Race D. Frequency-response characteristics of vascular resistance vessels. Am J Physiol 1968; 215:1397–1402.

7. Toska K, Eriksen M. Respiration-synchronous fluctuations in stroke volume, heart rate and arterial pressure in humans. J Physiol 1993; 472:501–512.

8. Macefield VG, Wallin BG. Modulation of muscle sympathetic activity during spontaneous and artificial ventilation and apnoea in humans. J Auton Nerv Syst 1995; 53:137–147.

9. Dornhorst AC, Howard P, Leathart GL. Respiratory variations in blood pressure. Circulation 1952; 6:553–558.

10. Dornhorst AC. Pulsus paradoxus. Int Care Med 1986; 12:387–388.

11. Katragadda S, Xie A, Puleo D, Skatrud JB, Morgan BJ. Neural mechanism of the pressor response to obstructive and nonobstructive apnea. J Appl Physiol 1997; 83: 2048–2054.

12. Bernardi L, Keller F, Sanders M, Reddy PS, Griffith B, Meno F, Pinsky MR. Respiratory sinus arrhythmia in the denervated human heart. J Appl Physiol 1989; 67: 1447–1455.

13. Iriuchijima J, Kumada M. Activity of single vagal fibers efferent to the heart. Jpn J Physiol 1964; 14:479–487.

14. McAllen RM, Spyer KM. Two types of vagal preganglionic motoneurones projecting to the heart and lungs. J Physiol 1978; 282:353–364.

15. Daly MDeB, Scott MJ. The effects of stimulation of the carotid body chemoreceptors on heart rate in the dog. J Physiol 1958; 144:148–166.

16. Angell-James JE, Daly M De B. The effects of artificial lung inflation on reflexly induced bradycardia associated with apnoea in the dog. J Physiol 1978; 274:349–366.

17. Daly M De B, Litherland AS, Wood LM. The reflex effects of inflation of the lungs on heart rate and hind limb vascular resistance in the cat. IRCS Med Sci Libr Compend 1983; 11:859–860.

18. Levy MN, Degeest, Zieske H. Effects of respiratory centre activity on the heart. Circ Res 1966; 18:67–78.

19. Snyder CD. A study of the causes of respiratory change of heart rate. Am J Physiol 1915; 37:104–117.

20. Shykoff BE, Naqvi SJ, Menon AS, Slutsky AS. Respiratory sinus arrhythmia in dogs. J Clin Invest 1991; 87:1621–1627.

21. Simon PM, Taha BH, Dempsey JA, Skatrud JB, Iber C. Role of vagal feedback from the lung in hypoxic-induced tachycardia in humans. J Appl Physiol 1995; 78: 1522–1530.

22. Fritsch JM, Smith ML, Simmons DT, Eckberg DL. Differential modulation of human vagal and sympathetic activity. Am J Physiol 1991; 260:R635–R641.

23. Horner R, Brooks D, Kozar LF, Gan K, Phillipson E. Respiratory-related heart rate variability persists during central apnea in dogs: mechanisms and implications. J Appl Physiol 1995; 78:2003–2013.

24. Melcher A. Respiratory sinus arrhythmia in man: a study in heart rate regulating mechanisms. Acta Physiol Scand Suppl 1976; 435:1–31.
25. Angell James JE, Daly M De B. Cardiovascular responses in apnoeic asphyxia: role of arterial chemoreceptors and the modification of their effects by a pulmonary vagal inflation reflex. J Physiol 1969; 201:87–104.
26. Gupta PD, Singh M. Carotid chemoreceptors and vagi in hypoxic and cyanide-induced tachycardia in the dog. Am J Physiol 1981; 240:H874–H880.
27. Kaufman MP, Iwamoto GA, Ashton JH, Cassidy SS. Responses to inflation of vagal afferents with endings in the lung of dogs. Circ Res 1982; 51:525–531.
28. Anrep GV, Pascual W, Rössler R. Respiratory variations in heart rate: II. The central mechanism of the respiratory arrhythmia and the inter-relations between the central and the reflex mechanisms. Proc R Soc Lond B Biol Sci 1936; 119B:218–232.
29. Haymet BT, McCloskey DI. Baroreceptor and chemoreceptor influences on heart rate during the respiratory cycle in the dog. J Physiol 1975; 245:699–712.
30. Gandevia SC, McCloskey DI, Potter EK. Inhibition of baroreceptors and chemoreceptor reflexes on heart rate by afferents from the lungs. J Physiol 1978; 276:369–381.
31. Davidson NS, Goldner S, McCloskey DI. Respiratory modulation of baroreceptor and chemoreceptor reflexes affecting heart rate and cardiac vagal efferent nerve activity. J Physiol 1976; 259:523–530.
32. Eckberg DL, Kifle YT, Roberts VL. Phase relationship between normal human respiration and baroreflex responsiveness. J Physiol 1980; 304:489–502.
33. Eckberg DL, Nerhed C, Wallin BG. Respiratory modulation of muscle sympathetic and vagal cardiac outflow in man. J Physiol 1985; 365:181–196.
34. Iber C, Simon P, Skatrud JB, Mahowald MW, Dempsey JA. The Breuer-Hering reflex in humans: effects of pulmonary denervation and hypocapnia. Am J Respir Crit Care Med 1995; 152:217–224.
35. Dempsey JA. Personal communication.
36. Hamilton RD, Winning AJ, Horner RL, Guz A. The effect of lung inflation on breathing in man during wakefulness and sleep. Respir Physiol 1988; 73: 145–154.
37. Daly M De B, Hazzledine JL, Ungar A. The reflex effects of alterations in lung volume on systemic vascular resistance in the dog. J Physiol 1967; 188:331–351.
38. Guyton AC, Lindsey AW, Abernathy B, Richardson T. Venous return at various right atrial pressures and the normal venous return curve. Am J Physiol 1957; 89: 609–615.
39. Linden RJ, Kappagoda CT. Atrial Receptors. Cambridge, UK: Cambridge University Press, 1982.
40. Keatinge WR. The effect of increased filling pressure on rhythmicity and atrioventricular conduction in isolated hearts. J Physiol 1959; 149:193–208.
41. Brooks CM, Lu HH, Lange G, Mangi R, Shaw RB, Geoly K. Effects of localized stretch of the sinoatrial node region of the dog heart. Am J Physiol 1966; 211: 1197–1202.
42. Goetz KL. Effect of increased pressure within a right heart cul-de-sac on heart rate in dogs. Am J Physiol 1965; 209:507–512.

43. Freyschuss U, Melcher A. Sinus arrhythmia in man: influence of tidal volume and oesophageal pressure. Scand J Clin Lab Invest 1975; 35:487–496.
44. Blaber AP, Hughson RL. Cardiorespiratory interactions during fixed-pace resistive breathing. J Appl Physiol 1996; 80:1618–1626.
45. Angell James JE. The effects of changes of extramural, "intrathoracic," pressure on aortic arch baroreceptors. J Physiol 1971; 214:89–103.
46. Fitzgerald RS, Robotham JL, Anand A. Baroreceptor output during normal and obstructed breathing and Mueller maneuvers. Am J Physiol 1981; 240:H721–H729.
47. Kato H, Menon AS, Slutsky AS. Mechanisms mediating the heart rate response to hypoxemia. Circulation 1988; 77:407–414.
48. Kato H, Menon AS, Chen F-J, Slutsky AS. Contribution of pulmonary receptors to the heart rate response to acute hypoxemia in rabbits. Circulation 1988; 78:1260–1266.
49. Scott MJ. The effects of hyperventilation on the reflex cardiac response from the carotid bodies of the cat. J Physiol 1966; 186:307–320.
50. Fagius J, Wallin BG. Sympathetic reflex latencies and conduction velocities in normal man. J Neurol Sci 1980; 47:433–448.
51. Gross PM, Whipp BJ, Davidson JT, Koyal SN, Wasserman K. Role of the carotid bodies in the heart rate response to breath holding in man. J Appl Physiol 1976; 41:336–340.
52. Honda Y, Hashizume I, Kimura H, Severinghaus JW. Bilateral carotid body resection in man enhances hypoxic tachycardia. Jpn J Physiol 1988; 38:917–928.
53. Band DM, McClelland M, Phillips DL, Saunders KB, Wolff CB. Sensitivity of the carotid body to within-breath changes in arterial P_{CO_2}. J Appl Physiol 1978; 45:768–777.
54. Goodman NW, Nail BS, Torrance RW. Oscillations in the discharge of single carotid chemoreceptor fibres of the cat. Respir Physiol 1974; 20:251–269.
55. Gardner WN. The pattern of breathing following step changes of alveolar partial pressures of CO_2 and O_2 in man. J Physiol 1980; 300:55–73.
56. Sant'Ambrogio FB, Mathew OP, Clark WD, Sant'Ambrogio G. Laryngeal influences on breathing pattern and posterior cricoarytenoid muscle activity. J Appl Physiol 1985; 58:1298–1304.
57. Nadel JA, Widdicombe JG. Reflex effects of upper airway irritation on total lung resistance and blood pressure. J Appl Physiol 1962; 17:861–865.
58. Tomori A, Widdicombe JG. Muscular, bronchomotor and cardiovascular reflexes elicited by mechanical stimulation of the respiratory tract. J Physiol 1969; 200:25–49.
59. Angell-James, Daly M De B. Some aspects of upper respiratory tract reflexes. Acta Otolaryngol 1975; 79:242–252.
60. Widdicombe JG. Respiratory reflexes in man and other mammalian species. Clin Sci 1961; 21:163–170.
61. Barman SM, Gebber GL. Basis for synchronization of sympathetic and phrenic nerve discharges. Am J Physiol 1976; 231:1601–1607.
62. Cohen MI, Gootman PM. Periodicities in efferent discharge of splanchnic nerve of the cat. Am J Physiol 1970; 218:1092–1101.
63. Boczek-Funcke A, Häbler H-J, Jänig W, Michaelis M. Respiratory modulation of

the activity in sympathetic neurones supplying muscle, skin, and pelvic organs in the cat. J Physiol 1992; 449:333–361.

64. Gilbey MP, Numao Y, Spyer KM. Discharge patterns of cervical sympathetic preganglionic neurones related to central respiratory drive in the rat. J Physiol 1986; 378:253–265.

65. Gregor M, Jänig W, Wiprich L. Cardiac and respiratory rhythmicities in cutaneous and muscle vasoconstrictor neurones to the cat's hindlimb. Pfliigers Arch 1977; 370:299–302.

66. Guyenet PG, Darnall RA, Riley TA. Rostral ventrolateral medulla and sympathorespiratory integration in rats. Am J Physiol 1990; 259:R1063–R1074.

67. Kimura N. Central rhythmic control of sympathetic nerve discharge: II. sympathetic nerve rhythms during morphine-induced phrenic nerve quiescence. Jikekai Med J 1988; 35:535–548.

68. Seals DR, Suwarno NO, Dempsey JA. Influence of lung volume on sympathetic nerve discharge in normal humans. Circ Res 1990; 67:130–141.

69. Seals DR, Suwarno NO, Joyner MJ, Iber C, Copeland JG, Dempsey JA. Respiratory modulation of muscle sympathetic nerve activity in intact and lung denervated humans. Circ Res 1993; 72:440–454.

70. Häbler H-J, Jänig W, Michaelis M. Respiratory modulation in the activity of sympathetic neurones. Prog Neurobiol 1994; 43:567–606.

71. Bachoo M, Polosa C. Properties of a sympatho-inhibitory and vasodilator reflex evoked by superior laryngeal nerve afferents in the cat. J Physiol 1985; 364:183–198.

72. Koepchen HP, Seller H, Polster J, Langhorst P. Über die Fein-Vasomotorik der Muskelstrohmbahn und ihre Beziehung zur Ateminnervation. Pflügers Arch 1968; 302:285–299.

73. Koizumi K, Seller H, Kaufman A, Brooks CM. Pattern of sympathetic discharges and their relation to baroreceptor and respiratory activities. Brain Res 1971; 27: 281–294.

74. Czyzyk MF, Fedorko L, Trzebski A. Pattern of the respiratory modulation of the sympathetic activity is species dependent: synchronization of the sympathetic outflow over the respiratory cycle in the rat. In: Ciriello J, Calaresu FR, Renaud LP, Polosa C, eds. Organization of the Autonomic Nervous System: Central and Peripheral Mechanisms. New York: Alan R Liss, 1987:143–152.

75. Numao Y, Koshiya N, Gilbey MP, Syper KM. Central respiratory drive-related activity in sympathetic nerves of the rat: the regional differences. Neurosci Lett 1987; 81:279–284.

76. Darnall RA, Guyenet P. Respiratory modulation of the pre- and postganglionic lumbar vasomotor sympathetic neurons in the rat. Neurosci Lett 1990; 119:148–152.

77. Häbler H-J, Jänig W, Krummell M, Peters OA. Respiratory modulation of the activity in postganglionic neurons supplying skeletal muscle and skin of the rat hindlimb. J Neurophysiol 1993; 70:920–930.

78. Bachoo M, Polosa C. Properties of the inspiration-related activity of sympathetic preganglionic neurones of the cervical trunk in the cat. J Physiol 1987; 385:545–564.

79. Richter DW, Spyer KM. Cardiorespiratory control. In: Loewy AD, Spyer KM, eds. Central Regulation of Autonomic Functions, New York: Oxford University Press, 1990:189–207.

80. Connelly CA, Wurster RD. Sympathetic rhythms during hyperventilation-induced apnea. Am J Physiol 1985; 249:R424–R431.

81. Zhong S, Zhou S, Gebber GL, Barman SM. Coupled oscillators account for the slow rhythms in sympathetic nerve discharge and phrenic nerve activity. Am J Physiol 1997; 272:R1314–R1324.

82. Trzebski A, Kubin L. is the central inspiratory activity responsible for P_{CO_2}-dependent drive of the sympathetic discharge? J Auton Nerv Sys 1981; 3:401–420.

83. Sant'Ambrogio G, Sant'Ambrogio FB. Reflexes from the upper airway, lungs, chest wall, and limbs. In: Crystal RG, West JB, Weibel ER, Barnes PJ, eds. The Lung. Vol 2. Philadelphia: Lippincott-Raven, 1997:1805–1819.

84. Daly M De B, Robinson BH. An analysis of the reflex systemic vasodilator response elicited by lung inflation in the dog. J Physiol 1968; 195:387–406.

85. Glick G, Wechsler AS, Epstein SE. Reflex cardiovascular depression produced by stimulation of pulmonary stretch receptors in the dog. J Clin Invest 1969; 48:467–473.

86. Salisbury PF, Galletti P-M, Lewin RJ, Rieben PA. Stretch reflexes from the dog's lung to the systemic circulation. Circulation Res 1959; 7:62–67.

87. Ott NT, Shepherd JT. Vasodepressor reflex from lung inflation in the rabbit. Am J Physiol 1971; 221:889–895.

88. Gerber U, Polosa C. Effects of pulmonary stretch receptor afferent stimulation on sympathetic preganglionic neuron firing. Can J Physiol Pharmacol 1978; 56:191–198.

89. Gootman PM, Feldman JL, Cohen MI. Pulmonary afferent influences on respiratory modulation of sympathetic discharge. In: Koepchen HP, Hilton SM, Trzebski A, eds. Central Interaction Between Respiratory and Cardiovascular Control Systems. Berlin: Springer-Verlag, 1980:172–178.

90. Yu J, Roberts AM, Joshua IG. Lung inflation evokes reflex dilation of microvessels in rat skeletal muscle. Am J Physiol 1990; 258:H939–H945.

91. Daly MDeB, Ward J, Wood LM. The peripheral chemoreceptors and cardiovascular-respiratory integration. In: Taylor EW, ed. The Neurobiology of the Cardiorespiratory System. Manchester, UK: Manchester University Press, 1987:342–368.

92. Hagbarth K-E, Vallbo ÅB. Pulse and respiratory grouping of sympathetic impulses in human muscle nerves. Acta Physiol Scand 1968; 74:96–108.

93. Paintal AS. Cardiovascular receptors. In: Neil E, ed. Handbook of Sensory Physiology. Vol. 3/1. Berlin: Springer-Verlag, 1972:1–45.

94. Linden RJ, Mary DASG, Weatherill D. The nature of the atrial receptors responsible for a reflex decrease in activity in renal nerves in the dog. J Physiol 1980; 300:31–40.

95. Karim F, Kidd C, Malpus CM, Penna PE. The effects of stimulation of the left atrial receptors on sympathetic efferent nerve activity. J Physiol 1972; 227:243–260.

96. Coleridge HM, Coleridge JCG, Kidd C. Cardiac receptors in the dog, with particular

reference to two types of afferent ending in the ventricular wall. J Physiol 1964; 174:323–339.

97. Aviado DM, Li TH, Kalow W, Schmidt CF, Turnbull GL, Peskin GW, Hess ME, Weiss AJ. Respiratory and circulatory reflexes from the perfused heart and pulmonary circulation of the dog. Am J Physiol 1951; 165:261–277.

98. Mason JM, Ledsome JR. Effects of obstruction of the mitral orifice or distension of the pulmonary vein-atrial junctions on renal and hindlimb vascular resistance in the dog. Circ Res 1974; 35:24–32.

99. Lloyd TC. Control of systemic vascular resistance by pulmonary and left heart baroreflexes. Am J Physiol 1972; 222:1511–1517.

100. Thames MD, Donald DE, Shepherd JT. Behavior of cardiac receptors with nomyelinated vagal afferents during spontaneous respiration in cats. Circ Res 1977; 41: 694–701.

101. Sagawa K. Baroreflex control of systemic arterial pressure and vascular bed. In: Shepherd JT, Abboud FM, eds. Handbook of Physiology: Section 2. The Cardiovascular System. Vol III, Part 2. Bethesda, MD: American Physiological Society, 1983: 453–496.

102. Summer WR, Permutt S, Sagawa K, Shoukas AA, Bromberger-Barnea B. Effects of spontaneous respiration on canine left ventricular function. Circ Res 1979; 45: 719–728.

103. Tang PC, Maire FW, Amassian VE. Respiratory influence on the vasomotor center. Am J Physiol 1957; 191:218–224.

104. Boczek-Funke A, Dembowsky K, Häbler H-J, Jänig W, Michaells M. Respiratory-related activity patterns in preganglionic neurones projecting into the cat cervical sympathetic trunk. J Physiol 1992; 457:277–296.

105. Morgan BJ, Denahan T, Ebert TJ. Neurocirculatory consequences of negative intrathoracic pressure vs asphyxia during voluntary apnea. J Appl Physiol 1993; 74: 2969–2975.

106. Saunders JS, Ferguson DW, Mark AL. Arterial baroreflex control of sympathetic nerve activity during elevation of blood pressure in normal man: dominance of aortic baroreflexes. Circulation 1988; 77:279–288.

107. Smith ML, Beightol LA, Fritsch-Yelle JM, Ellenbogen KA, Porter TR, Eckberg DL. Valsalva's maneuver revisited: a quantitative method yielding insights into human autonomic control. Am J Physiol 1996; 271:H1240–H1249.

108. Rowell LB, Johnson DG, Chase PB, Comess, KA, Seals DR. Hypoxemia raises muscle sympathetic nerve activity but not norepinephrine in resting humans. J Appl Physiol 1989; 66:1736–1743.

109. Katona PG, Dembowsky K, Czachurski J, Seller H. Chemoreceptor stimulation on sympathetic activity: dependence on respiratory phase. Am J Physiol 1989; 257: R1027–R1033.

110. Angell James, Daly M De B. Reflex respiratory and cardiovascular effects of stimulation of receptors in the nose of the dog. J Physiol 1972; 220:673–696.

111. McCloskey DI, Mitchell JH. Reflex cardiovascular and respiratory responses originating in exercising muscle. J Physiol 1972; 224:173–186.

112. Adreani CM, Hill JM, Kaufman MP. Responses of group III and IV muscle afferents to dynamic exercise. J Appl Physiol 1997; 82:1811–1817.

113. Hinsey JC, Hare K, Philips RA. Sensory components of the phrenic nerve of the cat. Proc Soc Exp Biol Med 1939; 41:411–414.

114. Duron B. Intercostal and diaphragmatic muscle afferents. In: Hornbein TF, ed. Regulation of Breathing. Part I. New York: Marcel Dekker, 1981:473–540.

115. Offner B, Dembowsky K, Czachurski J. Characteristics of sympathetic reflexes evoked by electrical stimulation of phrenic nerve afferents. J Auton Nerv Syst 1992; 41:103–112.

116. Szulczyk A, Szulczyk P, Zywuszko B. Analysis of reflex activity in cardiac sympathetic nerve induced by myelinated phrenic nerve afferents. Brain Res 1988; 447: 109–115.

117. Road JD, West NH, Van Vliet BN. Ventilatory effects of stimulation of phrenic afferents. J Appl Physiol 1987; 63:1063–1069.

118. Hussain SNA, Chatillon A, Comtois A, Roussos C, Magder S. Chemical activation of thin-fiber phrenic afferents: 2. Cardiovascular responses. J Appl Physiol 1991; 70:77–86.

119. Harms CA, Babcock MA, McClaran SR, Pegelow DF, Nickele GA, Nelson WB, Dempsey JA. Respiratory muscle work compromises leg blood flow during maximal exercise. J Appl Physiol 1997; 82:1573–1583.

120. Brown TE, Beightol LA, Koh J, Eckberg DL. Important influence of respiration on human R-R interval power spectra is largely ignored. J Appl Physiol 1993; 75: 2310–2317.

121. Batsel HL. Activity of bulbospinal neurons during passive hyperventilation. Exp Neurol 1967; 19:357–374.

122. Hayano J, Yasuma F, Okada A, Mukai S, Fujinami T. Respiratory sinus arrhythmia: a phenomenon improving pulmonary gas exchange and circulatory efficiency. Circulation 1996; 94:842–847.

123. Huikuri HV, Niemelä MJ, Ojala S, Rantala A, Ikäheimo MJ, Airaksinen KEJ. Circadian rhythms of frequency domain measures of heart rate variability in healthy subjects and patients with coronary artery disease. Circulation 1994; 90:121–126.

124. Vanoli E, Adamson PB, Lin B, Pinna GD, Lazzara R, Orr WC. Heart rate variability during specific sleep stages: a comparison of healthy subjects with patients with myocardial infarction. Circulation 1995; 91:1918–1922.

125. Bonsignore MR, Romano S, Marrone O, Insalaco G. Respiratory sinus arrhythmia during obstructive sleep apnoeas in humans. J Sleep Res 1995; 4(suppl 1):68–70.

126. Eckberg DL, Bastow H, Scruby AE. Modulation of human sinus node function by systemic hypoxia. J Appl Physiol 1982; 52:570–577.

127. Morgan BJ. Acute and chronic cardiovascular responses to sleep disordered breathing. Sleep 1996; 19:S206–S209.

2

Chemoreflex-Baroreflex Interactions in Cardiovascular Disease

DARREL P. FRANCIS and ANDREW J. S. COATS

Royal Brompton Hospital
London, England

PIOTR PONIKOWSKI

Military Hospital
Wroclaw, Poland

I. Introduction

Reflex feedback control mechanisms play important roles in the maintenance of homeostasis in many physiological systems. Physiologists have over the past few decades have acquired detailed information on the behavior of such reflexes in intact physiological states in regulating the cardiovascular and respiratory systems. In this chapter we survey these findings, and then address the state of knowledge of the interplay between these regulatory reflexes in health and in the presence of chronic heart failure.

II. Chemoreceptors: Anatomy, Physiology, Neuroanatomy, Clinical Tests, Pathophysiology

A. Peripheral Chemoreceptors and Hypoxia

The peripheral chemoreceptors are localized in the carotid and aortic bodies. They increase their firing rate primarily in response to hypoxia but also, to some extent, to hypercapnia.

Animal experiments, in which it is possible directly to sample chemorecep-

33

tor afferent firing rates, have suggested differential responses to hypoxia from the two peripheral chemoreceptor groups. A fall in arterial P_{O_2} causes a larger increment in the firing rate of carotid body chemoreceptors than of aortic body chemoreceptors (1). Chemoreception in the aortic body may well be more attuned to detecting changes in overall oxygen content than partial pressure, by virtue of its much higher blood flow (2).

The two chemoreceptor groups may also differ in their relative impact on respiratory rate and tidal volume, the two components that determine overall ventilation. Carotid body stimulation by hypoxia produces increases in both rate and depth of respiration, whereas aortic body stimulation leads to only a small increase in respiratory rate and little or no effect on depth (3).

The response of these peripheral chemoreceptors to different static levels of P_{O_2} has been extensively studied in animals. Some level of tonic chemoreceptor firing occurs even at very high P_{O_2} values, but only when Pa_{O_2} falls below a certain level does the rate of firing increase significantly. This level, which is the highest Pa_{O_2} at which chemoreception can be said to be occurring, is around 200 mmHg in cats (4). But only below about 100 mmHg does firing rise rapidly enough to be useful in fine respiratory control (5).

In humans, information about the differential response from the two chemoreceptor groups has been gleaned from work on patients who have undergone therapeutic bilateral carotid body resection (6–8). These studies indicate that the great majority of the human hypoxic response is dependent on the carotid body.

B. Adaptation to Hypoxia

Adaptation over time is another area of interest that is being developed. In humans facing a steep decline in oxygen saturation, there is an initial period of marked hyperpnea lasting about 10 minutes, after which the phenomenon of "hypoxic ventilatory decline" supervenes, and the patient returns to a minute ventilation rate that is only mildly elevated above normal. It is not known if this is a consequence of chemoreceptor habituation or a change in the central response to continuous chemoreceptor firing.

Animal studies have permitted detailed evaluation of chemoreceptor firing. In some species there is an attenuation of the firing response over time. For example in the rabbit, there is a loss of about one-third of the firing response to hypoxia after 1 hr (9). In contrast, the goat does not show this effect, and indeed, shows an increased sensitivity to hypoxia after 1 hr (5).

The most plausible explanation for the overall phenomenon of hypoxic ventilatory decline in humans is that increased firing of the peripheral chemoreceptors is responsible for the initial increase in ventilation, but that hypoxia eventually interferes with central brainstem function, resulting in a blunting of the ventilatory response after 10–30 min (10).

C. Clinical Tests

In the intact human, it is not practicable to measure directly the firing rate of chemoreceptors, of afferent nerves, or of brainstem activity. The most readily measured output parameter is total ventilation rate, which can be determined by spirometer (11) or pneumotachograph: this gives information about the total gain of the respiratory control system. The overall ventilation is the product of respiratory rate and tidal volume: it is the latter that is most markedly altered in response to chemoreceptor stimulation; some have therefore chosen to measure tidal volume as the output of the ventilatory system.

Measuring the stimulus to the peripheral chemoreceptors presents a further problem. The most direct physiological parameter to measure is arterial partial pressure of oxygen (P_{O_2}). Some workers have taken the approach of exposing the subject to a constant level of hypoxia for several minutes and then sampling arterial blood slowly while quantifying the ventilatory response. This allows accurate determination of both stimulus and response, during a (short) steady state. One problem with this approach is that hypoxia causes a rise in ventilation sufficient to depress the arterial P_{CO_2}. Therefore, as a further refinement, exogenous CO_2 can be added to the inspired air, at a rate controlled automatically or manually by the investigator, in order to keep the P_{CO_2} at a constant level, thereby avoiding any secondary ventilatory changes attributable to CO_2-sensitive reflex responses.

An alternative approach has been to consider the dynamic response of the ventilatory control system to transient stimuli (12), which has the advantage of being safe enough to apply not only with normal subjects but also in patients with disease. In chronic heart failure, the peripheral hypoxic response as measured by this method has been found to be enhanced (13), showing at least its sensitivity in detecting disease-associated alterations in chemoreceptor responses.

D. Hypercapnia—Central Sensors

The major part of the ventilatory response to carbon dioxide is independent of the peripheral sensors we have discussed. From the early 1950s, evidence had been accumulating that pH changes in the cerebrospinal fluid of the cerebral ventricles could have a dramatic effect on ventilation (14,15). More focal application of these acid stimuli subsequently identified the ventrolateral medulla as the site of greatest sensitivity (16); within this, there is a rostral area (of Mitchell) and a caudal area (of Loeschke), as reviewed by Natie (17). The broad spread of electrophysiological and immunohistochemical evidence pointing to these areas includes observational and interventional experiments on a variety of species (18).

Among the neurons of the superficial medulla, several workers have identified numerous tonically active units whose firing rates, while independent of respiration itself, vary with the P_{CO_2} in the overlying cerebrospinal fluid (19). While these are clearly chemosensitive cells, it should not be overlooked that the presence of a response to pH does not prove that they are the key central chemoreceptive neurons whose output modulates respiration.

Focal injections of nanoliter volumes of acetazolamide solution, which have been shown to produce zones of acidosis with radius less than 350 μm, are able to stimulate respiration at numerous sites within the ventrolateral medulla (20). The most sensitive locations include not only the superficial areas of Mitchell and Loeschke but also deeper sites near the nucleus of the solitary tract and the locus cereleus. A further consideration is that not all areas of the brainstem undergo the same tissue pH change following an alteration in arterial pH: identification of sites whose pH falls significantly after injection of CO_2-rich saline into the vertebral artery (21) may also contribute usefully to the task of defining the true central chemoreceptive neurons.

How exactly is hypercapnia sensed? Several experiments have pointed out that ventilation responds to changes in both CSF pH and P_{CO_2}. These imply two possibilities. First, there could be independent sensory mechanisms for pH and P_{CO_2}. Second, there could be a common sensor that detects pH in an intracellular compartment: CO_2 from the extracellular fluid can easily enter the cell and lower its pH, while bicarbonate cannot cross so easily. This could explain why some (in vitro) studies show that if medullary tissue P_{CO_2} is kept constant while the bicarbonate is decreased, although tissue pH falls, there is no response by the neurons (22).

One further observation is that the response to hypoxia together with hypercapnia is much larger than the sum of the effects of each alone (23); that is, there is a positive synergy between the two stimuli.

III. Baroreceptors

The arterial baroreceptors, located at the carotid sinuses and aortic arch, are sensitive to changes in arterial blood pressure. Signals from them are carried to the cardiovascular control center in the brainstem, from which vagal efferent regulate the activity of the sinoatrial node of the heart. By this baroreflex mechanism, a rise in blood pressure leads to a prompt widening of the RR interval, with a latency of approximately 1 sec. Although the RR interval response saturates at extremes, over a wide range it is linearly related to arterial blood pressure: the slope of this relationship (in milliseconds per millimeter of mercury) is defined as the baroreflex sensitivity.

Two main methods have been used to measure baroreflex sensitivity in humans. The neck chamber technique (24) involves applying negative pressure to a flexible collar around the neck while heart rate and arterial pressure are measured. However, it is never possible to exclude a direct psychological effect on heart rate following the sensation of pressure changes around the neck, which would interfere with determination of true reflex sensitivity.

More widely used now are techniques based on the administration of vasoactive agents (25), such as the pressors angiotensin and phenylephrine or the vasodilator glyceryl trinitrate. Blood pressure can now be measured continuously and noninvasively using infrared photoplethysmography.

The pharmacological blood pressure stimuli offer the advantage of eliminating subject awareness. In humans, a typical bolus dose of 50–150 μg of phenylephrine, the α-adrenoceptor agonist, causes a prompt and progressive rise in blood pressure of 20–30 mmHg. Alternatively, a continuous infusion may be used to maintain an elevated blood pressure and the infusion rate changed to bring about a different degree of elevation.

Disease is known to affect baroreflex sensitivity in humans. Hypertension (26) and chronic heart failure (27,28) are both associated with a chronically reduced baroreflex gain. Acute myocardial infarction results in depressed baroreflex sensitivity in the first few days, but the sensitivity returns to normal in many patients within 2–3 months (29). The degree of depression of the baroreflex is not well correlated to the degree of depression of left ventricular ejection and has been proposed as a useful independent prognostic indicator of sudden cardiac death after myocardial infarction (30).

IV. Respiratory Effects of Cardiovascular Regulators

A. Effect of Blood-Pressure Changes on Ventilation

It has long been known that changes in arterial blood pressure affect ventilation. Experiments from the first quarter of the century demonstrated that pharmacological elevation of blood pressure using adrenaline reduces minute ventilation (31). Conversely, lowering blood pressure in the cat by inducing a hemorrhage leads to a rise in ventilation (32). Several mechanisms have been proposed.

One initially attractive proposition (33) was that the change in blood pressure causes a change in blood flow through the chemoreceptive tissues, which, in turn, alters the dynamic equilibrium concentrations of oxygen and carbon dioxide in the fluid bathing the chemoreceptors. Under this hypothesis, the effect is exerted peripherally.

However, direct measurements of discharge frequency of chemoreceptor afferents (34) have shown that in the range of 60 to 160 mmHg, arterial blood pressure has only a small effect on chemoreceptor firing, which is inadequate to explain the magnitude of the changes in ventilation.

An alternative theory is that the rise in blood pressure is sensed by arterial baroreceptors and the afferent signal feeds into the ventilatory system at the level of the brainstem. This idea led to experiments involving direct baroreceptor stimulation in the cat (35), which showed more significant effects on thoracic and abdominal respiration.

B. Central Effect of Norepinephrine on Ventilation

An association between elevated plasma norepinephrine levels and sleep apnea syndrome in humans has long been recognized (36). While it may well be that the episodic arterial oxygen desaturation causes increased norepinephrine release, we should not forget the possibility that norepinephrine itself may contribute by having an inhibitory effect on ventilation.

In goats, intracarotid injections of norepinephrine have been shown to have a respiratory depressant effect (37).

More detailed experiments using intravenous injections in dogs (38) have confirmed this phenomenon. They show that norepinephrine causes not only a rise in blood pressure but also a fall in respiration, alongside a fall in arterial O_2 and a small rise in arterial CO_2. Moreover, even when the dog was mechanically ventilated at a constant rate, norepinephrine injection still led to a fall in arterial O_2 and a rise in arterial CO_2. Finally, electrical stimulation of the nucleus reticularis parvocellularis, a known brainstem vasopressor site, led to a respiratory response similar to that seen with norepinephrine, which suggests that this may be norepinephrine's site of action on the respiratory system.

C. Angiotensin II and Vasopressin

Several animal studies have looked at the central respiratory effects of two cardiovascular peptide hormones: vasopressin and angiotensin II. Both are well known to cause an increase in arterial blood pressure. Vasopressin causes a small decrease in ventilation, a response that is ablated by the administration of sodium nitroprusside to restore blood pressure to baseline.

In contrast, administration of angiotensin II alone does not cause an change in ventilation, but if the rise in blood pressure is eliminated by the use of nitroprusside, a marked rise in ventilation is unmasked (39). Measurements of baroreceptor activity (40) and studies of baroreceptor denervation (41) point to a central site of action of angiotensin II on the respiratory system.

V. Cardiovascular Consequences of Chemoreceptor Stimulation

While the chemoreceptor reflexes play an important role in regulating ventilation, they also have profound effects on the cardiovascular control centers.

By the late 1950s, it had been established that the main cardiovascular effects of systemic hypoxia were tachycardia, hypertension, positive inotropy, and veno- and vasoconstriction. Yet several workers had reported that local carotid body hypoxia caused bradycardia rather than tachycardia.

In 1961, Downing et al. (42) addressed this issue. They administered hypoxic stimuli (venous blood with P_{O_2} ~30 mmHg) to the *isolated* carotid body of anesthetized dogs, and found marked reductions in heart rate (from 134 to 81 beats per minute). Blood pressure was almost unchanged and cardiac output fell slightly. When the hypoxic carotid body stimuli were repeated after vagotomy, the bradycardic effects were much milder (from 150 to 131 beats per minute) and the blood pressure showed a small rise. In contrast, application of *systemic* hypoxia (by inhalation of nitrogen) led to tachycardia, hypertension, and increased cardiac output.

Furthermore, Downing et al. studied left ventricular and aortic pressure and aortic flow. These measurements demonstrated that while both isolated carotid body hypoxia and systemic hypoxia caused peripheral vasoconstriction, the isolated hypoxic stimulus caused a positive inotropic response while systemic hypoxia caused negative inotropy. In summary, the authors found that despite the effect of local hypoxia on the carotid bodies being a vagally mediated bradycardia and a positive inotropy, the response of the whole animal to systemic hypoxia was in fact a reproducible tachycardia and negative inotropy. Only the vasoconstrictive effects of the two stimuli coincided. They concluded that the cardiovascular chemoreflex response (unlike the ventilatory response) might be dependent on chemoreceptors outside the carotid body.

The central hemodyamic effects of carotid chemoreceptor stimulation have been found to include bradycardia and a negative inotropic effect on the ventricular myocardium (43). In contrast, aortic chemoreceptor stimulation has been shown to cause a positive inotropic effect and an increase in heart rate (44). The physiological significance of this dichotomy is not clear. In disease states, differential changes in the sensitivity of the two receptor areas may change the net effect of chemoreceptor-generated responses to alterations in arterial blood gases.

It is important to bear in mind that chemoreflex stimulation leads to an increase in ventilation: this has an effect on heart rate and blood pressure, which confounds the observation of the direct chemoreceptor-to-cardiovascular reflex (45). In the left panel of Figure 1, a dog shows little change in blood pressure or heart rate on to chemoreceptor stimulation by intracarotid nicotine. However, once the lungs are denervated by a brief steam inhalation and then ventilated artificially (right panel), there is clear bradycardia and hypertension in response to the same chemostimulant.

A wealth of evidence from early 1960s established that the major peripheral response to hypoxia is vasoconstriction. Efforts have been made to delineate the mechanism of the vascular responses to chemoreceptor stimulation by separately measuring the vasoconstrictor response in the gracilis muscle and the paw (46). The results show an interesting divergence: alongside the immediate bradycardia, there is vasoconstriction in the muscle and a (weaker) vasodilatation in the paw; overall systemic arterial pressure is little changed (Fig. 2).

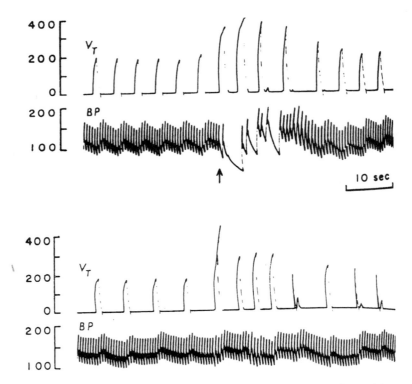

Figure 1 Effects on respiration (VT, ml), blood pressure (BP, mmHg) and heart rate of intracarotid injection of 10 μg of nicotine in a dog. (Top) The dog is breathing spontaneously, while injection (bottom) was performed after a steam inhalation that denervated the lung. (From Ref. 42.)

The investigators established that vagal stimulation to cause the same amount of bradycardia did *not* bring about these vasomotor changes, and that the responses were dependent on intact innervation of the carotid body area and of the muscle bed. This implied that the vasomotor phenomena are a neurological reflex loop and are independent of the heart rate effects of chemoreceptor stimulation. Administration of phentolamine abolished the muscle vasoconstriction, indicating that it occurred by withdrawal of sympathetic tone. In contrast, paw vasodilatation was unaffected by the α-adrenoceptor antagonist phentolamine, the β-adrenoceptor antagonist propranolol, the cholinergic antagonist atropine, or the histaminergic antagonist tripelennamine.

Human studies have shown that moderate hypercapnia causes an increase in blood pressure and a tachycardia, with more marked effects if the experiment is carried out in hypoxia than in hyperoxia (47). Indirect evidence, from experi-

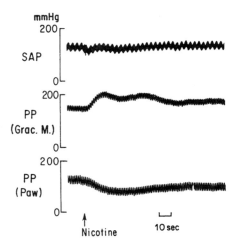

Figure 2 Reflex responses in muscle and paw. Stimulation of right carotid chemorecep- tors by intracarotid injection of 10 microgram of nicotine. SAP = systemic arterial pres- sure; PP (Grac. M.) = perfusion pressure in gracilis muscle; PP (Paw) = perfusion pres- sure in paw. (From Ref. 46.)

ments involving constant hyperventilation with normal and subnormal alveolar P_{CO_2} levels, suggests that these cardiovascular effects are not dependent on changes in ventilation (48).

What is the physiological significance of the tachycardia and muscle vaso- constriction seen during hypoxia or hypercapnia? It has been speculated that these responses are an attempt to compensate for the reduction in quality of blood by diverting blood away from the more metabolically active tissue such as the mus- cle, allowing a relatively greater quantity of blood to be delivered to key vascular beds in the coronary and cerebral circulation.

VI. Chemoreflex-Baroreflex Interactions in Dogs

While there has been extensive research on the responses of the ventilatory sys- tem to changes in gas tension and of the cardiovascular system to changes in blood pressure and considerable data on the effect of stimulation of each system on the resting state of the other, there is much less literature concentrating on the interplay of reflexes in the two systems, at least in one direction: a baroreflex effect on chemoreceptor sensitivity.

In a series of detailed experiments in dogs (49), the Iowa group analyzed the change in chemoreflex sensitivity with alterations in arterial blood pressure levels. Carotid chemoreceptors were activated by intracarotid injections of nicotine, while the change in ventilation and end-tidal P_{CO_2} were measured. This procedure was carried out at different blood pressures: resting, low (using artificial hemorrhage) or high (by transiently inflating a cuff around the abdominal aorta). They found that lowering the arterial pressure from 117 to 57 mmHg caused an enhancement of the ventilatory response (to 1 µg of nicotine) from 3.1 to 5.7 L/min. Furthermore, elevation of the blood pressure to 140 mmHg caused a depression of the nicotine-induced ventilatory response to 0.9 L/min. Ventilation–blood pressure slopes at three levels of chemoreceptor stimulation are plotted in Figure 3. This shows that chemoreceptor stimulation causes a rise in ventilation in all circumstances, but the size of the increment falls as the carotid blood pressure is raised.

While this demonstrated a strong effect, there was still the question of whether this reflex interaction was occurring at the level of the chemoreceptor itself or in the central nervous system. They therefore went on to isolate (and perfuse independently) both carotid bifurcations. This allowed them to measure the chemoreflex response to stimulation of chemoreceptors on one side, while they could alter the blood pressure sensed by the baroreceptors on the *other* side

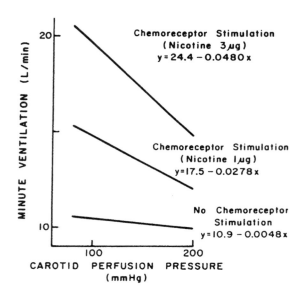

Figure 3 Relationship between carotid perfusion pressure and minute ventilation in the presence or absence of carotid chemoreceptor stimulation by nicotine. Slopes calculated from data from eight dogs with vagus nerves intact. Slopes during chemoreceptor stimulation are significantly different from slope with no chemoreceptor stimulation. (From Ref. 49.)

of the neck. They found that elevating the blood pressure on one side from 81 to 199 mmHg led to an attenuation of the nicotine-induced chemoreflex response of the contralateral chemoreceptors from 4.1 to 1.1 L/min.

Clearly the interplay between the reflexes was not dependent on the chemo- and barostimuli coinciding in place, but this did not necessarily prove that the interaction was a central one. It was still conceivable that the rise in blood pressure was leading via a brainstem reflex to a change in neural activation of the contralateral chemoreceptors. So bilateral low cervical vagotomies were carried out: this eliminated sympathetic outflow to the carotid bodies. Even in these conditions, the chemoreflex response was attenuated (3.5–1.6 L/min) by elevated blood pressure (82–190 mmHg): further evidence of a central interaction between these two reflexes.

The group also looked at the cardiovascular efferent arm of the chemoreflex (50), using a similar protocol. While the stimulus to the chemoreceptors remained intracarotid infusion of nicotine, the response being measured was vasoconstriction (as quantified by perfusion pressure in the innervated gracilis muscle). Again the experiment was carried out starting from different baseline blood pressures. At a baseline blood pressure of 102 mmHg, a 10-μg nicotine stimulus caused a 20-mmHg increase in gracilis perfusion pressure. When the blood pressure was raised to 132 mmHg, the same stimulus led to a greatly attenuated vasoconstrictor response: 4 mmHg. Conversely, experiments with hemorrhagic hypotension showed falls in blood pressure from 127 to 73 and then 46 mmHg caused enhancement in the nicotine-induced gracilis vasoconstrictor response from 7 to 20 and then 32 mmHg.

The investigators moved on to study the effect of chemoreceptor stimulation at one carotid while the blood pressure at the *other* carotid sinus was controlled: again a rise in carotid pressure caused an attenuation in vasoconstrictor response to chemoreceptor stimulation on the other side. Finally, they established that the change in blood pressure applied to one carotid did not affect P_{O_2}, P_{CO_2}, and pH in the blood perfusing the other carotid and therefore could not directly interfere with the chemoreceptor input, which was evidence of a genuine baroreflex-chemoreflex interaction.

Other studies have considered the cardiovascular chemoreflex response when the baroreflex input is at extreme values (51). In ventilated dogs, the carotid chemoreceptors were stimulated by a local infusion of blood with P_{O_2} below 40 mmHg, P_{CO_2} above 70 mmHg, and pH below 7.15: these values had been previously determined to achieve maximal chemoreceptor stimulation (52). The procedure was repeated at different carotid sinus pressures: low (50 mmHg), intermediate (129 mmHg) and high (212 mmHg). In each case, aortic pressure and blood flow in the hindlimb and kidney were monitored: these were normalized by comparison to the control values (129 mmHg before chemoreceptor stimulation).

The experiment showed first that both chemoreceptor stimulation and lowering the carotid sinus pressure had similar cardiovascular effects: a rise in aortic pressure, a marked fall in hindlimb blood flow, and a smaller decline in renal blood flow. Elevating the carotid sinus pressure had the opposite effect. The key results, however, were that at low or high carotid sinus perfusion pressures, maximal chemoreceptor stimulation had little or no effect on aortic pressure, hindlimb, or renal blood flow. This effect persisted even after cutting the cervical vagosympathetic efferent fibers (which could have allowed the vasomotor center to directly modulate the chemoreceptors). Baroreceptor denervation eliminated this effect, which excluded the possibility that the pressure changes were being sensed by the chemoreceptors themselves.

The same authors (53) went on to address the question of why chemoreceptor stimulation fails to add to sympathetic output when carotid sinus pressure is low: is it simply because sympathetic output is already maximal, or is there further reserve? By interrupting the afferents from the low-pressure mechanoreceptors of the atria and great veins, they were able to uncover further vasoconstrictive reserve. In other words, the magnitude of the chemoreflex-induced cardiovascular response is constrained by some limit; atrial mechanoreceptor–induced cardiovascular responses are not.

From these animal experiments, we could surmise that the central interaction between these two reflexes is "proximal" in the final common pathway.

VII. Chemoreflex-Baroreflex Interactions in Humans

The study of chemoreflex-baroreflex interactions in humans began with investigations of the reflex response to diving. Bradycardia has long been recognized to accompany diving. Changes in vascular tone had been a subject of much dispute until a key study compared the effects of simple breath-holding and facial immersion on heart rate, intra-arterial blood pressure, and forearm blood flow (54) (Fig. 4).

The authors found that both stimuli resulted in qualitatively similar effects: bradycardia, a rise in blood pressure, and a fall in forearm blood flow. The combination of the latter two effects implied vasoconstriction. The immersion stimulus, however, caused a larger effect in all of these parameters than did the breath-hold, as well as a more abrupt fall in flow.

What is the mechanism of this fall in blood flow? Direct measurement of sympathetic nerve activity in the peroneal nerve have been made in humans during hypoxic stress (55). Hypoxia alone led to a significant increase in sympathetic activity, but this change was greatly enhanced when the patient was asked to briefly hold his or her breath at the end of expiration (thereby eliminating the confounding effect of hyperventilation). A further consideration was that there was a tendency to hypocapnia as a result of the hyperventilatory response to

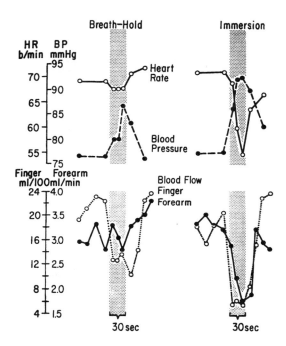

Figure 4 Average values of heart rate, mean arterial blood pressure, and blood flow to the finger and forearm before, during (shaded area), and after breath holding and immersion in 10 subjects. (From Ref. 54.)

hypoxia. Addition of CO_2 to the inspired gas mixture allowed the formation of an isocapnic hypoxic state. In this state, sympathetic activity was again elevated, and interestingly showed a larger rise in response to apnea than it did during hypocapnic hypoxia. The conclusion was that when chemoreceptors are stimulated, the antisympathetic effect of the reflex ventilatory response markedly attenuates the direct sympathoexcitatory effect (Fig. 5).

The two main chemoreflex stimulants are not equipotent in their respiratory and cardiovascular effects: hypercapnia has been found to have a much larger increase in ventilation and sympathetic nerve activity than hypoxia (56). Even for equivalent levels of increase in ventilation, the hypercapnic stimulus caused a larger increment in sympathetic nerve activity than hypoxia. This implied that the (central) CO_2 chemoreceptors were more closely tied to the sympathetic outflow than the (peripheral) hypoxic chemoreceptors. However, when the subjects maintained voluntary apnea, the relationship was reversed: hypoxia caused a much larger increase in sympathetic nerve activity than hypercapnia. The authors

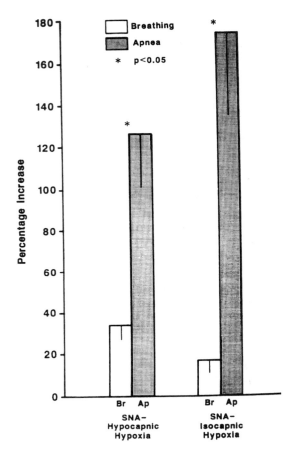

Figure 5 Group data for 11 subjects that compare percentage increase in sympathetic nerve activity (SNA) with (left) hypocapnic hypoxia and (right) isocapnic hypoxia, during breathing and apnea. (From Ref. 55.)

speculate that this phenomenon is caused by pulmonary afferents whose signals inhibit peripheral chemoreceptor afferent signals in the nucleus tractus solitarius: in normal breathing the hypoxic effect is therefore attenuated; during apnea, the full hypoxic effect is uncovered (Fig. 6).

The same group moved on to study the combined effect on sympathetic nerve activity of baroreceptor stimulation (using a phenylephrine infusion to raise the blood pressure by at least 10 mmHg) and chemoreceptor stimulation (57). Hypoxia alone raised sympathetic nerve activity from 255 to 354 U/min; in contrast, when hypoxia was applied to subjects receiving a phenylephrine infusion, there was *no* rise in activity (87 to 50 U/min). A different picture was obtained with the other chemoreceptor stimulant: hypercapnia alone raised sympathetic nerve activity from 116 to 234 U/min; on a background of baroreceptor activation by phenylephrine there was still a rise from 32 to 61 U/min ($p < 0.05$) (Fig. 7).

From these data, it appears that *peripheral* hypoxic chemoreceptor afferent signals experience inhibition by baroreceptor signals in a way that does not apply, or applies less, to *central* hypercapnic chemoreceptor afferents.

We have seen that chemoreflex activation causes sympathetic activation, tachycardia, and hypertension, but what is the effect of all of these on the sensitivity of the baroreflex itself? In an early study from Oxford (47), changes in alveolar P_{CO_2} had no significant effect on baroreflex sensitivity (as assessed by phenylephrine injection) (Fig. 8). A limitation of this study is that the maximum elevation of alveolar P_{CO_2} studied was only 10 mmHg (1.3 kPa).

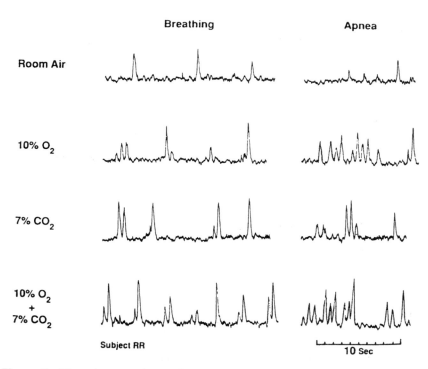

Figure 6 Direct intraneural recordings of sympathetic nerve activity measured during exposures to room air, isocapnic hypoxia (10% O_2, 90% N_2, titrated CO_2), during (left) spontaneous breathing and (right) end-expiratory apnea. (From Ref. 56.)

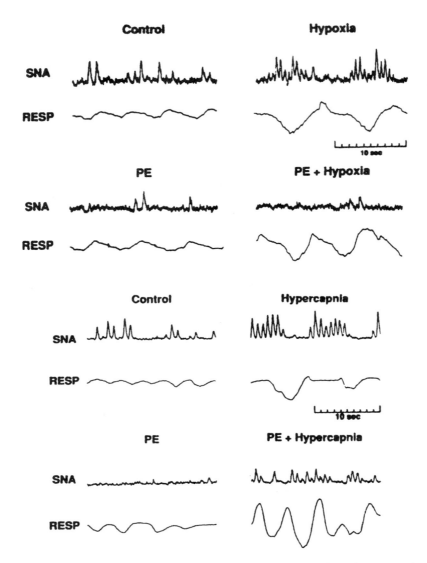

Figure 7 Recordings of sympathetic nerve activity (SNA) and respiratory tracings (RESP). (Top) The effect on a single subject of hypercapnia and phenylephrine infusion (PE) given separately and together. (Bottom) The effect on a single subject of hypoxia and phenylephrine infusion (PE) given separately and together. (From Ref. 57. Copyright American Society for Clinical Investigation.)

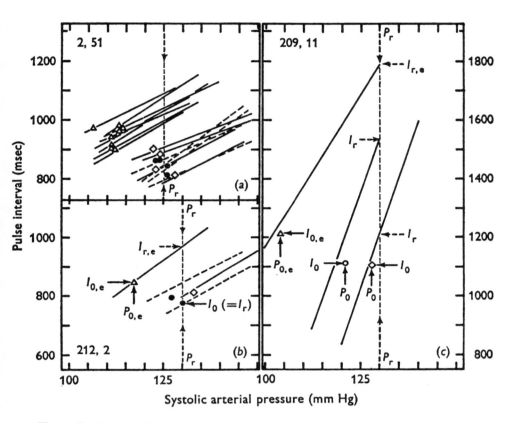

Figure 8 Results of three experiments showing the relationships between pulse interval (I) and systolic arterial pressure (P) during the pressure rises following drug injection, for which periods only the regression lines are shown. Plotted points (I_0 and P_0) are the mean I and P for the eight heartbeats immediately preceding the drug-induced rises of P. Triangles represent measurements at normal alveolar gas concentrations. Measurements were also taken when the alveolar CO_2 was raised by 5 mmHg (open circles), 10 mmHg (open diamonds), and 5 mmHg with coexisting hypoxia (closed circles). (From Ref. 47.)

In further studies (48), Bristow's group went on to use a wider range of alveolar P_{CO_2} (35–50 mmHg), with which they were able to establish a significant trend toward attenuation of the baroreflex gain (deltaI/deltaP) at higher P_{CO_2} levels (open circles in Fig. 9). However, when patients mimicked, with normal alveolar P_{CO_2}s, the hyperventilation that would normally arise when the PCO_2 rises, there was no comparable change in baroreflex gain ("+" in Fig. 9).

From these data, we can conclude that there is an attenuation of the baro-

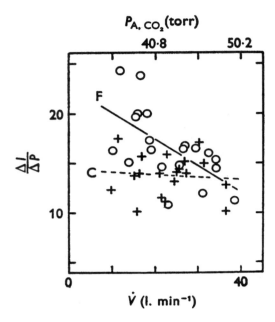

Figure 9 The effect of varying ventilation on baroreflex sensitivity ($\Delta I/\Delta P$) during free breathing (O, line F) and mimicked free breathing (+, line C). (From Ref. 48.)

reflex with increasing chemoreflex stimulation and that this effect is not dependent on the changes in ventilation that are normally also seen.

VIII.   Clinical Correlations

Pulling together data from disparate realms of research, animal and human, using isolated organs and complete organisms, we can extract some generalizations.

First, although we frequently consider the cardiovascular and respiratory systems as separate entities, with specific modes of interaction, in fact the control pathways of both systems are heavily intertwined (Fig. 10).

Chemoreceptor stimulation causes a marked increase in ventilation and sympathetic nerve activity, while baroreceptor activation causes a mild decrease in ventilation and a sharp reduction in sympathetic activity.

Baroreflex activation in the human has a particularly potent inhibitory effect on the sensitivity to peripheral chemoreceptor stimulation, with little (if any) inhibitory effect on the sensitivity to central chemoreceptor firing.

Increases in ventilation cause a complex cascade of pulmonary and cardiovascular effects, including activation of lung stretch receptors and an elevation in arterial blood pressure: these make it difficult to isolate the direct cardiovascular effects of chemostimuli in a spontaneously breathing subject.

Nevertheless, despite their complexity, these interrelationships appear to form a stable network, which in normals allows each subsystem to be adequately regulated, while allowing appropriate cross-talk between systems. In disease states, such as in chronic heart failure, there is a breakdown of the normal magnitude (and in some cases, direction) of the cardiorespiratory reflexes, which can lead to potentially maladaptive feedback loops.

A. Reflex Disturbances in Hypertension

Hypertension is associated with impaired baroreflex sensitivity in humans (26) and in animal models. There are abnormalities of ventilatory control also: in human hypertensives, the ventilatory response to hypoxic chemoreceptor stimulus is approximately doubled (58). Studies in spontaneously hypertensive rats

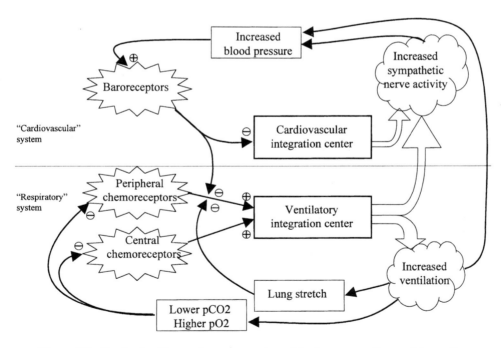

Figure 10 Synthesis of interactions among some of the important reflexes of the cardiovascular and respiratory systems.

(59) have identified tonic hyperactivity of chemoreceptor afferents, which is alleviated by the administration of 100% oxygen.

It has been speculated that the depressed baroreflex sensitivity of hypertension, through a reduction in the usual inhibition of chemoreceptor activity, may contribute to enhanced chemoreceptor activity (60). Of course, the converse is also plausible: that hyperactive chemoreflex could stimulate the sympathetic nervous system, which would be expected to depress the baroreflex.

B.   Reflex Disturbances in Chronic Heart Failure

In patients with chronic heart failure, a key symptom is shortness of breath on mild exertion or even at rest. Alongside this, there is often objective hyperventilation at rest and a higher degree of exercise hyperpnea than is seen in normals (61). The sensitivities of both the peripheral (13) and central (62) chemoreceptor systems are enhanced in chronic heart failure.

The hypothesis that the elevation in chemoreceptor sensitivity could be a contributory factor to the increased ventilation at rest and during exercise has received support from studies showing them to be positively correlated (63).

In chronic heart failure, the fine-detail short-term oscillations in heart rate and blood pressure are attenuated (or even disappear) and are replaced by prominent, discrete, very low frequency oscillations whose origins are incompletely understood. These large, slow fluctuations are observed more frequently in patients with enhanced chemoreflex sensitivity and they are reduced when oxygen is administered (64), giving grounds for believing in a chemoreflex harmonic oscillation as the source of this phenomenon.

Patients with a more prominently enhanced chemoreflex sensitivity also have more severely depressed baroreflexes (see Fig. 11) (65). It is possible that, in chronic heart failure, there is a vicious circle (see Fig. 12) of overactive chemoreflex, which suppresses the baroreflex, which in turn uncovers a further enhancement of chemoreflex. One of the mechanisms by which the chemoreflex exerts its effect could be by constitutively activating the sympathetic nervous system: this continuous high sympathetic outflow not only further sensitizes the chemoreflex but also prevents the baroreflex from operating efficiently. All of these components have the potential to trigger other elements in the cascade of detrimental neurohormonal changes that are now recognized in chronic heart failure (66) (Fig. 12).

We are now aware that attenuation of baroreflex sensitivity is a negative prognostic indicator in patients who have suffered a myocardial infarction (67). However, despite understandable enthusiasm for its use in clinical risk assessment, estimation of baroreflex sensitivity is beset by many difficulties in cardiac patients: it is impossible in patients with atrial fibrillation or pacemaker dependency, it is often attenuated by the ravages of autonomic neuropathy in diabetics, and it is technically difficult in patients with frequent extrasystoles.

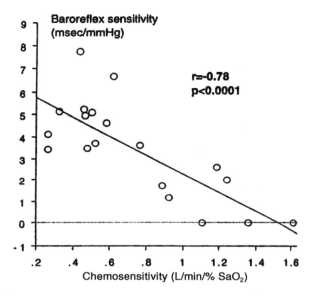

Figure 11 Inverse correlation between chemosensitivity and baroreflex sensitivity in patients with chronic heart failure. (From Ref. 65.)

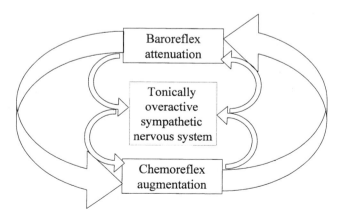

Figure 12 Potential vicious circles of reflex derangements in chronic heart failure.

None of these pathologies prevents assessment of chemoreflex sensitivity. Moreover, the chemoreflex is *enhanced* in patients with more severe disease and is consequently easier to measure accurately, in contrast with the baroreflex, which, as it is attenuated, tends to be submerged beneath the background noise.

Finally, measurement is less invasive for chemoreflex than baroreflex, and the equipment needed is readily available from a variety of suppliers. In the future, chemoreflex assessment is likely to take its place alongside baroreflex assessment in the evaluation of prognosis in patients with heart disease.

C. Very Low Frequency Rhythms

During sleep, recordings of ventilation and oxygen saturation show marked oscillations in some patients. These fluctuations may be purely a result of chemoreflex-pulmonary resonances called periodic breathing, or, when severe enough to cause frank apnea, Cheyne-Stokes respiration (CSR), or they may involve episodic upper airways collapse—obstructive sleep apnea (OSA). OSA is endemic with a prevalence of a few percent in the general population, while CSR is particularly frequent in patients with congestive heart failure.

Alongside these rhythmical changes, with period 40–60 sec, in ventilation and blood gas concentrations, there are corresponding stereotyped patterns of oscillation in heart rate and blood pressure. When analyzed in the frequency domain, these fall into the very low frequency band. In heart failure, this frequency band can become the predominant one because of the failure of intrinsic harmonic baroreflex oscillation and of respiratory sinus arrhythmia to generate the usual levels of low-frequency and high-frequency power, respectively.

In CSR, there is a rise in blood pressure in association with the hypoxemia (and hypercarbia). In chronic heart failure patients, this generally coincides with a dramatic rise in heart rate, which may be attributable to the powerful sympathoexcitatory effects of chemoreceptor stimulation in the presence of only weak sympathoinhibitory baroreflexes. Such a pattern is shown in Figure 13, where RR represents the RR interval, which is the reciprocal of the heart rate; ILV represents instantaneous lung volume and IMV represents instantaneous minute volume (in arbitrary units).

The resulting simultaneous tachycardia, acute rise in blood pressure, and arterial hypoxia constitute a potentially maladaptive combination for the supply-demand balance of the myocardium. This may be a consequence of the combination of attenuated baroreflexes and enhanced chemoreflexes seen in chronic heart failure (Fig. 14).

During one night, this vigorous integrated cardiorespiratory challenge may be repeated over 400 times; the whole sequence may recur night after night. While the direct consequences of this are currently unknown, it is interesting to note that this pattern of nocturnal respiration is associated with an increase in daytime blood pressure (68) and may carry a higher overall mortality (69).

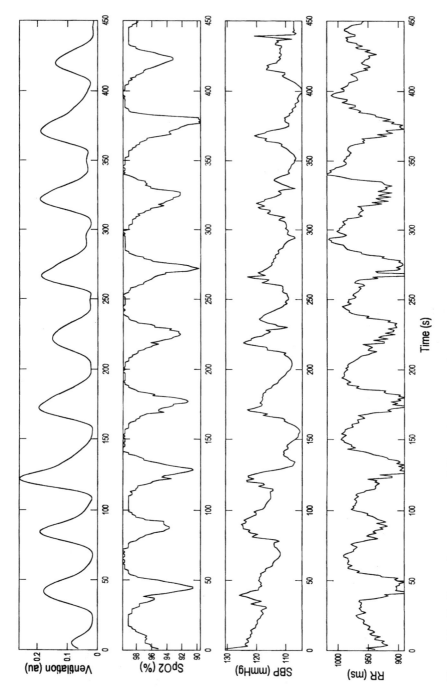

Figure 13 Cardiovascular counterparts of Cheyne-Stokes respiration.

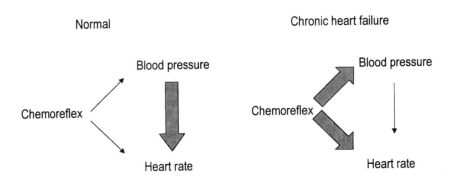

Figure 14 Altered balance between chemoreflex and baroreflex control of heart rate in chronic heart failure.

D. Chemoreflex-Baroreflex Interactions in Sleep-Disordered Breathing

Sleep-disordered breathing is very common in patients with CHF (70), and may worsen symptoms, impair cardiorespiratory function, and unfavorably influence outcome (69). Although the mechanisms are not yet completely elucidated, it is now becoming accepted that patients with periodic breathing patterns have not only enhanced chemoreflex sensitivity but also depressed baroreflex sensitivity (71).

A parallel situation may exist in OSA, in which recent work has established that the blood pressure increase induced by hypoxia is markedly exaggerated (72). These findings illuminate the observation that untreated sleep apneics rarely manifest the normal dip in blood pressure during the night (73), since the repetitive sympathetic stimuli are an upward influence on nocturnal blood pressure. Moreover, these chemoreflex effects may reset the baroreceptors to a higher set point, which could contribute to the daytime hypertension that can be seen in these patients (74,75).

References

1. Lahiri S, Nishino A, Mulligan E, Nishino T. Comparison of aortic and carotid chemoreceptor response to hypercapnia and hypoxia. J Appl Physiol 1981; 51:55–61.
2. Lahiri S. Role of arterial O_2 flow in peripheral chemoreceptor excitation. Fed Proc 1980; 39:2648–2652.
3. Hopp FA, Seagard JL, Bajic J, Zuperku EJ. Respiratory responses to aortic and carotid chemoreceptor activation in the dog. J Appl Physiol 1991; 70:2359–2550.
4. Biscoe TJ, Purves MS, Sampson SR. The frequency of nerve impulses in single carotid body chemoreceptor afferent fibres recorded in vivo with intact circulation. J Physiol (Lond) 1970; 208:121–131.

5. Nielsen AM, Bisgard GE, Vidruk EH. Carotid chemoreceptor activity during acute and sustained hypoxia in goats. J Appl Physiol 1988; 65:1796–1802.

6. Lugliani R, Whipp BJ, Seard C, Wasserman K. Effect of bilateral carotid body resection on ventilatory control at rest and during exercise in man. N Engl J Med 1971; 285:1105–1111.

7. Swanson GD, Whipp BJ, Kaufman RD, Aqleh KA, Winter B, Belville JW. Effect of hypercapnia on hypoxic ventilatory drive in normal and carotid body-resected man. J Appl Physiol 1978; 45:971–977.

8. Honda Y, Watanabe S, Hashizume I, Satomura Y, Hata N, Sakakibara Y, Severinghaus JW. Hypoxic chemosensitivity in asthmatic patients two decades after carotid body resection. J Appl Physiol 1979; 46:632–638.

9. Li K, Ponte JL, Sadler CL. Carotid body chemoreceptor response to prolonged hypoxia in the rabbit: effects of domperidone and propranolol. J Physiol (Lond) 1990; 430:1–11.

10. Mortola JP, Gautier H. Interaction between metabolism and ventilation: effects of respiratory gases and temperature. In: Dempsey JA, Pack AI, eds. Regulation of Breathing. New York: Marcel Dekker, 1995.

11. Kronenberg R, Hamilton FN, Gabel R, Hickey R, Read DJC, Severinghaus J. Comparison of three methods for quantitating respiratory response to hypoxia in man. Respir Physiol 1972; 16:109–125.

12. Edelman NH, Epstein PE, Lahiri S, Cherniack NS. Ventilatory responses to transient hypoxia in man. Respir Physiol 1973; 17:302–314.

13. Chua TP, Ponikowski P, Webb-Peploe K, Harrington D, Anker S, Piepoli M, Coats AJS. Clinical characteristics of chronic heart failure patients with augmented peripheral chemoreflex. Eur Heart J 1997; 18:480–486.

14. Leusen IR. Chemosensitivity of the respiratory center: influence of CO_2 in the cerebral ventricles on respiration. Am J Physiol 1954; 176:39–44.

15. Pappenheimer JR, Fencl V, Heisey SR, Held D. Role of cerebral fluids in control of respiration as studied in unanesthetised goats. Am J Physiol 1965; 208:436–450.

16. Mitchell RA, Loeschke HH, Massion WH, Severinghaus JW. Respiratory responses mediated through superficial chemosensitive areas on the medulla. J Appl Physiol 1963; 18:523–533.

17. Nattie EE. Central chemoreception. In: Dempsey JA, Pack AI, eds. Regulation of Breathing. New York: Marcel Dekker, 1995.

18. Nattie EE, Li A, Coates EL. Central chemoreceptor location and the ventrolateral medulla. In: Trouth CO, Millis RM, Kiwull-Schöne HF, Schlafke ME, eds. Ventral Brainstem Mechanisms and Control of Respiration and Blood Pressure. New York: Marcel Dekker, 1995.

19. Lipscomb WT, Boyarski LL. Neurophysiological investigation of medullary chemosensitive areas of respiration. Respir Physiol 1972; 16:362–376.

20. Coats EL, Li A, Natie EE. Widespread sites of brainstem ventilatory chemoreceptors. J Appl Physiol 1993; 75:5–14.

21. Arita H, Ichikawa K, Kuwana S, Kogo N. Possible locations of pH-dependent central chemoreceptors: intramedullary regions with acidic shift of extracellular fluid pH during hypercapnia. Brain Res 1989; 485:285–293.

22. Neubauer JA, Gonsalves SF, Chou W, Geller HM, Edelman NH. Chemosensitiv-

ity of medullary neurons in explant tissue cultures. Neuroscience 1991; 45:701–708.

23. Lahiri S, DeLaney RG. Stimulus interaction in the responses of carotid body chemoreceptor single afferent fibers. Respir Physiol 1975; 24:249–266.

24. Ludbrook J, Mancia G, Ferrari A, Zanchetti A. The variable-pressure neck-chamber method for studying the carotid baroreflex in man. Clin Sci Mol Med 1977; 53:165–171.

25. Smyth HS, Sleight P, Pickering GW. Reflex regulation of arterial pressure during sleep in man: a quantitative method of assessing baroreflex sensitivity. Circ Res 1969; 24(1):109–121.

26. Bristow JD, Honour AJ, Pickering GW, Sleight P, Smyth HS. Diminished baroreflex sensitivity in high blood pressure. Circulation 1969; 39(1):48–54.

27. Eckberg DL, Drabinski M, Braunwald E. Defective cardiac parasympathetic control in patients with heart disease. N Engl J Med 1971; 285:877–883.

28. Mancia G, Seravalle G, Giannattasio C, Bossi M, Preti L, Cattaneo BM, Grassi G. Reflex cardiovascular control in congestive cardiac failure. Am J Cardiol 1992; 69:17G–23G.

29. Schwartz PJ, Zaza A, Pala M, Locati E, Beria G, Zanchetti A. Baroreflex sensitivity and its evolution during the first year after myocardial infarction. J Am Col Cardiol 1988; 12(3):629–636.

30. Farrell TG, Odemuyiwa O, Bashir Y, Cripps TR, Malik M, Ward DE, Camm AJ. Prognostic value of baroreflex sensitivity testing after acute myocardial infarction. Br Heart J 1992; 67(2):129–137.

31. Wright S. Action of adrenaline and related substances on respiration. J Physiol (Lond) 1930; 69:493–499.

32. D'Silva JL, Gill D, Mendel D. The effects of acute haemorrhage on respiration in the cat. J Physiol (Lond) 1966; 298:369–377.

33. Landgren S, Neil E. Chemoreceptor impulse activity following haemorrhage. Acta Physiol Scand 1951; 23:158–167.

34. Biscoe TJ, Bradley GW, Purves MJ. The relation between carotid body chemoreceptor discharge, carotid sinus pressure and carotid body venous flow. J Physiol (Lond) 1970; 208:99–120.

35. Bishop B. Carotid baroreceptor modulation of diaphragm and abdominal muscle activity in the cat. J Appl Physiol 1974; 36:12–19.

36. Eisenberg E, Zimlichman R, Lavie P. Plasma norepinephrine levels in patients with sleep apnea syndrome. N Engl J Med 1990; 322:932–933.

37. Pizarro J, Warner MM, Ryan M, et al. Intracarotid norepinephrine infusions inhibit ventilation in goats. Respir Physiol 1992; 90:299–300.

38. Millis RM, Trouth CO, Johnson SM, Wood DH, Dehkordi O, Wray SR. Arterial oxygen desaturation and respiratory failure associated with sympathetic overactivity. In: Trouth CO, Millis RM, Kiwull-Schöne HF, Schlafke ME, eds. Ventral Brainstem Mechanisms and Control of Respiration and Blood Pressure. New York: Marcel Dekker, 1995.

39. Ohtake PJ, Jennings DB. Angiotensin II stimulates respiration in awake dogs and antagonises baroreceptor stimulation. Respir Physiol 1991; 85:289–304.

40. Schmid PG et al. Different aspects of vasopressin and angiotensin II on baroreflexes. Fed Proc 1985; 44:2388–2392.

41. Potter EK, McCloskey DI. Respiratory stimulation by angiotensin II. Respir Physiol 1979; 36:367–373.
42. Downing SE, Remensnyder JP, Mitchell JH. Cardiovascular responses to hypoxic stimulation of the carotid bodies. Circ Res 1962; 10:676–685.
43. Hainsworth R, Karim F, Sofola OA. Left ventricular inotropic responses to stimulation of carotid body chemoreceptors in anaesthetised dogs. J Physiol (Lond) 1979; 287:455–466.
44. Karim F, Hainsworth R, Sofola OA, Wood LM. Responses of the heart to stimulation of aortic body chemoreceptors in dogs. Circ Res 1980; 46:77–83.
45. Hainsworth R, Jacobs L, Comro JH Jr. Afferent lung denervation by brief inhalation of steam. J Appl Physiol 1973; 34:708–714.
46. Calvelo MG, Abboud FM, Ballard DR, Abdel-Sayed W. Reflex vascular responses to stimulation of chemoreceptors with nicotine and cyanide. Circ Res 1970; 27:259–276.
47. Bristow JD, Brown EB, Cunningham DJC, Goode RC, Howson MG, Sleight P. The effects of hypercapnia, hypoxia and ventilation on the baroreflex regulation of the pulse interval. J Physiol 1971; 216:281–302.
48. Bristow JD, Brown EB, Cunningham JDC, Howson MH, Lee MJR, Pickering TG, Sleight P. The effects of raising alveolar P_{CO_2} and ventilation separately and together on the sensitivity and setting of the baroreceptor cardiodepressor reflex in man. J Physiol 1974; 243:401–425.
49. Heistad DD, Abboud FM, Mark AL, Schmid PG. Effect of baroreceptor activity on ventilatory response to chemoreceptor stimulation. J Appl Physiol 1975; 39(3):411–416.
50. Heistad DD, Abboud FM, Mark AL, Schmid PG. Interaction of baroreceptor and chemoreceptor reflexes. J Clin Invest 1974; 53:2336–1236.
51. Mancia G. Influence of carotid baroreceptors on vascular responses to carotid chemoreceptor stimulation in the dog. Circ Res 1975; 36:270–276.
52. Pelletier CL. Circulatory responses to graded stimulation of the carotid chemoreceptors in the dog. Circ Res 1972; 31:431–443.
53. Mancia G, Shepherd JT, Donald DE. Interplay among carotid sinus, cardiopulmonary, and carotid body reflexes in dogs. Am J Physiol 1976; 230(1):19–24.
54. Heistad DD, Abboud FM, Eckstein JW. Vasoconstrictor response to simulated diving in man. J Appl Physiol 1968; 25(5):542–549.
55. Somers VK, Mark AL, Zavala DC, Abboud FM. Influence of ventilation and hypocapnia on sympathetic responses to hypoxia in normal humans. J Appl Physiol 1989; 67(5):2095–2100.
56. Somers VK, Mark AL, Zavala DC, Abboud FM. Contrasting effects of hypoxia and hypercapnia on ventilation and sympathetic activity in humans. J Appl Physiol 1989; 67(5):2101–2106.
57. Somers VK, Mark AL, Abboud FM. Interaction of baroreceptor and chemoreceptor reflex control of sympathetic nerve activity in normal humans. J Clin Invest 1991; 87:1953–1957.
58. Somers VK. Mark AL. Abboud FM. Potentiation of sympathetic nerve responses to hypoxia in borderline hypertensive subjects. Hypertension 1988; 11(6 pt 2):608–612.
59. Przybylski J, Trzebski A, Czyzewski T, Jodkowski J. Responses to hyperoxia, hypoxia, hypercapnia and almitrine in spontaneously hypertensive rats. Bull Eur Physiopathol Respir 1982; 18:145–154.

60. Narkiewicz K. Somers VK. The sympathetic nervous system and obstructive sleep apnea: implications for hypertension. J Hypertens 1997; 15(12 Pt 2):1613–1619.

61. Clark AL, Volterrani M, Swan JW, Coats AJ The increased ventilatory response to exercise in chronic heart failure: relation to pulmonary pathology. Heart 1997; 77(2): 138–46.

62. Andreas S, Morguet AJ, Werner GS, Kreutzer H. Ventilatory response to exercise and to carbon dioxide in patients with heart failure. Eur Heart J 1996; 17:750–755.

63. Chua TP, Clark AL, Amadi AA, Coats AJ. Relation between chemosensitivity and the ventilatory response to exercise in chronic heart failure. J Am Coll Cardiol 1996; 27(3):650–657.

64. Ponikowski P, Chua TP, Piepoli M, Amadi AA, Harrington D, Webb-Peploe K, Volterrani M, Colombo R, Mazzuero G, Giordano A, Coats AJ. Chemoreceptor dependence of very low frequency rhythms in advanced chronic heart failure. Am J Physiol 1997; 272(1 pt 2):H438–H447.

65. Ponikowski P, Chua TP, Piepoli M, Ondusova D, Webb-Peploe K, Harrington D, Anker SD, Volterrani M, Colombo R, Mazzuero G, Giordano A, Coats AJ. Augmented peripheral chemosensitivity as a potential input to baroreflex impairment and autonomic imbalance in chronic heart failure. Circulation 1997; 96(8):2586–2594.

66. Packer M. The neurohormonal hypothesis: a theory to explain the mechanism of disease progression in heart failure. J Am Coll Cardiol 1992; 20:248–254.

67. La Rovere MT, Bigger JT Jr, Marcus FI, Mortara A, Schwartz PJ. Baroreflex sensitivity and heart-rate variability in prediction of total cardiac mortality after myocardial infarction. Lancet 1998; 351(9101):478–484.

68. Bradley TD, Floras JS. Pathophysiologic and therapeutic implications of sleep apnea in congestive heart failure. J Cardiac Failure 1996; 2(3):223–240.

69. Hanly PJ, Zuberi-Khokhar NS. Increased mortality associated with Cheyne-Stokes respiration in patients with congestive heart failure. Am J Respir Crit Care Med 1996; 153(1):272–276.

70. Javaheri S, et al. Sleep apnea in 81 ambulatory male patients with stable heart failure: types and their prevalences, consequences, and presentations. Circulation 1998; 97: 2154–2159.

71. Ponikowski P, et al. Oscillatory breathing patterns during wakefulness in patients with chronic heart failure: clinical implications and role of augmented peripheral chemosensitivity. Circulation 1999; 100:2418–2424.

72. Narkiewicz K, et al. Selective potentiation of peripheral chemoreflex sensitivity in obstructive sleep apnea. Circulation 1999; 99:1183–1189.

73. Somers VK, et al. Sympathetic neural mechanism in obstructive sleep apnea. J Clin Invest 1995; 96:1897–1904.

74. Ziegler MG, et al. The effect of hypoxia on baroreflexes and pressor sensitivity in sleep apnea and hypertension. Sleep 1995; 18:859–865.

75. Carlson JT, et al. Depressed baroreflex sensitivity in patients with obstructive sleep apnea. Am J Respir Crit Care Med 1996; 154:1490–1496.

3

Lower Brainstem Mechanisms of Cardiorespiratory Integration

PATRICE G. GUYENET

University of Virginia School of Medicine
Charlottesville, Virginia

I. Introduction

Patients with obstructive sleep apnea (OSA) experience repeated surges in sympathetic nerve discharge (SNA) that are especially intense at the end of each apneic episode (1). OSA patients also have a chronic increase in SNA, which is presumed to be a major risk factor for cardiovascular diseases (1). The acute and recurrent sympathoactivation associated with each apneic episode is attributed to three main factors. One is the activation of peripheral and central chemoreceptors due to CO_2 accumulation and blood O_2 desaturation. Another is the loss of mechanical feedback from the lungs (1). The final one is arousal itself.

This review begins with a description of the spinomedullary network that regulates SNA and cardiovagal efferent activity. This first section also describes the control of this circuitry by monoamines whose release increases abruptly on awakening and could be involved in the sympathetic surges of OSA. The second part describes the effect of respiration on sympathetic and cardiovagal activity, with special emphasis on the central pathway of the peripheral and central chemoreflexes. The biology of cardiopulmonary sensory afferents, including peripheral chemoreceptors, is not reviewed.

II. Medullospinal Circuits that Control Sympathetic Tone and Cardiovagal Efferent Activity

Sympathetic tone is generated by a complex network of neurons located within the lower brainstem. A major convergence point of this system is a group of ventrolateral medullary neurons that project directly to the intermediolateral cell column of the spinal cord (IML). These cells [rostral ventrolateral medulla (RVLM) presympathetic neurons, C1, and non-C1 cells in Fig. 1] drive sympathetic preganglionic neurons (SPGNs) via a largely monosynaptic connection (Fig. 1). These are essential relays for all known supraspinal sympathetic reflexes, two of which (baroreflex and chemoreflex) are reviewed below.

The central neural mechanisms responsible for generating the cardiovagal tone are also described in this section, though they are far less understood.

A. Sympathetic Tone Generation: Spinal Mechanisms

Location and Phenotype of SPGNs That Control the Heart and Blood Vessels

SPGNs are located mostly in the lateral horn (also known as the intermediolateral cell column, or IML) from the lower cervical to the upper lumbar level (e.g.,

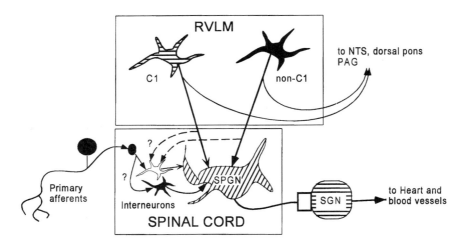

Figure 1 The core bulbospinal network for control of sympathetic vasomotor tone. RVLM, rostral ventrolateral medulla; C1, neurons containing all the enzymes necessary for the synthesis of adrenaline; non-C1, noncatecholaminergic bulbospinal neurons presumed to release glutamate; SPGN, sympathetic preganglionic neuron; SGN, sympathetic ganglionic neuron.

caudal C8 to L3-L5 in rat). SPGNs are also found in lateral and medial extensions of the IML (the lateral funicular area and the intercalated cell group) and around the central canal (central autonomic nucleus) (2). The exact proportion of SPGNs that control vascular smooth muscles and the myocardium as opposed to other cellular targets is not known. Myocardial control originates from SPGNs located in upper thoracic segments (T1 to T3 in rat). This innervation is somewhat lateralized (3,4). The right side of the spinal cord controls rate preferentially, while ventricular contractility is regulated preferentially by SPGNs located on the left side (3,4). This anatomical segregation suggests that the brain could have the ability to fine-tune the activity of sympathetic efferents governing cardiac rate independently of those regulating contractility, but, at present, there is no physiological evidence that such a differential regulation occurs. Vasoconstrictor SPGNs that control skin and muscle flow are presumably dispersed throughout the IML. Splanchnic, renal and adrenal SPGNs are confined to specific albeit overlapping sets of thoracic segments. All SPGNs regardless of function are cholinergic, and the vast majority contain high levels of NO-synthase. The release of NO by the soma or dendrites of SPGNs may serve as a retrograde signal that enhances the presynaptic release of both excitatory and inhibitory transmitters from as yet unidentified spinal inputs (5,6). This enhancement is mediated via cGMP accumulation (5,6). The physiological context in which NO may be released by SPGNs is unknown. Elsewhere in the brain, NO production is generally activated by calcium entry, often via *N*-methyl-D-aspartate (NMDA) receptor channels. This mechanism could be present in SPGNs because they most likely have NMDA receptors (7–9). Although all SPGNs are cholinergic and most contain NO-synthase, they display considerable phenotypical heterogeneity. For instance, at least four different neuropeptides have been detected in mammalian SPGNs by immunohistochemistry (enkephalin, somatostatin, neurotensin, and substance P) (10). SPGNs are also heterogeneous in their expression of several calcium-binding proteins. For instance calretinin is present in SPGNs that innervate norepinephrine-releasing adrenal chromaffin cells but it is absent from SPGNs that control their adrenergic counterparts (11). Also, calbindin D28K is present only in SPGNs that contact NPY-negative (secretomotor and pilomotor) sympathetic ganglionic neurons (SGNs) (12). These differences suggest that the secondary phenotype of SPGNs (peptide, calcium-binding protein) could relate to their function (e.g., vasomotor vs. other) and/or to their specific anatomical targets.

Intrinsic Properties of SPGNs

The intrinsic properties of adult SPGNs recorded in vitro appear fairly homogeneous, but all experiments have been performed on randomly sampled SPGNs. This limitation would severely reduce the opportunity to identify differences between functional classes, especially if these differences were quantitative rather than qualitative. The repolarizing phase of the action potential of SPGNs has a marked calcium hump and the neurons have a large calcium-mediated afterhyperpolarization (AHP). SPGNs express at least five types of potassium conductances (A-current, transient and persistent Ca-activated currents, inward rectifier, delayed rectifier) many of which are probably regulated by G protein–coupled receptors (13). The major differences between individual SPGNs in vitro seem related to development. In the neonate, a significant proportion of SPGNs recorded in vitro are electrically coupled and some of those are also spontaneously active (14,15). These characteristics are not seen in the adult.

Spinal Interneurons

Many (perhaps all) SPGNs have inputs from spinal cord interneurons (16–20) (Fig. 1). Segmental interneurons are generally located in close vicinity to the SPGNs (laminae V and VII) (16). However, SPGNs may also be contacted by propriomedullary interneurons located as far as the cervical level (21). Electrophysiological data in vitro indicate that many of the segmental interneurons use gamma-aminobutyric acid (GABA), glycine, or glutamate as fast transmitters (7,22–26). Between one-third and one-half of the synaptic inputs of SPGNs that project to the superior cervical ganglion or to the adrenal medulla are GABAergic (27). The figures for SPGNs that control arterial tone or the heart are unknown, and so is the relative contribution of spinal vs. supraspinal inputs to this GABAergic innervation.

The major excitatory drive to vasoconstrictor, adrenal, renal, and cardio-accelerator SPGNs originates in the medulla oblongata (RVLM, Fig. 1), and is generally thought to be due to monosynaptic excitatory inputs. The exact role of spinal interneurons in vasomotor control remains somewhat of a mystery and is probably grossly underrated in our present understanding. A potential role in spinal nociceptive reflexes is suggested by the observation that electrical stimulation of thoracic dorsal roots in acutely spinalized preparation elevates arterial pressure and heart rate. Mechanoreceptors and other receptors from the chest wall could well control sympathetic tone to the heart via these interneurons. Because sensory afferents do not project monosynaptically to SPGNs, the spinal component of the sympathetic reflexes must be mediated by interneurons (28). However, the importance of these spinal reflexes is uncertain in individuals with an intact neuraxis, and nociceptive sympathetic reflexes are generally believed to involve long loops through the lower brainstem (29). Still, recent evidence suggests that the baroreceptor-mediated inhibition of SPGNs in vivo may be mediated at least in part by the activation of spinal glycinergic or GABAergic interneurons (30–32). It is therefore possible that descending medullary pathways control a "spinal sympathetic network" via projections both to SPGNs and to their antecedent interneurons along the lines illustrated in Figure 1. Spinal sympathetic pressor reflexes are dramatically exacerbated after spinal injury in animals and humans, such that even relatively innocuous stimulations may cause severe hypertensive episodes (33,34). This exacerbation of spinal reflexes is attributed to synaptic reorganization (35,36).

Effects of Catecholamines on SPGNs

Catecholamines have multiple pre- and postsynaptic actions on SPGNs. The IML region receives its catecholaminergic inputs from several brainstem sites, including the ventrolateral medulla (C1 neurons), the ventrolateral pons (A5 neurons), and the hypothalamus (Fig. 2).

The postsynaptic effects of catecholamines, though complex and variable from cell to cell, are understood the best. At rest in slices, α_1-receptor agonists depolarize most SPGNs by closing a resting K conductance (37–39). In a smaller percentage of neurons, α_2-receptor agonists produce opposite effects (37,40), while many SPGNs exhibit both responses. Catecholamines also reduce calcium currents through voltage-operated channels. By analogy with other neurons, this action is probably mediated by α_2-adrenergic receptors, though this, to our knowledge, has not been actually reported for SPGNs. Interestingly this particular α_2-

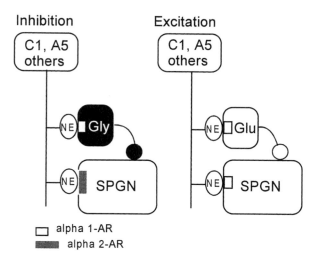

Figure 2 Differential control of sympathetic efferents by catecholamines at the spinal level. Catecholamines may either excite or inhibit sympathetic efferents depending on the type of receptor present on the SPGNs and on the type of interneuron that is simultaneously activated. SPGNs that control the heart appear predominantly activated by catecholamines.

mediated effect could, in fact, increase responsiveness of SPGNs to excitatory synaptic inputs by reducing the Ca-induced K conductance, which contributes to the late AHP. Finally, in some SPGNs, α_1-adrenergic agonists produce an afterdepolarization mediated by a Ca-activated Na conductance, which further raises the responsiveness of the neurons to excitatory inputs. In summary, most known postsynaptic effects of norepinephrine (NE) on SPGNs except the α_2-mediated increase in K conductance are likely to increase the responsiveness of these cells to synaptic inputs.

SPGNs are also influenced indirectly by catecholamines via local interneurons. For example α_1-adrenergic agonists commonly increase the frequency of glycinergic PSPs (41). This effect is most probably due to an increase in the rate of discharge of the interneurons and therefore it is likely to be due to the presence of α_1-receptors on the somata or dendrites on these interneurons. Catecholamines are also likely to exert direct presynaptic effects on terminals that impinge on SPGNs, although this has not yet been demonstrated. For instance, presynaptic inhibitory control of transmitter release by α_2-adrenergic receptors is most likely operating in the case of the C1 cells since somatodendritic high-voltage-activated (HVA) calcium currents are inhibited by α_2-adrenergic agonists in the somata of these cells (42).

In summary, the multiplicity of potentially opposing actions of catecholamines in the region of the IML precludes predicting a single "overall effect" of catecholamines on SPGN activity in vivo. The final effect of catecholamines on a given SPGN will depend on the type of postsynaptic receptor present on the cell. It will also depend on whether the SPGN is active or at rest and finally on whether interneurons are also simultaneously targeted by the catecholamine. Figure 2 depicts two anatomically plausible synaptic arrangements that would result in massive excitation by catecholamines in one case or powerful inhibition in the other. This complexity suggests that activation of a given catecholaminergic input to the autonomic region of the thoracic cord may produce patterns of response whereby some types of SPGNs may be excited while some others may be inhibited. Stimulation of the A5 noradrenergic neurons that project both to SPGNs and to spinal interneurons may produce such a differentiated response because it causes splanchnic constriction and lumbar vasodilation (43).

The SPGNs that control myocardial function are probably among those that have strong α_1-receptor–mediated responses because microinjection of exogenous α_1-adrenergic agonists at the T2-T3 level increases cardiac rate and contractility (44). Based on this information, one would surmise that physiological conditions generally associated with an increased release of brain NE release—such as transition from sleep to waking state, stress, or CO_2 accumulation due to apnea—could increase cardiac sympathetic activity at least in part via increased NE release in the IML.

B. Supraspinal Mechanisms: Role of the RVLM in the Generation of Sympathetic Tone

Sympathoexcitatory Role of RVLM

The ventrolateral medulla (VLM) is a division of the reticular formation that extends from the caudal end of the facial motor nucleus to the spinomedullary junction. Following the suggestion of Dampney and his collaborators (45), the VLM can be roughly subdivided into three rostrocaudal segments: RVLM, intermediate VLM (IVLM), and the caudal VLM (CVLM) (Fig. 3). The rostral part (RVLM, 0–800 µm behind the caudal end of the facial motor nucleus in the rat, FN in Fig. 3) is characterized by the presence of C1 neurons (containing tyrosine-hydroxylase, TH, dopamine β-hydroxylase, DBH, and phenylethanolamine *N*-methyl transferase, PNMT) with projection directed toward the IML but not toward the hypothalamus or basal forebrain. Dorsal to these C1 neurons lies a region of the RVLM containing the expiration-related Botzinger neurons. These cells are late expiratory interneurons involved in respiratory rhythmogenesis and/ or pattern generation. The RVLM contains no noradrenergic neurons. The IVLM (Fig. 3) extends to the rostral end of the lateral reticular nucleus (800–1600 µm behind facial motor nucleus in rat). Its lower part is defined by the presence of

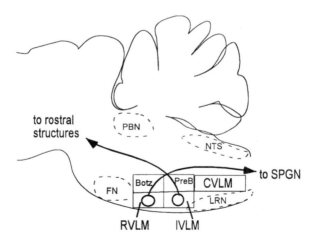

Figure 3 Principal functional subdivisions of the ventrolateral medulla. The ventrolateral medulla contains the core neural network responsible for cardiorespiratory integration. This network receives information from cardiopulmonary afferents via the nucleus of the solitary tract (NTS) and spinoreticular pathways. Botz, Botzinger neurons; FN, facial motor nucleus; LRN, lateral reticular nucleus; PreB, pre-Botzinger nucleus; PBN, parabrachial nuclei; NTS, nucleus of the solitary tract.

C1 neurons, which project to the midbrain and hypothalamus but not to the cord. This region also contains the bulk of the GABAergic propriomedullary interneurons responsible for the sympathetic baroreflex to be described below. The dominant cardiovascular effect produced by microinjections of excitatory amino acids into the IVLM is sympathoinhibition due to the activation of these interneurons, hence the name of medullary *depressor area* also given to this region by prior investigators (46). The dorsal half of IVLM, also called the pre-Botzinger nucleus (PreB in Fig. 3), contains the "kernel" of the respiratory rhythm-generating network (47,48). The IVLM also contains few noradrenergic neurons except at its very caudal end (A1 neurons). The third and last component of the VLM (CVLM) extends from the rostral tip of the lateral reticular nucleus to the medullospinal junction. It is characterized by the presence of A1 noradrenergic neurons and by the absence of C1 cells. This region contains multiple types of respiratory neurons, including the bulk of the respiratory pre–motor neurons that innervate phrenic and other spinal motor neurons involved in respiration.

In anesthetized animals, arterial pressure drops sharply and SNA virtually disappears after microinjection into the RVLM of transmitters or drugs that reduce neuronal activity (e.g., the $GABA_A$ agonist muscimol, opioid peptides, or α_2-adrenergic agonists). Hypotensive effects of this magnitude are not observed when the same agents are microinjected elsewhere in the brainstem (including the IVLM or CVLM). These data indicate that the RVLM exerts a globally excitatory influence on sympathetic efferents that control circulation (see 49–53 for reviews). Though RVLM projects widely throughout the lower brainstem, the prevailing opinion is that its excitatory control over vasomotor and cardiac sympathetic efferents is exerted mostly via a direct neuronal projection to the IML (Fig. 1). Consistent with this theory, the projection of the RVLM to the thoracic spinal cord consists mostly of neurons whose pattern of discharge is very similar to that of single sympathetic efferents innervating the heart and vasculature (see 52 and 54 for recent reviews). Their defining characteristics are an ongoing activity at resting levels of blood pressure, generally strong inhibition by activation of arterial baroreceptors, a pulse-related discharge, and a respiratory modulation similar to that of sympathetic nerves recorded under the same experimental conditions (Fig. 4). Recent results indicate that two-thirds of the bulbospinal RVLM exhibiting these neurophysiological characteristics are C1 neurons, while the rest are not (55–63). The spinally project-ing C1 neurons also innervate several other brainstem structures such as the NTS, other parts of the ventrolateral medulla, the dorsolateral and ventrolateral pons, the PAG and the locus ceruleus (64) (Fig. 1). Whether these projections constitute alternative and more indirect routes for the control of SPGNs is un-known.

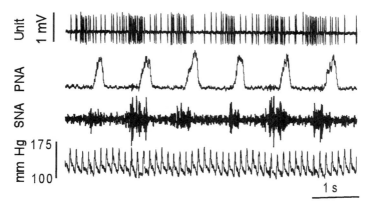

Figure 4 Sympathetic nerve discharge (SNA) is largely determined by the activity of the sympathoexcitatory neurons of the RVLM (top trace). Note the similarity between the unit discharge pattern and SNA. Note also the synchronization of SNA and of the unit activity with the discharge of the phrenic nerve (PNA, rectified and integrated). (Unpublished data of P. M. McCulloch and P. Guyenet from a chloralose-anesthetized rat.)

Functional Heterogeneity of RVLM Sympathoexcitatory Neurons: The Organotopy Hypothesis

The pattern of discharge of bulbospinal and barosensitive RVLM neurons is not uniform. For instance, in the rat, this class of neuron exhibits one of two distinctive respiratory patterns found also in SGNs (65). Also, some of these RVLM neurons are very barosensitive and have powerful chemoreceptor inputs like muscle vasoconstrictor or cardiac SGNs while others are only modestly barosensitive and are selectively inhibited by raising hypothalamic temperature (66). The latter are thus more reminiscent of the vasoconstrictor neurons that innervate cutaneous arterioles. These observations suggest the possibility that subgroups of RVLM sympathoexcitatory neurons might control specific cardiovascular targets. The organization appears to be "organotopic" (Fig. 5), by which is meant that a given RVLM neuron may target selectively a functional group of SPGNs (e.g., SPGNs that control selectively muscle arterioles rather than skin arterioles) irrespective of their specific anatomical location in the spinal cord (67,68). The theory is also supported by functional exploration of the RVLM with very small injections of glutamate. For instance, this approach suggests that bulbospinal neurons, which regulate cardiac function, might be preferentially located at the rostral tip of the RVLM (69).

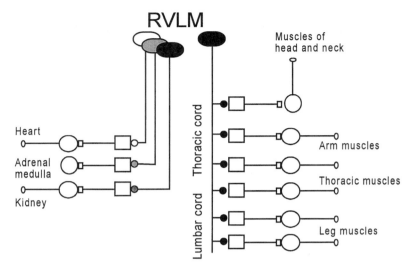

Figure 5   Organotopic anatomical arrangement of RVLM bulbospinal sympathoexcitatory neurons. RVLM sympathoexcitatory cells are probably organized into functional subgroups that control the heart or specific vascular beds.

How Do RVLM Bulbospinal Neurons Excite SPGNs?

The prevailing opinion is that RVLM bulbospinal neurons drive SPGNs predominantly via a monosynaptic excitatory input to SPGNs using glutamate as main
transmitter (Fig. 1). Additional polysynaptic routes via spinal interneurons are
suspected but not fully demonstrated (Fig. 1). Whether glutamate is released by
C1 cells remains unsettled.

   The fact that some C1 cells project monosynaptically to SPGNs is demonstrated by electron microscopy (62), but this evidence does not exclude that C1
cells might also innervate interneurons that reside in close vicinity of SPGNs.
The spinal sites of termination of the nonaminergic component of the RVLM
projection are not precisely known because there is no specific histological
marker for them.

   The hypothesis that the RVLM to IML projection uses glutamate is supported by the presence of a high concentration of terminals immunoreactive for
this amino acid in the IML and by the fact that glutamate immunoreactivity in
the IML is reduced caudal to spinal cord lesions (70). This evidence is very
suggestive but not definitive, because spinal lesions also lead to a massive pruning
of the dendrites of SPGNs and the drop-off of glutamate immunoreactivity in the
IML could be related to the retraction of the dendrites of SPGNs (36). However,

electrophysiological data also suggest that glutamate is the major transmitter re-leased in the IML when RVLM bulbospinal neurons are activated (70–72). Again the data are very suggestive but not definitive because the results are also compat-ible with the possibility that RVLM neurons might activate spinal glutamatergic interneurons by releasing unidentified transmitters. It is conceivable that gluta-mate could be the major transmitter released by all RVLM bulbospinal neurons regardless of whether they express the catecholaminergic phenotype (C1 cells), but this hypothesis remains untested at present.

The bulbospinal projection of RVLM includes cells that are immunoreac-tive for peptides, at least after treatment with colchicine [substance P, VIP, en-kephalins, somatostatin, NPY (57–60,73)]. Some of these peptides (opioids, so-matostatin, NPY) exert mostly inhibitory effects elsewhere in the central nervous system (CNS) (74), suggesting that the particular subgroups of C1 cells that ex-press them may inhibit some of their targets (SPGNs or others). A critical unan-swered question is whether these inhibitory peptides are present in the C1 cells that subserve a vasomotor or cardioaccelerator function.

In summary, the RVLM projects at least in part monosynaptically to SPGNs, but projections to local interneurons are not excluded. The pattern of activity of RVLM bulbospinal neurons mirrors that of sympathetic nerves, sug-gesting that the function of these cells is to provide an excitatory drive to SPGNs. The RVLM projection includes nonaminergic glutamatergic neurons intermixed with C1 cells, which make and presumably release catecholamines plus a variety of peptides transmitters. The possibility that C1 cells also release glutamate re-mains unproven.

What Regulates the Discharge of RVLM Sympathoexcitatory Neurons in Vivo?

RVLM sympathoexcitatory neurons (C1 and non-C1) receive convergent infor-mation from a very large number of brain areas and play a key role in virtually all sympathetic reflexes (summarized in Fig. 6). Excitatory and inhibitory inputs from the raphe and the lateral tegmental field (LTF in Fig. 6) converge on these neurons and tend to synchronize their discharge at various low frequencies that are also observed in sympathetic nerves (4–6 Hz, 10 Hz, etc.) (75–77). Most inputs to RVLM sympathoexcitatory neurons appear to use either glutamate or GABA as primary transmitters. For example, the excitation of RVLM sympa-thoexcitatory neurons by stimulation of peripheral chemoreceptors or by activa-tion of somatosensory or vagal afferents is attenuated or blocked by microinjec-tion of glutamate receptor antagonist in RVLM or by iontophoretic application of the same agents (29,78,79). Conversely, sympathoinhibitory reflexes are usually attenuated by introducing GABA antagonists into RVLM. In agreement with these in vivo data, work in slices or in brainstem–spinal cord preparations indi-

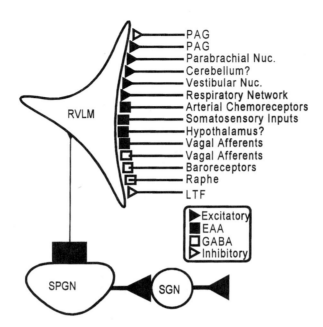

Figure 6 Convergence of sympathetic reflexes and central inputs on RVLM sympathoexcitatory neurons. RVLM sympathoexcitatory neurons play an important role in most cardiopulmonary reflexes and receive inputs from the major brain nuclei involved in cardiovascular control.

cates that, in the RVLM, most fast PSCs, either spontaneous or evoked by focal stimulation, are mediated by glutamate, GABA or, more rarely, by glycine (80,81). This result is not unexpected, given that the overwhelming majority of synapses in the brainstem and cord (>94%) seem to contain one of these three transmitters (27,82).

What is more surprising is that injections of glutamate receptor antagonists into RVLM should consistently fail to change resting sympathetic tone and arterial pressure (see, for example, 83–85). This observation has been variously interpreted. One interpretation is that inotropic glutamate transmission is not needed for the resting discharge (2–30 Hz) of RVLM sympathoexcitatory neurons in vivo because these cells are autoactive and/or are controlled by excitatory transmitters other than glutamate. Another interpretation is that the discharge of RVLM sympathoexcitatory neurons results from a balance between glutamate inputs and inhibitory inputs from interneurons located in RVLM or its immediate vicinity (85). Proponents of this second theory interpret the ineffectiveness of glutamate receptor antagonists injected in RVLM on resting sympathetic tone to the fact that these blockers also reduce the activity of inhibitory interneurons and thus produce as much disinhibition of the bulbospinal neurons as disfacilitation. Experimental evidence supports both viewpoints—namely, that RVLM sympathoexcitatory neurons may be intrinsically active and also that they receive a tonic barrage of excitatory and inhibitory inputs.

In slices (neonate rat up to 21 days of age), RVLM bulbospinal neurons are indeed spontaneously active due to intrinsic membrane properties (86,87). Their intrinsic discharge rate can be up- or down-regulated by a large variety of neurohormones acting on G protein–coupled postsynaptic receptors (noradrenaline, angiotensin, vasopressin, substance P) (86–92). All these substances have been identified by electron microscopy (EM) in synaptic inputs to C1 cells (93–98), though the physiological context in which they are released is unknown. Collectively, these observations suggest that the resting discharge of RVLM sympathoexcitatory neurons in vivo could derive at least in part from the intrinsic properties of these cells. They also emphasize the potential role of slow transmitters (neurohormones) in this system. For instance, the pronounced hypotension produced by microinjection of the antagonist sarthran in chloralose-anesthetized rats supports the possibility that under certain circumstances angiotensin II might be critical to maintain the discharge of RVLM sympathoexcitatory neurons (99).

Lipski and collaborators have provided evidence that the discharge of RVLM sympathoexcitatory neurons in vivo might be also triggered by synaptic events (100). In this study (adult rats), the action potentials of the cells were commonly triggered by events that these authors interpreted as large, fast excitatory PSPs (EPSPs) (100) though other interpretations of these events such as membrane oscillations remain possible (87). Also the depolarizing events identified by Lipski et al. were not identified as glutamatergic. Alternate possibilities include ACh or ATP because nicotinic and P2X receptors are also present on RVLM sympathoexcitatory neurons (101,102).

Though the extent and chemical nature of the excitatory synaptic drives of RVLM sympathoexcitatory neurons remain controversial, there is no doubt that these neurons are under strong tonic inhibitory control in vivo. This is indicated by the presence of numerous fast PSPs, with polarity reversed by chloride injection (100). Most of this tonic inhibition seems to be GABAergic, judged from the strong excitatory effect of iontophoretically applied GABA$_A$ receptor antagonists and the lack of effect of strychnine similarly applied (100,103). A large part of the tonic GABAergic inhibition of RVLM sympathoexcitatory neurons originates from propriobulbar interneurons that are activated by arterial baroreceptors and are concentrated in the IVLM (104).

ACh, NE, and serotonin are implicated in sleep stages. Thus the effect of these substances on RVLM neurons is potentially important for understanding the cardiovascular pathology of sleep disorders. In the neonate in vitro (3–21 days), the only catecholamine receptors detectable on bulbospinal RVLM neurons are of the α_2-adrenergic (α_2-AR) type. Histological data indicate that this receptor is of the α_{2A} variety (105). Stimulation of these α_2-ARs produces a modest amount of outward current that is mediated by the opening of inwardly rectifying K channels and normally suppresses the spontaneous activity of the neurons. Stimulation of α_2-ARs also inhibits current through voltage-activated calcium channels (mostly P/Q and N) in the same neurons (42). This effect does not appear to change neuronal accommodation detectably and its role remains undetermined. One possibility is that calcium channel inhibition serves to inhibit transmitter release from dendrites or terminals. α_2-ARs are also located presynaptically to RVLM bulbospinal neurons, and their activation by agonists depresses excitatory and inhibitory synaptic inputs to RVLM bulbospinal neurons (unpublished results from A. Hayar and P. Guyenet).

The serotonin input to RVLM sympathoexcitatory neurons probably originates from cells in the pontomedullary raphe (106). Iontophoretic application of serotonin excites RVLM sympathoexcitatory neurons via a 5HT-2–like receptor while higher concentrations of 5-HT or 5-HT-1A agonists produce inhibition (107,108). These effects have not been examined in vitro at the cellular level and may have both pre- and postsynaptic components. Excitatory 5-HT2 receptors are also present on SPGNs (109), which are also innervated by serotonergic fibers (110,111). Thus one would surmise that the activity of serotonergic medullary raphe neurons may have a globally excitatory influence on sympathetic tone generation. In agreement with this view, stimulation of the medullary raphe under anesthesia activates the sympathetic outflow (111,112). The discharge of serotonergic neurons within the medullary raphe is state-dependent. Highest during heightened states of vigilance, it is the lowest during rapid-eye-movement (REM) sleep (113). Arousal from non-REM (NREM) or REM sleep is therefore expected to increase the activity of medullary raphe serotonergic cells, which, in turn, ought to enhance sympathetic activity by activating SPGNs and their excitatory inputs from the RVLM. This mechanism could contribute to the cardiovascular pathology associated with sleep apnea.

The RVLM receives its extrinsic cholinergic input from the pedunculopontine tegmental nucleus (PPT), a structure also involved in the generation of sleep stages (114). PPT cholinergic neurons are believed to be active during waking and REM sleep but inactive during NREM sleep. The medial edge of RVLM also contains neurons that are immunoreactive for choline-acetyl transferase and whose physiological role is unknown (115). Increasing the release of acetylcholine (ACh) in RVLM either by microinjection or by reducing hydrolysis with an inhibitor of acetylcholinesterase (AChE) augments arterial pressure and sympathetic tone (116) via a predominantly muscarinic mechanism (117,118). The synaptic mechanism responsible for the activation of RVLM sympathoexcitatory neurons by ACh is not fully elucidated (102,119). In any case, the data clearly indicate that the release of ACh within the RVLM causes sympathoactivation.

Current understanding of the physiology of the PPT suggests that ACh could be released in the RVLM at the transition between sleep and waking, which could contribute to the pathology of sleep apnea.

C. Supraspinal Mechanisms: Sympathoinhibitory Pathways in the Cord and Medulla Oblongata

The existence of descending inhibitory pathways that control the sympathetic outflow is suspected, but these pathways are still poorly characterized, perhaps because they utilize complex polysynaptic routes that are difficult to study under anesthesia. The hypothetical possibilities compatible with experimental data are represented in Figure 7.

Electrical stimulation or microinjection of excitatory amino acids in several brainstem regions (raphe, gigantocellular "depressor" area) can produce decreases in AP and sympathoinhibition (51,120–124). However, these methods lack cellular resolution and cannot resolve whether a descending inhibitory input has been activated or whether the sympathoinhibition is due to inhibition of the sympathoexcitatory neurons of the RVLM (124,125).

The most persuasive evidence in favor of a monosynaptic inhibitory input to SPGNs is that stimulation of the rostral medullary region elicits GABAergic inhibitory PSPs (IPSPs) in many SPGNs in the neonate (126). However, because

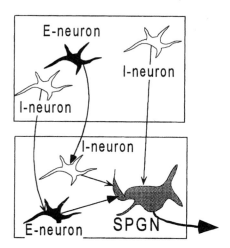

Figure 7 Other pathways that regulate sympathetic preganglionic neurons. Schematic representation of some of the medullary pathways that may be functionally inhibitory to SPGN activity. The existence of these pathways is not fully demonstrated and the exact location of the bulbospinal neurons is still debated.

electrical stimulation provides mediocre spatial resolution, especially in the neonate, the precise location of the GABAergic neurons responsible for this monosynaptic inhibition remains uncertain.

Various types of data suggest that bulbospinal E or I neurons (as defined in Fig. 7) may be present in the raphe (76,127–130), the gigantocellular field (120,122), or even the RVLM itself (131,132). The raphe neurons implicated in sympathetic control probably include nonserotonergic cells (20,59,133). Finally, a heavy innervation of the IML from the caudal NTS has also been described (61,134). This constitutes the shortest conceivable pathway for reflex control of sympathetic tone, but there is yet no evidence that this pathway controls circulation.

In summary, recent evidence suggests that several brainstem areas within and outside RVLM may provide descending inhibitory inputs to SPGNs, most probably of a GABAergic nature. Each of these hypotheses requires more definitive evidence.

D. Baroreflexes

Stimulation of arterial baroreceptors inhibits the sympathetic outflow to the heart, the kidney, and most of the vasculature (muscle, splanchnic). It also activates the cardiovagal outflow (cardiovagal baroreflex) and depresses the phrenic nerve discharge (barorespiratory reflex) (135). In contrast to the sympathetic baroreflex, the barorespiratory reflex is usually weak under anesthesia, and it is overridden by the activation of chemoreceptors. It is thus clearly observed only when the respiratory drive is small. Figure 8 illustrates the simultaneous inhibition of the activity of the splanchnic nerve (30–3000 Hz bipolar recording) and of a phrenic nerve (rectified and integrated with low-pass filter) by intravenous administration of phenylephrine in a chloralose-anesthetized rat (unpublished results of P. McCulloch and P. G. Guyenet). Figure 9 depicts a hypothetical wiring diagram of the three baroreflexes (respiratory, cardiovagal, and sympathetic). In this diagram, the sympathetic and, to a lesser degree, the cardiovagal pathways are based on considerable neurophysiological and neuroanatomical evidence (see 49, 52, and 136 for reviews). The pathway of the barorespiratory reflex remains an educated guess.

Sympathetic Baroreflex

This polysynaptic reflex involves three stages: the NTS, the ventrolateral medulla (specifically the intermediate part called here IVLM), and the RVLM (see 50, 53, and 136 for prior review). The circuit includes an excitatory, presumably glutamatergic projection from the NTS to the IVLM, which drives inhibitory GABAergic projections from IVLM to the sympathetic premotoneurons of the RVLM (137). The central role of the IVLM is inferred from four types of con-

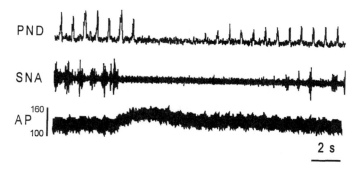

Figure 8   Two facets of the baroreflex: sympathoinhibition and inhibition of respiration. This experiment performed in chloralose-anesthetized rats (McCulloch and Guyenet, unpublished) shows that elevating arterial pressure with an i.v. injection of phenylephrine silences the activity of the splanchnic nerve (SNA) and the discharge of the phrenic nerve (PNA). The effect on PNA (barorespiratory reflex) is observed only when central respiratory drive is low. It is shunted out if P_{CO_2} is increased to increase respiratory drive.

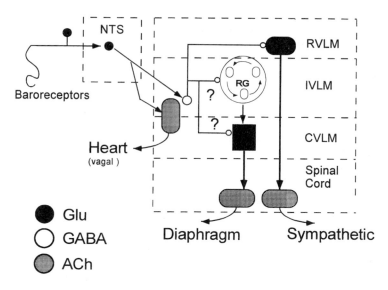

Figure 9   Pathway of the baroreflexes. In this representation, the pathway of the sympathetic and cardiovagal reflexes elicited by stimulation of arterial baroreceptors is based on considerable experimental data. The pathway of the cardiorespiratory baroreflex is an educated guess. For abbreviations, see Figures 1 and 3.

verging information. First, bilateral inhibition of the IVLM by microinjection into this region of $GABA_A$ receptor agonists (e.g., muscimol) or broad-spectrum GLU receptor antagonists (e.g., kynurenic acid) blocks the baroreflex (46,138). Second, sustained elevations of AP cause neuronal expression of c-Fos in this region (139), including within GABAergic cells that project to or through RVLM (137). Third, IVLM contains propriomedullary neurons that display an appropriate discharge pattern in response to baroreceptor stimulation (excitatory response and pulse-modulated firing) (140,141). Finally, activation of baroreceptors inhibits RVLM presympathetic neurons via a postsynaptic GABAergic, bicuculline-sensitive, input (100,103). Considerable uncertainty surrounds the first stage of the reflex (i.e., the processing of baroreceptor afferent information within the NTS). Though many NTS neurons have been shown to respond to synchronous electrical activation of baroreceptor afferents by inhibition or excitation (reviewed in 142), the NTS neurons that normally convey baroreceptor information to the ventrolateral medulla have not been clearly identified. There is reason to believe that these projection neurons may not receive monosynaptic inputs from baroreceptors but could represent higher-order cells (143). This issue is addressed below in the context of the cardiovagal baroreflex.

Cardiovagal Baroreflex

Our understanding of the central networks that control cardiovagal motoneurons (CVMs, Fig. 10) is based on neuroanatomy and an uncommonly small amount of neurophysiological data considering the importance of this system for cardiovascular regulation. Chronotropic, dromotropic, and negative inotropic control operates through largely distinct postganglionic neurons clustered in separate cardiac ganglia (144–146). These classes of postganglionic neurons also appear to be controlled by separate populations of CVMs located mostly in nucleus ambiguus (Fig. 10) and, to a smaller degree, in the dorsal motor nucleus of the vagus (144–146). The neuronal inputs to CVMs are best known from the pattern of retrograde labeling that follows infection of cardiac ganglia with pseudorabies virus (147,148). This work suggests that a majority of the monosynaptic inputs to CVMs originates from interneurons located in the ventrolateral medulla, while a smaller number are located in the ventrolateral aspect of the NTS. The latter region is not known to receive significant numbers of baroreceptor afferent terminals, and it is only at a later stage of viral infection that the NTS contains numerous labeled neurons in its dorsal aspect, which does receive the bulk of baroreceptor afferents. These anatomical data suggest several possibilities, two of which are illustrated in Figure 10. Option A is that first-order baroreceptor neurons (the cells that receive monosynaptic inputs from baroreceptors) drive CVMs indirectly via interneurons located in the ventrolateral medulla. These interneurons would have to be excitatory, since baroreceptor activation produces chloride-indepen-

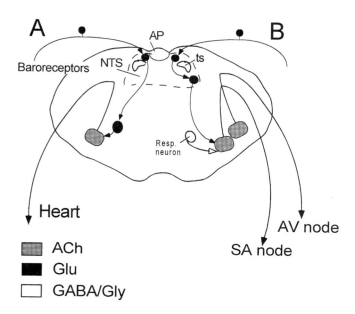

Figure 10   Neural control of cardiovagal motoneurons. NTS, nucleus of the solitary tract; ts, solitary tract; AP, area postrema.

dent depolarizing potentials in CVMs (149). Experiments in slices tend to argue against the need for a two-neuron chain between NTS and CVMs because electrical stimulation of the NTS excite these cells in apparently monosynaptic fashion via the release of glutamate (150). The importance of glutamate transmission for excitation of CVMs by baroreceptors is supported by experiments demonstrating that microinjection of glutamate receptor blockers in their vicinity blocks the cardiovagal baroreflex (138) and by intracellular recording showing pulse-synchronous, chloride-independent depolarizing potentials in CVMs in vivo (149). Work from the latter authors also demonstrated that CVMs are inhibited during the phrenic nerve discharge (inspiration) via a postsynaptic chloride-dependent increase in membrane conductance which shunts the depolarizing effect of the baroreceptor input (149). The chloride dependence of the postsynaptic inhibition suggests in turn that it must be mediated by either GABA or glycine (reviewed in 151). In summary, the bulk of the evidence supports scheme B whereby CVMs receive a glutamatergic excitatory input from second- or higher-order barosensory neurons via the NTS. This input is probably essential to sustain the activity of CVMs, and it is responsible for their pulse-related discharge. The second major input to CVM is inhibitory and originates from ventrolateral medullary interneurons that are active during inspiration. CVMs, like many CNS neurons, also receive inputs from brainstem serotonergic and substance P–containing neurons (152). At present the pathway responsible for the effect of nonadapting lung-stretch receptors on the cardiovagal outflow is completely unknown.

E. Control of Sympathetic Efferent Activity by Respiration

In humans and all mammals examined, SNA fluctuates in synchrony with the breathing cycle (Fig. 4 illustrates the case of a chloralose-anesthetized rat). Some of these fluctuations are due to cardiopulmonary reflexes, principally the arterial baroreflex described above. The baroreflex produces a respiratory oscillation of SNA simply because arterial pressure and hence the discharge of arterial baroreceptors oscillates during the breathing cycle. Other receptors such as chest proprioreceptors, peripheral chemoreceptors, lung, cardiac, and airway receptors—whose discharge pattern is also modulated or caused by respiratory movements—probably also contribute to the respiratory rhythmicity of the sympathetic outflow (for review see 153).

The second major cause of respiratory fluctuations in the sympathetic nerve discharge is central cardiorespiratory coupling. This phenomenon can be isolated and studied in anesthetized animals in which baroreceptors and other known sources of sensory feedback have been eliminated by surgical and other means. In this case SNA still fluctuates in synchrony with the phrenic nerve discharge (e.g., 65, 154). Typically, the respiratory oscillations of SNA are superimposed on a high resting level of discharge that resists hyperventilation to phrenic apnea, and the amplitude of the respiratory oscillations is roughly proportional to that of the phrenic nerve discharge (65).

F. Central Cardiorespiratory Coupling

The Common Cardiorespiratory Network Theory

This theory, refined in 1990 by Richter and Spyer (155), holds that the various respiratory outflows (to diaphragm, chest and abdominal muscles, and airways) as well as the sympathetic vasomotor and the cardiovagal outflows receive synaptic inputs from a common pool of lower brainstem interneurons whose discharge pattern is synchronized to respiration. The theory (Fig. 11) views these interneurons as multipurpose cells, whose role is neither specifically respiratory nor cardiovascular. For lack of a better word, these still largely unidentified cells may be called *cardiorespiratory interneurons*. They could be either inhibitory or excitatory and their activity, fairly stereotyped in all mammals examined, is thought to belong to one of three respiratory patterns commonly found in the medulla (inspiratory, postinspiratory, or expiratory) (156). These multipurpose interneurons would owe their respiratory pattern of discharge to inputs from a small core

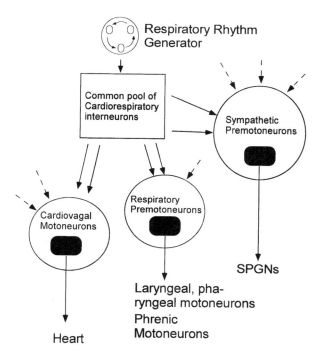

Figure 11 Organization of the medullary cardiorespiratory network. This schema, inspired by the vision of Richter and Spyer (155), illustrates the notion that cardiovagal motor neurons, sympathetic vasomotor efferents, and the respiratory motor neurons may be regulated by a common pool of cardiorespiratory interneurons whose function is neither purely respiratory nor purely cardiovascular. These neurons would derive their on-off respiratory pattern from a respiratory rhythm generator, perhaps located within the pre-Botzinger nucleus (PreB in Fig. 3). Sympathetic pre–motor neurons and cardiovagal motor neurons, however, receive a majority of their inputs from other systems (arrows with dotted lines).

of neurons dedicated specifically to respiratory rhythm generation (RG in Figs. 9 and 11). The latter may be confined to the pre-Botzinger nucleus of the IVLM (Figs. 3 and 9) (48,156).

This broad concept is consistent with the anatomical proximity between identified neurons that regulate the lungs, the upper airways, and cardiovascular performance within the medulla oblongata and pons (48,157–160). It provides a plausible working hypothesis to explain how an increase in respiratory drive could generate the appropriate increase in cardiac output needed to increase O_2 delivery to the tissues. However, putting this theory to the test will require investigators to identify the location, phenotype, and input-output properties of the postulated cardiorespiratory interneurons that control sympathetic and cardiovagal efferents. This is a goal that has been notably elusive so far.

Role of RVLM Presympathetic Neurons in Cardiorespiratory Coupling

It is probable that the bulbar respiratory network modulates the sympathetic outflow via the bulbospinal sympathoexcitatory neurons of the RVLM. This conclusion derives in large part from the close similarity between the discharge probability of these RVLM cells during the respiratory cycle and that of individual postganglionic units in deafferented preparations (buffer and vagus nerves cut). In the rat, for example, one finds the same three respiratory patterns in RVLM cells with putative vasomotor function as in postganglionic neurons of the lumbar chain (65,161–163). The predominant pattern consists of an increased firing probability during the postinspiratory phase with or without a dip during early inspiration. A second type of neuron exhibits a pattern that is the mirror image of the first (peak during early inspiration, nadir during postinspiration), while other neurons seem to be influenced little or not at all by respiration. In those RVLM neurons that are markedly respiration-synchronous, the magnitude of the respiratory fluctuations is similar to that present in single ganglionic cells. The existence of respiratory patterns in many RVLM vasomotor neurons indicates that these cells receive inputs from brainstem neurons with discharges synchronized with the network that generates the respiratory rhythm. The multiplicity of pattern indicates that various types or combinations of cardiorespiratory interneurons must impinge on RVLM vasomotor neurons. The existence of more than one pattern also indicates that the respiratory network modulates sympathetic efferents selectively. Finally the fact that RVLM vasomotor neurons retain a high basal level of discharge even when the activity of the central respiratory network is silenced by hyperventilation also suggests that the vasomotor neurons receive only a portion of their excitatory input from this network.

The synaptic mechanisms responsible for the increased discharge probability of RVLM sympathoexcitatory neurons during specific phases of the respiratory cycle (excitation, disinhibition, etc.) have not been examined. Also, the location and phenotype of the cardiorespiratory interneurons that convey this respiratory pattern to RVLM sympathoexcitatory neurons is not precisely known. In the rat, the Botzinger neurons, respiratory interneurons that discharge during expiration (see location of these cells in Fig. 3), have axonal collaterals that make close appositions with the dendrites of some C1 neurons (164). These close appositions may represent synaptic contacts. However a postsynaptic input from Botzinger neurons could not increase the activity of RVLM sympathoexcitatory cells when respiration is enhanced but, at best, could reduce their activation during late expiration. Indeed the discharge rate of Botzinger neurons increases in direct proportion to the respiratory drive, and these cells clearly release an inhibitory transmitter, probably GABA or glycine (165). The respiratory control of RVLM sympathoexcitatory neurons is further complicated by the fact that different types of cardiorespiratory interneurons may be recruited in different species to activate the sympathetic outflow (for a review of these species differences, see 153).

From a functional and pathological point of view, it is important to note that cardiac sympathetic efferents are among those that receive a marked excitatory drive from the CRG (77). This strong input must play a major role in coordinating cardiac contractility and rate (hence cardiac output) with pulmonary gas exchanges. During OSA, it seems highly probable that the central respiratory drive would be enhanced due to CO_2 buildup, resulting in an increased activity of cardiac sympathetic nerves. It seems logical to assume that the increased sympathetic discharge could contribute to the ischemic events or arrhythmias associated with this type of pathology.

G. The Peripheral Chemoreflex

Effects Produced by Activation of Peripheral Chemoreceptors

Activation of carotid chemoreceptors produces complex effects on autonomic outflows in which secondary reflexes triggered by the increase in breathing play a major part (reviewed in 166). The major contributing factors to the overall response are summarized in Figure 12. During chemoreceptor stimulation, CVMs are subjected to three major influences: a primary activation (pathway 1, responsible for the so-called primary bradycardia observed when changes in ventilation are not allowed to take place) and two inhibitory inputs. Input 2 is the inspiratory inhibition normally responsible for sinus arrhythmia. What little is known of its cellular mechanism has been described above. This input is assumed to be magnified during chemoreceptor stimulation due to the increase in central respiratory drive. Input 3 is a negative feedback from nonadapting lung stretch receptors. Its magnitude is species-specific and increases along with the degree of respiratory activation. The integration of inputs 1–3 defines the overall effect on CVM activity, which may vary from excitation to inhibition, depending on the anesthesia, species, and intensity of chemoreceptor stimulation. The overall effect on heart rate mirrors the change in CVM activity to the extent that parasympathetic tone dominates. For instance, in the dog under anesthesia, when chemoreceptor stimulation is mild, bradycardia driven by pathway 1 dominates, but tachycardia is present when respiration is more strongly activated.

Most evidence suggests that activation of carotid chemoreceptors produces a more or less generalized increase in sympathetic tone, including to the heart. This excitation is the result of three major converging influences (4–6) which, if the stimulus is hypoxia, may later be counteracted by a reduction in central chemoreceptor activity due to hyperventilation (pathway 7). Pathway 6, the sym-

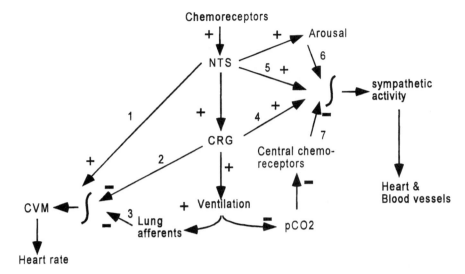

Figure 12 Major effects produced by stimulation of chemoreceptors. This schematic summarizes the various types of cardiovascular changes elicited by stimulation of chemoreceptors. The precise central neural mechanisms underlying most of these responses is largely unknown.

pathoexcitation associated with arousal, would seem a priori especially important in the context of sleep apnea. Chemoreceptor stimulation in awake or unanesthetized, decorticate animal preparations produces strong aversive behaviors associated with hypertension and an autonomic pattern associated with the defense reaction (pupillary dilatation, increased heart rate and AP, and visceral and cardiac sympathetic activation, with shunting of blood flow through muscles) (166,167).

Central Pathways That Mediate the Effect of Peripheral Chemoreceptors on Autonomic Outflows

Chemoreceptor afferents terminate within the NTS from the level of the area postrema to the caudal commissural NTS (168). There is considerable overlap between the sites of termination of chemoreceptor and baroreceptor afferents, though chemoreceptor projections appear heavier more caudally in the commissural subnucleus. In some studies, introduction of retrograde tracers into the carotid body has also produced the appearance of terminal labeling ventromedial to the NTS in a strip of tissue extending to the nucleus ambiguus. These data suggest the possibility of direct innervation of the ventrolateral medullary region by chemoreceptor afferents (for review see 169, p. 124). The nucleus ambiguus also sends an efferent projection to the carotid sinus (168).

Beyond the NTS, the neuronal substrate of pathway 1 (primary bradycardic response) is unknown. Pathway 3 is also uncharted. The initial step must involve the NTS, since slowly adapting pulmonary stretch receptors terminate exclusively within specific subnuclei of the NTS (170). Integration between afferent information from chemoreceptor and stretch receptors could occur within the NTS—but, if so, this is likely to occur at the level of third- or higher-order interneurons, since the majority of NTS neurons that receive inputs from peripheral chemoreceptors do not receive inputs from pulmonary stretch receptors or display a respiratory rhythm (171).

Peripheral chemoreceptor stimulation activates the sympathetic outflow in bursts synchronized with the phrenic nerve discharge. The sympathoactivation is mediated in large part by activation of the RVLM bulbospinal projection to SPGNs, as shown by unit recording (172,173). Under anesthesia, the response is unchanged by complete transection of the brainstem rostral to the pons (174). However, without anesthesia, strong chemoreceptor stimulation produces aversive effects and defense reaction–type responses that are likely to involve suprapontine structures. Inhibiting neurons within the pre-Botzinger area/IVLM (Fig. 13) eliminates respiratory outflows and replaces the phasic bursts of sympathoactivation caused by stimulation of carotid chemoreceptors by a continuous sympathoactivation (172). Whereas massive bilateral lesions of the dorsolateral pons

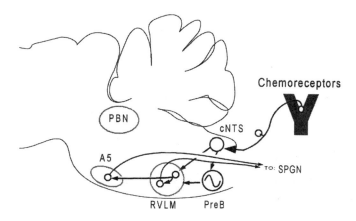

Figure 13 Pathway responsible for the increase in sympathetic nerve activity caused by stimulation of peripheral chemoreceptors. PBN, parabrachial nuclei; A5, ventrolateral pontine noradrenergic cell group and its surrounding region; PreB, pre-Botzinger nucleus; cNTS, caudal part of nucleus of the solitary tract.

(PBN) (Fig. 13) disrupt the phrenic response to chemoreceptor stimulation they do not affect the sympathetic response (174). Finally, unit recording and other data suggest that activation of the A5 noradrenergic neurons of the ventrolateral pons (Fig. 13) may be required for full expression of the sympathoactivation (175). These neurophysiological observations have been integrated into the tentative wiring diagram showed in Figure 13. This diagram incorporates evidence that the NTS contains neurons that convey chemoreceptor information exclusive of other sensory modalities (baroreceptor, stretch receptor, etc.) to the ventrolateral medulla (176). It is hypothesized that these neurons are capable of activating the respiratory network at the level of the ventrolateral medulla and that the sympathoexcitatory neurons of RVLM and ventrolateral pons (A5) can also be activated by these inputs independently of the respiratory system (pathway 5 in Fig. 12).

Stimulation of central or peripheral chemoreceptors may also increase sympathetic activity by reducing baroreflex inhibition, although this interaction has not been detected by all investigators and therefore must be either small or very sensitive to anesthesia (e.g., 177). In rats, inhibition of RVLM sympathoexcitatory neurons by stimulation of the aortic depressor nerve is somewhat more effective during inspiration than during expiration or postinspiration, periods of the respiratory cycle during which these neurons are generally more active (178). The authors postulated the existence of a nonlinear postsynaptic summation of the two inputs on RVLM sympathoexcitatory neurons, but the data are equally compatible with an interaction between baro- and chemoreflex inputs upstream from the RVLM (i.e., within the IVLM or the NTS).

H. Central Chemoreceptors: Effects on Sympathetic and Cardiovagal Outflows

Hypoventilation or apnea causes an increase in P_{CO_2} that is primarily sensed within the medulla oblongata, causing an increase in respiratory drive and activation of the sympathetic outflow to the heart and blood vessels. This textbook knowledge derives from experiments on anesthetized animals with severed vagus and buffer nerves in which phrenic nerve discharge and sympathetic tone were simultaneously recorded (for a recent reference, see, e.g., 154). The general observation is that sympathetic activation occurs in bursts synchronized with the respiratory cycle (during inspiration or postinspiration, depending on the species), suggesting that this activation is driven by elements of the central respiratory network. There is some rather indirect evidence that the sympathetic outflow can be activated by central chemoreceptors independently of their effect on the respiratory system (discussed in 153, p. 341). Some of these experiments suggest that high CO_2 levels can activate sympathetic tone in acutely spinally transected animals (179).

The synchronization of SNA with the respiratory cycle is very similar when central or peripheral chemoreceptors are activated, suggesting that common mechanisms are recruited to activate the sympathetic outflow in both cases. These hypothetical mechanisms have been discussed in detail above apropos of the peripheral chemoreflex. In fact, very little is known of the pathway leading from central chemoreceptors to SPGNs except that it involves the activation of RVLM sympathoexcitatory neurons (65,153).

I. Central Hypoxia and Sympathetic Tone

Is the RVLM an oxygen sensor? Sun and Reis have proposed that RVLM sympathoexcitatory neurons have oxygen-sensing capability. Hypoxia would activate these cells directly, causing an increased sympathetic tone and stimulating circulation and oxygen delivery to the body (180). The theory is based on the following observations (180–183). Hypoxia increases sympathetic tone even in animals without peripheral chemoreceptors. The increase in sympathetic tone is associated with an activation of RVLM sympathoexcitatory neurons. The direct hypoxic activation of these cells is not due to the release of glutamate, contrary to the effect of peripheral chemoreceptors, and it can be mimicked by iontophoretic application of metabolic poisons such as cyanide in their vicinity. Finally, hypoxia or cyanide activates RVLM neurons in slices in part by increasing an inward current through calcium channels (184). The main problem with the theory is that the P_{O_2} below which direct hypoxic activation of RVLM neurons is triggered has not been determined. At present, it appears probable that the mechanism described by Sun and Reis accounts for the sympathoactivation associated with anoxia such as occurs during cerebral ischemia (185). It appears somewhat unlikely that the oxygen-sensing capability of the RVLM could play a role in the sympathoactivation associated with apneic episodes.

III. Summary and Conclusion

Sympathetic tone is generated by a complex network of neurons located within the lower brainstem. This network converges within the rostral ventrolateral medulla on a group of neurons (RVLM sympathoexcitatory neurons). These cells provide the bulk of the excitatory drive to the sympathetic preganglionic neurons that regulate the heart and blood vessels. They are activated by peripheral and central chemoreceptors via lower brainstem circuits that are very imperfectly understood at present. The transition from sleep to waking state is associated with the release of modulators such as catecholamines, serotonin, and ACh, which exert generally stimulatory effects at multiple points along the spinomedullary network that generates the sympathetic tone to the heart and blood vessels.

References

1. Narkiewicz K, Somers VK. The sympathetic nervous system and obstructive sleep apnea: implications for hypertension. J Hypertens 1997; 15:1613–1619.

2. Cabot JB. Sympathetic preganglionic neurons: cytoarchitecture, ultrastructure, and biophysical properties. In: Loewy AD, Spyer KM, eds. Central Regulation of Autonomic Functions. London: Oxford University Press, 1990:44–67.

3. Murugaian J, Sundaram K, Krieger A, Sapru H. Relative effects of different spinal autonomic nuclei on cardiac sympathoexcitatory function. Brain Res Bull 1990; 24:537–542.

4. Sundaram K, Murugaian J, Sapru H. Cardiac responses to the microinjections of excitatory amino acids into the intermediolateral cell column of the rat spinal cord. Brain Res 1989; 482:12–22.

5. Wu SY, Dun SL, Förstermann U, Dun NJ. Nitric oxide and excitatory postsynaptic currents in immature rat sympathetic preganglionic neurons in vitro. Neuroscience 1997; 79:237–245.

6. Wu SY, Dun NJ. Potentiation of IPSCs by nitric oxide in immature rat sympathetic preganglionic neurones in vitro. J Physiol (London) 1996; 495:479–490.

7. Dun NJ, Wu SY, Shen E, Miyazaki T, Dun SL, Ren C. Synaptic mechanisms in sympathetic preganglionic neurons. Can J Physiol Pharmacol 1992; 70(suppl): S86–S91.

8. Shen E, Mo N, Dun NJ. APV-sensitive dorsal root afferent transmission to neonate rat sympathetic preganglionic neurons in vitro. J Neurophysiol 1990; 64:991–999.

9. Bazil MK, Gordon FJ. Spinal NMDA receptors mediate pressor responses evoked from the rostral ventrolateral medulla. Am J Physiol 1991; 260:H267–H275.

10. Krukoff TL, Ciriello J, Calaresu FR. Segmental distribution of peptide-like immunoreactivity in cell bodies of the thoracolumbar sympathetic nuclei of the cat. J Comp Neurol 1985; 240:90–102.

11. Edwards SL, Anderson CR, Southwell BR, McAllen RM. Distinct preganglionic neurons innervate noradrenaline and adrenaline cells in the cat adrenal medulla. Neuroscience 1996; 70:825–832.

12. Grkovic I, Anderson CR. Calbindin D28K-immunoreactivity identifies distinct subpopulations of sympathetic pre- and postganglionic neurons in the rat. J Comp Neurol 1997; 386:245–259.

13. Miyazaki T, Dun NJ, Kobayashi H, Tosaka T. Voltage-dependent potassium currents of sympathetic preganglionic neurons in neonatal rat spinal cord thin slices. Brain Res 1996; 743:1–10.

14. Logan SD, Pickering AE, Gibson IC, Nolan MF, Spanswick D. Electrotonic coupling between rat sympathetic preganglionic neurones in vitro. J. Physiol. (Lond) 1996; 495:491–502.

15. Shen E, Wu SY, Dun NJ. Spontaneous and transmitter-induced rhythmic activity in neonatal rat sympathetic preganglionic neurons in vitro. J Neurophysiol 1994; 71:1197–1205.

16. Cabot JB, Alessi V, Carroll J, Ligorio M. Spinal cord lamina V and lamina VII

interneuronal projections to sympathetic preganglionic neurons. J Comp Neurol 1994; 347:515–530.

17. Bogan N, Mennone A, Cabot JB. Light microscopic and ultrastructural localization of GABA-like immunoreactive input to retrograde labeled sympathetic preganglionic neurons. Brain Res 1989; 505:257–270.

18. Cabot JB, Alessi V, Bushnell A. Glycine-like immunoreactive input to sympathetic preganglionic neurons. Brain Res 1992; 571:1–18.

19. Strack AM, Sawyer WB, Hughes JH, Platt KB, Loewy AD. A general pattern of CNS innervation of the sympathetic outflow demonstrated by transneuronal pseudorabies viral infections. Brain Res 1989; 491:156–162.

20. Strack AM, Sawyer WB, Platt KB, Loewy AD. CNS cell groups regulating the sympathetic outflow to adrenal gland as revealed by transneuronal cell body labeling with pseudorabies virus. Brain Res 1989; 491:274–296.

21. Jansen ASP, Loewy AD. Neurons lying in the white matter of the upper cervical spinal cord project to the intermediolateral cell column. Neuroscience 1997; 77: 889–898.

22. Mo N, Dun NJ. Is glycine an inhibitory transmitter in rat lateral horn cells? Brain Res 1987; 400:139–144.

23. Dun NJ, Mo N. Inhibitory postsynaptic potentials in neonatal rat sympathetic preganglionic neurones in vitro. J Physiol (Lond) 1989; 410:267–281.

24. Mo N, Dun NJ. Excitatory postsynaptic potentials in neonatal rat sympathetic preganglionic neurons: possible mediation by NMDA receptors. Neurosci Lett 1987; 77:327–332.

25. Cammack C, Logan SD. Excitation of rat sympathetic preganglionic neurones by selective activation of the NK_1 receptor. J Auton Nerv Syst 1996; 57:87–92.

26. Spanswick D, Pickering AE, Gibson IC, Logan SD. Inhibition of sympathetic preganglionic neurons by spinal glycinergic interneurons. Neuroscience 1994; 62:205–216.

27. Llewellyn-Smith IJ, Minson JB, Pilowsky PM, Arnolda LF, Chalmers JP. The one hundred percent hypothesis: glutamate or GABA in synapses on sympathetic preganglionic neurons. Clin Exp Hypertens 1995; 17:323–333.

28. Sato A, Schmidt RF. Somatosympathetic reflexes: afferent fibers, central pathways, discharge characteristics. Physiol Rev 1973; 53:916–947.

29. Sun MK, Spyer KM. Nociceptive inputs into rostral ventrolateral medulla spinal vasomotor neurones in rats. J Physiol (Lond) 1991; 436:685–700.

30. Lewis DI, Coote JH. Mediation of baroreceptor inhibition of sympathetic nerve activity via both a brainstem and spinal site in rats. J Physiol (Lond) 1994; 481: 197–205.

31. Lewis DI, Coote JH. Chemical mediators of spinal inhibition of rat sympathetic neurones on stimulation in the nucleus tractus solitarii. J Physiol (Lond) 1995; 486: 483–494.

32. Lewis DI, Coote JH. Baroreceptor-induced inhibition of sympathetic neurons by GABA acting at a spinal site. Am J Physiol Heart Circ Physiol 1996; 270:H1885–H1892.

33. Osborn JW, Taylor RF, Schramm LP. Chronic cervical spinal cord injury and autonomic hyperreflexia in rats. Am J Physiol 1990; 258:R169–R174.

34. Chau D, Kim NJ, Schramm LP. Sympathetically correlated activity of dorsal horn neurons in spinally transected rats. J Neurophysiol 1997; 77:2966–2974.
35. Hong YG, Cechetto DF, Weaver LC. Spinal cord regulation of sympathetic activity in intact and spinal rats. Am J Physiol 1994; 266:H1485–H1493.
36. Krassioukov AV, Weaver LC. Morphological changes in sympathetic preganglionic neurons after spinal cord injury in rats. Neuroscience 1996; 70:211–225.
37. Inokuchi H, Yoshimura M, Polosa C, Nishi S. Adrenergic receptors (alpha 1 and alpha 2) modulate different potassium conductances in sympathetic preganglionic neurons. Can J Physiol Pharmacol 1992; 70(suppl):S92–S97.
38. Yoshimura M, Polosa C, Nishi S. Slow EPSP and the depolarizing action of noradrenaline on sympathetic preganglionic neurons. Brain Res 1987; 414:138–142.
39. Yoshimura M, Polosa C, Nishi S. Noradrenaline-induced afterdepolarization in cat sympathetic preganglionic neurons in vitro. J Neurophysiol 1987; 57:1314–1324.
40. Yoshimura M, Polosa C, Nishi S. Slow IPSP and the noradrenaline-induced inhibition of the cat sympathetic preganglionic neuron in vitro. Brain Res 1987; 419: 383–386.
41. Coote JH, Lewis DI. Bulbospinal catecholamine neurones and sympathetic pattern generation. J Physiol Pharmacol 1995; 46:259–271.
42. Li YW, Guyenet PG, Bayliss DA. Voltage-dependent calcium currents in bulbospinal neurons of neonatal rat rostral ventrolateral medulla: modulation by α_2-adrenergic receptors. J Neurophysiol 1998; 79:583–594.
43. Huangfu D, Hwang LJ, Riley TA, Guyenet PG. Splanchnic nerve response to A5-area stimulation in rats. Am J Physiol 1992; 263:R437–R446.
44. Sundaram K, Murugaian J, Sapru H. Microinjections of norepinephrine into the intermediolateral cell column of the spinal cord exert excitatory as well as inhibitory effects on the cardiac function. Brain Res 1991; 544:227–234.
45. Hirooka Y, Polson JW, Potts PD, Dampney RAL. Hypoxia-induced Fos expression in neurons projecting to the pressor region in the rostral ventrolateral medulla. Neuroscience 1997; 80:1209–1224.
46. Willette RN, Punnen S, Krieger AJ, Sapru HN. Interdependence of rostral and caudal ventrolateral medullary areas in the control of blood pressure. Brain Res 1984; 321:169–174.
47. Smith JC, Funk GD, Johnson SM, Feldman JL. Cellular and synaptic mechanisms generating respiratory rhythm: insights from in vitro and computational studies. In: Trouth CO, Millis RM, Kiwull-Schone H, Schlafke M, eds. Ventral Brainstem Mechanisms and Control of Respiration and Blood Pressure. New York: Marcel Dekker, 1995:463–496.
48. Smith JC, Ellenberger HH, Ballanyi K, Richter DW, Feldman JL. Pre-Botzinger complex—a brainstem region that may generate respiratory rhythm in mammals. Science 1991; 254:726–729.
49. Dampney RAL. The subretrofacial vasomotor nucleus: anatomical, chemical and pharmacological properties and role in cardiovascular regulation. Prog Neurobiol 1994; 42:197–228.
50. Dampney RAL. Functional organization of central pathways regulating the cardiovascular system. Physiol Rev 1994; 74:323–364.
51. Guyenet PG. Role of the ventral medulla oblongata in blood pressure regulation.

In: Loewy AD, Spyer KM, eds. Central Regulation of Autonomic Functions. New York: Oxford University Press, 1990:145–167.

52. Guyenet PG, Koshiya N, Huangfu D, Baraban SC, Stornetta RL, Li YW. Role of medulla oblongata in generation of sympathetic and vagal outflows. In: Holstege G, Bandler R, Saper CB, eds. The Emotional Motor System. Amsterdam: Elsevier, 1996:127–144.

53. Sun MK. Central neural organization and control of sympathetic nervous system in mammals. Prog Neurobiol 1995; 47:157–233.

54. Sun MK. Pharmacology of reticulospinal vasomotor neurons in cardiovascular regulation. Pharmacol Rev 1996; 48:465–494.

55. Lipski J, Kanjhan R, Kruszewska B, Smith M. Barosensitive neurons in the rostral ventrolateral medulla of the rat in vivo: morphological properties and relationship to C1 adrenergic neurons. Neuroscience 1995; 69:601–618.

56. Schreihofer AM, Guyenet PG. Identification of C1 presympathetic neurons in rat rostral ventrolateral medulla by juxtacellular labeling ''in vivo.'' Comp Neurol 1997; 387:524–536.

57. Jansen AS, Farwell DG, Loewy AD. Specificity of pseudorabies virus as a retrograde marker of sympathetic preganglionic neurons: implications for transneuronal labeling studies. Brain Res 1993;617:103–112.

58. Schramm LP, Strack AM, Platt KB, Loewy AD. Peripheral and central pathways regulating the kidney: a study using pseudorabies virus. Brain Res 1993; 616:251–262.

59. Jansen ASP, Wessendorf MW, Loewy AD. Transneuronal labeling of CNS neuropeptide and monoamine neurons after pseudorabies virus injections into the stellate ganglion. Brain Res 1995; 683:1–24.

60. Jansen ASP, Nguyen XV, Karpitskiy V, Mettenleiter TC, Loewy AD. Central command neurons of the sympathetic nervous system: basis of the fight- or flight response. Science 1995; 270:644–646.

61. Amendt K, Czachurski J, Dembowsky K, Seller H. Bulbospinal projections to the intermediolateral cell column: a neuroanatomical study. J Auton Nerv Syst 1979; 1:103–107.

62. Milner TA, Morrison SF, Abate C, Reis DJ. Phenylethanolamine N-methyltransferase-containing terminals synapse directly on sympathetic preganglionic neurons in the rat. Brain Res 1988; 448:205–222.

63. Zagon A, Smith AD. Monosynaptic projections from the rostral ventrolateral medulla oblongata to identified sympathetic preganglionic neurons. Neuroscience 1993; 54:729–743.

64. Haselton JR, Guyenet PG. Ascending collaterals of medullary barosensitive neurons and C1 cells in rats. Am J Physiol 1990; 258:R1051–R1063.

65. Haselton JR, Guyenet PG. Central respiratory modulation of medullary sympathoexcitatory neurons in rat. Am J Physiol 1989; 256:R739–R750.

66. McAllen RM, May CN. Effects of preoptic warming on subretrofacial and cutaneous vasoconstrictor neurons in anaesthetized cats. J Physiol (Lond) 1994; 481:719–730.

67. McAllen RM, May CN, Shafton AD. Functional anatomy of sympathetic premotor cell groups in the medulla. Clin Exp Hypertens 1995; 17:209–221.

68. Dampney RA, McAllen RM. Differential control of sympathetic fibres supplying hindlimb skin and muscle by subretrofacial neurones in the cat. J Physiol (Lond) 1988; 395:41–56.

69. Campos RR, McAllen RM. Cardiac sympathetic premotor neurons. Am J Physiol Regul Integr Comp Physiol 1997; 272:R615–R620.

70. Morrison SF, Callaway J, Milner TA, Reis DJ. Glutamate in the spinal sympathetic intermediolateral nucleus: localization by light and electron microscopy. Brain Res 1989; 503:5–15.

71. Deuchars SA, Morrison SF, Gilbey MP. Medullary-evoked EPSPs in neonatal rat sympathetic preganglionic neurones in vitro. J Physiol (Lond) 1995; 487:453–463.

72. Morrison SF, Emsberger P, Milner TA, Callaway J, Gong A, Reis DJ. A glutamate mechanism in the intermediolateral nucleus mediates sympathoexcitatory responses to stimulation of the rostral ventrolateral medulla. Prog Brain Res 1989; 81:159–169.

73. Minson JB, Llewellyn-Smith IJ, Pilowsky PM, Chalmers JP. Bulbospinal neuropeptide Y-immunoreactive neurons in the rat; comparison with adrenaline synthesizing neurons. J Auton Nerv Syst 1994; 47:233–244.

74. Colmers WF, Bleakman D. Effects of neuropeptide Y on the electrical properties of neurons. Trends Neurosci 1994; 17:373–379.

75. Barman SM, Orer HS, Gebber GL. Caudal ventrolateral medullary neurons are elements of the network responsible for the 10-Hz rhythm in sympathetic nerve discharge. J Neurophysiol 1994; 72:106–120.

76. Barman SM, Gebber GL. Subgroups of rostral ventrolateral medullary and caudal medullary raphe neurons based on patterns of relationship to sympathetic nerve discharge and axonal projections. J Neurophysiol 1997; 77:65–75.

77. Zhong S, Zhou SY, Gebber GL, Barman SM. Coupled oscillators account for the slow rhythms in sympathetic nerve discharge and phrenic nerve activity. Am J Physiol 1997; 272:R1314–R1324.

78. Sun MK, Guyenet PG. Arterial baroreceptor and vagal inputs to sympathoexicitatory neurons in rat medulla. Am J Physiol 1987; 252:R699–R709.

79. Sun M-K, Reis DJ. NMDA receptor-mediated sympathetic chemoreflex excitation of RVL-spinal vasomotor neurones in rats. J Physiol (Lond) 1995; 482:53–68.

80. Lin HH, Wu SY, Lai CC, Dun NJ. GABA- and glycine-mediated inhibitory postsynaptic potentials in neonatal rat rostral ventrolateral medulla neurons in vitro. Neuroscience 1998; 82:429–442.

81. Hayar A, Guyenet PG. Pre- and postsynaptic inhibitory actions of methionine-enkephalin on identified bulbospinal neurons of the rat rostral ventrolateral medulla. J Neurophysiol 1998; 80:2003–2014.

82. Örnung G, Ottersen OP, Cullheim S, Ulfhake B. Distribution of glutamate-, glycine- and GABA-immunoreactive nerve terminals on dendrites in the cat spinal motor nucleus. Exp Brain Res 1998; 118:517–532.

83. Kiely JM, Gordon FJ. Role of rostral ventrolateral medulla in centrally mediated pressor responses. Am J Physiol 1994; 267:H1549–H1556.

84. Koshiya N, Huangfu D, Guyenet PG. Ventrolateral medulla and sympathetic chemoreflex in the rat. Brain Res 1993; 609:174–184.

85. Ito S, Sved AF. Tonic glutamate-mediated control of rostral ventrolateral medulla and sympathetic vasomotor tone. Am J Physiol 1997; 273:R487–R494.
86. Kangrga IM, Loewy AD. Whole-cell recordings from visualized C1 adrenergic bulbospinal neurons: ionic mechanisms underlying vasomotor tone. Brain Res 1995; 670:215–232.
87. Li YW, Bayliss DA, Guyenet PG. C1 neurons of neonatal rats: Intrinsic beating properties and α_2-adrenergic receptors. Am J Physiol 1995; 269:R1356–R1369.
88. Li YW, Guyenet PG. Angiotensin II decreases a resting K^+ conductance in rat bulbospinal neurons of the C1 area. Circ Res 1996; 78:274–282.
89. Li YW, Guyenet PG. Effect of substance P on C1 and other bulbospinal cells of the RVLM in neonatal rats. Am J Physiol Regul Integr Comp Physiol 1997; 273: R805–R813.
90. Sun MK, Guyenet PG. Excitation of rostral medullary pacemaker neurons with putative sympathoexcitatory function by cyclic AMP and beta-adrenoceptor agonists in vitro. Brain Res 1990; 511:30–40.
91. Sun MK, Young BS, Hackett JT, Guyenet PG. Rostral ventrolateral medullary neurons with intrinsic pacemaker properties are not catecholaminergic. Brain Res 1988; 451:345–349.
92. Sun MK, Hackett JT, Guyenet PG. Sympathoexcitatory neurons of rostral ventrolateral medulla exhibit pacemaker properties in the presence of a glutamate-receptor antagonist. Brain Res 1988; 438:23–40.
93. Milner TA, Pickel VM, Reis DJ. Tyrosine hydroxylase and enkephalin in the rostral ventrolateral medulla: major synaptic contacts from opioid terminals on catecholaminergic neurons. Prog Clin Biol Res 1990; 328:195–198.
94. Milner TA, Reis DJ, Giuliano R. Afferent sources of substance P in the C1 area of the rat rostral ventrolateral medulla. Neurosci Lett 1996; 205:37–40.
95. Milner TA, Pickel VM, Abate C, Joh TH, Reis DJ. Ultrastructural characterization of substance P-like immunoreactive neurons in the rostral ventrolateral medulla in relation to neurons containing catecholamine-synthesizing enzymes. J Comp Neurol 1988; 270:427–445.
96. Milner TA, Pickel VM, Guiliano R, Reis DJ. Ultrastructural localization of choline acetyltransferase in the rat rostral ventrolateral medulla: evidence for major synaptic relations with non-catecholaminergic neurons. Brain Res 1989; 500:67–89.
97. Milner TA, Pickel VM, Chan J, Massari VJ, Oertel WH, Park DH, Joh TH, Reis DJ. Phenylethanolamine N-methyltransferase-containing neurons in the rostral ventrolateral medulla: II. Synaptic relationships with GABAergic terminals. Brain Res 1987; 411:46–57.
98. Milner TA, Pickel VM, Abate C, Joh TH, Reis DJ. Ultrastructural characterization of substance P-like immunoreactive neurons in the rostral ventrolateral medulla in relation to neurons containing catecholamine-synthesizing enzymes. J Comp Neurol 1988; 270:402–405, 427–445.
99. Ito S, Sved AF. Blockade of angiotensin receptors in rat rostral ventrolateral medulla removes excitatory vasomotor tone. Am J Physiol 1996; 270:R1317–R1323.
100. Lipski J, Kanjhan R, Kruszewska B, Rong WF. Properties of presympathetic neurones in the rostral ventrolateral medulla in the rat: An intracellular study in vivo. J Physiol (Lond) 1996; 490:729–744.

101. Sun MK, Wahlestedt C, Reis DJ. Action of externally applied ATP on rat reticulo-spinal vasomotor neurons. Eur J Pharmacol 1992; 224:93–96.
102. Huangfu D, Schreihofer AM, Guyenet PG. Effect of cholinergic agonists on bulbo-spinal C1 neurons in rats. Am J Physiol 1997; 272:R249–R258.
103. Sun MK, Guyenet PG. GABA-mediated baroreceptor inhibition of reticulospinal neurons. Am J Physiol 1985; 249:R672–R680.
104. Minson JB, Llewellyn-Smith IJ, Chalmers JP, Pilowsky PM, Arnolda LF. c-fos identifies GABA-synthesizing barosensitive neurons in caudal ventrolateral me-dulla. Neuroreport 1997; 8:3015–3021.
105. Guyenet PG, Stornetta RL, Riley T, Norton FR, Rosin DL, Lynch KR. Alpha(2A)-adrenergic receptors are present in lower brainstem catecholaminergic and seroton-ergic neurons innervating spinal cord. Brain Res 1994; 638:285–294.
106. Gao KM, Mason P. Somatodendritic and axonal anatomy of intracellularly labeled serotonergic neurons in the rat medulla. J Comp Neurol 1997; 389:309–328.
107. Wang WH, Lovick TA. Excitatory 5-HT2-mediated effects on rostral ventrolateral medullary neurones in rats. Neurosci Lett 1992; 141:89–92.
108. Wang WH, Lovick TA. Inhibitory serotonergic effects on rostral ventrolateral med-ullary neurons. Pflugers Arch Eur J Physiol 1992; 422:93–97.
109. Ma RC, Dun NJ. Excitation of lateral horn neurons of the neonatal rat spinal cord by 5-hydroxytryptamine. Dev Brain Res 1986; 24:89–98.
110. Jensen I, Llewellyn-Smith IJ, Pilowsky P, Minson JB, Chalmers J. Serotonin inputs to rabbit sympathetic preganglionic neurons projecting to the superior cervical gan-glion or adrenal medulla. J Comp Neurol 1995; 353:427–438.
111. Chalmers JP, Pilowsky PM, Minson JB, Kapoor V, Mills E, West MJ. Central serotonergic mechanisms in hypertension. Am J Hypertens 1988; 1:79–83.
112. Huangfu DH, Hwang LJ, Riley TA, Guyenet PG. Role of serotonin and catechol-amines in sympathetic responses evoked by stimulation of rostral medulla. Am J Physiol 1994; 266:R338–R352.
113. Jacobs BL, Fornal CA. Serotonin and motor activity. Curr Opin Neurobiol 1997; 7:820–825.
114. Yasui Y, Cechetto DF, Saper CB. Evidence for a cholinergic projection from the pedunculopontine tegmental nucleus to the rostral ventrolateral medulla in the rat. Brain Res 1990; 517:19–24.
115. Ruggiero DA, Giuliano R, Anwar M, Stornetta R, Reis DJ. Anatomical substrates of cholinergic-autonomic regulation in the rat. J Comp Neurol 1990; 292:1–53.
116. Giuliano R, Ruggiero DA, Morrison S, Ernsberger P, Reis DJ. Cholinergic regula-tion of arterial pressure by the C1 area of the rostral ventrolateral medulla. J Neu-rosci 1989; 9:923–942.
117. Sapru HN. Cholinergic mechanisms subserving cardiovascular function in the me-dulla and spinal cord. Prog Brain Res 1989; 81:171–179.
118. Punnen S, Willette RN, Krieger AJ, Sapru HN. Medullary pressor area: site of action of intravenous physostigmine. Brain Res 1986; 382:178–184.
119. Kubo T, Taguchi K, Sawai N, Ozaki S, Hagiwara Y. Cholinergic mechanisms re-sponsible for blood pressure regulation on sympathoexcitatory neurons in the rostral ventrolateral medulla of the rat. Brain Res Bull 1997; 42:199–204.
120. Aicher SA, Reis DJ, Ruggiero DA, Milner TA. Anatomical characterization of a

novel reticulospinal vasodepressor area in the rat medulla oblongata. Neuroscience 1994; 60:761–779.

121. Aicher SA, Reis DJ, Nicolae R, Milner TA. Monosynaptic projections from the medullary gigantocellular reticular formation to sympathetic preganglionic neurons in the thoracic spinal cord. J Comp Neurol 1995; 363:563–580.

122. Aicher SA, Reis DJ. Gigantocellular vasodepressor area is tonically active and distinct from caudal ventrolateral vasodepressor area. Am J Physiol 1997; 272:R731–R742.

123. Coleman MJ, Dampney RAL. Powerful depressor and sympathoinhibitory effects evoked from neurons in the caudal raphe pallidus and obscurus. Am J Physiol 1995; 268:R1295–R1302.

124. McCall RB. Central neurotransmitters involved in cardiovascular regulation. In: Antonaccio MJ, ed. Cardiovascular Pharmacology. Vol. 3. New York: Raven Press, 1990:161–200.

125. McCall RB. GABA-mediated inhibition of sympathoexcitatory neurons by midline medullary stimulation. Am J Physiol 1988; 255:R605–R615.

126. Deuchars SA, Spyer KM, Gilbey MP. Stimulation within the rostral ventrolateral medulla can evoke monosynaptic GABAergic IPSPs in sympathetic preganglionic neurons in vitro. J Neurophysiol 1997; 77:229–235.

127. Barman SM, Gebber GL. The axons of raphespinal sympathoinhibitory neurons branch in the cervical spinal cord. Brain Res 1988; 441:371–376.

128. Morrison SF, Gebber GL. Raphe neurons with sympathetic-related activity: baroreceptor responses and spinal connections. Am J Physiol 1984; 246:R338–R348.

129. Morrison SF, Gebber GL. Axonal branching patterns and funicular trajectories of raphe spinal sympathoinhibitory neurons. J Neurophysiol 1985; 53:759–772.

130. Pilowsky PM, Miyawaki T, Minson JB, Sun QJ, Arnolda LF, Llewellyn-Smith IJ, Chalmers JP. Bulbospinal sympatho-excitatory neurons in the rat caudal raphe. J Hypertens 1995; 13:1618–1623.

131. Zagon A, Spyer KM. Stimulation of aortic nerve evokes three different response patterns in neurons of rostral VLM of the rat. Am J Physiol 1996; 271:R1720–R1728.

132. Miura M, Takayama K, Okada J. Distribution of glutamate- and GABA-immunoreactive neurons projecting to the cardioacceleratory center of the intermediolateral nucleus of the thoracic spinal cord of SHR and WKY rats: a double-labeling study. Brain Res 1994; 638:139–150.

133. Loewy AD. Raphe pallidus and raphe obscurus projections to the intermediolateral cell column in the rat. Brain Res 1981; 222:129–133.

134. Mtui EP, Anwar M, Gomez R, Reis DJ, Ruggiero DA. Projections from the nucleus tractus solitarius to the spinal cord. J Comp Neurol 1993; 337:231–252.

135. Maass-Moreno R, Katona PG. Species dependence of baroreceptor effects on ventilation in the cat and the dog. J Appl Physiol 1989; 67:2116–2124.

136. Kumada M, Terui N, Kuwaki T. Arterial baroreceptor reflex: its central and peripheral neural mechanisms. Prog Neurobiol 1990; 35:331–361.

137. Chan RKW, Sawchenko PE. Organization and transmitter specificity of medullary neurons activated by sustained hypertension: implications for understanding baroreceptor reflex circuitry. J Neurosci 1998; 18:371–387.

138. Guyenet PG, Filtz TM, Donaldson SR. Role of excitatory amino acids in rat vagal and sympathetic baroreflexes. Brain Res 1987; 407:272–284.

139. Li YW, Dampney RAL. Expression of Fos-like protein in the brain following sustained hypertension and hypotension in conscious rabbits. Neuroscience 1994; 61: 613–634.

140. Jeske I, Morrison SF, Cravo SL, Reis DJ. Identification of baroreceptor reflex interneurons in the caudal ventrolateral medulla. Am J Physiol 1993; 264:R169–R178.

141. Terui N, Masuda N, Saeki Y, Kumada M. Activity of barosensitive neurons in the caudal ventrolateral medulla that send axonal projections to the rostral ventrolateral medulla in rabbits. Neurosci Lett 1990; 118:211–214.

142. Spyer KM. Annual review prize lecture: central nervous mechanisms contributing to cardiovascular control. J Physiol (Lond) 1994; 474:1–20.

143. Spyer KM. Central nervous mechanisms contributing to cardiovascular control. J Physiol (Lond) 1994; 474:1–19.

144. Massari VJ, Johnson TA, Gatti PJ. Cardiotopic organization of the nucleus ambiguus? An anatomical and physiological analysis of neurons regulating atrioventricular conduction. Brain Res 1995; 679:227–240.

145. Gatti PJ, Johnson TA, Massari VJ. Can neurons in the nucleus ambiguus selectively regulate cardiac rate and atrio-ventricular conduction? J Auton Nerv Syst 1996; 57:123–127.

146. Gatti PJ, Johnson TA, McKenzie J, Lauenstein JM, Gray A, Massari VJ. Vagal control of left ventricular contractility is selectively mediated by a cranioventricular intracardiac ganglion in the cat. J Auton Nerv Syst 1997; 66:138–144.

147. Standish A, Enquist LW, Schwaber JS. Innervation of the heart and its central medullary origin defined by viral tracing. Science 1994; 263:232–235.

148. Standish A, Enquist LW, Escardo JA, Schwaber JS. Central neuronal circuit innervating the rat heart defined by transneuronal transport of pseudorabies virus. J Neurosci 1995; 15:1998–2012.

149. Gilbey MP, Jordan D, Richter DW, Spyer KM. Synaptic mechanisms involved in the inspiratory modulation of vagal cardio-inhibitory neurones in the cat. J Physiol (Lond) 1984; 356:65–78.

150. Willis A, Mihalevich M, Neff RA, Mendelowitz D. Three types of postsynaptic glutamatergic receptors are activated in DMNX neurons upon stimulation of NTS. Am J Physiol 1996; 271:R1614–R1619.

151. Spyer KM. The central nervous organization of reflex circulatory control. In: Loewy AD, Spyer KM, eds. Central Regulation of Autonomic Functions. New York: Oxford University Press, 1990:168–188.

152. Massari VJ, Johnson TA, Llewellyn-Smith IJ, Gatti PJ. Substance P nerve terminals synapse upon negative chronotropic vagal motoneurons. Brain Res 1994; 660:275–287.

153. Guyenet PG, Koshiya N. Respiratory-sympathetic integration in the medulla oblongata. In: Kunos G, Ciriello J, eds. Central Neural Mechanisms in Cardiovascular Regulation. Vol. II. Boston: Birkhauser, 1992:226–247.

154. Millhorn DE. Neural respiratory and circulatory interaction during chemoreceptor stimulation and cooling of ventral medulla in cats. J Physiol (Lond) 1986; 370: 217–231.

155. Richter DW, Spyer KM. Cardiorespiratory control. In: Loewy AD, Spyer KM, eds. Central Regulation of Autonomic Functions. New York: Oxford University Press, 1990:189–207.

156. Schwarzacher SW, Wilhelm Z, Anders K, Richter DW. The medullary respiratory network in the rat. J Physiol (Lond) 1991; 435:631–644.

157. Dobbins EG, Feldman JL. Brainstem network controlling desending drive to phrenic motoneurons in rat. J Comp Neurol 1994; 347:64–86.

158. Feldman JL, Smith JC, Ellenberger HH, Connelly CA, Liu GS, Greer JJ, Lindsay AD, Otto MR. Neurogenesis of respiratory rhythm and pattern: emerging concepts. Am J Physiol 1990; 259:R879–R886.

159. Smith JC, Morrison DE, Ellenberger HH, Otto MR, Feldman JL. Brainstem projections to the major respiratory neuron populations in the medulla of the cat. J Comp Neurol 1989; 281:69–96.

160. Duffin J, Ezure K, Lipski J. Breathing rhythm generation: Focus on the rostral ventrolateral medulla. News Physiol Sci 1995; 10:133–140.

161. Guyenet PG, Haselton JR, Sun MK. Sympathoexcitatory neurons of the rostroventrolateral medulla and the origin of the sympathetic vasomotor tone. Prog Brain Res 1989; 81:105–116.

162. Guyenet PG, Darnall RA, Riley TA. Rostral ventrolateral medulla and sympatho-respiratory integration in rats. Am J Physiol 1990; 259:R1063–R1074.

163. Darnall RA, Guyenet P. Respiratory modulation of pre- and postganglionic lumbar vasomotor sympathetic neurons in the rat. Neurosci Lett 1990; 119:148–152.

164. Sun QJ, Minson J, Llewellyn-Smith IJ, Arnolda L, Chalmers J, Pilowsky P. Botzinger neurons project towards bulbospinal neurons in the rostral ventrolateral medulla of the rat. J Comp Neurol 1997; 388:23–31.

165. Jiang C, Lipski J. Extensive monosynaptic inhibition of ventral respiratory group neurons by augmenting neurons in the Botzinger complex in the cat. Exp Brain Res 1990; 81:639–648.

166. Marshall JM. Peripheral chemoreceptors and cardiovascular regulation. Physiol Rev 1994; 74:543–594.

167. Hilton SM, Marshall JM. The pattern of cardiovascular response to carotid chemoreceptor stimulation in the cat. J Physiol (Lond) 1982; 326:495–513.

168. Housley GD, Martin-Body RL, Dawson NJ, Sinclair JD. Brain stem projections of the glossopharyngeal nerve and its carotid sinus branch in the rat. Neuroscience 1987; 22:237–250.

169. Blessing WW. The Lower Brainstem and Bodily Homeostasis. New York: Oxford University Press, 1997.

170. Kalia M, Richter D. Morphology of physiologically identified slowly adapting lung stretch receptor afferents stained with intra-axonal horseradish peroxidase in the nucleus of the tractus solitarius of the cat: I. A light microscopic analysis. J Comp Neurol 1985; 241:503–520.

171. Mifflin SW. Absence of respiration modulation of carotid sinus nerve inputs to nucleus-tractus-solitarius neurons receiving arterial chemoreceptor inputs. J Auton Nerv Syst 1993; 42:191–200.

172. Koshiya N, Guyenet PG. Tonic sympathetic chemoreflex after blockade of respiratory rhythmogenesis in the rat. J Physiol (Lond) 1996; 491:859–869.

173. Sun MK. Pharmacology of reticulospinal vasomotor neurons in cardiovascular regulation. Pharmacol Rev 1996; 48:465–494.

174. Koshiya N, Guyenet PG. Role of the pons in the carotid sympathetic chemoreflex. Am J Physiol 1994; 267:R508–R518.

175. Koshiya N, Guyenet PG. A5 noradrenergic neurons and the carotid sympathetic chemoreflex. Am J Physiol 1994; 267:R519–R526.

176. Koshiya N, Guyenet PG. NTS neurons with carotid chemoreceptor inputs arborize in the rostral ventrolateral medulla. Am J Physiol 1996; 270:R1273–R1278.

177. Boczek-Funcke A, Habler HJ, Janig W, Michaelis M. Rapid phasic baroreceptor inhibition of the activity in sympathetic preganglionic neurones does not change throughout the respiratory cycle. J Auton Nerv Syst 1991; 34:185–194.

178. Miyawaki T, Pilowsky P, Sun QJ, Minson J, Suzuki S, Arnolda L, Llewellyn-Smith I, Chalmers J. Central inspiration increases barosensitivity of neurons in rat rostral ventrolateral medulla. Am J Physiol 1995; 268:R909–R918.

179. Zhang TX, Rohlicek CV, Polosa C. Responses of sympathetic preganglionic neurons to systematic hypercapnia in the acute spinal cat. J Auton Nerv Syst 1982; 6: 381–390.

180. Sun MK, Reis DJ. Central neural mechanisms mediating excitation of sympathetic neurons by hypoxia. Prog Neurobiol 1994; 44:197–219.

181. Sun MK, Reis DJ. Hypoxia selectively excites vasomotor neurons of rostral ventrolateral medulla in rats. Am J Physiol 1994; 266:R245–R256.

182. Reis DJ, Golanov EV, Ruggiero DA, Sun M-K. Sympatho-excitatory neurons of the rostral ventrolateral medulla are oxygen sensors and essential elements in the tonic and reflex control of the systemic and cerebral circulations. J Hypertens 1994; 12(suppl 10):S159–S180.

183. Sun M-K, Reis DJ. Decerebration does not alter hypoxic sympathoexcitatory responses in rats. J Auton Nerv Syst 1995; 53:77–81.

184. Sun MK, Reis DJ. Hypoxia-activated $Ca2+$ currents in pacemaker neurones of rat rostral ventrolateral medulla in vitro. J Physiol (Lond) 1994; 476:101–116.

185. Guyenet PG, Brown DL. Unit activity in nucleus paragigantocellularis lateralis during cerebral ischemia in the rat. Brain Res 1986; 364:301–314.

4

Mechanical Interactions Between the Respiratory and Circulatory Systems

JOHN V. TYBERG and ISRAEL BELENKIE

The University of Calgary
Calgary, Alberta, Canada

I. Introduction

Heart-lung interaction has become increasingly interesting due to the investigations of Bradley and his collaborators. In one of their studies of sleep apnea, they examined 5 patients with chronic, stable, congestive heart failure who also had Cheyne-Stokes respiration during sleep (1). When these patients were treated with nasal continuous positive airway pressure (CPAP), not only did the respiratory abnormality disappear but, unexpectedly, ejection fraction improved, cardiac dyspnea was alleviated, and the patients improved [from New York Heart Association (NYHA) functional class III or IV to II]. These authors subsequently studied a group of patients with congestive heart failure and found two different responses to CPAP. In those in whom mean pulmonary capillary wedge pressure (PCWP) was less than 12 mmHg, cardiac index fell as expected. However, in those in whom PCWP exceeded 12 mmHg, CPAP increased both cardiac output and stroke volume. Thus, they concluded that CPAP has salutary effects in the subset of heart failure patients with worse hemodynamics and higher PCWPs (2). It appears that CPAP is emerging as an effective treatment in heart failure, but the mechanism(s) by which it works may not be adequately explained by the calculated decrease in LV afterload (3).

99

These observations are consistent with the earlier work of Schulman et al., who studied a group of patients on PEEP and found that it increased LV end-diastolic and end-systolic volumes in those whose hemodynamic indices were worse (4). They may also prove to be consistent with other work from these investigators, who found that the response to PEEP was dependent on RV performance (5) or LV ischemia (4), PEEP increasing LV volume in patients with severely depressed biventricular function.

Because of these provovative findings and the questions that remain unanswered, in this chapter we describe the salient principles that form the basis of our understanding of heart-lung interaction, present a hypothesis to be tested clinically, and provide a critique of that hypothesis.

II. Principles

A. The Frank-Starling Law

A frequently quoted form of the law was stated in 1914 by Patterson, Piper, and Starling (6): "The mechanical energy set free on passage from the resting to the contracted state depends on the area of 'chemically active surfaces,' i.e., on the length of the muscle fibres." This is equivalent to the simple statement that the strength of systolic contraction depends upon end-diastolic volume. As outlined by Guz (3), this principle was anticipated by several cardiovascular physiologists much earlier—indeed, beginning with Hales in 1740. Perhaps more remarkable is the fact that the relevance of the Frank-Starling law has been the subject of sometimes bitter debate through much of this century. As our understanding of the issue evolved, it became more clear that the debate has hinged on the meaning of "effective filling pressure." Almost all investigators have affirmed the Frank-Starling law when defined in terms of end-diastolic dimensions. Effective venous pressure was defined by Henderson and Barringer in 1913 as the difference between the pressure in the veins and that outside the heart (7). As a means of measuring the pressure outside the heart and thus establishing effective atrial pressure, Wiggers and co-workers (8) developed a multiple-side-hole cannula to measure intrathoracic pressure in the vicinity of the heart. Using this cannula in experiments on conscious animals, Rushmer and Thal (9) concluded that "the diastolic size of the ventricular chambers is determined by the effective filling pressure only under abnormal conditions such as cardiac decompensation and heart-lung preparations." However, using a model of pericardial tamponade caused by air in the pericardium, Sarnoff and collaborators defined effective ventricular filling pressures as the differences between atrial pressures and pericardial pressure. They showed that RV and LV stroke work could be predicted by their respective "effective filling pressures," but not by the intracavitary pressures (10). Thus, they justified the Frank-Starling law (10–12). The essence of our own work on the pericardium (13–22) has been to reaffirm this principle by measuring pericardial pressure with a flat, liquid-containing balloon located between the pericardium and the heart, when the pericardial cavity does not contain abnormal amounts of fluid (23). We believe that this technique measures pericardial and, indeed, pleural constraint more accurately than any conventional open-catheter system. Thus, in anesthetized animals, Sarnoff and collaborators and we have shown that many variations in ventricular performance can be predicted accurately from changes in transmural end-diastolic pressure (end-diastolic intracavitary pressure minus pericardial pressure) as well as from changes in end-diastolic volume (with which changes in transmural end-diastolic pressure are closely correlated). This conclusion is consistent with the 1955 statement of L. N. Katz, who observed that "Even the use of end-diastolic pressure as an index of end-diastolic volume is not justified. . . . Furthermore, if the expansion of the heart is limited, for example by the pericardium, changes in end-diastolic pressure lose much of their meaning in terms of change in end-diastolic volume" (24).

However, in conscious, intact animals and in human subjects, the relation between effective filling pressure and end-diastolic volume (and, so, the relevance of the Frank-Starling law) remains less well established. Boettcher et al. (25) studied the end-diastolic pressure-volume relation in intact dogs in which blood volume had been expanded by saline infusion and concluded that the Frank-Starling law is not important in the normal animal because end-diastolic volume is nearly maximal at rest and does not increase further (in fact, a decrease was demonstrated) despite large increases in LV end-diastolic pressure (to ~30 mmHg). In a comparable way, Jardin et al. infused saline into patients with chronic obstructive lung disease and observed similar PCWP–LV volume relations: at the highest pressures (i.e., 20 mmHg), LV end-diastolic volume decreased (26). It is entirely possible (but as yet unproved) that the increases in LV end-diastolic pressure are accompanied by large increases in pericardial pressure, such that effective filling pressures—transmural LV end-diastolic pressures—actually decrease to explain the decreases in end-diastolic volume. Because we are seldom able to achieve transmural LV end-diastolic pressures greater than 10 to 12 mmHg in experimental animals, this explanation would be consistent with the findings of Parker and Case, who demonstrated that LV stroke work does not increase substantially in patients by increasing end-diastolic pressure above 10 mmHg (27). This explanation would also seem to be consistent with the findings of Crexells et al., who, in patients with acute myocardial infarction, concluded that the optimal LV filling pressure (mean PCWP) was 14 to 18 mmHg, which corresponded to a right atrial pressure of approximately 8 mmHg (28). We have shown that pericardial pressure approximates right atrial pressure during acute volume loading in experimental animals (16,29) and in patients (14), suggesting that the optimal transmural LV end-diastolic pressure should have been approximately 10 mmHg in Crexells' patients. Also, while changing the level of PEEP, Smiseth et al. (30) measured pleural, pericardial, and right atrial pressures in patients during surgery. They showed that pericardial pressure approximated right atrial pressure and that PCWP minus right atrial pressure provided a useful estimate of transmural LV end-diastolic pressure and, thus, end-diastolic size.

Thus, in the volume-loaded human subject, we suggest that pericardial pressure may vary and sometimes be high, which, in turn, would imply significant pericardial constraint. Subtracting these high pericardial pressures from the intracavitary pressures would yield transmural pressures that would be substantially lower than the intracavitary pressures. Presumably, the changes in transmural pressure would correlate closely with the changes in LV end-diastolic volume. Therefore, there may be no particular reason to invoke alterations in contractility to account for changes in systolic performance during many maneuvers that tend to affect ventricular and pericardial pressures, and changes in LV systolic performance may correspond to changes in LV end-diastolic volume, as predicted by the Frank-Starling law.

B. How Changing External Constraint Affects the Assessment of Ventricular Performance

As presented by Glantz and Parmley in 1978 (31), when LV end-diastolic pressure (or its surrogates, PCWP and left atrial pressure) is used as the preload parameter in the construction of a ventricular function curve, the assessment of LV contractility may be profoundly influenced by changes in LV "diastolic compliance" (i.e., as assessed by the position of the LV diastolic pressure–volume relation). We have clearly demonstrated this phenomenon in two experimental models.

Grant et al. studied the effects of ventilation on heart-lung interaction, LV diastolic compliance, and the ventricular function curve in anesthetized term lambs that had been instrumented before interruption of the placental circulation (32). Consistent with the prediction of Glantz and Parmley, we found that ventilation shifted the LV end-diastolic pressure–dimension relation rightward and the stroke work–end-diastolic pressure relation upward, respectively, suggesting that diastolic compliance and LV contractility had increased. Opening the chest and pericardium shifted the relations further in the same direction. The transmural LV end-diastolic–pressure dimension, the LV stroke work–transmural end-diastolic pressure, and the LV stroke work–end-diastolic dimension relations all remained unchanged throughout these maneuvers, indicating that neither "true myocardial compliance" (i.e., the transmural LV end-diastolic pressure–dimension relation) nor "true myocardial contractility" (i.e., the LV stroke work–end-diastolic dimension relation) were changed. The misleading relations, those involving intracavitary pressure, could now be fully accounted for by considering the effect of changes in pericardial pressure. Thus, the Frank-Starling law—in terms of both end-diastolic dimensions and transmural end-diastolic pressure—fully explained the observed changes in LV performance.

This principle is illustrated by Figure 1 (22), which is based on observations of Belenkie et al. We studied the effects of pulmonary embolization (autologous clots) and volume loading on LV diastolic compliance and the ventricular function curve in anesthetized, closed-chest, closed-pericardium dogs (16–18). As shown schematically in the upper left panel, after several incremental embolizations, volume loading (venous infusion of a blood-saline mixture) increased LV end-diastolic pressure and *decreased* end-diastolic volume (assessed as the product of minor-axis diameters), thus indicating that the pressure-volume relation was shifted progressively leftward (i.e., "diastolic compliance" was decreased). LV stroke work also decreased progressively as end-diastolic pressure increased (upper right panel), thus indicating that the stroke work–end-diastolic volume relation was shifted progressively downward and rightward, implying that LV contractility had decreased: However, when we evaluated LV preload in terms

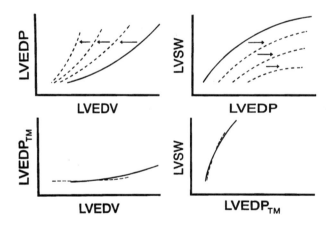

Figure 1 A schematic diagram derived from experimental data showing how pulmonary embolism and acute volume loading affect diastolic compliance (left panel) and ventricular function (right panel). The top panel represents the conventional approaches that define compliance and ventricular function in terms of left ventricular end-diastolic pressure (LVEDP). In contrast, the bottom panel employs transmural LVEDP (LVEDP$_{TM}$). According to the conventional analyses, pulmonary embolism decreases LV diastolic compliance [i.e., the LVEDP-LVEDV (volume) relations shift leftward] and contractility [i.e., the LVSW (stroke work)–LVEDP relations shift to the right and downward]. When transmural LVEDP is used, there is no change in either diastolic compliance or contractility. Therefore, LV hypovolemia, in turn caused by increased external constraint, is a sufficient explanation for the profound decrease in ventricular performance (i.e., LV stroke work). (Modified from Ref. 22. Copyright Pulsus Group Inc.)

of *transmural* end-diastolic pressure (bottom panels), neither the transmural LV end-diastolic pressure–volume relation nor the LV stroke work–end-diastolic pressure relation changed, indicating that neither "true diastolic compliance" (i.e., the transmural LV end-diastolic pressure–dimension relation) nor "true contractility" (i.e., the LV stroke work–end-diastolic transmural pressure relation) were changed. Thus, the Frank-Starling law—expressed either in terms of transmural end-diastolic pressure or end-diastolic dimensions—completely explained the observed changes in LV performance. Not shown are the LV stroke work data, plotted in terms of end-diastolic volume, which yielded the identical conclusion.

C. Ventricular Interaction

In the open-chest, open-pericardium experimental animal or (when the heart is so small that pericardial constraint is negligible) in the intact animal or subject, acute volume loading increases LV end-diastolic volume; therefore, according to the Frank-Starling law, it increases systolic performance. However, under conditions such as those illustrated in Figure 1, volume loading can *decrease* LV end-diastolic volume and so (equally according to the Frank-Starling law) *decrease* systolic performance. During acute volume loading or unloading, ventricular interaction may be responsible for such an apparently paradoxical effect. The concept can be clarified by referring to Figure 2, which is also derived from our studies of volume loading and pulmonary embolization, in the presence (17) and absence of the pericardium (18). However, this seemingly extreme manifestation of ventricular interaction may not be fundamentally different from accepted aspects of pericardium-mediated ventricular interaction. For instance, it has long been suggested that one of the normal functions of the pericardium is to equalize the outputs of the two ventricles; for example, if the output of the RV is excessive, the overfilled LV compresses the RV, thereby reducing its output (33–36).

To compare the results of the two series of experiments, we normalized both LV end-diastolic volume and stroke work in terms of transmural pressure. LV end-diastolic volume and stroke work were both defined to be 100% when LV transmural pressure was 5 mmHg. The relations shown on the paired left and right panels are identical; the thickened lines indicate the operating ranges of the relations with or without the pericardium. That is, in the presence of the pericardium (left panel), because transmural LV end-diastolic pressure did not exceed 10 mmHg, LV end-diastolic volume did not exceed 110% and stroke work was less than 200%. In the absence of the pericardium (right panel), because transmural LV end-diastolic pressure always exceeded 5 mmHg, LV end-diastolic volume and stroke work increased to much greater levels. In both panels, the paired arrows describing the sides of a triangle (the hypotenuse of which is a segment of the given relation) illustrate the typical effects of volume loading. With the

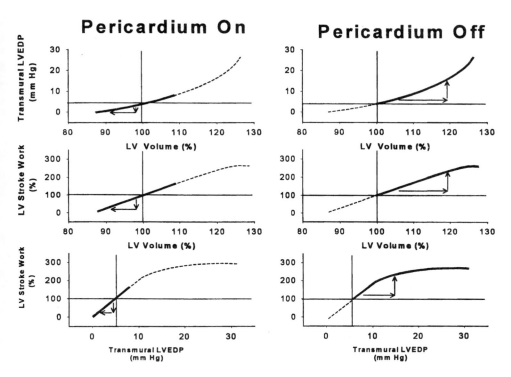

Figure 2 A schematic diagram illustrating ventricular interaction (left panel) and show-ing how the effects of volume loading after pulmonary embolism differ qualitatively, de-pending on whether the pericardium is present. In order to compare the results of two investigations (17,18); data were normalized such that LV end-diastolic volume and LV stroke work were set equal to 100% when transmural LVEDP (in the left panel, LVEDP minus pericardial pressure; in the right panel, LVEDP) was equal to 5 mmHg. The top panel shows diastolic compliance (transmural LVEDP vs. end-diastolic volume), the mid-dle panel left ventricular function (LV stroke work) in terms of LV end-diastolic volume, and the bottom panel LV function in terms of transmural LVEDP. The left and right paired relations are identical; the thickened lines indicate the operating regions of the relations, with or without the pericardium. In both panels, the paired arrows tending to describe the sides of a triangle describe the typical effects of volume loading. In the right panel, volume loading increases end-diastolic volume and transmural LVEDP (top panel), and the in-creases in LV stroke work are predicted by both the increases in end-diastolic volume (middle panel) and transmural LVEDP (bottom panel). In the left panel, volume loading decreases end-diastolic volume and transmural LVEDP (top panel), and the decreases in LV stroke work are predicted by both the decreases in end-diastolic volume and transmural LVEDP. (Modified from Ref. 18.)

pericardium off (right panel), the effects are predictable: volume loading always increases end-diastolic volume and transmural pressure (top panel), and the increases in LV stroke work are predicted by both the increases in end-diastolic volume (middle panel) and transmural pressure (bottom panel). With the pericardium on (left panel), the effects of ventricular interaction are paradoxical and surprising: volume loading decreases end-diastolic volume and transmural pressure (top panel), but once again the decreases in LV stroke work are predicted by the decreases in end-diastolic volume (middle panel) and transmural pressure (bottom panel).

Figure 2 does not show RV dimensions, but when the pericardium was intact (left panel), we consistently noted that changes in LV volume were proportional to changes in diameter from the septum to the LV free wall. In turn, changes in this diameter were reciprocally related to changes in the diameter from the septum to the RV free wall (i.e., when former diameter is increased, the latter diameter is decreased, and vice versa). These reciprocal relations were not observed when the pericardium was open (right panel). Thus, we conclude that, in the presence of the degree of ventricular interaction illustrated in the left panel, as RV volume increased, LV volume decreased.

It is important to point out the the pulmonary arterial circulation had been embolized to a substantial degree before the interactions schematized in Figure 2 occurred. Although the effects of volume loading shown in the right panel are predictable and not likely to be in any way dependent on the presence of pulmonary hypertension, the effects shown in the left panel may occur *only* under such particular conditions (i.e., when increased RV afterload has raised RV diastolic pressure, which increases pericardial pressure and shifts the septum toward the LV in diastole). Thus, ventricular interaction to the degree illustrated here may or may not occur in the absence of pulmonary hypertension.

We suggest that our recent clinical study (37) also demonstrates critical elements of such ventricular interaction. In patients with severe chronic congestive heart failure, Atherton et al. demonstrated that causing blood to pool peripherally *may increase* LV volume (37), an observation that may prove to be the most significant implication of pericardium-mediated ventricular interaction. We measured LV volume using a nuclear technique while we applied lower-body negative pressure (LBNP). In the normal control subjects and in the patients with less severe heart failure, LBNP decreased LV volume as expected. However, in the patients with more severe failure, LBNP increased LV volume. Although we have long realized that the pericardium may minimize the decrease in LV end-diastolic volume caused by nitrates, because most of the decrease in intracavitary end-diastolic pressure may be due to the decrease in pericardial pressure (15,38,39), there was no such direct, compelling evidence that, in heart failure, an increase in capacitance might actually increase LV volume in some patients (40). Atherton's observation may explain the paradoxical arteriolar vasodilation seen in response to LBNP in patients with heart failure (41–44). It is also consistent with the view that the excessive neurohumoral stimulation characteristic of heart failure is due to decreased LV baroreceptor stimulation (45), which is ultimately due to decreased transmural end-diastolic pressure(46). It is recognized that, while Atherton's study demonstrated certain critical elements of the ventricular interaction illustrated in Figure 2, no measurements of LV performance (e.g., cardiac output, stroke volume, or stroke work) were made to see if an increase in LV volume was accompanied by a Frank-Starling–mediated increase in systolic performance. Although cardiac output may well have increased, such a demonstration of the effect is critical.)

LBNP-induced paradoxical vasodilatation is completely consistent with Wang's findings in our laboratory—that LV distention and therefore vagal C-fiber activity is a function of LV transmural pressure, not intracavitary pressure per se (46). While recording C-fiber activity directly, we opened the pericardium and observed that, at the same intracavitary LV end-diastolic pressure, C-fiber activity was greater after the pericardium had been opened. This implies that cardiac baroreceptor activity and its consequences are subject to the complexities of ventricular interaction.

Wang also linked vagal C-fiber activity and venous capacitance (47), an association that may also prove to be important to heart-lung interaction. In our model of coronary embolization–induced ischemic heart failure in which venous capacitance is decreased, we observed that intrapericardial administration of lidocaine or vagotomy caused capacitance to decrease further. This implied that increased vagal C-fiber activity tends to increase capacitance. Thus, LV baroreceptors tend to offset the decrease in capacitance that accompanies heart failure. In the context of ventricular interaction, if volume unloading (however mediated) increases LV volume, there will be a further augmenting (i.e., volume unloading) effect due to the increased venous capacitance.

Other studies also suggest that, in patients with severe heart failure, interventions that reduce central blood volume may increase end-diastolic volume and sometimes LV systolic performance, in contrast to these same interventions decreasing end-diastolic volume (i.e., preload) and performance in normal individuals. It has been very recently reported that, in patients awaiting cardiac transplantation, vigorous application of nitrates, increased angiotensin-converting enzyme (ACE) inhibitor dosages, and diuresis led to long-term (8-month) reductions in wedge pressure (early reduction, 24 to 15 mmHg; late, 12 mmHg) and systemic vascular resistance (early reduction, 1650 to 1200 dynes/s/cm^5, late, 1000 dynes/s/cm^5) (48), presumably as a result of improved systolic performance. In a remarkable paper of two generations ago, Howarth, McMichael, and Sharpey-Schafer showed that cardiac output increased when right atrial pressure was lowered by venesection in patients with severe low-output heart failure (49). Although an explanation based on a descending limb of the Starling curve was proposed, the observation would seem to lack none of the features of ventricular interaction.

In summary, the Frank-Starling law appears to apply broadly when effective filling pressure is considered as the true filling pressure. Of course, changes in contractility may complicate analyses of hemodynamic changes. However, in the absence of factors that clearly affect myocardial function, such as ischemia or inotropic agents, altered ventricular interaciton often accounts for the changes in performance. Therefore, ventricular interaction must be considered in the analysis of the complex changes that are associated with the use of pressure-assisted ventilation as well.

III. Hypothesis

When CPAP is administered to patients in heart failure, the increase in intrathoracic pressure tends to displace blood from the thorax to the periphery. The result of this displacement is to decrease RV volume and, by the mechanism outlined above, reciprocally increase LV end-diastolic volume. This increased LV preload increases systolic performance, as predicted by the Frank-Starling law.

IV. Critique

In a series of recent investigations using sedated, chronically instrumented pigs, Genovese and Scharf and their colleagues have studied the hemodynamic effects of CPAP in both pacing-induced heart failure (50) and acute hypervolemia (51). In both cases, although CPAP increased stroke volume and cardiac output consistent with clinical experience, it did not increase (but tended to decrease) LV end-diastolic volume. There may prove to be important deficiencies in this experimental model (e.g., the pericardium was not closed and the porcine mediastinum might be different from that in human subjects), but it must be granted that the best available evidence in experimental animals fails to support our hypothesis.

However, in our judgment, no satisfactory hemodynamic explanation for the promising therapeutic effects of CPAP has yet been advanced. Because there are deficiencies in all animal models and because the results of all experimental investigations require confirmation in patients, we urge that our hypothesis be tested directly in clinical studies. Atherton's remarkable results (37) require confirmation by other investigators; when those studies are undertaken, the consequences of any increase in LV volume must be measured accurately in terms of changes in LV stroke volume. If our hypothesis is verified by clinical studies, experimental studies should be undertaken to elucidate the hemodynamic mechanism in detail. For example, why does the LV fill ''preferentially'' as overall heart size presumably decreases? What is the role of the septum in the mechanism? And what is the possible contribution of CPAP-induced changes in pulmonary vascular resistance?

V. Conclusion

The encouraging therapeutic effects of CPAP and the unexpected, potentially important results of administering LBNP to patients in heart failure demand satisfactory hemodynamic explanations. Ventricular interaction may or may not be the correct explanation, but a coordinated series of clinical and experimental investigations designed to test this hypothesis should help us better understand why CPAP seems to be an effective treatment for patients with heart failure.

Acknowledgments

Dr. Tyberg is a Medical Scientist of the Alberta Heritage Foundation for Medical Research (Edmonton). Investigations cited in this chapter were supported in part by operating grants to Dr. Tyberg from the Heart and Stroke Foundation of Alberta (Calgary) and from the Medical Research Council of Canada (Ottawa) and to Dr. Belenkie from the Heart and Stroke Foundation of Alberta. The authors gratefully acknowledge the editorial assistance of Dr. Naomi Anderson.

REFERENCES

1. Takasaki Y, Orr D, Popkin J, Rutherford R, Liu P, Bradley TD. Effect of nasal continuous positive airway pressure on sleep apnea in congestive heart failure. Am Rev Respir Dis 1989; 140:1578–1584.
2. Bradley TD, Holloway RM, McLaughlin PR, Ross BL, Walters J, Liu PP. Cardiac output response to continuous positive airway pressure in congestive heart failure. Am Rev Respir Dis 1992; 145:377–382.
3. Guz A. Chairman's introduction. In: Porter R, Fitzsimons DW, eds. The Physiological Basis of Starling's Law of the Heart. Amsterdam: Elsevier, 1974:1–5.
4. Schulman DS, Biondi JW, Matthay RA, Zaret BL, Soufer R. Differing responses in right and left ventricular-filling, loading and volumes during positive end-expiratory pressure. Am J Cardiol 1989; 64:772–777.
5. Schulman DS, Biondi JW, Matthay RA, Barash PG, Zaret BL, Soufer R. Effect of positive end-expiratory pressure on right ventricular performance: importance of baseline right ventricular function. Am J Med 1988; 84:57–67.
6. Patterson SW, Piper H, Starling EH. The regulation of the heart beat. J Physiol Lond 1914; 48:465–513.
7. Henderson Y, Barringer TBJ. The relation of venous pressure to cardiac efficiency. Am J Physiol 1913; 13: 352–369.

8. Wiggers CJ, Levy MN, Graham G. Regional intrathoracic pressures and their bearing on calculation of effective venous pressures. Am J Physiol 1947; 151:1–12.

9. Rushmer RF, Thal N. Factors influencing stroke volume: a cinefluorographic study of angiocardiography. Am J Physiol 1952; 168:509–521.

10. Isaacs JP, Berglund E, Sarnoff SJ. The pathologic physiology of acute cardiac tamponade studied by means of ventricular function curves. Am Heart J 1954; 48:66–76.

11. Sarnoff SJ, Berglund E. Ventricular function: 1. Starling's law of the heart studied by means of simultaneous right and left ventricular function curves in the dog. Circulation 1954; 9:706–718.

12. Sarnoff SJ. Myocardial contractility as described by ventricular function curves: observations on Starling's law of the heart. Physiol Rev 1955; 35:107–122.

13. Tyberg JV, Misbach GA, Glantz SA, Moores WY, Parmley WW. A mechanism for the shifts in the diastolic, left ventricular, pressure-volume curve: the role of the pericardium. Eur J Cardiol 1978; 7 (suppl):163–175.

14. Tyberg JV, Taichman GC, Smith ER, Douglas NWS, Smiseth OA, Keon WJ. The relation between pericardial pressure and right atrial pressure: an intraoperative study. Circulation 1986; 73:428–432.

15. Kingma I, Smiseth OA, Belenkie I, Knudtson ML, MacDonald RPR, Tyberg JV, Smith ER. A mechanism for the nitroglycerin-induced downward shift of the left ventricular diastolic pressure-diameter relationship of patients. Am J Cardiol 1986; 57:673–677.

16. Belenkie I, Dani R, Smith ER, Tyberg JV. Ventricular interaction during experimental acute pulmonary embolism. Circulation 1988; 78:761–768.

17. Belenkie I, Dani R, Smith ER, Tyberg JV. Effects of volume loading during experimental acute pulmonary embolism. Circulation 1989; 80:178–188.

18. Belenkie I, Dani R, Smith ER, Tyberg JV. The importance of pericardial constraint in experimental pulmonary embolism and volume loading. Am Heart J 1992; 123:733–742.

19. Tyberg JV, Smith ER. An evaluation of the pericardial hypothesis: The relevance of transmural right ventricular end-diastolic pressure. Coronary Artery Dis 1991; 2:717–722.

20. Traboulsi M, Scott-Douglas NW, Smith ER, Tyberg JV. The right and left ventricular intracavitary and transmural pressure-strain relationships. Am Heart J 1992; 123:1279–1287.

21. Hamilton DR, Dani RS, Semlacher RA, Smith ER, Kieser TM, Tyberg JV. Right atrial and right ventricular transmural pressures in dogs and humans: effects of the pericardium. Circulation 1994; 90:2492–2500.

22. Tyberg JV, Belenkie I, Manyari DE, Smith ER. Ventricular interaction and venous capacitance modulate left ventricular preload. Can J Cardiol 1996; 12:1058–1064.

23. Smiseth OA, Frais MA, Kingma I, Smith ER, Tyberg JV. Assessment of pericardial constraint in dogs. Circulation 1985; 71:158–164.

24. Katz LN. Analysis of the several factors regulating the performance of the heart. Physiol Rev 1955; 35:91–106.

25. Boettcher DH, Vatner SF, Heyndrickx GR, Braunwald E. Extent of utilization of

the Frank-Starling mechanism in conscious dogs. Am J Physiol Heart Circ Physiol 1978; 234:H338–H345.

26. Jardin F, Gueret P, Prost JF, Farcot JC, Ozier Y, Bourdarias JP. Two-dimensional echocardiographic assessment of left ventricular function in chronic obstructive pulmonary disease. Am Rev Respir Dis 1984; 129:135–142.

27. Parker JO, Case RB. Normal left ventricular function. Circulation 1979; 60:4–12.

28. Crexells C, Chatterjee K, Forrester JS, Dikshit K, Swan HJC. Optimal level of filling pressure in the left side of the heart in acute myocardial infarction. N Engl J Med 1973; 289:1263–1266.

29. Smiseth OA, Refsum H, Tyberg JV. Pericardial pressure assessed by right atrial pressure: a basis for calculation of left ventricular transmural pressure. Am Heart J 1983; 108:603–605.

30. Smiseth OA, Thompson CR, Ling H, Robinson M, Miyagishima RT. A potential clinical method for calculating transmural left ventricular filling pressure during positive end-expiratory pressure ventilation: an intraoperative study in humans. J Am Coll Cardiol 1996; 27:155–160.

31. Glantz SA, Parmley WW. Factors which affect the diastolic pressure-volume curve. Circ Res 1978; 42:171–180.

32. Grant DA, Kondo CS, Maloney JE, Walker AM, Tyberg JV. Changes in pericardial pressure during the perinatal period. Circulation 1992; 86:1615–1621.

33. Shabetai R. The Pericardium. New York: Grune & Stratton, 1981:34–37.

34. Henderson Y, Prince AL. The relative systolic discharges of the right and left ventricles and their bearing on pulmonary congestion and depletion. Heart 1914; 5:217–226.

35. Hamilton WF. Role of the Starling concept in regulation of the normal circulation. Physiol Rev 1955; 35:161–168.

36. Wiggers CJ. Cardiac output, stroke volume, and stroke work. In: Luisada AA, ed. Cardiovascular Functions. New York: McGraw Hill, 1962:81–91.

37. Atherton JJ, Moore TD, Lele SS, Thomson HL, Galbraith AJ, Belenkie I, Tyberg JV, Frenneaux MP. Diastolic ventricular interaction in chronic heart failure. Lancet 1997; 349:1720–1724.

38. Tyberg JV, Misbach GA, Parmley WW, Glantz SA. Effects of the pericardium on ventricular performance. In: Baan J, Yellin EL, Arntzenius AC, eds. Cardiac Dynamics. The Hague and Boston: Martinus Nijhoff, 1980:159–168.

39. Smith ER, Smiseth OA, Kingma I, Manyari D, Belenkie I, Tyberg JV. Mechanism of action of nitrates: role of changes in venous capacitance and in the left ventricular diastolic pressure-volume relation. Am J Med 1984; 76(6A):14–21.

40. Dupuis J, LaLonde G, Lebeau R, Bichet D, Rouleau JL. Sustained beneficial effect of a seventy-two hour intravenous infusion of nitroglycerin in patients with severe chronic congestive heart failure. Am Heart J 1990; 120:625.

41. Ferguson DW, Abboud FM, Mark AL. Selective impairment of baroreflex mediated vasoconstrictor responses in patients with ventricular dysfunction. Circulation 1984; 69:451–460.

42. Kassis E, Jacobsen TN, Mogensen F, Amtorp O. Sympathetic reflex control of skeletal muscle blood flow in patients with congestive heart failure: evidence of β-adrenergic circulatory control. Circulation 1986; 74:929–938.

43. Atherton JJ, Moore TD, Frenneaux MP. Low-pressure baroreceptor abnormalities in heart failure: role of pericardial constraint. Eur J Cardiac Pacing Electrophysiol 1995; 5:188–195.
44. Eckberg DL. Baroreflexes and the failing human heart. Circulation 1997; 96:4133–4137.
45. Abboud FM. Ventricular syncope: is the heart a sensory organ? N Engl J Med 1989; 320:390–392.
46. Wang SY, Sheldon RS, Bergman DW, Tyberg JV. Effects of pericardial constraint on left ventricular mechanoreceptor activity in cats. Circulation 1995; 92:3331–3336.
47. Wang SY, Manyari DE, Tyberg JV. Cardiac vagal reflex modulates intestinal vascular capacitance and ventricular preload in dogs with acute myocardial infarction. Circulation 1996; 94:529–533.
48. Steimle AE, Stevenson LW, Chelimsky-Fallick C, Fonarow GC, Hamilton MA, Moriguchi JD, Kartashov A, Tillisch JH. Sustained hemodynamic efficacy of therapy tailored to reduce filling pressures in survivors with advanced heart failure. Circulation 1997; 96:1165–1172.
49. Howarth S, McMichael J, Sharpey-Schafer EP. Effects of venesection in low output heart failure. Clin Sci 1946; 6:41–50.
50. Genovese J, Huberfeld S, Tarasiuk A, Moskowitz M, Scharf SM. Effects of CPAP on cardiac output in pigs with pacing-induced congestive heart failure. Am J Respir Crit Care Med 1995; 152:1847–1853.
51. Genovese J, Moskowitz M, Tarasiuk A, Graver LM, Scharf SM. Effects of continuous positive airway pressure on cardiac output in normal and hypervolemic unanesthetized pigs. Am J Respir Crit Care Med 1994; 150:752–758.

5

Physiological Effects of Sleep on the Cardiovascular System

RICHARD L. HORNER

University of Toronto
Toronto, Ontario, Canada

I. Introduction and Overview

This chapter summarizes the effects of wakefulness, non-rapid-eye-movement (NREM) sleep, and REM sleep on the cardiovascular system. In addition, the changes in autonomic nervous system activities that occur between these sleep-wake states are reviewed, with particular emphasis on the transient effects observed at arousal from sleep. Particular attention is focused on the cardiovascular responses to arousal, because of the increasing realization that arousal mechanisms are important in the acute and chronic cardiovascular consequences of common sleep-related breathing disorders, such as obstructive sleep apnea (OSA) and central sleep apnea (1–3). For example, in OSA patients, the repetitive large brief surges in heart rate (HR) and blood pressure (BP) associated with arousal from sleep and resolution of apneas are thought to increase the risk for development of adverse cardiovascular events such as angina, myocardial infarction, stroke, and systemic hypertension (1,3). The presence of nighttime OSA can also produce sustained daytime hypertension (3). Given that the clinical syndrome of OSA affects 2–4% of the middle-aged population (4), the cardiovascular effects of arousal from sleep and OSA are a major public health burden (5,6). The ad-

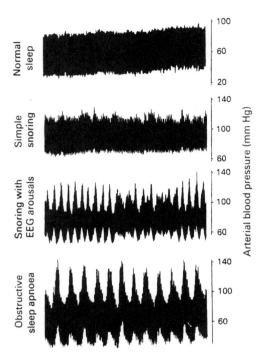

Figure 1   Figure showing the significant role of sleep disturbance on the nighttime blood pressure profile. Arterial blood pressure profiles are shown in 1) a normally sleeping subject, 2) a snorer, 3) a snorer whose sleep is disrupted by repetitive arousals, and 4) a patient with obstructive sleep apnea. Each trace shows about 10 min of recording. (From Ref. 86 with permission of BMJ Publishing Group.)

verse impact of sleep-disordered breathing events on the nighttime BP profile is highlighted in Figure 1.

II. Cardiovascular Outputs in Periods of Established Wakefulness and Sleep

Figure 2 illustrates the overall changes in HR and BP between periods of established wakefulness, NREM sleep, and REM sleep. NREM sleep is generally associated with reductions in HR and BP compared to established wakefulness. Tonic REM sleep is associated with further decreases, whereas phasic REM sleep events produce characteristic phasic increases in HR and BP. The direction of these overall changes is generally applicable across species (7,8). It is important to

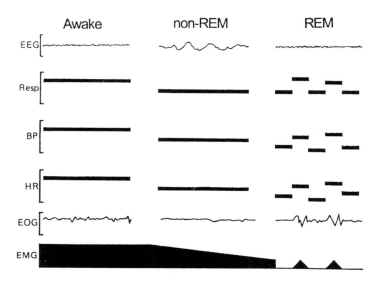

Figure 2 Schema showing overall changes in mean blood pressure (BP), heart rate (HR), and respiration (Resp) between established periods of wakefulness, NREM sleep and REM sleep. The general changes in appearance of the electroencephalogram (EEG), electro-oculogram (EOG), and neck electromyogram (EMG) are also shown schematically for the different sleep-wake states. Note the phasic changes in cardiorespiratory outputs associated with phasic REM events (i.e., eye movements and muscle twitches). (Adapted from Ref. 8 with permission of Company of Biologists Ltd.)

note, however, that whether there is an overall change in the mean levels of HR and BP in REM sleep compared to non-REM sleep or waking depends in large part on the relative amounts of phasic versus tonic REM sleep and whether both these REM phases are included in the comparison with the other sleep-wake states. The mechanisms involved in producing these overall changes in HR and BP in periods of established sleep and wakefulness are summarized below.

A. Hemodynamic Changes Across Sleep-Wake States

Following the pioneering work of Mancia and colleagues (see 7 for review), there has been much progress in delineating the mechanisms underlying the changes in HR and BP in sleep and wakefulness, in large part because animal studies allow the use of invasive techniques to make measurements that are either technically difficult or not feasible in humans. Figure 3 shows data from chronically instrumented, naturally sleeping cats that highlight the major factors contributing to the hemodynamic changes occurring across sleep-wake states. Cardiac output

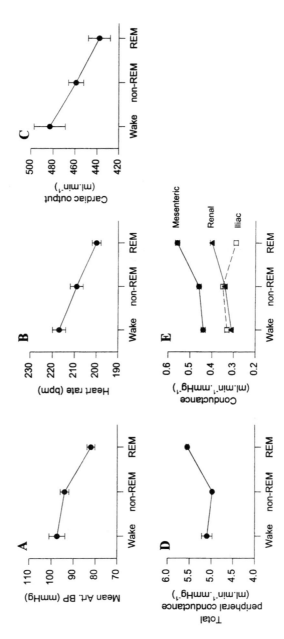

Figure 3 Changes in (A) mean arterial blood pressure—Art. BP, (B) heart rate, (C) cardiac output, (D) total peripheral conductance, and (E) regional conductances in the mesenteric, renal and iliac vascular beds across sleep-wake states. Data obtained in chronically instrumented, naturally sleeping cats. (Plotted from data in Ref. 7.)

decreases upon progression from wakefulness to NREM and REM sleep—a change primarily caused by the decreased HR because of the minimal changes in stroke volume (7,8). The minimal change in total peripheral conductance between waking and NREM sleep observed in this, and several other studies (e.g., 9,10; and for review see 7,8), has been taken to indicate that a decreased HR, and hence cardiac output, is the major factor contributing to the decreased BP in NREM sleep.

In such studies in chronically instrumented cats, REM sleep is associated with increased total peripheral conductance compared to the other states, a change that is indicative of a *net* vasodilatation (Fig. 3D). This net vasodilatation, coupled with a further decrease in cardiac output in REM sleep, is thought to be responsible for the overall decrease in BP. In subsequent studies, however, it was shown that there are *regional* changes in vascular conductance in REM sleep that are not apparent upon inspection of total peripheral conductance. For example, there is vasodilatation in the mesenteric and renal vascular beds in REM sleep but decreased conductance in the ileac circulation (Fig. 3E). Further experiments attributed this localized decrease in conductance to a vasoconstriction in the skeletal muscle circulation (7,8). The skeletal muscle vasculature is also thought to play an important role in producing the phasic increases in BP that typically occur during phasic REM events, such as eye movements and muscle twitches. Although the autonomic mechanisms producing these transient BP surges in phasic REM sleep are discussed in more detail below, these events are associated with phasic decreases in total peripheral conductance in the skeletal muscle vasculature due to transient vasoconstriction (7,8,11).

It should be noted, however, that the magnitude of the change in BP from NREM to REM sleep observed in Figure 3 is larger than that observed in most other studies (e.g., compare with 7,8,12). It appears that this larger effect of REM sleep on BP may be related to the time that these chronically instrumented cats were studied postoperatively (12,13). Nevertheless, the mechanisms that affect HR and BP at the transition from NREM sleep to REM are generally applicable across species. Their contribution, however, may vary in magnitude between species and within individuals such that the overall mean levels of HR and BP may change to a varying degree from NREM sleep to REM, although variability is typically increased during REM. The autonomic mechanisms responsible for the overall effects of sleep-wake state on HR, BP, and regional vascular conductances are discussed below.

B. Autonomic Nervous System Changes Across Sleep-Wake States

The changes in HR and BP observed across sleep-wake states are largely dependent upon intact vagal and sympathetic innervations (9,14). Determination of the precise autonomic mechanisms involved in mediating these effects of sleep on

HR and BP has been facilitated by those studies documenting the actual changes in sympathetic and parasympathetic outputs. In some studies, direct recording of autonomic nervous system activity has been performed; e.g., microneurography has been used extensively to document sleep-related changes in muscle sympathetic nerve activity in humans (15–17). Chronic recordings of renal sympathetic activity have been performed in animals (e.g., 18). In contrast, other studies have inferred state-related changes in autonomic activity by observing changes in BP and HR with blockade of one (or other) branch of the autonomic nervous system (e.g., 19–22). Spectral analysis techniques have also been useful in determining sleep-related changes in autonomic output (e.g., 23,24).

Although each of these different approaches has yielded valuable information, each technique has its own advantages and disadvantages. For example, interpretation of changes in autonomic nervous system activity from microneurographic recordings from muscle sympathetic nerve is somewhat limited because only one branch of the autonomic nervous system is recorded and because this branch shows characteristic differences across sleep-wake states compared to the sympathetic output to other vascular beds. For example in REM sleep, sympathetic nerve output to muscle blood vessels is increased (15–17), whereas the sympathetic output to the renal vasculature is decreased (18). Confirmation of this differential effect of REM sleep on vasomotor tone in different vascular beds has been obtained in studies that have recorded blood flow in several vascular beds at the same in time in REM sleep (Fig. 3) (7,8). Figure 4 shows an example of the changes in muscle sympathetic nerve activity across sleep-wake states, in particular the increased activity in REM sleep. An example of decreased sympathetic activity in the renal nerve in REM is shown in Fig. 5. A differential distribution of sympathetic output to different vascular beds has also been observed in a pharmacological model of REM sleep; in this model, the REM-like state was associated with increased sympathetic output to vasoconstrictor fibers of hindlimb skeletal muscle but decreased output to the cardiac, renal, splanchnic, and lumbar sympathetic nerves (25). Depending on the magnitude of this differential distribution of sympathetic output in REM, the overall balance of vasodilation and vasoconstriction in the major resistance vessels will determine the net change in BP in REM sleep (see above).

Spectral analysis of HR variability has also been used to determine the prevailing balance of sympathetic and parasympathetic activities (26,27), and this approach has been applied to sleep (e.g., 23,24). However, the results of such studies, performed during spontaneous breathing, are somewhat complicated because interpretation relies on the validity of several assumptions that may be affected by the influences of sleep and its disturbance (27). In particular, changes in sleep-wake state are associated with changes in other physiological variables—e.g., blood gases, lung volume, breathing pattern and respiratory effort (28,29)—each of which can independently influence sympathetic and parasympathetic out-

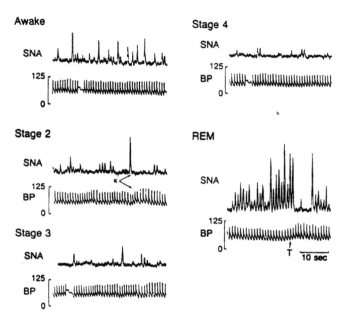

Figure 4 Muscle sympathetic nerve activity (SNA) and blood pressure (BP) recorded across sleep-wake states in a human subject. Note the progressive decrease in SNA from waking to the deeper stages of NREM sleep (stages 2 to 4). Note also the high and variable SNA in REM sleep. (From Ref. 17. Copyright © 1993 Massachusetts Medical Society. All rights reserved.)

flow (27,30–32) and therefore obscure the primary state-dependent effects on autonomic activity. However, most important for studies during sleep, particularly in patients with sleep-related breathing disorders, are the wide fluctuations in respiratory rate that accompany sleep onset and arousals from sleep. In these cases, interpretation becomes complicated because these fluctuations can fully encompass the frequency ranges used to separate the sympathetic and parasympathetic components of HR variability (27).

Despite these caveats, the results of studies using the variety of techniques described above, in a variety of species, suggest that established wakefulness exerts a tonic stimulatory effect on the sympathetic output to the heart and blood vessels (15–17,19,23,24). This is similar to the tonic stimulating effects on respiratory, and nonrespiratory, motor activity (28,33–35), and may be attributable to the same "wakefulness stimulus."

In contrast to the documented effects of wakefulness on sympathetic drive, the effects of waking on parasympathetic activity are less clear-cut. Several stud-

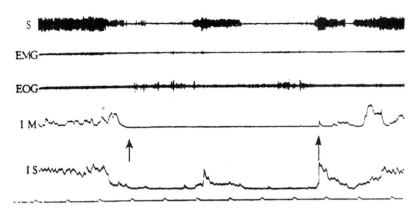

Figure 5 Decrease in renal sympathetic nerve activity in REM sleep recorded in a chronically instrumented cat, with phasic increases associated with phasic REM sleep events. S, raw sympathetic nerve activity; IS, integrated sympathetic nerve activity; IM, integrated neck muscle activity. Other abbreviations as for Figure 2. (From Ref. 18.)

ies in animals and humans suggest that established wakefulness is associated with a tonic withdrawal of parasympathetic drive to the heart, and that this is an important factor contributing to the increased HR when awake (20,21,23,36; see 7,8,12 for reviews). However, a major factor contributing to this parasympathetic withdrawal in established wakefulness is probably secondary to a change in breathing. For example, upper airway resistance typically increases in sleep (29,37–40), leading to increased respiratory efforts in response to the load (29). Increased respiratory efforts themselves can lead to an increased vagal contribution to HR variability by the central mechanisms associated with respiratory sinus arrhythmia (41–44). The respiratory slowing observed in some individuals during sleep (e.g., 45) would also increase the magnitude of the vagal contribution to sinus arrhythmia in these individuals (46).

That sleep-related changes in blood gases, breathing pattern, and effort can importantly contribute to the parasympathetic control of HR was demonstrated by a recent study in dogs, in which breathing rate and depth and blood gases were controlled by constant mechanical ventilation, while HR changes were monitored during spontaneous fluctuations in sleep-wake state with blockade of the cardiac sympathetic innervation (19). Under these conditions, there was a minimal change in the parasympathetic influence on HR between NREM sleep and steady-state established wakefulness (Fig. 6), showing that changes in breathing pattern importantly contribute to the vagal withdrawal and increased HR when awake (19). However, vagal influences make major contributions to the HR acceleration

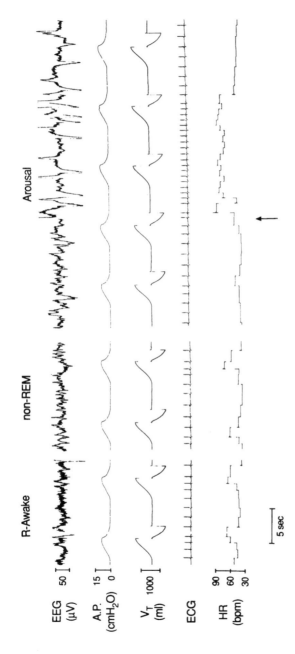

Figure 6 Example showing the differential effects of established wakefulness vs. transitions into wakefulness on the parasympathetic control of heart rate. The traces show changes in heart rate 1) between periods of established relaxed wakefulness (R-Awake) and non-REM sleep (left panels), and 2) at the transition from non-REM sleep to wakefulness (right panels, point of awakening indicated by arrow). The traces are from a dog undergoing constant mechanical ventilation with blockade of the cardiac sympathetic innervation—i.e., leaving only the parasympathetic innervation active. Mean heart rate changed minimally between steady-state wakefulness and NREM sleep, but awakening from sleep produced significant vagal withdrawal and large increases in heart rate. No body movements or evidence of overt behavioral arousal were noticeable at awakening; the large voltage deflections on the EEG trace are artifacts due to eye movements. The swings in airway pressure (A.P.) are produced by mechanical ventilation. EEG, electroencephalogram; V_T, tidal volume; ECG, electrocardiogram. (From Ref. 19.)

at arousal from sleep, even in the absence of changes in breathing pattern (see below). In addition, bursts of cardiac vagal efferent activity can also contribute to HR deceleration in REM (22).

III. Transient Effects of Arousal from Sleep on the Cardiovascular System

As summarized above, there have been several detailed studies into the mechanisms involved in mediating the changes in HR and BP between periods of established sleep and wakefulness. Comparatively little attention, however, has been focused on the mechanisms underlying the large, brief surges in HR and BP accompanying arousal from sleep. This neglect is somewhat surprising given that the repetitive surges in HR and BP at arousal from sleep are thought to predispose to increased risk for development of adverse cardiovascular events in patients with sleep-related breathing disorders (see Section I and 1–3,5,6). This section summarizes the changes in atuonomic nervous system activity that occur at arousal from sleep.

A. Autonomic Nervous System Responses to Arousal from Sleep

One study in intact, chronically instrumented cats has reported that spontaneous arousals from NREM sleep are associated with large increases in renal sympathetic nerve activity (18). In humans, the occurrence of K complexes during sleep is associated with transient increases in muscle sympathetic nerve activity, HR, and BP (15–17,47). An example of such a response is shown in Figure 7. Since K complexes during sleep are thought to be markers of an endogenous arousal/ alerting response (48), these observations are consistent with the suggestion that arousal-related mechanisms lead to sympathetic activation. The decrease in cardiac vagal activity after presentation of ''natural arousing stimuli'' in cats (14) is often taken as evidence that arousal from sleep leads to vagal withdrawal. However, the number and types of stimuli applied to how many cats is unclear in that study, as is whether the stimuli were applied in wakefulness or sleep.

Overall, these studies show that compared to what is known regarding the effects of established wakefulness and sleep on the autonomic nervous system outputs to the cardiovascular system (summarized in Section II), there is a relative lack of studies systematically investigating the acute effects of arousal from sleep on sympathetic and parasympathetic activities. Moreover, it is not known how the effects observed at arousal from sleep are physiologically different compared to subsequent established wakefulness. Therefore, the aim of a recent study was to systematically determine the effects of arousal from sleep on sympathetic and parasympathetic outputs to the cardiovascular system and compare these effects with those in subsequent periods of established wakefulness (19). Measurements of HR were made in awake and sleeping dogs with and without blockade of the

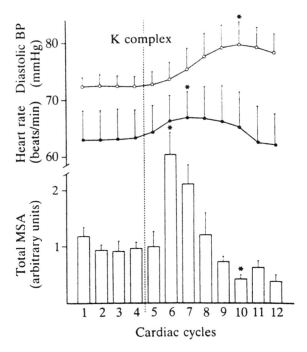

Figure 7 Cardiovascular consequences of a K complex in humans. Mean diastolic blood pressure (BP), heart rate, and muscle sympathetic nerve activity (MSA) are shown for several cardiac cycles before and after a K complex (indicated by vertical dashed line). Note the transient excitation of MSA, heart rate, and blood pressure after the K complex. (From Ref. 15 with permission of Oxford University Press.)

cardiac sympathetic and parasympathetic innervations. Studies were performed during spontaneous breathing and when breathing was controlled by constant mechanical ventilation at levels just below resting arterial P_{CO_2}. Mechanical ventilation was used to identify the independent effects of the arousal from sleep *per se* on the HR changes—i.e., in the absence of confounding influences such as changes in breathing pattern, lung volume, and blood gases which in themselves can lead to changes in cardiac autonomic output and obscure the primary effect of the state change (27,30–32). Under these controlled conditions, wake onset was associated with large, transient increases in HR compared to NREM sleep (mean increase = 30%, 20 beats per minute), and this was subsequently found to be due to both phasic sympathetic activation and parasympathetic withdrawal (19). However, subsequent periods of established wakefulness (i.e., periods separated by at least 30 sec from wake onset) were associated with smaller tonic increases in HR (mean increase = 6%, 4 beats per minute), and this was due to sympathetic activation with a minimal change in parasympathetic output (19). These changes reflect the primary effects of changes in sleep-wake state on cardiac sympathetic and parasympathetic outputs, because this study was performed with constant mechanical ventilation to hold level the respiratory influences on autonomic activity. In addition, these conditions serve to highlight the profound transient effects of normal spontaneous arousals from sleep on HR and autonomic nervous system outputs. As can be observed in Figure 6, the HR at spontaneous arousal from sleep can even increase to the levels observed during mild exercise, despite no evidence of overt behavioral arousal such as body movements. Overall, the large transient parasympathetic withdrawal to the heart (19) and the increased sympathetic drive to the heart and blood vessels (18,19,47) would explain the large, brief HR and BP responses at arousal from sleep.

B. Model to Explain the Large, Brief Surges in HR and BP at Arousal from Sleep

Despite the documented effects of arousal from sleep on sympathetic and parasympathetic activities to the heart and blood vessels (summarized above), there is currently no model that been put forward to explain why such large, brief changes in autonomic output occur at wake onset compared to subsequent established wakefulness. However, a component of these autonomic changes may be explained by a model similar to the one used to account for the stimulatory effects of arousal from sleep on pulmonary ventilation. This ventilatory model is described here briefly in order to highlight how similar reasoning may apply to the cardiovascular system. In the ventilatory model, the surge in ventilation at arousal from sleep is explained by differences in both the set point for Pa_{CO_2} and the hypercapnic ventilatory response between sleep and wakefulness. In sleep compared to waking, there is reduced ventilation and increased Pa_{CO_2} because of 1) an increase in the Pa_{CO_2} required to maintain spontaneous breathing (28,49,50), 2) reduced ventilatory responses to the increased Pa_{CO_2} (51), 3) increased upper airway resistance (37,52), 4) reduced compensatory responses to this respiratory load (38,53), and 5) decreased tonic drive to respiratory neurons (54) and motor neurons (35). However, an important consequence of the increased Pa_{CO_2} in sleep is that upon arousal, the arterial CO_2 is initially higher than the levels normally encountered in wakefulness. This discrepancy drives ventilation to a level determined by the waking CO_2 response curve and produces a transient surge in ventilation (28,55,56).

Similar reasoning applied to the control mechanisms for HR and BP may explain a component of the hemodynamic consequences of arousal from sleep. In this scheme, the decreased muscle sympathetic nerve activity observed in NREM sleep compared to wakefulness, in association with a decreased HR and BP (15–17), suggests that sleep is associated with a change in baroreceptor function (compare the sleep-related changes in the control of ventilation mentioned above). Indeed, there are other data suggesting that there is a downward resetting of the baroreflex in NREM sleep compared to wakefulness, and this appears to be accompanied by increased baroreflex sensitivity (57,58), although this latter effect is not observed consistently (59) and needs to be systematically reinvestigated. Figure 8 illustrates how changes in the set point and sensitivity of the baroreflex between wakefulness and sleep could explain a component of the in-

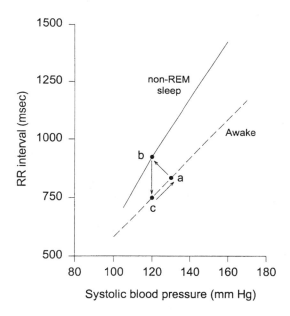

Figure 8 Hemodynamic model that may explain some of the increased heart rate and blood pressure at awakening from sleep. This model is based on the differences between wakefulness and sleep in the set point and sensitivity of the baroreflex. Points a and b indicate typical changes in heart rate (plotted as RR interval) and blood pressure between wakefulness and NREM sleep; the dashed and solid lines represent baroreflex sensitivities in these states. (From Ref. 57.) Systolic pressure is shown on the abscissa because this is typically used to quantify baroreflex responses (e.g., 57–59). Upon arousal from sleep (at point b), the level of systolic pressure will initially represent a hypotensive stimulus compared to the levels normally encountered in wakefulness, and this inappropriate level will drive compensatory mechanisms to increase blood pressure (i.e., from c to a). There will also be some increase in heart rate due to differences in the set point of the baroreflex curves between sleep and wakefulness. In this model, the transient nature of the blood pressure and heart rate change at awakening is explained in terms of a difference in the set point of the baroreflex between wakefulness and sleep and possibly an overshoot of the waking set point.

creased HR and BP at arousal from sleep. In this model, because the set point for mean arterial BP is lower during sleep and the sensitivity of the baroreflex may be higher (57,58), the BP upon a sudden awakening from sleep will initially represent a hypotensive stimulus compared to the levels normally encountered in wakefulness. This inappropriately low BP will drive compensatory mechanisms to increase BP, and there will also be some increase in HR due to differences in the set point of the responses between sleep and wakefulness (Fig. 8). In this model, the transient nature of the BP and HR surge at awakening would have to be explained in terms of a difference in the baroreflex set point between wakefulness and sleep and possibly an overshoot of the waking set point.

C. Limitations of the Hemodynamic Model to Explain the Surge in HR and BP at Arousal from Sleep

Explaining the acute stimulatory effects of arousal from sleep on HR and BP simply in terms of baroreflex responses has certain limitations. Indeed, these limitations (discussed below) make this model unlikely to be able to fully explain the magnitude of the transient surges in HR and BP at arousal. For example, changes in HR and BP occur in baroreceptor-denervated animals awake and asleep (60), indicating that major state-dependent influences on cardiac autonomic activity and vasomotor tone can occur independently of the baroreflex. Furthermore, that HR and BP changes are larger after baroreceptor denervation than before (60) suggests that the baroreflex normally buffers the hemodynamic effects of a change in sleep-wake state. Moreover, HR increases dramatically at arousal from sleep at a time when BP also increases significantly. The large increase in HR, despite the surge in BP, suggests that the baroreflex may even be uncoupled at arousal from sleep. That pharmacologically induced BP increases produce typical baroreflex-induced decreases in HR during sleep unless sleep is disturbed by a K complex (57) supports this suggestion. Indeed, following the K complex, BP continues to increase, but this is now accompanied by a significant rise in HR. Spontaneous K complexes during sleep themselves often lead to significant increases in HR and BP that occur concomitantly with increased muscle sympathetic nerve activity (15–17,47).

Taken together, these data suggest that phasic arousal reactions may uncouple baroreflex-induced slowing of the heart. Arousals associated with the defense reaction (61,62) and mental activity (58) have a similar effect. This concept is especially relevant because there is evidence for spontaneous activation of a distinct, transiently heightened awake state at wake onset compared to subsequent wakefulness (63–66; see 67 for review). As such, these data suggest that arousal from sleep is likely accompanied by transient uncoupling of the baroreflex, and this contributes to the transient surges in HR and BP at wake onset compared to subsequent wakefulness. These effects would occur via concomitant sympathetic activation and vagal withdrawal described previously. The inhibitory effects of wakefulness on the baroreflex control of HR may explain why only about 15%

of spontaneous fluctuations in RR intervals and arterial pressures follow the directions predicted by the baroreflex (68).

IV. Summary and Unanswered Questions

This chapter describes the autonomic nervous system changes that occur between states of wakefulness and sleep, with particular emphasis on the transient effects observed at arousal from sleep. Determination of these mechanisms assumes special importance given the relevance of the hemodynamic consequences (both transient and chronic) of arousal from sleep in patients with sleep-related breathing disorders that lead to increased risk for angina, myocardial infarction, stroke, left ventricular impairment, and systemic hypertension (1–3).

One of the next major challenges is to uncover the nature of the relationship between the changes in activity of sleep-wake–related neurons with effects on autonomic outputs, such as those producing the large brief surges in HR and BP at arousal from sleep in excess of subsequent wakefulness. For example, it needs to be determined if arousal from sleep, from a neurophysiological viewpoint, represents a state of being "more awake" (i.e., a more intense activation of state-related nuclei at wake onset compared to subsequent wakefulness), or whether there is a transient activation of neural pathways at wake onset (e.g., activation of the fight or flight response), which then become inactive in later periods of wakefulness.

Although the latter hypothesis has yet to be investigated, the firing patterns upon awakening of monoaminergic neurons in the dorsal raphe and locus ceruleus nuclei would support the former hypothesis. These neuronal groups are integral to the reticular activating system, and large transient increases in discharge have been noted for most serotonergic dorsal raphe neurons at spontaneous awakening from REM sleep (65,66) and for most noradrenergic locus ceruleus neurons at awakening from NREM sleep (64), with the levels of discharge far exceeding those in later wakefulness. Given the evidence that locus ceruleus and dorsal raphe neurons are important in modulating sensory (69) and motor responsiveness (70), respectively, their bursts of activity at awakening may serve a protective function by preparing an animal to respond immediately to any potentially threatening stimuli. Viewed in this context, the abrupt changes in EEG pattern and increases in postural muscle tone, accompanied by the large cardiorespiratory changes at arousal from sleep, would be appropriate physiological responses. Recent studies using the acoustic startle reflex, and its modulation by sensory inputs, also support the hypothesis that the moments just after awakening are neurophysiologically distinct compared to subsequent established wakefulness (63; reviewed in 67). Given the evidence that the "wakefulness stimulus" exerts powerful stimulatory effects on sympathetic outflow and produces transient vagal withdrawal, a transiently aroused awake state at wake onset would be expected to exert major influences on HR and BP compared to subsequent waking.

As mentioned, the mechanisms and pathways underlying the influence of this transient arousal state on the cardiovascular system at wake onset needs to be determined and are at present not well understood (71). For example, although changes in locus ceruleus neuronal activity parallel changes in sympathetic tone across sleep-wake states in cats (72), the nature of this association and its relevance to sleep-related cardiovascular control needs to be established. Similar considerations hold for the postulated influences of sleep-wake–related serotonergic neurons on sympathetic output (71). Indeed, it has been shown that serotonergic medullary raphe neurons, like the dorsal raphe neurons that are intimately involved in sleep regulation, have higher discharge in wakefulness (66,73–76) and project to sympathetic preganglionic neurons (71,77,78), where 5-HT depolarizes those neurons and can increase BP (79–81). However, although such effects provide appropriate circuitry and an attractive mechanism to explain state-dependent changes in sympathetic outputs, the actual relevance of these mechanisms to the effects of sleep on BP needs to be established.

It also remains to be determined if the neuronal systems engaged at arousal from sleep are altered by disturbances in the physiological variables that accompany repetitive apneas—e.g., hypoxia and hypercapnia—and whether these effects produce long-term sequelae (e.g., chronic sympathetic activation). Indeed, it is relevant to note that exposure to repetitive hypoxia in humans leads to elevated sympathetic activation after removal of the hypoxic stimulus (82) and leads to chronic hypertension in rats (83). Discharge of locus ceruleus neurons is increased by increased Pa_{CO_2} and decreased Pa_{O_2}, and these effects are associated with increased sympathetic output (84,85). Raphe neurons also increase their firing rates with increased levels of inspired CO_2 (76). Further studies into the basic neuronal mechanisms engaged at arousal from sleep, the modulation of these activities by changes in chemical respiratory stimuli associated with sleep-disordered breathing, and the role of central neuronal processes in modulating autonomic outputs will improve understanding of the mechanisms underlying the large HR and BP responses at arousal from sleep and the clinical consequences.

Acknowledgments

The author is a Parker B. Francis Fellow in Pulmonary Research.

REFERENCES

1. Shepard JW Jr. Hypertension cardiac arrhythmias myocardial infarction and stroke in relation to obstructive sleep apnea. Clin Chest Med 1992; 13:437–458.
2. Bradley TD. Right and left ventricular functional impairment and sleep apnea. Clin Chest Med 1992; 13:459–479.

3. Brooks D, Horner RL, Kozar LF, Render-Teixeira CL, Phillipson EA. Obstructive sleep apnea as a cause of systemic hypertension: evidence from a canine model. J Clin Invest 1997; 99:106–109.
4. Young T, Palta M, Dempsey J, Skatrud J, Badr S. The occurrence of sleep-disordered breathing among middle-aged adults. N Engl J Med 1993; 328:1230–1235.
5. Phillipson EA. Sleep apnea: a major public health problem. N Engl J Med 1993; 328:1271–1273.
6. Dempsey JA. Sleep apnea causes daytime hypertension (editorial). J Clin Invest 1997; 99:1–2.
7. Mancia G, Zanchetti A. Cardiovascular regulation during sleep In: Orem J, Barnes CD, eds. Physiology in Sleep. New York: Academic Press, 1980:1–55.
8. Coote JH. Respiratory and circulatory control during sleep. J Exp Biol 1982; 100: 223–244.
9. Baccelli G, Guazzi M, Mancia G, Zanchetti A. Neural and non-neural mechanisms influencing circulation during sleep. Nature 1967; 223:184–185.
10. Khatri IM, Fries ED. Hemodynamic changes during sleep. J Appl Physiol 1967; 22: 867–873.
11. Mancia G, Baccelli G, Adams DB, Zanchetti A. Vasomotor regulation during sleep in the cat. Am J Physiol 1971; 220:1086–1093.
12. Parmeggiani PL. The autonomic nervous system in sleep. In: Kryger MH, Roth T, Dement WC, eds. Principles and Practice of Sleep Medicine. Philadelphia: WB Saunders, 1994:194–203.
13. Sei H, Sakai K, Kanamori N, Salvert D, Vanni-Mercier G, Jouvet M. Long-term variations of arterial blood pressure during sleep in freely moving cats. Physiol Behav 1994; 55:673–679.
14. Baust W, Bohnert B. The regulation of heart rate during sleep. Exp Brain Res 1969; 7:169–180.
15. Hornyak M, Cejnar M, Elam M, Wallin BG. Muscle sympathetic nerve activity during sleep in man. Brain 1991; 114:1281–1295.
16. Okada H, Iwase S, Mano T, Sugiyama Y, Watanabe T. Changes in muscle sympathetic nerve activity during sleep in humans. Neurology 1991; 41:1961–1966.
17. Somers VK, Dyken ME, Mark AL, Abboud FM. Sympathetic-nerve activity during sleep in normal subjects. N Engl J Med 1993; 328:303–307.
18. Baust W, Weidinger H, Kirchner F. Sympathetic activity during natural sleep and arousal. Arch Ital Biol 1968; 106:379–390.
19. Horner RL, Brooks D, Kozar LF, Tse S, Phillipson EA. Immediate effects of arousal from sleep on cardiac autonomic outflow in the absence of breathing in dogs. J Appl Physiol 1995; 79:151–162.
20. Zemaityte D, Varoneckas G, Sokolov E. Heart rhythm control during sleep. Psychophysiology 1984; 21:279–289.
21. Kirby DA, Verrier RL. Differential effects of sleep stage on coronary hemodynamic function. Am J Physiol 1989; 256:H1378–H1383.
22. Verrier RL, Lau TR, Wallooppillai U, Quattrochi J, Nearing BD, Moreno R, Hobson JA. Primary vagally mediated decelerations in heart rate during tonic rapid eye movement sleep in cats. Am J Physiol 1998; 274:R1136–R1141.
23. Furlan R, Guzzetti S, Crivellaro W, Dassi S, Tinelli M, Baselli G, Cerutti S, Lombardi F, Pagani M, Malliani A. Continuous 24-hour assessment of the neural regula-

tion of systemic arterial pressure and RR variabilities in ambulant subjects. Circulation 1990; 81:537–547.

24. Berlad I, Shlitner A, Ben-Haim S, Lavie P. Power spectrum analysis and heart rate variability in Stage 4 and REM sleep: evidence for state specific changes in autonomic dominance. J Sleep Res 1993; 2:88–90.

25. Futuro-Neto HA, Coote JH. Changes in sympathetic activity to heart and blood vessels during desynchronized sleep. Brain Res 1982; 252:259–268.

26. Askelrod S, Gordon D, Madwed JB, Snidman NC, Shannon DC, Cohen RJ. Hemodynamic regulation: investigation by spectral analysis. Am J Physiol 1985; 249: H867–H875.

27. Novak V, Novak P, De Champlain J, Le Blanc AR, Martin R, Nadeau R. Influence of respiration on heart rate and blood pressure fluctuations. J Appl Physiol 1993; 74:617–626.

28. Phillipson EA, Bowes G. Control of breathing during sleep. In: Cherniack NS, Widdicombe JG, eds. Handbook of Physiology: The Respiratory System. Sec. 3, Vol. 2, Part 2. Bethesda, MD: American Physiological Society, 1986:649–689.

29. Henke KG, Badr MS, Skatrud JB, Dempsey JA. Load compensation and respiratory muscle function during sleep. J Appl Physiol 1992; 72:1221–1234.

30. Kollai M, Koizumi K. Reciprocal and non-reciprocal action of the vagal and sympathetic nerves innervating the heart. J Auton Nerv Syst 1979; 1:33–52.

31. Seals DR, Suwarno NO, Dempsey JA. Influence of lung volume on sympathetic nerve discharge in normal humans. Circ Res 1990; 67:130–141.

32. Somers VK, Mark AL, Zavala DC, Abboud FM. Influence of ventilation and hypocapnia on sympathetic nerve responses to hypoxia in normal humans. J Appl Physiol 1989; 67:2095–2100.

33. Glenn LL, Foutz AS, Dement WC. Membrane potential of spinal motoneurons during natural sleep in cats. Sleep 1978; 1:199–204.

34. Orem J. Respiratory neurons and sleep. In: Kryger MH, Roth T, Dement WC, eds. Principles and Practice of Sleep Medicine. Philadelphia: WB Saunders, 1994:177–193.

35. Horner RL, Kozar LF, Kimoff RJ, Phillipson EA. Effects of sleep on the tonic drive to respiratory muscle and the threshold for rhythm generation in the dog. J Physiol 1994; 474:525–537.

36. George CF, Kryger MH. Sleep and control of heart rate. Clin Chest Med 1985; 6: 595–601.

37. Skatrud JB, Dempsey JA. Airway resistance and respiratory muscle function in snorers during NREM sleep. J Appl Physiol 1985; 59:328–335.

38. Hudgel DW, Mulholland M, Hendricks C. Neuromuscular and mechanical responses to inspiratory resistive loading during sleep. J Appl Physiol 1987; 63:603–608.

39. Hudgel DW. Role of upper airway anatomy and physiology in obstructive sleep apnea. Clin Chest Med 1992; 13:383–398.

40. Orem J, Netick A, Dement WC. Increased upper airway resistance to breathing during sleep in the cat. Electroencephalogr Clin Neurophysiol 1977; 43:14–22.

41. Anrep GV, Pascual W, Rossler R. Respiratory variations of the heart rate: II. The central mechanism of the respiratory arrhythmia and the inter-relations between the central and the reflex mechanisms. Proc R Soc London B Biol Sci 1936; 119:218–230.

42. De Burgh Daly M. Interactions between respiration and circulation. In: Cherniack NS, Widdicombe JG, eds. Handbook of Physiology: The Respiratory System. Sec. 3, Vol. 2, Part 2. Bethesda, MD:American Physiological Society, 1986:529–594.

43. Shykoff BE, Naqvi SSJ, Menon AS, Slutsky AS. Respiratory sinus arrhythmia in dogs: effects of phasic afferents and chemostimulation. J Clin Invest 1991; 87:1621–1627.

44. Horner RL, Brooks D, Kozar LF, Gan K, Phillipson EA. Respiratory-related heart rate variability persists during central apnea in dogs: mechanisms and implications. J Appl Physiol 1995; 78:2003–2013.

45. Shea SA. Behavioural and arousal-related influences on breathing in humans. Exp Physiol 1996; 81:1–26.

46. Hirsch JA, Bishop B. Respiratory sinus arrhythmia in humans: how breathing pattern modulates heart rate. Am J Physiol 1981; 241:H620–H629.

47. Morgan BJ, Crabtree DC, Puleo DS, Badr MS, Toiber F, Skatrud JB. Neurocirculatory consequences of abrupt change in sleep-state in humans. J Appl Physiol 1996; 80:1627–1636.

48. Halasz P. Arousals without awakening—dynamic aspect of sleep. Physiol Behav 1993; 54:795–802.

49. Skatrud JB, Dempsey JA. Interaction of sleep state and chemical stimuli in sustaining rhythmic ventilation. J Appl Physiol 1983; 55:813–822.

50. Datta AK, Shea SA, Horner RL, Guz A. The influence of induced hypocapnia and sleep on the endogenous respiratory rhythm in humans. J Physiol 1991; 440:17–33.

51. Phillipson EA, Murphy E, Kozar LF. Regulation of respiration in sleeping dogs. J Appl Physiol 1976; 40:688–693.

52. Hudgel DW, Martin RJ, Johnson B, Hill P. Mechanics of the respiratory system and breathing pattern during sleep in normal humans. J Appl Physiol 1984; 56:133–137.

53. Weigand L, Zwillich CW, White DP. Sleep and the ventilatory response to resistive loading in normal men. J Appl Physiol 1988; 64:1186–1195.

54. Orem J, Osorio I, Brooks E, Dick T. Activity of respiratory neurons during NREM sleep. J Neurophysiol 1985; 54:1144–1156.

55. Phillipson EA. Sleep disorders. In: Murray JF, Nadel JA, eds. Textbook of Respiratory Medicine. Philadelphia: WB Saunders, 1988:1841–1860.

56. Bradley TD, Phillipson EA. Central sleep apnea. Clin Chest Med 1992; 13:493–505.

57. Smyth HS, Sleight P, Pickering GW. Reflex regulation of arterial pressure during sleep in man. Circ Res 1969; 24:109–121.

58. Conway J, Boon N, Vann Jones J, Sleight P. Involvement of the baroreceptor reflexes in the changes in blood pressure with sleep and mental arousal. Hypertension 1983; 5:746–748.

59. Bristow JD, Honnour AJ, Pickering TG, Sleight P. Cardiovascular and respiratory changes during sleep in normal and hypertensive subjects. Cardiovasc Res 1969; 3:476–485.

60. Guazzi M, Zanchetti A. Blood pressure and heart rate during natural sleep of the cat and their regulation by carotid sinus and aortic reflexes. Arch Ital Biol 1965; 103:789–817.

61. Hilton SM. The defence-arousal system and its relevance for circulatory and respiratory control. J Exp Biol 1982; 100:159–174.
62. Hilton SM. Ways of viewing the central nervous control of the circulation—old and new. Brain Res 1975; 87:213–219.
63. Horner RL, Sanford LD, Pack AI, Morrison AR. Activation of a distinct arousal state immediately after spontaneous awakening from sleep. Brain Res 1997; 778: 126–133.
64. Aston-Jones G, Bloom FE. Activity of norepinephrine-containing locus coeruleus neurons in behaving rats anticipates fluctuations in the sleep-waking cycle. J Neurosci 1981; 1:876–886.
65. Trulson ME, Jacobs BL. Raphe unit activity in freely moving cats: correlation with level of behavioral arousal. Brain Res 1979; 163:135–150.
66. Jacobs BL, Azmitia EC. Structure and function of the brain serotonin system. Phys Rev 1992; 72:165–229.
67. Horner RL. Arousal mechanisms and autonomic consequences. In: Pack AI, ed. Pathogenesis, Diagnosis and Treatment of Sleep Apnea. New York: Marcel Dekker. Submitted.
68. Eckberg DL, Sleight P. Human baroreflexes in health and disease. Monogr Physiol Soc 1992; 43:79–119.
69. Foote SL, Bloom FE, Aston-Jones G. Nucleus locus coeruleus: new evidence of anatomical and physiological specificity. Phys Rev 1983; 63:844–914.
70. Jacobs BL, Fornal CA. Activation of 5-HT neuronal activity during motor behavior. Semin Neurosci 1995; 7:401–408.
71. Guyenet PG. Role of the ventral medulla oblongata in blood pressure regulation. In: Loewy AD, Spyer KM, eds. Central Regulation of Autonomic Functions. New York: Oxford University Press, 1990:145–167.
72. Reiner PB. Correlational analysis of central noradrenergic neuronal activity and sympathetic tone in behaving cats. Brain Res 1986; 378:86–96.
73. Heym J, Steinfels GF, Jacobs BL. Activity of serotonin-containing neurons in the nucleus raphe pallidus of freely moving cats. Brain Res 1982; 251:259–276.
74. Trulson ME, Trulson VM. Activity of nucleus raphe pallidus neurons across the sleep-waking cycle in freely moving cats. Brain Res 1982; 237:232–237.
75. Fornal C, Auerbach S, Jacobs BL. Activity of serotonin-containing neurons in nucleus raphe magnusin freely moving cats. Exp Neurol 1985; 88:590–608.
76. Veasey SG, Fornal CA, Metzler CW, Jacobs BL. Response of serotonergic caudal raphe neurons in relation to specific motor activities in freely moving cats. J Neurosci 1995; 15:5346–5359.
77. Loewy AD. Raphe pallidus and raphe obscurus projections to the intermediolateral cell column in the rat. Brain Res 1981; 211:146–152.
78. Coote JH. Bulbospinal serotonergic pathways in the control of blood pressure. J Cardiovasc Pharmacol 1990; 15(S7):S35–S41.
79. McCall RB. Evidence for a serotonergically mediated sympathoexcitatory response to stimulation of medullary raphe nuclei. Brain Res 1984; 311:131–139.
80. Pilowsky PM, Kapoor V, Minson JB, West MJ, Chalmers JP. Spinal cord serotonin release and raised blood pressure after brainstem kainic acid injection. Brain Res 1986; 366:354–357.

81. Pickering AE, Spanswick D, Logan SD. 5-Hydroxytryptamine evokes depolarizations and membrane potential oscillations in rat sympathetic preganglionic neurons. J Physiol 1994; 480:109–121.
82. Morgan BJ, Crabtree DC, Palta M, Skatrud JB. Combined hypoxia and hypercapnia evokes long-lasting sympathetic activation in humans. J Appl Physiol 1995; 79:205–213.
83. Fletcher EC, Lesske J, Qian W, Miller CC III, Unger T. Repetitive, episodic hypoxia causes diurnal elevation of blood pressure in rats. Hypertension 1992; 19:555–561.
84. Elam M, Yao T, Thorén P, Svensson TH. Hypercapnia and hypoxia: chemoreceptor-mediated control of locus coeruleus neurons and splanchnic sympathetic nerves. Brain Res 1981; 222:373–381.
85. Guyenet PG, Koshiya N, Huangfu D, Verberne AJM, Riley TA. Central respiratory control of A5 and A6 pontine noradrenergic neurons. Am J Physiol 1993; 264: R1035–R1044.
86. Davies RJO, Crosby J, Vardi-Visy K, Clarke M, Stradling JR. Non-invasive beat to beat arterial blood pressure during non-REM sleep in obstructive sleep apnoea and snoring. Thorax 1994; 49:335–339.

6

Influence of Sleep and Sleep Apnea on Autonomic Control of the Cardiovascular System

KRZYSZTOF NARKIEWICZ

Medical University of Gdansk
Gdansk, Poland

BRADLEY G. PHILLIPS

University of Iowa College of Pharmacy
Iowa City, Iowa

VIREND K. SOMERS

Mayo Clinic and Mayo Foundation
Rochester, Minnesota

I. Introduction

Normal sleep is accompanied by distinct alterations in blood pressure and heart rate. These alterations are dependent upon sleep stage and appear to be mediated primarily by changes in autonomic circulatory control. It has become increasingly clear that sleep does not consist of a homogenous autonomic cardiovascular profile but rather represents a dynamic and organized modulation of neural circulatory control. The spectrum of autonomic regulation during normal sleep includes sympathetic inhibition, bradycardia, and lower blood pressures during synchronized non-rapid-eye-movement (NREM) sleep, and sympathetic activation with intermittent surges in blood pressure and heart rate during REM sleep. In patients with obstructive sleep apnea, the normal sleep stage–related changes in sympathetic activity and blood pressure are opposed by chemoreflex-mediated responses to hypoxemia and hypercapnia. These chemoreflex-mediated responses frequently overwhelm the modulatory effects of normal sleep on neural circulatory control.

Several approaches have been used in studying the role of the autonomic nervous system in regulating heart rate and blood pressure during sleep. Our understanding of these regulatory mechanisms has been advanced by the recent application of measurements of heart rate variability and of direct intraneural measurements of sympathetic nerve traffic to muscle blood vessels (muscle sympathetic nerve activity, or MSNA) and to skin (skin sympathetic nerve activity, or SSNA). This chapter seeks to review autonomic physiology and pathophysiology during normal sleep and in sleep apnea, with an emphasis on more recent developments. The potential links between autonomic changes in sleep and sleep apnea and cardiovascular events are addressed. Because of limitations of space, only few references relevant to specific areas can be included.

II. Normal Sleep

A. Neural Circulatory Responses to Normal Sleep

Blood Pressure and Heart Rate

Studies in animals have demonstrated that NREM or synchronized sleep is accompanied by a fall in blood pressure, mediated in part by a reduction in cardiac output and a decrease in total peripheral resistance (1). REM sleep is accompanied by intermittent surges in blood pressure and heart rate, with occasional irregularity in respiration (2–5). Changes in heart rate and blood pressure during normal sleep are modest. Overall, heart rate and blood pressure decline progressively from stages I through to IV of NREM sleep. During REM, blood pressure and heart rate are similar to levels recorded during quiet wakefulness.

Heart Rate Variability

Studies of heart rate variability during different stages of normal sleep have utilized spectral analysis to quantify the oscillatory powers of fluctuations in heart rate at low frequency (LF) and high frequency (HF) (6). The LF oscillation lies between 0.04 and 0.1 Hz and the HF oscillation occurs at the frequency of respiration (usually about 0.25 Hz). It is generally assumed that the LF oscillatory power of heart rate variability increases in association with increased sympathetic modulation of heart rate within the same subject. Similarly, it is thought that within-subject increases in HF oscillatory power of heart rate variability are associated with an increased vagal modulation of heart rate. In order to compensate for variations in total power of heart rate variability, a normalization procedure (the LF/HF ratio) is often used.

   Using spectral analysis of heart rate variability during quiet wakefulness and during the different sleep stages, a number of studies have consistently demonstrated similar results (7–10). The LF oscillatory component of heart rate variability decreases progressively during synchronized sleep, with an associated decrease in the LF/HF of heart rate variability (Figs. 1 and 2). During REM sleep, however, there is an increase in the LF component of heart rate variability and

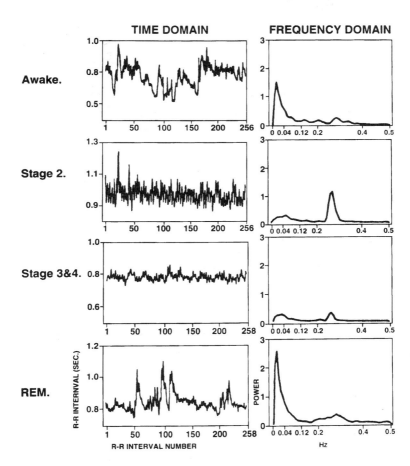

Figure 1 Representative data from one patient illustrating the time domain and frequency domain plots for wakefulness, stages II, III, and IV, and REM sleep. Time-domain axis is plotted RR interval number versus RR interval time in seconds. The frequency domain is plotted frequency in hertz versus power. Note the similarities between time-domain and frequency-domain representations in REM sleep and in wakefulness. During REM, there is an increase in absolute heart rate variability and an increased power of the low-frequency oscillation of heart rate. By contrast during stages II, III, and IV of NREM sleep, the high frequency oscillatory component of RR variability is increased. (From Ref. 9.)

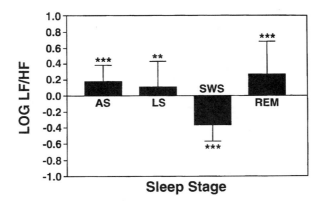

Figure 2 Log of low frequency/high frequency (LF/HF) in normal subjects during wakefulness (AS), light sleep (LS), slow-wave sleep (SWS), and REM sleep. The LF/HF declines during NREM sleep, particularly during slow-wave sleep. This ratio, however, increases during REM sleep. The increase in LF/HF of RR interval during REM is consistent with an increase in sympathetic modulation of heart rate. (From Ref. 7.)

an increase in the LF/HF ratio (Figs. 1 and 2). These findings from spectral analysis are consistent with a reduction in sympathetic heart rate modulation during synchronized sleep and an increased sympathetic modulation of heart rate during REM sleep.

Nevertheless, the assumption that heart rate during REM is governed exclusively by a dominance of sympathetic activity is challenged by reports of intermittent increases in vagal activity during REM sleep. Verrier et al. (11) have demonstrated that during tonic REM sleep in cats, primary deceleration in heart rate may occur, which is neither preceded nor followed by increases in heart rate or arterial pressure. These brief episodes of heart rate slowing are eliminated by glycopyrrolate, suggesting that the cardiac decelerations are secondary to changes in central regulation of cardiac autonomic control, namely a bursting or cardiac vagal efferent activity (11).

Pathophysiological conditions may also significantly alter measurements of heart rate variability during sleep. Vanoli et al. (8) have demonstrated that the heart rate variability patterns described above may be severely disrupted in patients after myocardial infarction. In eight patients following a recent myocardial infarction, LF/HF increased during NREM sleep, significantly different from the decrease in LF/HF of RR interval evident during NREM in normal control subjects. During REM, LF/HF increased further in postinfarct patients to levels even greater than those recorded during wakefulness. These investigators suggested that myocardial infarction was accompanied by a loss of the capacity for cardiac vagal activation during sleep, so that sleep in these patients was associated with sympathetic dominance. They hypothesized that the loss of sleep-related vagal activation may be implicated in nocturnal sudden death in patients after myocardial infarction.

Muscle Sympathetic Nerve Activity

Microneurographic measurements of sympathetic nerve traffic have increased our insight into the sympathetic mechanisms regulating blood pressure during the different sleep stages. This technique involves the insertion of a tungsten micro-electrode directly into the sympathetic nerve fascicles of a peripheral nerve (usually the peroneal or tibial nerves in the leg and occasionally the median nerve in the arm). These recordings allow direct intraneural measurements of multifiber sympathetic nerve traffic. MSNA measurements are quantifiable, particularly within the same subject during the same session. In contrast to measurements of plasma norepinephrine, MSNA recordings provide a moment-by-moment representation of sympathetic nerve traffic and in a sense serve as a "window" on the sympathetic nervous system. Utilizing these recordings, several investigators have demonstrated similar patterns of changes in MSNA during daytime sleep (12,13), after sleep deprivation (12), and during normal nighttime sleep (13,14).

From stages I through IV of NREM sleep, reductions in heart rate and blood pressure are accompanied by a progressive reduction in MSNA (Fig. 3). During NREM sleep, arousal stimuli elicit K complexes on the electroencephalogram (EEG), which are accompanied by bursts of sympathetic nerve activity and transient increases in blood pressure. This response of MSNA to arousal is strikingly different from the MSNA–arousal relationship during wakefulness. During wakefulness, arousal stimuli do not increase sympathetic nerve traffic to muscle but do increase sympathetic activity involving skin (15). Arousal stimuli do, however, increase sympathetic traffic to muscle after spinal cord injury (16) or anesthesia of the vagal or glossopharyngeal nerves (which carry baroreceptor reflex afferent impulses) (17). Therefore, during normal sleep, there appears to be a change in the neural processing of auditory and possibly other arousal stimuli.

The synchronous reduction in heart rate, blood pressure, and sympathetic nerve traffic during NREM sleep is suggestive of a profound resetting of the arterial baroreflex. Normally the baroreflex responds to reductions in blood pressure during wakefulness by increasing both heart rate and MSNA. During NREM sleep, the baroreflex likely plays a permissive role in allowing the simultaneous reduction of heart rate and MSNA together with blood pressure. Because of alter-

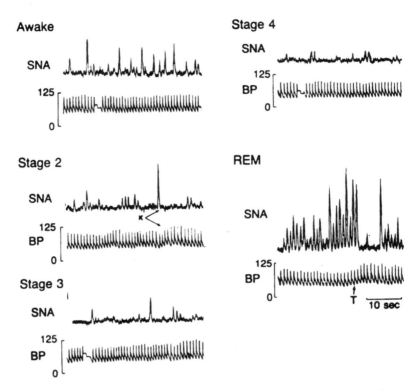

Figure 3 Recordings of sympathetic nerve activity (SNA) and mean blood pressure (BP) in a single subject while awake and while in stages II, III, IV, and REM sleep. As NREM sleep deepens (stages II through IV), sympathetic nerve activity gradually decreases and blood pressure and variability in blood pressure are gradually reduced. Arousal stimuli elicited K complexes on the electroencephalogram (not shown), which were accompanied by increases in sympathetic nerve activity and blood pressure (indicated by the arrows, stage II sleep). In contrast to the changes during NREM sleep, heart rate, blood pressure, and blood pressure variability increased during REM sleep, together with a profound increase in sympathetic nerve activity. There was a frequent association between REM twitches (momentary periods of restoration of muscle tone, denoted by T on the tracing) and abrupt inhibition of sympathetic nerve discharge and increases in blood pressure. (From Ref. 14. © 1993, Massachusetts Medical Society. All rights reserved.)

ations in absolute levels of blood pressure and heart rate during sleep, studies of baroreflex function during different sleep stages are not easily interpreted. Nevertheless, several investigators have shown that the gain of the arterial barore-ceptor reflex increases during sleep (18,19). Power spectral analysis of heart rate and blood pressure during sleep support the notion of an increase in baroreflex gain during NREM sleep (20).

During REM sleep, however, MSNA increases to about twice the levels seen during wakefulness, with blood pressure and heart rate on average similar to levels during wakefulness (Figs. 3 and 4) (14). The increase in MSNA during REM primarily occurs during phasic REM—i.e., during the episodes of rapid eye movements—and is associated with intermittent surges in blood pressure and heart rate fluctuations. The blood pressure increase due to sympathetic mediated vasoconstriction in skeletal muscle during REM is opposed by vasodilation in mesenteric and renal vascular beds. The increase in MSNA during REM appears to be linked to a loss of postural muscle tone, suggesting that the loss of muscle tone during REM is a disinhibitory (or excitatory) stimulus to sympathetic activa-tion. REM "twitches" or brief periods of return of muscle tone induce surges in blood pressure and sympathetic inhibition.

Skin Sympathetic Nerve Activity

While studies of MSNA during sleep have demonstrated distinct sleep-related changes, the same is not true for studies of skin SNA during sleep. Takeuchi and colleagues (21) measured both muscle and skin sympathetic activity using a dou-ble recording microneurographic technique in 8 healthy volunteers during poly-somnographic monitoring during NREM sleep. Their data suggested that both skin SNA and muscle SNA were centrally suppressed during light sleep. Arousal stimuli during sleep induced K complexes and increases in both MSNA and SSNA (Fig. 5). Similar multiunit recordings of skin sympathetic activity together with recordings of electrical skin resistance and skin blood flow in sleep-deprived healthy subjects were conducted by Noll and colleagues (22). These investigators reported that NREM sleep was always associated with an increase in skin resis-tance. Skin blood flow also increased during sleep. No significant difference in mean skin SNA was found between wakefulness and NREM sleep, although during REM sleep, skin SNA was relatively greater compared to the preceding stage II sleep period. These investigators also found an association between K complexes and bursts of skin SNA, followed by transient changes in skin resis-tance, blood flow, and arterial pressure. Interestingly, they noted that bursts of skin SNA were followed by brief increases in skin blood flow within the innerva-tion area of the impaled fascicle, suggesting the existence of specific sympathetic vasodilator fibers in skin that are activated during sleep.

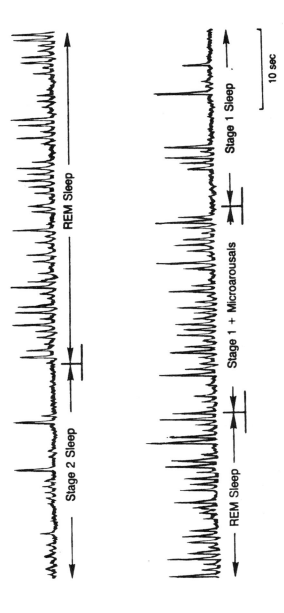

Figure 4 Changes in sympathetic nerve discharge frequency and amplitude are shown during the transition from stage II sleep to REM sleep (upper tracing) and the transition from REM sleep to stage I sleep, with frequent "microarousals," and then to established stage I sleep (lower tracings). (From Ref. 14. © 1993, Massachusetts Medical Society. All rights reserved.)

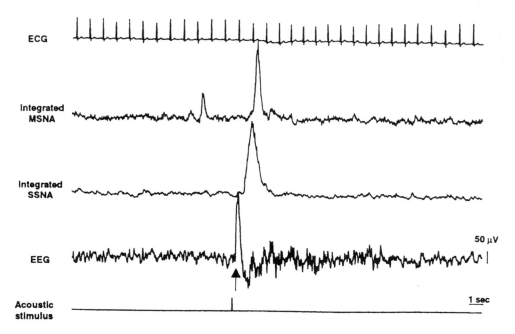

Figure 5   Recordings of the electrocardiogram (ECG), muscle sympathetic nerve activity (MSNA), skin sympathetic nerve activity (SSNA) and electroencephalogram (EEG) during sleep in a normal subject. Also shown is the response to an acoustic stimulus with the associated K complex and increases in SSNA and MSNA. A similar response of skin and muscle SNA is evident during spontaneous K complexes. (From Ref. 21.)

B. Clinical Relevance of Autonomic Neural Circulatory Control During Sleep

There is increasing evidence of a circadian rhythm in cardiovascular events, including in sudden death. This concept is covered in greater detail elsewhere (23). The mechanisms underlying the circadian rhythm in cardiovascular events are not clear. The predominance of REM sleep in the early hours of the morning before awakening and the sympathetic and hemodynamic alterations during REM may conceivably be implicated in increased platelet aggregability, plaque rupture, and coronary vasospasm, thus acting as a trigger mechanism for thrombotic events that may present clinically only after arousal (24–27).

While regulation of autonomic function and hemodynamics during sleep may be directly relevant to understanding cardiovascular phenomena such as circadian rhythms in cardiovascular disease, neural circulatory effects of arousal may also have important implications. Arousal from NREM sleep is accompanied by increases in heart rate, blood pressure, and MSNA (28). Using measurements of blood pressure and RR interval, van de Borne and colleagues (20) have shown that arterial baroreflex sensitivity is markedly reduced during arousal from sleep and is accompanied by a reduction in the HF oscillatory component of RR interval and an increase in the LF oscillatory component. The data regarding baroreflex sensitivity are consistent with earlier findings from Conway et al. (18), suggesting that mental arousal after sleep is linked to a decrease in baroreflex gain. Arousal-related surges in blood pressure and heart rate may be potentiated in the setting of baroreflex impairment. Thus, these hemodynamic responses may be linked to initiation of vascular events in patients with preexisting cardiovascular disease.

Reductions in sympathetic activation during stage IV sleep, with consequent decreases in blood pressure, may be associated with clinically significant hypotension and consequent end-organ ischemia (29–31). This synchronized sleep-related hypotension may be especially relevant in patients with underlying cerebral vascular disease, bilateral carotid artery stenoses, and patients on multiple antihypertensive medications who also have coexistent autonomic dysfunction. In these patients, impaired perfusion secondary to iatrogenic nocturnal hypotension may be amplified by stenoses in conduit vessels and impaired autoregulation in parenchymal brain blood vessels. Dysfunctional autonomic regulation—for example, in diabetics—will potentiate nocturnal hypotension in the face of multiple antihypertensive medications.

III. Neural Circulatory Regulation in Obstructive Sleep Apnea

A. Autonomic Responses to Hypoxia, Hypercapnia, and the Mueller Maneuver

The autonomic effects of obstructive sleep apnea reflect an integrated response to several powerful stimuli. These include hypoxia, hypercapnia, apnea, the Mueller maneuver, and the effects of sleep. Direct and reflex effects of these stimuli are further modulated by other reflex mechanisms, such as the baroreflex. Identifying the individual effects of each of the above stimuli helps in understanding the integrated response to obstructive apneas and variations of the response in different pathophysiological conditions.

Sympathetic Responses to Apnea During Hypoxic Hypercapnia

Both hypoxia and hypercapnia result in local vasodilation (32). The vasodilatory action is opposed by chemoreflex-mediated sympathetic vasoconstriction. Hypoxia acts primarily on peripheral chemoreceptors in the carotid bodies (33,34). Hypercapnia acts primarily on central chemoreceptors in the brainstem (35). Both these stimuli elicit increases in minute ventilation and efferent sympathetic vasoconstrictor activity. Increased ventilation acts via thoracic afferents to inhibit sympathetic responses to both hypoxia and hypercapnia (36,37). Thus, during apnea, when the inhibitory influence of thoracic afferents is eliminated, the sympathetic neural responses to hypoxia and hypercapnia are potentiated. During episodes of sleep apnea, subjects are exposed to simultaneous hypoxia, hypercapnia, and apnea. Simultaneous hypoxia and hypercapnia result in synergistic increases in sympathetic traffic. Coexisting apnea further potentiates the sympathetic response. Thus, it would be expected that in patients with obstructive sleep apnea, hypoxia, hypercapnia, and the absence of lung inflation will result in marked increases in sympathetic nerve traffic (38). This sympathetic activation would be opposed by the normal mechanisms governing neural circulatory regulation during the different sleep stages, as described earlier.

Responses in Hypertension

There is an increased incidence of hypertension in patients with sleep apnea (39,40). An additional and important consideration in understanding responses to sleep apnea, particularly in sleep-apneic patients with hypertension, is that the sympathetic response to hypoxia and apnea may be markedly potentiated in hypertensive patients. In spontaneously hypertensive rats, chemoreflex afferent activity is increased during normoxia and is attenuated by chemoreflex deactivation by 100% oxygen (41). Hypertensive patients have an increased ventilatory response to a hypoxic stress (42). In untreated mild hypertensives, the sympathetic response to hypoxia is about twice that seen in matched controls (43). During apnea, the increase in sympathetic activity in the hypertensive patients is about 12-fold the response seen in normal subjects (43). Thus, in those patients with obstructive sleep apnea who also have hypertension, the sympathetic response to obstructive apneas during sleep may be exacerbated.

Baroreflex-Chemoreflex Interactions

The mechanism underlying the potentiated sympathetic response in hypertensives may be linked to baroreflex dysfunction. The baroreflexes exert a powerful inhibitory influence on chemoreflex responses (44,45). During hypoxia in normal subjects, simultaneous activation of the baroreceptors by intravenous phenylephrine infusion attenuates the sympathetic response to hypoxia (45). In patients with hypertension, in whom there may be underlying baroreflex impairment, the sympathetic response to chemoreflex activation may be increased, with a consequent increase in the pressor response to apneic episodes. A similar consideration is applicable to heart failure patients with sleep apnea, since heart failure is also linked to baroreflex impairment (46,47).

The Mueller Maneuver

While studies of chemoreflex involvement in sleep apnea have simulated sleep apnea using voluntary apnea together with hypoxia and hypercapnia, actual obstructive apneic events do not involve central apneas but rather consist of repetitive brief periods of inspiration against an obstructed airway. This generates significant changes in intrathoracic pressure, resulting in distortion of cardiac chamber geometry (48,49). This cardiac distortion during inspiration against an occluded airway (the Mueller maneuver) may itself result in significant neural and circulatory changes. The initial phase (first 10 sec) of a Mueller maneuver results in marked hypotension and a paradoxical reduction in sympathetic activity. Toward the end of the Mueller maneuver, however, sympathetic activity gradually increases, as does blood pressure (50). Thus, in seeking to understand sympathetic responses to prolonged obstructive apneic events, the response to the Mueller maneuver (which opposes the initial sympathetic excitatory response to hypoxia) needs to be considered.

Bradycardia During Apnea

The primary response to hypoxia is bradycardia. During hyperventilation, the vagally mediated bradycardia is prevented by the vagolytic effects of hyperventilation. However, with apnea during hypoxia, when the effect of ventilation is eliminated, chemoreflex-mediated vagal bradycardia becomes evident. The combined apnea response—consisting of sympathetic-mediated vasoconstriction in peripheral blood vessels (not including the cerebral and coronary circulations) and vagal bradycardia—constitutes part of the diving reflex (51,52).

The intensity of bradycardia during apnea varies considerably between individuals. One important determinant may be the sensitivity of baroreflex. As described earlier, the baroreflex has a powerful inhibitory influence on chemoreflex-mediated vasoconstriction (44,45). The baroreflexes may also influence chemoreflex-mediated bradycardia, such that in those clinical conditions where the baroreflex is impaired, vagal bradycardia may be potentiated (53). Neck suction and consequent baroreflex activation during apnea would normally be expected to increase the bradycardia during the apnea. However, baroreflex activation during apnea actually prevents chemoreflex-mediated bradyarrhythmias, suggesting that the inhibitory influence of baroreflex activation on chemoreflex responses extends not only to the sympathetic response but also to the vagal bradycardic response (53).

B. Autonomic Function in Wakefulness in Patients with Sleep Apnea

Several studies have demonstrated consistently that patients with obstructive sleep apnea have high levels of norepinephrine (54–56). These patients also have elevated MSNA recorded during quiet normoxic wakefulness (57,58). Increased MSNA is present in sleep-apneic patients of both genders and is evident whether or not patients are hypertensive (Fig. 6). Furthermore, high levels of sympathetic traffic in patients with obstructive sleep apnea are not explained by obesity, since obese patients proven not to have sleep apnea do not have markedly elevated levels of MSNA (59). In studies of unmedicated and otherwise healthy patients with obstructive sleep apnea, in comparison to sex- and body-mass index–matched healthy subjects in whom sleep apnea has been excluded by overnight polysomnography, several abnormalities in daytime neural circulatory control have become apparent (60). First, patients with severe sleep apnea have faster heart rates. These are associated with a marked reduction in overall heart rate variability but a relative increase in the LF oscillatory component of RR variability (Figs. 7 and 8). In patients with overt cardiovascular disease, reduced heart rate variability may be linked to adverse cardiovascular outcomes (6). Even though the sleep apnea patients studied were normotensive, with blood pressures very similar to those seen in control subjects, there was a marked increase in blood pressure variability. Thus, otherwise healthy patients with obstructive sleep apnea who are normotensive have faster heart rates, increased LF of RR, decreased RR variability, and increased blood pressure variability. These abnormal-

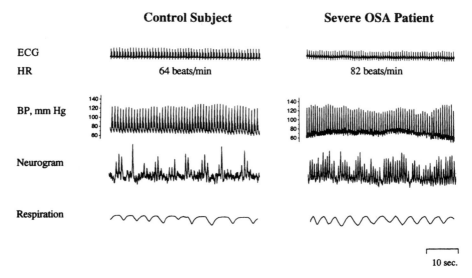

Figure 6 Electrocardiogram (ECG), blood pressure (BP), sympathetic neurograms, and respiration in a control subject (left) and in a patient with severe obstructive sleep apnea (OSA) (right), showing faster heart rate (HR), increased BP variability, and markedly elevated MSNA in the patient with OSA. Spectral analysis recordings for these subjects are shown in Figure 7. (From Ref. 60.)

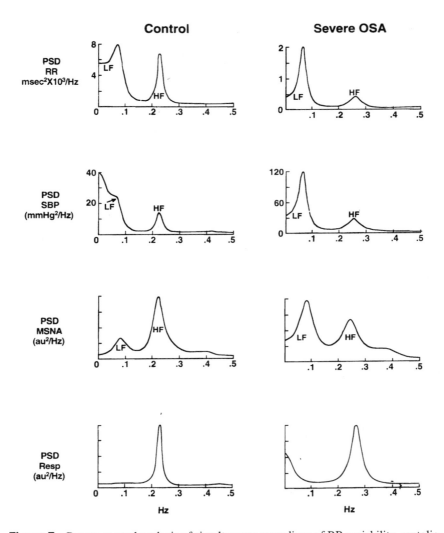

Figure 7 Power spectral analysis of simultaneous recordings of RR variability, systolic blood pressure (SBP) variability, muscle sympathetic nerve activity (MSNA) variability, and respiration (Resp) in the control subject (left) and in the patient with obstructive sleep apnea (OSA) (right) shown in Figure 6. RR variance is decreased and SBP variance is increased in the patient with OSA compared to the control subject. There is a relative predominance of the LF component over the HF component of RR interval in the patient with OSA. LF components are clearly present in the MSNA variability profiles of both subjects. PSD, power spectral density; au, arbitrary units. (From Ref. 60.)

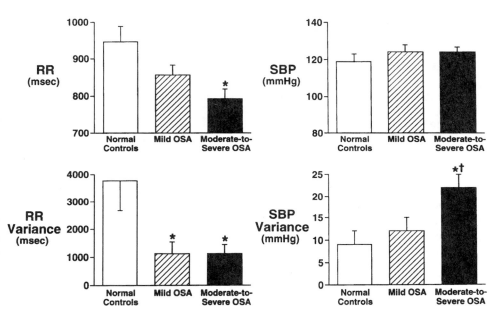

Figure 8 RR interval, systolic blood pressure (SBP), and their variances in control subjects ($n = 16$), patients with mild obstructive sleep apnea (OSA) ($n = 18$), and patients with moderate-to-severe OSA ($n = 15$). RR interval was reduced in the patients with moderate-to-severe OSA compared with the control subjects. Patients with mild OSA and those with moderate-to-severe OSA had an attenuated RR variance in comparison to that in the control subjects. SBP variance was markedly increased in patients with moderate-to-severe OSA compared to either control subjects or patients with mild OSA. * $p < 0.05$ versus controls subjects; † $p < 0.05$ versus mild OSA. Data are means ± SEM. (From Ref. 60.)

ities of neural control in sleep apnea are strikingly similar to the abnormalities in neural control evident in patients with essential hypertension. Increased blood pressure variability in hypertensive patients is associated with an increased likelihood of target-organ damage (61,62), independent of the absolute blood pressure level. Thus it may be that the abnormalities in neural control described above precede the development of sustained hypertension in sleep-apneic patients.

The mechanism underlying the derangement in neural control in sleep apnea is unknown. Abnormalities in chemoreflex function may be implicated. The arterial chemoreceptors may exert important influences on neural control even during normoxia. Elimination of the influence of arterial chemoreceptors using room air and 100% oxygen in a double-blind study showed that in patients with sleep apnea, suppression of the chemoreflexes slowed heart rate, lowered blood pressure, and decreased MSNA (Fig. 9) (63). Thus, potentiated chemoreflex function may contribute to the abnormalities in hemodynamics and in autonomic function described above.

C. Autonomic Function During Sleep in Patients with Sleep Apnea

Sympathetic and Hemodynamic Responses

We have described the effects of chemoreflex activation on sympathetic activity and that the sympathetic excitatory effect of hypoxia, hypercapnia, and apnea would be expected to oppose the sleep stage–related changes in hemodynamics and sympathetic traffic. Indeed, in patients with sleep apnea, there is a marked disruption of the tightly regulated changes in hemodynamics and sympathetic activity evident during the different stages of normal sleep (58). By contrast, the sympathetic nerve and blood pressure profile during sleep in sleep apneic patients

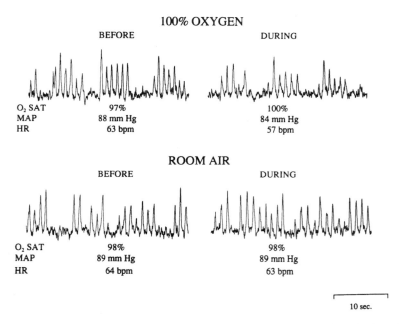

Figure 9 Recordings of muscle sympathetic nerve activity (MSNA) in a single patient with obstructive sleep apnea (OSA) during administration of 100% oxygen (top) and room air (bottom). MSNA, mean arterial pressure (MAP), and heart rate (HR) decreased during administration of 100% oxygen but did not change during administration of room air. (From Ref. 63.)

is dominated by responses to episodes of obstructive sleep apnea that occur continuously throughout sleep. Apneic episodes result in progressive increases in sympathetic nerve activity, these increases being most marked toward the end of apnea (Fig. 10) (58). At cessation of apnea and resumption of breathing, there is an abrupt termination of sympathetic activity and an increase in blood pressure. The duration of apnea and the level of oxygen desaturation are key factors in determining sympathetic activation during the episodes of obstructive sleep apnea. The surge in blood pressure and the end of apnea are explained in part by the increase in cardiac output, secondary to the increased venous return, which occurs during breathing after apnea. In addition, the severely vasoconstricted peripheral vasculature, together with the increased cardiac output, results in the marked increases in blood pressure. Other factors, such as increased muscle tone

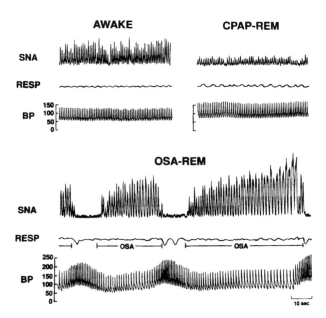

Figure 10 Recordings of sympathetic nerve activity (SNA), respiration (RESP), and intra-arterial blood pressure (BP) in the same subject when awake, with obstructive sleep apnea during REM sleep, and with elimination of obstructive apnea by CPAP therapy during REM sleep. SNA is very high during wakefulness but increases even further secondary to obstructive apnea during REM. BP increases from 130/65 mmHg when awake to 256/110 mmHg at the end of apnea. Elimination of apneas by CPAP results in decreased nerve activity and prevents BP surges during REM sleep. (From Ref. 58. © 1995, American Society for Clinical Investigation.)

and arousal, may also contribute to increased blood pressure at the end of apnea (64,65).

Bradycardia and Sleep Apnea

The chemoreflex-mediated vagal activation described earlier is frequently evident in clinical situations involving patients with sleep apnea. A number of studies have characterized the spectrum of bradyarrhythmic responses to obstructive sleep apnea, and these extend from sinus bradycardia to prolonged periods of cardiac asystole (66–68). Atropine prevents sleep apnea–induced bradycardia (69). From a clinical perspective, it is important that patients with nocturnal bradyarrhythmias evident on Holter monitoring be evaluated for obstructive sleep apnea, since CPAP rather than pacemaker implantation would be the preferred initial therapy. Furthermore, in those patients in whom bradyarrhythmias are also evident during the daytime, it is important to ensure that these patients do not fall asleep with consequent obstructive apnea during the daytime hours. While it may be appropriate to exclude thyroid hypofunction in sleep-apneic patients generally, this is particularly true for those with apnea-related bradyarrhythmias.

Sleep Apnea and "Nondippers"

Blood pressure and sympathetic activity in sleep-apneic patients are highest during REM sleep, since it is during this sleep stage that apneas are most prolonged (58). The reduction in muscle tone during REM may influence muscle tone in the upper airway, thus potentiating the likelihood of airway obstruction. Because of repetitive vasoconstriction and blood pressure surges, blood pressure overall does not fall during sleep in patients with sleep apnea. This blood pressure response to sleep in sleep-apneic patients may be important in understanding the absence of nocturnal hypotension in the subgroup of hypertensive patients termed "nondippers." Hypertensive patients in whom there is an absence of a nocturnal pressure decline (nondippers) are at increased risk for cardiac and vascular events (62,70,71). The nocturnal blood pressure profile in nondipper hypertensive patients is strikingly similar to that described in studies of 24 hr blood pressure measurements in patients with sleep apnea. Pankow et al. (72) have shown that nondipping of nocturnal blood pressure in patients with sleep apnea is related to apnea severity. Lavie et al. (73) have also reported that blood pressure during sleep correlated significantly with the apnea hypopnea index. In a study directed specifically at male nondippers with essential hypertension, Portaluppi and colleagues (74) concluded that hypertensive nondippers had a high probability of coexisting sleep-disordered breathing. Thus, obstructive sleep apnea and the consequent cardiovascular effects of repetitive hypoxemia, hypercapnia, respiratory acidosis, and blood pressure surges may be involved in the increased cardiovascular morbidity that characterizes those hypertensive patients in whom there is an absence of a nocturnal blood pressure decline.

Effects of Therapy with CPAP

Treatment with CPAP, when effective, results in a significant reduction in sympathetic nerve traffic and blunts blood pressure surges during sleep (Fig. 10). This effect is secondary to attenuation of apneic episodes by CPAP. Studies of ambulatory blood pressure report that nasal CPAP also reduces daytime blood pressure in patients with sleep apnea (75,76). Uncontrolled studies of the effects of CPAP on daytime sympathetic activity suggest that sympathetic drive may be reduced by regular CPAP use (77,78).

D. Clinical Relevance of Autonomic Responses to Obstructive Sleep Apnea

There is increasing evidence that obstructive sleep apnea is linked to cardiovascular morbidity and mortality. Autonomic mechanisms may be implicated. High sympathetic drive and abnormalities in cardiovascular variability, evident even during wakefulness, may precede and perhaps predispose to cardiovascular dysfunction, particularly to hypertension. During sleep, repetitive hypoxemia with consequent chemoreflex activation, sympathetic excitation, and blood pressure surges may be involved in cardiovascular events in sleep-apneic patients. In the setting of severe hypoxia, bradyarrhythmias (in particular prolonged asystole) may predispose to cerebral hypoperfusion as well as to dispersion of cardiac refractoriness and consequent life-threatening arrhythmias. Sleep apnea may also be an important factor in determining the increased cardiovascular risk in hypertensive nondippers. Given the morbidity associated with both sleep apnea and with obesity and the high incidence of occult sleep apnea in apparently asymptomatic obese subjects (79), the cardiovascular stigmata accompanying obstructive sleep apnea may be implicated in the cardiovascular risk that is associated with morbid obesity.

Acknowledgments

Krzysztof Narkiewicz was a recipient of a Fogarty International Research Fellowship from the NIH. Virend Somers is an Established Investigator of the American Heart Association. He and Bradley Phillips are Sleep Academic Awardees of the NIH and are supported by grant HL14388 from the NIH. We thank Linda Bang for typing of this manuscript. We also extend our appreciation to those colleagues who contributed to the work described in this review.

REFERENCES

1. Mancia G, Baccelli G, Adams DB, Zanchetti A. Vasomotor regulation during sleep in the cat. Am J Physiol 1971; 220:1086–1093.
2. George CF, Kryger MH. Sleep and control of heart rate. Clin Chest Med 1985; 6: 595–601.
3. Coccagna G, Mantovani M, Brignani F, Manzini A, Lugaresi E. Laboratory note: arterial pressure changes during spontaneous sleep in man. Electroencephalogr Clin Neurophysiol 1971; 31:277–281.
4. Khatri IM, Freis ED. Hemodynamic changes during sleep. J Appl Physiol 1967; 22: 867–873.
5. Snyder F, Hobson JA, Morrison DF, Goldfrank F. Changes in respiration, heart rate and systolic blood pressure in human sleep. J Appl Physiol 1964; 19:417–422.
6. Task Force of the European Society of Cardiology and the North American Society of Pacing and Electrophysiology. Heart rate variability: standards of measurement, physiological interpretation, and clinical use. Circulation 1996; 93:1043–1065.
7. Baharav A, Kotagal S, Gibbons V, Rubin BK, Pratt G, Karin J, Akselrod S. Fluctuations in autonomic nervous activity during sleep displayed by power spectrum analysis of heart rate variability. Neurology 1995; 45:1183–1187.
8. Vanoli E, Adamson PB, Ba-Lin MPH, Pinna GD, Lazzara R, Orr WC. Heart rate variability during specific sleep stages: a comparison of healthy subjects with patients after myocardial infusion. Circulation 1995; 91:1918–1922.
9. Vaughn BV, Quint SR, Messenheimer JA, Robertson KR. Heart period variability in sleep. Electroencephalogr Clin Neurophysiol 1995; 94:155–162.
10. Scholz UJ, Bianchi AM, Cerutti S, Kubicki S. Vegetative background of sleep: spectral analysis of the heart rate variability. Physiol Behav 1997; 62:1037–1043.
11. Verrier RL, Lau TR, Wallooppillai U, Quattrochi J, Nearing BD, Moreno R, Hobson JA. Primary vagally mediated decelerations in heart rate during tonic rapid eye movement sleep in cats. Am J Physiol 1998; 274:R1136–R1141.
12. Homyak M, Cejnar M, Elam M, Matousek M, Wallin BG. Sympathetic muscle nerve activity during sleep in man. Brain 1991; 114:1281–1295.
13. Okada H, Iwase S, Mano T, Sugiyama Y, Watanabe T. Changes in muscle sympathetic nerve activity during sleep in humans. Neurology 1991; 41:1961–1966.
14. Somers VK, Dyken ME, Mark AL, Abboud FM. Sympathetic-nerve activity during sleep in normal subjects. N Engl J Med 1993; 328:303–307.
15. Mark AL. Regulation of sympathetic nerve activity in mild human hypertension. J Hypertens 1990; 8 (suppl 7):S67–S75.
16. Stjernberg L, Blumberg H, Wallin BG. Sympathetic activity in man after spinal cord injury: outflow to muscle below the lesion. Brain 1986; 109:695–715.
17. Fagius J, Wallin BG, Sundlof G, Nerhed C. Englesson S. Sympathetic outflow in man after anaesthesia of the glossopharyneal and vagus nerves. Brain 1985; 108: 423–438.
18. Conway J, Boon N, Jones JV, Sleight P. Involvement of the baroreceptor reflexes in the changes in blood pressure with sleep and mental arousal. Hypertension 1983; 5:746–748.

19. Smyth HS, Sleight P, Pickering GW. Reflex regulation of arterial pressure during sleep in man: a quantitative method of assessing baroreflex sensitivity. Circ Res 1969; 24:109–121.
20. van de Borne P, Nguyen H, Biston P, Linkowski P, Degaute J-P. Effects of wake and sleep stages on the 24-h autonomic control of blood pressure and heart rate in recumbent men. Am J Physiol 1994; 266:H548–H554.
21. Takeuchi S, Iwase S, Mano T, Okada H, Sugiyama Y, Watanabe Y. Sleep-related changes in human muscle and skin sympathetic nerve activities. J Auton Nerv Syst 1994; 47:121–129.
22. Noll G, Elam M, Kunimoto M, Karlsson T, Wallin BG. Skin sympathetic nerve activity and effector function during sleep in humans. Acta Physiol Scand 1994; 151:319–329.
23. Muller JE, Tofler GH, Stone PH. Circadian variation and triggers of onset of acute cardiovascular disease. Circulation 1989; 79:733–743.
24. Nowlin JB, Troyer WG Jr, Collins WS, Silverman G, Nichols CR, McIntosh HD, Estes EH Jr, Bogdanoff MD. The association of nocturnal angina pectoris with dreaming. Ann Intern Med 1965; 63:1040–1046.
25. King MJ, Zir LM, Kaltman AJ, Fox AC. Variant angina associated with angiographically demonstrated coronary artery spasm and REM sleep. Am J Med Sci 1973; 265:419–422.
26. Kirby DA, Verrier RL. Differential effects of sleep stage on coronary hemodynamic function during stenosis. Physiol Behav 1989; 45:1017–1020.
27. Tofler GH, Brezinski D, Schafer AI, Czeisler CA, Rutherford JD, Willich SN, Gleason RE, Williams GH, Muller JE. Concurrent morning increase in platelet aggregability and the risk of myocardial infarction and sudden cardiac death. N Engl J Med 1987; 316:1514–1518.
28. Morgan BJ, Crabtree DC, Puleo DS, Badr MS, Toiber F, Skatrud JB. Neurocirculatory consequences of abrupt changes in sleep state in humans. J Appl Physiol 1996; 80:1627–1636.
29. Mancia G. Autonomic modulation of the cardiovascular system during sleep. N Engl J Med 1993; 328:347–349.
30. Hayreh SS, Zimmerman MB, Podhajsky P, Alward WL. Nocturnal arterial hypotension and its role in optic nerve head and ocular ischemic disorders. Am J Ophthalmol 1994; 117:603–624.
31. Kario K, Motai K, Mitsuhashi T, Suzuki T, Nakagawa Y, Ikeda U, Matsuo T, Nakayama T, Shimada K. Autonomic nervous system dysfunction in elderly hypertensive patients with abnormal diurnal variation: relation to silent cerebrovascular disease. Hypertension 1997; 30:1504–1510.
32. Daugherty RM Jr, Scott JB, Dabney JM, Haddy FJ. Local effects of O_2 and CO_2 on limb, renal, and coronary vascular resistances. Am J Physiol 1967; 213:1102–1110.
33. Wade JG, Larson Jr CP, Hickey RF, Ehrenfeld WK, Severinghaus JW. Effect of carotid endarterectomy on carotid chemoreceptor and baroreceptor function in man. N Engl J Med 1970; 282:823–829.
34. Lugliani RB, Whipp BJ, Seard C, Wasserman K. Effect of bilateral carotid-body resection on ventilatory control at rest and during exercise in man. N Engl J Med 1971; 285:1105–1111.

35. Gelfand R, Lambertsen CJ. Dynamic respiratory response to abrupt change of in-spired CO_2 at normal and high PO_2. J Appl Physiol 1973; 35:903–913.
36. Somers VK, Zavala DC, Mark AL, Abboud FM. Contrasting effects of hypoxia and hypercapnia on ventilation and sympathetic activity in humans. J Appl Physiol 1989; 67:2101–2106.
37. Somers VK, Zavala DC, Mark AL, Abboud FM. Influence of ventilation and hypo-capnia on sympathetic nerve responses to hypoxia in normal humans. J Appl Physiol 1989; 67:2095–2100.
38. Somers VK, Abbound FM. Chemoreflexes—responses, interactions and implica-tions for sleep apnea. Sleep 1993; 16:S30–S34.
39. Kales A, Cadieux RJ, Shaw LC, Vela Bueno A, Bixler EO, Schneck DW, Locke TW, Soldatos CR. Sleep apnoea in a hypertensive population. Lancet 1984; 2:1005–1008.
40. Young T, Peppard P, Palta M, Hla KM, Finn L, Morgan B, Skatrud J. Population-based study of sleep-disordered breathing as a risk factor for hypertension. Arch Intern Med 1997; 157:1746–1752.
41. Przybylski J, Trzebski A, Czyzewski T, Jodkowski J. Responses to hyperoxia, hy-poxia, hypercapnia and almitrine in spontaneously hypertensive rats. Bull Eur Physi-opathol Respir 1982; 18:145–154.
42. Trzebski A, Tafil M, Zoltowski M, Przybylski J. Increased sensitivity of the arterial chemoreceptor drive in young men with mild hypertension. Cardiovasc Res 1982; 16:163–172.
43. Somers VK, Mark AL, Abboud F. Potentiation of sympathetic nerve responses to hypoxia in borderline hypertensive subjects. Hypertension 1988; 11:608–612.
44. Heistad DD, Abboud FM, Mark AL, Schmid PG. Interaction of baroreceptor and chemoreceptor reflexes: modulation of the chemoreceptor reflex by changes in baro-receptor activity. J Clin Invest 1974; 53:1226–1236.
45. Somers VK, Mark AL, Abboud FM. Interaction of baroreceptor and chemoreceptor reflex control of sympathetic nerve activity in normal humans. J Clin Invest 1991; 87:1953–1957.
46. Rea RF, Berg WJ. Abnormal baroreflex mechanisms in congestive heart failure: recent insights. Circulation 1990; 81:2026–2027.
47. Ferguson DW, Berg WJ, Roach PJ, Oren RM, Mark AL. Effects of heart failure on baroreflex control of sympathetic neural activity. Am J Cardiol 1992; 69:523–531.
48. Condos WR, Latham RD, Hoadley SD, Pasipoularides A. Hemodynamics of the Mueller maneuver in man: right and left heart micromanometry and Doppler echo-cardiography. Circulation 1987; 76:1020–1028.
49. Scharf SM, Brown R, Warner KG, Khuri S. Intrathoracic pressures and left ventricu-lar configuration with respiratory maneuvers. J Appl Physiol 1989; 66:481–491.
50. Somers VK, Dyken ME, Skinner JL. Autonomic and hemodynamic responses and introduction during the Mueller maneuver in humans. J Auton Nerv Syst 1993; 44: 253–259.
51. de Burgh Daly M, Angell-James JE, Elsner R. Role of carotid-body chemoreceptors and their reflex interactions in bradycardia and cardiac arrest. Lancet 1979; 1:764–767.
52. de Burgh Daly M, Scott MJ. An analysis of the primary cardiovascular reflex effects

of stimulation of the carotid body chemoreceptors in the dog. Am J Physiol 1962; 162:555–573.

53. Somers VK, Dyken ME, Mark AL, Abboud FM. Parasympathetic hyperresponsiveness and bradyarrhythmias during apnoea in hypertension. Clin Auton Res 1992; 2: 171–176.

54. Baruzzi A, Riva R, Cirignotta F, Zucconi M, Cappelli M, Lugaresi E. Atrial natriuretic peptide and catecholamines in obstructive sleep apnea syndrome. Sleep 1991; 14:83–86.

55. Dimsdale JE, Coy T, Ziegler MG, Ancoli-Israel S, Clausen J. The effect of sleep apnea on plasma and urinary catecholamines. Sleep 1995; 18:377–381.

56. Fletcher EC, Miller J, Schaaf JW, Fletcher JG. Urinary catecholamines before and after tracheostomy in patients with obstructive sleep apnea and hypertension. Sleep 1987; 10:35–44.

57. Carlson JT, Hedner J, Elam M, Ejnell H, Sellgren J, Wallin BG. Augmented resting sympathetic activity in awake patients with obstructive sleep apnea. Chest 1993; 103:1763–1768.

58. Somers VK, Dyken ME, Clary MP, Abboud FM. Sympathetic neural mechanisms in obstructive sleep apnea. J Clin Invest 1995; 96:1897–1904.

59. Narkiewicz K, van de Borne PJH, Cooley RL, Dyken ME, Somers VK. Sympathetic activity in obese subjects with and without obstructive sleep apnea. Circulation 1998; 98:772–776.

60. Narkiewicz K, Montano N, Cogliati N, van de Borne PJH, Dyken ME, Somers VK. Altered cardiovascular variability in obstructive sleep apnea. Circulation 1998; 98: 1071–1077.

61. Frattola A, Parati G, Cuspidi C, Albini F, Mancia G. Prognostic value of 24-hour blood pressure variability. J Hypertens 1993; 11:1133–1137.

62. Palatini P, Penzo M, Racioppa A, Zugno E, Guzzardi G, Anaclerio M, Pessina AC. Clinical relevance of nighttime blood pressure and of daytime blood pressure variability. Arch Intern Med 1992; 152:1855–1860.

63. Narkiewicz K, van de Borne PJH, Montano N, Dyken M, Phillips BG, Somers VK. The contribution of tonic chemoreflex activation to sympathetic activity and blood pressure in patients with obstructive sleep apnea. Circulation 1998; 97:943–945.

64. Pinto JM, Garpestad E, Weiss JW, Bergau DM, Kirby DA. Hemodynamic changes associated with obstructive sleep apnea followed by arousal in a porcine model. J Appl Physiol 1993; 75:1439–1443.

65. Narkiewicz K, Somers VK. The sympathetic nervous system and obstructive sleep apnea: implications for hypertension. J Hypertens 1997; 15:1613–1619.

66. Guilleminault C, Connolly S, Winkle R, Melvin K, Tilkian A. Cyclical variation of the heart rate in sleep apnoea syndrome: mechanisms, and usufulness of 24 h electrocardiography as a screening technique. Lancet 1984; 1:126–131.

67. Guilleminault C, Connolly SJ, Winkle RA. Cardiac arrhythmia and conduction disturbances during sleep in 400 patients with sleep apnea sydrome. Am J Cardiol 1983; 52:490–494.

68. Tilkian AR, Guilleminault C, Schroeder JS, Lehrman KL, Simmons BL, Dement WC. Sleep induced apnea syndrome: relevance of cardiac arrhythmias and their reversal after tracheostomy. Am J Med 1977; 63:348–358.

69. Zwillich C, Devlin T, White D, Douglas N, Weil J, Martin R. Bradycardia during sleep apnea. J Clin Invest 1982; 69:1286–1292.

70. Verdecchia P, Schillaci G, Guerrieri M, Gatteschi C, Benemio G, Boldrini F, Porcellati C. Circadian blood pressure changes and left ventricular hypertrophy in essential hypertension. Circulation 1990; 81:528–536.

71. Verdecchia P, Schillaci G, Gatteschi C, Zampi I, Battistelli M, Bartoccini C, Porcellati C. Blunted nocturnal fall in blood pressure in hypertensive women with future cardiovascular morbid events. Circulation 1993; 88:986–992.

72. Pankow W, Nabe B, Lies A, Becker H, Kohler U, Kohn F-V, Lohmann FW. Influence of sleep apnea on 24-hour blood pressure. Chest 1997; 112:1253–1258.

73. Lavie P, Yoffe N, Berger I, Peled R. The relationship between the severity of sleep apnea syndrome and 24-h blood pressure values in patients with obstructive sleep apnea. Chest 1993; 103:717–721.

74. Portaluppi F, Provini F, Cortelli P, Plazzi G, Bertozzi N, Manfredini R, Fersini C, Lugaresi E. Undiagnosed sleep-disordered breathing among male nondippers with essential hypertension. J Hypertension 1997; 15:1227–1233.

75. Wilcox I, Grunstein RR, Hedner JA, Doyle J, Collins FL, Fletcher PJ, Kelly DT, Sullivan CE. Effect of nasal continuous positive airway pressure during sleep on 24-hour blood pressure in obstructive sleep apnea. Sleep 1993; 16:539–544.

76. Suzuki M, Otsuka K, Guilleminault C. Long-term nasal continuous positive airway pressure administration can normalize hypertension in obstructive sleep apnea patients. Sleep 1993; 16:545–549.

77. Stenlof K, Grunstein R, Hedner J, Sjostrom L. Energy expenditure in obstructive sleep apnea: effects of treatment with continuous positive airway pressure. Am J Physiol 1996; 271:E1036–E1043.

78. Waradekar NV, Sinoway LI, Zwillich CW, Leuenberger UA. Influence of treatment on muscle sympathetic nerve activity in sleep apnea. Am J Respir Crit Care Med 1996; 153:1333–1338.

79. Vgontzas AN, Tan TL, Bixler EO, Martin LF, Shubert D, Kales A. Sleep apnea and sleep disruption in obese patients. Arch Intern Med 1994; 154:1705–1711.

7

Mechanisms of Acute and Chronic Blood Pressure Elevation in Animal Models of Obstructive Sleep Apnea

C. D. SCHAUB, H. SCHNEIDER, and C. P. O'DONNELL

Johns Hopkins University
Baltimore, Maryland

I. Introduction

Human obstructive sleep apnea (OSA) is associated with an increased risk of cardiovascular morbidity and mortality (1–6). The existence of a direct link between the sleep and respiratory disturbances of OSA and adverse cardiovascular outcomes is a matter of considerable debate. What it is agreed, however, is that obstruction of the upper airway during sleep produces acute surges in systemic and pulmonary artery pressures that match the periodicity of the apnea (7–11). These acute cardiovascular events at night may be responsible for the development of cardiovascular morbidity and mortality in OSA patients.

Despite strong associations between OSA and adverse cardiovascular outcomes in humans, a cause-and-effect relationship has yet to be established. The presence of confounding and comorbid conditions in humans with OSA complicates the interpretation of clinical studies. This has led several investigators to develop animal models to investigate cardiovascular outcomes in OSA (12–18).

Animal models can closely simulate the sleep, respiratory, and cardiovascular disturbances of OSA. In particular, experimentally inducing upper airway obstructions in a sleeping dog can accurately reproduce the acute surges in systemic and pulmonary artery pressures present in human OSA (19–21). A recent study has examined the cardiovascular consequences of chronic OSA in a canine model, demonstrating that several weeks of nighttime OSA in normal animals results in chronic daytime hypertension (22). Thus, the development of an animal model has established a cause-and-effect relationship between OSA and cardiovascular morbidity.

A further advantage of animal models is their ability to provide mechanistic insight. It is possible to control and independently manipulate many of the primary disturbances in sleep and breathing that characterize OSA. At the same time, invasive techniques can be used to measure cardiovascular parameters not possible in OSA patients. Thus, animal models allow systematic manipulation and control of the primary events of OSA while examining multiple cardiovascular outputs.

Classic physiological studies have examined individually the effects of many of the components of apnea, such as the effects of intrathoracic pressure (ITP) swings and hypoxia, on cardiovascular parameters. In Section II, we discuss the insights that can be gained by reviewing classic physiological literature. However, studying the effects of each component of apnea in isolation may fail to fully characterize the cardiovascular changes taking place during OSA. Instead, an integrated approach may be necessary to accurately determine the acute and chronic cardiovascular responses to airway occlusion during sleep. The major focus of this chapter is to review how studies from animal models of OSA have provided mechanistic insight into the cardiovascular disturbances of OSA. In particular, we build a case for hypoxia playing a dominant role in the acute and chronic cardiovascular abnormalities of OSA.

II. Obstructive Sleep Apnea: A Mueller Maneuver, a Breath-Hold/Diving Reflex, and a State Change?

Three separate areas of physiological study overlap to simulate the disturbances taking place in OSA. The first is that of the mechanical interactions that can occur between the heart and lungs during the obstructed inspiratory efforts that characterize OSA. The Mueller maneuver (i.e., voluntary inspiratory efforts against a closed glottis) is a classic method for studying such mechanical effects of respiration on the circulation (23). The second is the development of a progressive hypoxic/hypercapnic stimulus in the absence of ventilation that is characteristic of the breath-hold or diving reflex (24,25). Finally, the perpetual cycling of sleep and arousal will produce distinct cardiovascular changes associated with transitions between sleep-wake states (26–29). Immediately below, we discuss what is understood about the cardiovascular consequences of OSA from each of these three separate areas of physiology.

The Mueller maneuver provides a simplified model of the mechanical effects of OSA on the circulation. In a Mueller maneuver, large decreases in ITP cause decreases in left ventricular stroke volume (LVSV) and increases in right ventricular stroke volume (RVSV) (23,30–32). As a result of these opposite yet simultaneous changes in stroke volume, blood pools in the pulmonary circulation (23). We would expect that the ITP swings during OSA would cause similar alterations in LVSV and RVSV. However, in OSA, unlike the Mueller maneuver, it is possible that the blood pooled in the pulmonary circulation redistributes itself during the "expiratory" phase between the brief obstructed inspiratory efforts. Thus, the Mueller maneuver may model obstructed breathing during sleep in important ways, but it does not fully characterize the relationship between breathing and the circulation during apneic sleep.

Features of the breath-hold and diving reflex can simplify our understanding of the cardiovascular events taking place during OSA. These responses are characterized by a hypoxic stimulus coincident with an inability to move air. These circumstances lead to a unique situation in which an increase in sympathetic nerve activity to the peripheral vasculature causes a vasoconstriction (24,25), while an increase in parasympathetic activity to the heart causes a marked bradycardia (24). This acts to maintain blood flow to the heart and brain and to decrease the metabolic demands of the heart. However, at apnea termination, there is an abrupt change from obstructed to non-obstructed breathing in the face of a continuing chemical stimulus and a transient arousal from sleep. Thus, like the Mueller maneuver, the breath-hold/diving reflex provides a basis for understanding the cardiovascular disturbances taking place during OSA, but important questions about events unique to OSA must still be addressed.

OSA is associated with recurrent changes in sleep-wake states (33). At apnea termination, patients progress from either non–rapid-eye-movement (NREM) or rapid-eye-movement (REM) sleep to an aroused state of transient wakefulness (33,34). The transition to wakefulness is accompanied by tachycardia and elevated blood pressure (26–29). However, at the time of arousal, immediately after the apneic period, many other factors, such as hypoxia or the resumption of ventilation, may also produce cardiovascular disturbances.

Clearly, OSA is more complicated than the Mueller maneuver, the breath-hold/diving reflex models, and the state change we employed to simplify the situation. The interactions of large negative ITP swings, blood gas disturbances, arousal, and sleep obscures the role that each plays in the hemodynamic changes occurring in response to an apneic event. Because of the complexity of OSA, animal models have been used to control for these factors unique to apnea in order to understand the physiological and pathophysiological effects on the heart and circulation.

III. Cardiovascular Responses in Animal Models of OSA

Significant advancements have recently been made in understanding the cardiovascular responses to the physiological stresses caused by OSA. In reviewing literature that has examined the cardiovascular effects of OSA, we focus in particular on animal models of OSA, because they can simulate human OSA while

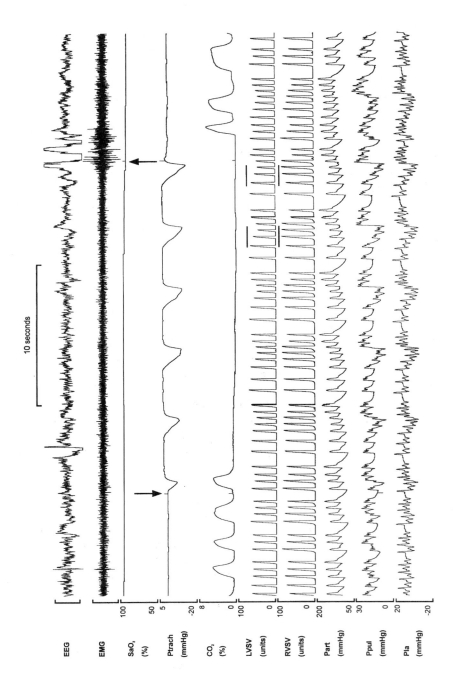

allowing us to examine specific physiological mechanisms in the absence of confounding variables. Such mechanisms include large negative ITP swings, hypoxia, hypercapnia, arousal, and hormonal alterations. All of these factors can affect hemodynamic homeostasis and may in some way contribute to detrimental effects of OSA on the cardiovascular system.

A. Intrathoracic Pressure Swings

It is well known that purely mechanical factors associated with respiration have a significant impact on the heart and circulation (35). Only recently have the effects of large negative swings in pleural pressure on cardiac and hemodynamic parameters during OSA been elucidated (15,21,36,37). Intrathoracic pressure swings in OSA, like the Mueller maneuver, disrupt left and right ventricular outputs as well as systemic and pulmonary arterial pressures. However, because ITP swings are only a transient component of an obstructive event during sleep, the evidence presented below indicates that mechanical factors of respiration play only a minor role in the hemodynamic changes taking place in OSA.

Cardiac Effects of Negative Swings in Intrathoracic Pressure

The mechanical effects of the Mueller maneuver are known to increase output from the right heart while decreasing output from the left heart (23,30–32). During a Mueller maneuver, the pressure gradient for blood to return to the heart from the peripheral vasculature increases as the pressure in the thorax decreases, leading to an increase in venous return (23,32,37). In contrast, the decrease in pleural pressure leads to an increase in left ventricular transmural pressure as the pressure gradient against which the heart must pump to expel blood from the thorax increases (35). The increase in transmural pressure can be characterized as an increase in left ventricular afterload and results in a decrease in output from the left heart (35). Thus, studies of the cardiovascular effects of the Mueller maneuver suggest that the large negative swings in ITP that occur in OSA would affect cardiac performance.

Our group used a canine model of OSA to examine the effects of upper airway obstruction during sleep on ventricular output (21). We showed that inspiratory efforts against an obstructed airway, like the Mueller maneuver, are accompanied by large and opposite fluctuations in LVSV and RVSV (Fig. 1) (21). The

---

Figure 1 Computer-generated sample trace from one animal during a single period of induced upper airway obstruction (between arrows) in NREM sleep showing EEG and nuchal EMG activity, arterial hemoglobin saturation (Sa_{O2}), tracheal pressure (Ptr), expired carbon dioxide (CO_2), left ventricular stroke volume (LVSV), right ventricular stroke volume (RVSV), systemic arterial pressure (Part), pulmonary arterial pressure (Ppul), and left atrial pressure (Pla). Horizontal lines on LVSV and RVSV traces mark the last two obstructed inspiratory efforts, during which LVSV falls and RVSV rises. (From Ref. 21.)

swings in negative pleural pressure during an obstructed inspiration decreased LVSV by a maximum of $33.8 \pm 1.0\%$ while increasing RVSV by a maximum of $14.2 \pm 6.0\%$. This is consistent with the finding of Tarasiuk and Scharf (38) that right heart blood volume increases during an obstructive apnea. On the other hand, the decrease in LVSV as pleural pressure falls (21) is presumably due to increased afterload (39) and a decreased end-diastolic volume associated with ventricular interdependence (32). Thus, during the transient periods of obstructed inspiration in OSA, the increases in RVSV and decreases in LVSV are consistent with cardiac responses to the Mueller maneuver.

As noted earlier, the mechanical heart-lung interactions of OSA are not comparable to a sustained Mueller maneuver. Rather, OSA is best modeled as a series of transient Mueller maneuvers separated by an "expiratory" phase during which ITP returns to normal. It is possible that during this expiratory phase, the increase in RVSV and decrease in LVSV that occurred during the previous obstructed inspiration could be reversed or counterbalanced. Indeed, when stroke volumes were averaged over the course of an entire respiratory cycle during an obstructive apnea, LVSV and RVSV changed identically (21). These data indicate that while the Mueller maneuver can model the cardiac changes that occur during the transient periods of obstructed inspiration, the mechanical effects on cardiac function over the course of an apnea are more complicated.

Over the course of an apneic event, there is an overall trend for LVSV and RVSV to decrease (21). This pattern of a fall in LVSV and RVSV is consistent with those reported in OSA patients (40–43). The exact mechanisms by which stroke volume falls over the course of an apnea remains to be elucidated. One likely mechanism may involve increased afterload, resulting from the peripheral vasoconstriction that develops progressively throughout the apnea. Such a hypothesis is supported by the studies of Chen and Scharf (44), who evaluated the role of ITP swings on the cardiac effects of apneas in sedated pigs. They argued that if ITP swings were significantly contributing to the cardiac effects of sleep apnea, we would expect to see more profound changes in LV function and mean arterial pressure in obstructive apneas than in central apneas, since the former are associated with swings in airway pressure. However, the authors found that indexes of LV afterload, such as LV end-systolic myocardial segment length and mean arterial pressure (MAP), increased more in central than in obstructive apnea (44). This finding implies that neural rather than mechanical factors increase LV afterload and could account for the fall in stroke volume over the course of an obstructive apnea. In summary, mechanical heart-lung interactions account for transient, opposite, and reversible changes in LVSV and RVSV during obstructed inspiratory efforts but do not appear to play a role in the overall decrease in stroke volume that occurs over the course of an entire apneic event.

Vascular Effects of Negative Intrathoracic Pressure Swings

In addition to their effect on LVSV and RVSV, ITP swings have also been implicated in blood pressure responses to obstructed breathing during sleep. Consider that during an obstructed inspiratory effort, blood pools in the pulmonary arterial circuit as venous return and left ventricular afterload both increase simultaneously (35). When the obstruction is released, the blood that has been shifted to the central compartment is discharged back into peripheral compartments, thus potentially contributing to a surge in systemic arterial pressure. Tarasiuk and Scharf (37) examined whether the combined effects of increased venous return and left ventricular afterload induced the expected increase in mean arterial pressure during obstructive apneas. They concluded that changes in venous return were not related to shifts in blood volume from peripheral to central circulations (37). This suggested that large negative decreases in ITP do not play a major role in the increase in mean arterial pressure associated with obstructive apneas.

Several other studies support the concept that changes in ITP over the course of an obstructive apnea do not contribute to an overall increase in systemic arterial pressure (17,20,44,45). In particular, Goodnight White et al. (17) examined the effect of obstructed and nonobstructed breathing on the acute systemic arterial blood pressure response to apnea in chloralose-anesthetized baboons. They found that systolic and diastolic blood pressure increased progressively over the course of an apnea to the same degree in both obstructive and nonobstructive apneas. Thus, the presence of ITP swings does not influence the degree of acute hypertension associated with an apnea.

Swings in Intrathoracic Pressure and Sustained Hypertension

The above discussion argues that the transient changes in ITP do not play a major role in contributing to the hemodynamic changes that occur in response to a single apnea. It would, therefore, be unlikely that ITP changes during sleep with obstructed breathing would significantly contribute to sustained hemodynamic changes in response to multiple or chronic apneas. However, no study to date has attempted to examine whether repetitive, transient ITP changes at nighttime, in the absence of blood gas disturbances and arousals, can produce sustained hypertension. Such a study is perhaps unattractive in view of the positive evidence relating hypoxemia to nighttime and daytime hypertension discussed in Section III.B.

B. Hypoxia

It is well known that OSA patients become progressively more hypoxic throughout the duration of an obstructed apnea (9). In fact, episodic hypoxia is one of the defining characteristics of OSA. Animal models of OSA have demonstrated a strong cause-and-effect relationship between hypoxia and acute (45) and chronic (46) blood pressure elevations. In particular, Fletcher et al. have developed a rat model of exposure to intermittent hypoxia for 7 hr per day. These rats develop sustained daytime hypertension within just a few weeks (46). A chronic canine model of OSA also developed sustained daytime hypertension (Fig. 2) (22) in a time period comparable to the rat model of intermittent hypoxia. Taken together, these two animal models provide a strong argument that the intermittent hypoxia of OSA leads to systemic hypertension. In the discussion that follows, we detail the pathways and mechanisms by which hypoxia causes cardiac and vascular disturbances in response to OSA.

Hypoxia and Peripheral Chemoreceptors

Several lines of evidence suggest that hypoxia causes vasoconstriction of the systemic vasculature by stimulating peripheral chemoreceptors. The linear relationship between Sa_{O_2} and blood pressure during apnea in the sleeping dog (19) suggests that chemoreceptor stimulation is an important mechanism in the apnea-associated blood pressure elevation. To more directly determine the afferent mechanisms that modulate sympathetic nerve activity (SNA) to the vasculature, we measured neural output from the peripheral chemoreceptors during apnea in the anesthetized cat (18). We found that apnea increased carotid sinus nerve activity from the carotid chemoreceptors in the cat concomitantly with an increase in renal SNA and systemic blood pressure. Hypoxia was the dominant factor stimulating the carotid chemoreceptors, since apneas induced in the presence of

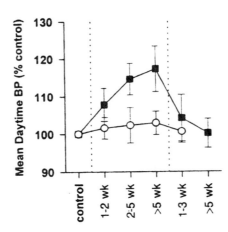

Figure 2 Mean daytime arterial BP during periods of OSA (filled squares) and sleep fragmentation (open circles) in four dogs. The dashed lines represent the beginning and end of either the OSA or sleep fragmentation phase. (From Ref. 22. Copyright 1997 American Society for Clinical Investigation.)

100% oxygen reduced both sinus nerve output and renal SNA by approximately 80% and abolished the acute hypertensive response (18). Thus peripheral chemoreceptor stimulation by hypoxia during apnea is associated with an acute increase in blood pressure.

If hypoxia affects blood pressure through the carotid chemoreceptors, we would predict that denervating the carotid chemoreceptors should eliminate the hypertensive response to apnea. Fletcher et al. (47) examined the chronic effects of episodic hypoxia on MAP in rats that had undergone bilateral carotid denervation. Rats with sectioned carotid sinus nerves exhibited no increase in MAP above baseline after 35 days of episodic hypoxia. This provided evidence that episodic hypoxia can induce hypertension via peripheral chemoreceptor neuronal pathways. An important note is that it is the administration of episodic as opposed to chronic, continuous hypoxia that increases MAP. Other animal studies, such as that by Henley and Tucker (48), show that chronic exposure to a hypoxic stimulus can actually prevent the development of systemic hypertension in spontaneously hypertensive rats. Episodic hypoxia also reflects better than continuous hypoxia the intermittent oxygen desaturation experienced by OSA patients. Thus, the findings of the Fletcher group extend the results of short-term studies by demonstrating that, over a period of weeks, continuous, episodic hypoxia can chronically elevate MAP by acting through carotid chemoreceptors.

Hypoxia and Stimulation of the Autonomic Nervous System (ANS)

Hypoxia acts through the ANS to produce acute increases in systemic arterial blood pressure. We have made direct measurements of renal SNA to dissect the afferent mechanisms that modulate sympathetic activity to the peripheral vasculature during and after apnea in anesthetized cats (18) (Fig. 3). Apneas were induced with the animal breathing either room air or 100% oxygen. We demonstrated that breathing hyperoxia caused large decreases in the renal SNA and blood pressure response to apnea. Thus, hypoxic stimulation of the carotid chemoreceptors caused the large increase in renal SNA and blood pressure during apnea. This excitatory stimulus to renal SNA from the chemoreceptors overwhelms simultaneous inhibitory input from arterial baroreceptors as blood pressure rises over the course of the apnea. At apnea termination, however, renal SNA falls precipitously in the presence of an elevated systemic blood pressure. The sudden fall in SNA after apnea results from a unique interaction between sustained inhibitory input from arterial baroreceptors and a sudden withdrawal of excitatory input from chemoreceptors (Fig. 3). Hypoxic stimulation of chemoreceptors, therefore, is the dominant afferent input increasing renal SNA in response to apnea.

Hypoxia also acts through the ANS to chronically elevate blood pressure in response to episodic hypoxia (49). Fletcher and colleagues extended this work

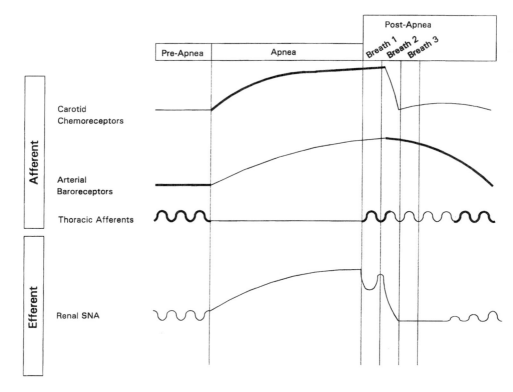

Figure 3 Schematic representation of the effect of afferent input from carotid chemore-ceptors, arterial baroreceptors, and thoracic afferents on efferent renal sympathetic nerve activity (SNA) before, during, and after a 60-sec period of apnea induced at end-expiration in the paralyzed, anesthetized cat breathing room air. The thick black line indicates over which periods each of these three afferent inputs acts to modulate renal SNA. (From Ref. 18. Copyright 1996 American Lung Association.)

further by elucidating the contribution of the renal artery sympathetic nerves and adrenal medulla in the hypoxia-induced increases in diurnal blood pressure (50). Performing studies in rats that had undergone demedullation and renal artery denervation, they showed that episodic hypoxia did not increase diurnal MAP in rats lacking either renal artery nerves or an adrenal medulla. This implies that increases in renal SNA mediated by chemoreceptor stimulation require intact renal nerves and an adrenal medulla in order to elevate systemic blood pressure. Thus, hypoxic activation of the ANS can produce both acute and chronic eleva-tions of the systemic arterial pressure.

Hypoxia and Pulmonary Arterial Pressure

In addition to its effect on systemic arterial pressure, hypoxia also plays a central role in elevating pulmonary arterial pressure during an apnea. Iwase et al. (45) have employed an anesthetized canine model of OSA to demonstrate that the increases in pulmonary artery pressure during an apnea were qualitatively similar to increases in systemic arterial pressure. Oxygen administration eliminated the increase in pulmonary artery pressure in response to airway obstruction, and induced hypoxia, in the absence of apnea, increased pulmonary artery pressure to an extent comparable to that observed with airway obstruction. Thus hypoxemia plays a dominant role in elevations of both pulmonary and systemic arterial pressure during an apnea.

Hypoxia and Heart Rate

Heart rate is another cardiovascular parameter subject to the effects of hypoxic chemoreceptor stimulation over the course of an apnea. Hypoxic chemoreceptor stimulation produces a bradycardia when ventilation is maintained constant but induces a tachycardia when ventilation is allowed to increase (24). During obstructive and central apneas, heart rate (HR) decreases from preapnea to endapnea (38). This finding is consistent with the effect of hypoxia producing a bradycardia in the absence of an increase in ventilation (24). However, Tarasiuk and Scharf (38) showed that bradycardia was more pronounced during a central apnea compared to an obstructive apnea. This led the authors to conclude that the obstructive inspiratory efforts, while not producing ventilation, may attenuate the hypoxic bradycardia by stimulating pulmonary or chest wall afferents. Thus, the activation of these mechanoreceptors likely attenuates the HR decrease during an obstructive apnea compared to a central apnea.

At apnea termination, there is a sudden change in HR. In the chronic dog model of OSA, a significant tachycardia occurs in the period immediately after apnea (20). The two most likely physiological conditions producing this tachycardia are 1) hypoxia coincident with ventilation, as discussed above, or 2) arousal. Both these stimuli are present at the termination of an apnea. In the discussion on arousal to follow, we present evidence that it is arousal, not the hypoxic stimulus, that accounts for the rapid HR observed in the immediate postapneic period. Thus, during apnea, hypoxia causes a bradycardia that may be partially attenuated by mechanoreceptor inputs associated with obstructed inspiratory efforts. At apnea termination, the resumption of ventilation in the continuing presence of hypoxia can restore HR to preapnea levels but does not appear to account for the marked tachycardia that can occur at this time.

C. Hypercapnia

In obstructive apneas, there is some degree of CO_2 retention coincident with the presence of hypoxia. Given the potential for hypercapnia and hypoxia to work synergistically to increase muscle SNA in humans (51,52), we can reasonably suspect that hypercapnia can alter cardiovascular parameters over the course of an apnea. Our lab examined the relative contribution of hypercapnic and hypoxic stimulation of chemoreceptors in the increase in renal SNA that occurs during apnea in anesthetized cats (18). By administering 100% oxygen, we were able to remove the hypoxic stimulus during apnea. During a 20-sec apnea on 100% oxygen, we could match the Pa_{CO_2} to levels observed in apneas of the same duration on room air. Hyperoxia markedly attenuated but did not completely eliminate the SNA response to apnea (18). This small increase in renal SNA during apnea that remained after administration of 100% oxygen can potentially be ascribed to hypercapnic stimulation of chemoreceptors.

An Interaction Between Hypercapnia and Hypoxia

Although the above discussion highlights that hypercapnia alone is not a potent vasoconstricting stimulus, it may potentiate the hypoxic stimulus. Bao et al. (53) showed in their rat model of OSA that the addition of CO_2 to a hypoxic stimulus causes a greater increase in SNA and MAP as well as a larger decrease in heart rate compared with a hypocapnic hypoxic stimulus. In fact, in this study, the addition of CO_2 to a hypoxic stimulus increased the blood pressure threefold more than that observed under hypocapnic hypoxic conditions. This supports the hypothesis that an interaction between hypercapnic and hypoxic stimuli during apnea is an important contributor to the cardiovascular changes taking place in OSA.

In summary, the hypercapnic stimulation of chemoreceptors appears to play only a minor role in the nocturnal periodic hypertensive episodes that accompany apneas. However, hypercapnia can interact to exacerbate the hypoxic stimulus, and this may be particualarly important in apneas of longer duration. Thus, the consideration of mechanisms by which OSA elevates SNA and blood pressure should include a role for hypercapnia in augmenting the known potent vasoconstricting influences of hypoxia.

D. Arousal

The above discussion argues that animal studies have elucidated an important role for chemoreflexes in mediating the cardiovascular changes during OSA. However, human studies in OSA patients suggest that arousal from sleep alone can account for the majority of the acute hypertensive response to apnea. These studies employed auditory stimuli to arouse normal subjects (54) and OSA patients whose apnea was abolished by continuous positive airway pressure (55). The results indicated that auditory arousal produced a similar hypertensive response as that exhibited by patients with obstructive breathing during sleep (55). In animal studies similar techniques of induced auditory arousal have also been used to evaluate cardiovascular responses (56). In addition, experimental manipulations in a canine dog model of OSA allow a more direct evaluation of the role that specific apnea-induced arousal plays in cardiovascular responses to apnea (20,57). These animal studies discussed below suggest that arousal contributes to the acute surges in blood pressure during nighttime apneas, but arousal does not contribute to the sustained daytime hypertension of OSA.

Canine Model of OSA Separates Arousal from Other Neural Reflexes

Animal models have provided a means to separate blood pressure responses due to arousal from those due to neural reflexes (chemoreceptors) and mechanical factors (ITP swings). Our group has used a canine model of OSA to selectively eliminate the arousal response to obstructive apnea by controlling airway patency to induce apneas either with or without arousal. These apneas are identically matched for duration, changes in ITP, and arterial hemoglobin desaturation (20). As expected, the mean arterial pressure and HR responses between pre- and end-obstruction periods were not different between matched apneas terminated either with or without arousal. However, in the immediate postapneic period, the absence of arousal both significantly blunted the hypertensive response and eliminated the tachycardic response (Fig. 4) (20). Furthermore, we have shown in the same model that the arousal-induced tachycardia in the immediate postapneic period contributes to the fall in left and right ventricular stroke volume occurring at this time (57). Thus, the stimulation of respiratory afferents to induce arousal produces an important contribution to the acute cardiovascular changes that occur after apnea termination.

The efferent mechanism by which apnea-induced arousal produces tachycardia is withdrawal of parasympathetic activity to the heart. The tachycardia present after an induced apnea in the canine model could be completely eliminated by prior administration of atropine (57). Furthermore, atropine significantly attenuated the rise in systemic arterial pressure and the fall in stroke volume immediately after an apnea, suggesting that these two responses were dependent on the presence of a tachycardic response to apnea. Thus, arousal and the subsequent tachycardia represent important factors accounting for the acute hemodynamic responses in OSA.

A porcine model of OSA indicates that arousal may also increase peripheral vascular constriction (58). Furthermore, these authors have examined the central mechanisms that regulate changes in vascular resistance upon arousal. This work shows that specific regions of the brain may control changes in vascular tone in response to specific sleep events. They found that in pigs, administration of a β-adrenoreceptor antagonist (propranolol) into the lateral ventricle significantly attenuated the increase in total peripheral resistance and MAP normally seen in the arousal phase after a period of induced airway obstruction. Although not

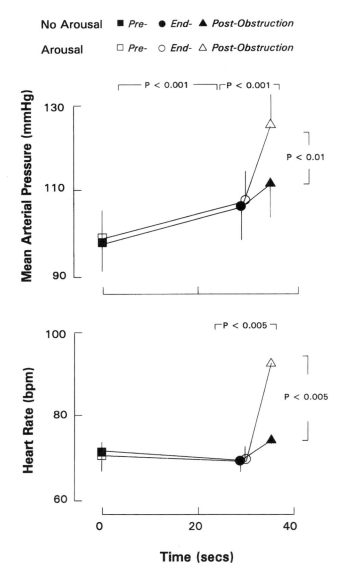

Figure 4   MAP (upper panel) and heart rate (lower panel) responses to airway obstruction with or without arousal during NREM sleep in pre-, end-, and postobstruction periods. (From Ref. 20.)

directly controlling for arousal, these data indicate that activation of β-receptors within the central nervous system (CNS) may contribute to regulation of the vascular resistance responses to arousal from sleep apnea.

While arousal plays an important role in acutely elevating blood pressure in response to sleep apnea, the work of Brooks et al. (22,56) suggests that arousal plays no significant role in sustained daytime hypertension. By controlling for postapneic arousal as a stimulus for arterial blood pressure surges, the study of Brooks et al. elucidated an important difference between the effect of OSA on daytime and nighttime hypertension. They found that while repetitive tone-induced arousals from sleep led to similar surges in nighttime blood pressure as induced airway obstruction, only OSA caused nighttime hypertension that was sustained in the daytime (22,56) (Fig. 2). This finding suggests that arousal from sleep plays an important role in transient increases in nighttime blood pressure. Thus, immediate postapneic blood pressure elevations can be largely accounted for by arousal from sleep, whereas hypoxic chemoreceptor stimulation appears capable of sustaining hypertension well beyond the termination of obstructed breathing.

E. Hormones

In the discussion so far we have addressed the mechanical and neural factors in OSA that alter cardiovascular homeostasis. It is possible that OSA could also have cardiovascular effects via hormonal pathways. It is most unlikely, however, that any vasoactive peptide could act within a single apnea to produce a cardiovascular effect. Any action of peptides in OSA would be expected to occur over hours or days. As such, the nighttime disturbances of OSA could potentially induce changes in vasoactive or volume-regulating hormones that may ramify into the following day to raise blood pressure or produce other cardiovascular abnormalities. Thus, hormones may provide a link between nighttime respiratory and sleep disturbances and sustained daytime cardiovascular morbidity.

Few animal data are available on the relationship between OSA and vasoactive hormones in animal models. Our group examined whether 12 hr of repetitive airway obstruction in a canine model could alter the plasma levels of vasoactive peptides (19). We found that the plasma levels of renin and atrial natriuretic peptide measured at 2-hr intervals did not change significantly in response to induced OSA, although renin did increase slightly in the morning after OSA was stopped. However, such a change was consistent with renin responding to rather than causing changes in blood pressure.

In clinical studies, hormone measurements have been made in OSA patients before and after treatment with continuous positive airway pressure (CPAP) (59–62). These studies suggest that OSA acts to raise atrial natriuretic peptide levels and to lower plasma renin, arginine vasopressin, and aldosterone levels (59–62).

The interpretation of these results is difficult, since CPAP will have effects on lung volume and blood volume shifts independent of removal of upper airway obstruction. The data from our canine model, which are free of any confounding effects of CPAP, indicate that vasoactive and volume-regulating hormones do not represent a major factor in the cardiovascular pathology of OSA. However, many questions remain unanswered and the use of animal models could significantly add to the data from clinical studies.

IV. Limitations of Animal Models of OSA

The limitations of animal models for the study of cardiovascular effects of OSA must also be acknowledged. These include studies performed under anesthesia (18,45), a state that does not represent sleep and can depress neural reflex loops. Some chronic animal models do not include measurements of sleep (46,47,49,50), a key variable in modifying cardiovascular responses. The porcine model of OSA appears able to sustain only relatively short periods of obstruction before arousal (58), leading one group making cardiovascular measurements in this model to perform studies after sedation (16,44). In the canine model, Kimoff et al. (13) acknowledge the potential criticism of inducing airway obstruction in the trachea and bypassing the upper airway, an area with significant implications in the development of human OSA. However, while such models may not necessarily elucidate the causes of OSA, they allow for important mechanistic studies examining the major hemodynamic consequences of OSA.

V. OSA and Confounding Disease States

Unfortunately, most people who experience obstructed breathing during sleep are not free of other comorbid conditions. Many also live with obesity, heart failure, and myocardial ischemia among other stresses to the heart. Only a small number of animal studies have attempted to examine the interaction between OSA and preexisting cardiovascular morbidity (15,16). Scharf and co-workers have shown that under conditions such as decreased coronary flow subsequent to stenosis, the hypoxia associated with an obstructive apnea leads to acute mycardial ischemia (15,16). As result of the coronary stenosis, it was not possible to increase coronary blood flow in order to compensate for hypoxic arterial blood associated with an apnea (16). This indicates how dangerous the cardiovascular consequences of OSA can be when imposed on an already impaired heart.

There are still many unanswered questions regarding the cardiovascular effects of OSA. In particular, we do not know to what extent comorbid factors such as obesity, congestive heart failure, lung disease, and primary pulmonary hypertension, for example, contribute to the harmful effects of OSA on the heart.

Animal models of OSA can provide a tool to examine these confounding variables and determine their contribution to the detrimental consequences of OSA.

VI. Summary

Obstructive sleep apnea is characterized by a unique set of physiological disturbances to the cardiovascular system. In this chapter we have examined the cardiovascular responses to the components of apnea such as hypoxia/hypercapnia, arousal, changes in intrathoracic pressure, and hormone levels. Because these disturbances overlap during an apnea, it was necessary to examine together their effects on the cardiovascular system. It appears that the neural response to hypoxia is the dominant factor in both the acute and chronic cardiovascular changes that occur during a continuous period of obstructive apneic events. Recently, the nighttime effects of OSA on mean arterial pressure has been shown to be a direct cause of daytime hypertension. Animal models of OSA will allow future studies to examine the role of comorbidity in exacerbating the detrimental cardiovascular effects of OSA.

REFERENCES

1. Hung J, Whitford EG, Parsons RW, Hillman DR. Association of sleep apnoea with myocardial infarction in men. Lancet 1990; 336:261–264.
2. Hedner J, Ejnell H, Caidahl K. Left ventricular hypertrophy independent of hypertension in patients with obstructive sleep apnoea. J Hypertens 1990; 8:941–946.
3. Guilleminault C, Connolly SJ, Winkle RA. Cardiac arrhythmia and conduction disturbances during sleep in 400 patients with sleep apnea syndrome. Am J Cardiol 1983; 52:490–494.
4. Bradley TD. Right and left ventricular functional impairment and sleep apnea. Clin Chest Med 1992; 13:459–479.
5. Peter JH, Koehler U, Grote L, Podszus T. Manifestations and consequences of obstructive sleep apnea. Eur Respir J 1995; 8:1572–1583.
6. Shepard JW Jr. Hypertension, cardiac arrhythmias, myocardial infarction, and stroke in relation to obstructive sleep apnea. Clin Chest Med 1992; 13:437–458.
7. Coccagna G, Mantovani M, Brignani F, Parchi C, Lugaresi E. Continuous recording of the pulmonary and systemic arterial pressure during sleep in syndromes of hypersomnia with periodic breathing. Bull Physiopathol Respir 1972; 8:1159–1172.
8. Tilkian AG, Guilleminault C, Schroeder JS, Lehrman KL, Simmons FB, Dement WC. Hemodynamics in sleep-induced apnea: studies during wakefulness and sleep. Ann Intern Med 1976; 85:714–719.
9. Shepard JW Jr. Hemodynamics in obstructive sleep apnea. In: Fletcher EC, ed. Abnormalities of Respiration During Sleep. Orlando, FL: Grune & Stratton, 1986:39–61.

10. Podszus T, Mayer J, Penzel T, Peter JH, von Wichert P. Nocturnal hemodynamics in patients with sleep apnea. Eur J Respir Dis 1986; 146:435–442.

11. Ringler J, Garpestad E, Basner RC, Weiss JW. Systemic blood pressure elevation after airway occlusion during NREM sleep. Am J Respir Crit Care Med 1994; 150: 1062–1066.

12. O'Donnell CP, King ED, Schwartz AR, Smith PL, Robotham JL. The effect of sleep deprivation on responses to airway obstruction in the sleeping dog. J Appl Physiol 1994; 77:1811–1818.

13. Kimoff RJ, Makino H, Horner RL, Kozar LF, Lue F, Slutsky AS, Phillipson EA. Canine model of obstructive sleep apnea: model description and preliminary application. J Appl Physiol 1994; 76:1810–1817.

14. Kirby DA, Verrier RL. Differential effects of sleep stage on coronary hemodynamic function. Am J Physiol 1989; 256:H1378–H1383.

15. Scharf SM, Graver LM, Balaban K. Cardiovascular effects of periodic occlusions of the upper airway in dogs. Am Rev Respir Dis 1992; 146:321–329.

16. Chen L, Scharf SM. Systemic and myocardial hemodynamics during periodic obstructive apneas in sedated pigs. J Appl Physiol 1998; 84:1289–1298.

17. Goodnight White S, Fletcher EC, Miller CC. Acute systemic blood pressure elevation in obstructive and nonobstructive breath hold in primates. J Appl Physiol 1995; 79:324–330.

18. O'Donnell CP, Schwartz AR, Smith PL, Robotham JL, Fitzgerald RS, Shirahata M. Reflex stimulation of renal sympathetic nerve activity and blood pressure in response to apnea. Am J Resp Crit Care Med 1996; 154:1763–1770.

19. O'Donnell CP, King ED, Schwartz AR, Robotham JL, Smith PL. The relationship between blood pressure and airway obstruction during sleep in the dog. J Appl Physiol 1994; 77:1819–1828.

20. O'Donnell CP, Ayuse T, King ED, Schwartz AR, Smith PL, Robotham JL. Airway obstruction during sleep increases blood pressure without arousal. J Appl Physiol 1996; 80:773–781.

21. Schneider H, Schaub CD, Andreoni KA, Schwartz AR, Smith PL, Robotham JL, O'Donnell, CP. Systemic and pulmonary hemodynamic responses to normal and obstructed breathing during sleep. J Appl Physiol 1997; 83:1671–1680.

22. Brooks D, Horner RL, Kozar LF, Render-Teixeira CL, Phillipson EA. Obstructive sleep apnea as a cause of systemic hypertension. J Clin Invest 1997; 99:106–109.

23. Robotham JL, Peters J. How changes in pleural and alveolar pressure cause changes in afterload and preload. In: Scharf SM, Cassidy SS, eds. Lung Biology in Health and Disease: Heart-Lung Interactions in Health and Disease. New York: Marcel Decker, 1989:251–283.

24. Daly M de B, Scott MJ. The effects of stimulation of the carotid body chemoreceptor on heart rate in the dog. J Physiol (Lond) 1958; 144:148–166.

25. Daly M de B, Scott MJ. The cardiovascular effect of hypoxia in the dog with special reference to the contribution of the carotid body chemoreceptors. J Physiol (Lond) 1962; 173:201–214.

26. Khatri IM, Freis ED. Hemodynamic changes during sleep. J Appl Physiol 1967; 22: 867–873.

27. Mancia G, Baccelli G, Adams AB, Zanchetti A. Vasomotor regulation during sleep in the cat. Am J Physiol 1971; 220:1086–1093.
28. Bristow JD, Honour AJ, Pickering TG, Sleight P. Cardiovascular and respiratory changes during sleep in normal and hypertensive subjects. Cardiovasc Res 1969; 3: 476–485.
29. Coccagna G, Mantovani M, Brignani F, Manzini A, Lugaresi E. Laboratory note: arterial pressure changes during spontaneous sleep in man. Electroencephalogr Clin Neurophysiol 1971; 31:277–281.
30. Robotham JL, Rabson J, Permutt S, Bromberger-Barnea B. Left ventricular hemodynamics during respiration. J Appl Physiol 1979; 47:1293–1303.
31. Scharf SM, Bianco JA, Tow DE, Brown R. The effects of negative intrathoracic pressure on left ventricular function in patients with coronary artery disease. Circulation 1981; 63:871–874.
32. Scharf SM, Brown R, Saunders N, Green LH. Effects of normal and loaded spontaneous inspiration on cardiovascular function. J Appl Physiol Respir Environ Exerc Physiol 1979; 47:582–590.
33. Guilleminault C. Sleep apnea syndrome: impact of sleep and sleep states. Sleep 1980; 3:227–234.
34. Ringler J, Basner RC, Shannon R, Schwartzstein R, Manning H, Weinberger SE, Weiss JW. Hypoxemia alone does not explain blood pressure elevations after obstructive apneas. J Appl Physiol 1990; 69:2143–2148.
35. Permutt S, Wise RA, Brower RG. How changes in pleural and alveolar pressure cause changes in afterload and preload. In: Scharf SM, Cassidy SS, eds. Lung Biology in Health and Disease: Heart-Lung Interactions in Health and Disease. New York: Marcel Decker, 1989:243–250.
36. Scharf SM, Graver LM, Khilnani S, Balaban K. Respiratory phasic effects of inspiratory loading on left ventricular hemodynamics in vagotomized dogs. J Appl Physiol 1992; 73:995–1003.
37. Tarasiuk A, Scharf SM. Effects of periodic obstructive apneas on venous return in closed-chest dogs. Am Rev Respir Dis 1993; 148:323–329.
38. Tarasiuk A, Scharf SM. Cardiovascular effects of periodic obstructive and central apneas in dogs. Am J Respir Crit Care Med 1994; 150:83–89.
39. Scharf SM, Brown R, Tow DE, Parisi AF. Cardiac effects of increased lung volume and decreased pleural pressure in man. J Appl Physiol Respir Environ Exerc Physiol 1979; 47:257–262.
40. Bonsignore MR, Marrone O, Romano S, Pieri D. Time course of right ventricular stroke volume and output in obstructive sleep apneas. Am J Respir Crit Care Med 1994; 149:155–159.
41. Stoohs R, Guilleminault C. Cardiovascular changes associated with obstructive sleep apnea syndrome. J Appl Physiol 1992; 72:583–589.
42. Garpestad E, Katayama H, Parker JA, Ringler J, Lilly J, Yasuda T, Moore RH, Strauss HW, Weiss JW. Stroke volume and cardiac output decrease at termination of obstructive apneas. J Appl Physiol 1992; 73:1743–1748.
43. Garpestad E, Parker JA, Katayama H, Lilly J, Yasuda T, Ringler J, Strauss HW, Weiss JW. Decrease in ventricular stroke volume at apnea termination is independent of oxygen desaturation. J Appl Physiol 1994; 77:1602–1608.

44. Chen L, Scharf SM. Comparative hemodynamic effects of periodic obstructive and simulated central apneas in sedated pigs. J Appl Physiol 1997; 83:485–494.

45. Iwase N, Kikuchi Y, Hida W, Miki H, Taguchi O, Satoh M. Effects of repetitive airway obstruction on O_2 saturation and systemic and pulmonary arterial pressure in anesthetized dogs. Am Rev Respir Dis 1992; 146:1402–1410.

46. Fletcher EC, Lesske J, Qian W, Miller CCI, Unger T. Repetitive, episodic hypoxia causes diurnal elevation of blood pressure in rats. Hypertension 1992; 19:555–561.

47. Fletcher EC, Lesske J, Behm R, Miller CCI, Stauss H, Unger T. Carotid chemoreceptors, systemic blood pressure, and chronic episodic hypoxia mimicking sleep apnea. J Appl Physiol Respir Environ Exerc Physiol 1992; 72:1978–1984.

48. Henley WN, Tucker A. Hypoxic moderation of systemic hypertension in the spontaneously hypertensive rat. Am J Physiol 1987; 252:R554–R561.

49. Fletcher EC, Lesske J, Culman J, Miller CC, Unger T. Sympathetic denervation blocks blood pressure elevation in episodic hypoxia. Hypertension 1992;20:612–619.

50. Bao G, Metreveli N, Li R, Taylor A, Fletcher EC. Blood pressure response to chronic episodic hypoxia: role of the sympathetic nervous system. J Appl Physiol 1997; 83:95–101.

51. Somers VK, Mark AL, Zavala DC, Abboud FM. Contrasting effects of hypoxia and hypercapnia on ventilation and sympathetic activity in humans. J Appl Physiol 1989; 67:2101–2106.

52. Ejnell HJ, Hedner J, Caidahl K, Sellgren J, Wallin G. Increased sympathetic activity as possible etiology of hypertension and left ventricular hypertrophy in patients with obstructive sleep apnea. In: Peter J, et al, eds. Sleep and Health Risk. Berlin: Springer-Verlag, 1991:341–347.

53. Bao G, Randhawa PM, Fletcher EC. Acute blood pressure elevation during repetitive hypocapnic and eucapnic hypoxia in rats. J Appl Physiol 1997; 82:1071–1078.

54. Davies RJ, Belt PJ, Roberts SJ, Ali NJ, Stradling JR. Arterial blood pressure responses to graded transient arousal from sleep in normal humans. J Appl Physiol 1993; 74:1123–1130.

55. Ringler J, Basner RC, Shannon R, Schwartzstein R, Manning H, Weinberger SE, Weiss JW. Hypoxemia alone does not explain blood pressure elevations after obstructive apneas. J Appl Physiol 1990; 69:2143–2148.

56. Brooks D, Horner RL, Kimoff RJ, Kozar LF, Render-Teixeira CL, Phillipson EA. Effect of obstructive sleep apnea versus sleep fragmentation on responses to airway occlusion. Am J Respir Crit Care Med 1997; 155:1609–1617.

57. Schneider H, Andreoni K, Chen CA, Schaub CD, Smith PL, Schwartz AR, Robotham, JL, O'Donnell, CP. Mechanisms of arousal induced arterial blood pressure increases in obstructive sleep apnea. Am J Respir Crit Care Med 1998; 157:A777.

58. Zinkovska S, Kirby DA. Intracerebroventricular propranolol prevented vascular resistance increases on arousal from sleep apnea. J Appl Physiol 1997; 82:1637–1643.

59. Ehlenz K, Peter JH, Dugi K, Firle K, Goubeaud R, Weber K, et al. Changes in volume- and pressure-regulating hormone systems during nasal CPAP therapy in patients with obstructive sleep apnea syndrome. In: Peter J, et al, eds. Sleep and Health Risk. Berlin: Springer-Verlag, 1991:518–531.

60. Ehlenz K, Peter JH, Schneider H, Elle T, Scheere B, von Wichert P, Kaffarnik H.

Renin secretion is substantially influenced by obstructive sleep apnea syndrome. Sleep 1990; 90:193–195.

61. Krieger J, Follenius M, Sforza E, Brandenberger G, Peter JD. Effects of treatment with nasal continuous positive airway pressure on atrial natriuretic peptide and arginine vasopressin release during sleep in patients with obstructive sleep apnoea. Clin Sci 1991; 80:443–449.

62. Follenius M, Krieger J, Krauth MO, Sforza F, Brandenberger G. Obstructive sleep apnea treatment: peripheral and central effects on plasma renin activity and aldosterone. Sleep 1991; 14:211–217.

8

Influence of Hypoxia, Chemoreceptors, and Sympathetic Activity in Chronic Hypertension in the Rat

EUGENE C. FLETCHER and GANG BAO

University of Louisville School of Medicine
Louisville, Kentucky

I. Introduction

As discussed in previous chapters of this text, systemic hypertension can be found in up to 90% of obstructive sleep apnea (OSA) patients (1–3). In Chapter 12, Young and Peppard address the prevalence of systemic hypertension associated with OSA in the general population. Several publications indicate that sleep apnea syndrome can be found in 30–35% of patients with primary systemic hypertension (4–7). While not all epidemiological studies agree, there is a growing consensus among sleep disorders investigators that OSA in a risk factor for systemic hypertension, independent of obesity and age.

In Chapters 5 and 6, the interaction of sleep with the cardiovascular system is discussed in detail. Acute apnea is accompanied by several autonomic responses, including marked increase in blood pressure (BP), tachycardia-bradycardia, elevation of intracranial pressure, and other hemodynamic and neurological changes. An analysis of the contributory mechanisms to the acute rise in BP is elegantly described by Schout and colleagues; the reader is referred to Chapter 7 in this text as well as a recent publication for further detailed reading (8). In both experimental animals as well as humans, closely repetitive apneas show not only an acute BP rise with each apnea but also a gradual rise in baseline BP, which is extended well beyond termination of the apneas (9). This, as well as epidemiological data, supports the conclusion that repetitive apneas can lead to a form of secondary systemic hypertension. Some even feel that snoring and repetitive sleep apnea are major contributors to the pool of patients labeled with "idiopathic systemic hypertension."

Both animal and human studies provide the opportunity for us to study in depth the relationship between apnea and its *acute* cardiovascular changes. On the other hand, it may take years for repetitive apnea to lead to sustained diurnal systemic hypertension in patients with this disease. Thus, several groups are now working on animal preparations in which recurrent events during sleep can be induced over a period of weeks or months to test the hypothesis that apnea/hypoxia leads to chronic sustained BP elevation. Horner has discussed one such model in the dog (10,11). This chapter discusses the use of an episodic hypoxia rat (EHR) preparation in which rats are exposed to recurrent short periods of episodic hypoxia (EH) for 8 hr per day over a 35-day period to induce sustained elevation of daytime BP. Of note is that, currently, 70% of hypertension research is carried out in rodents because of the many similarities of BP and cardiovascular response between these animals and humans. Given the short life span of a rat, many of the models of chronic renal and endocrine hypertension paralleling human clinical disease can be studied in greater depth in these animals than is possible in humans.

II. The Chronic Episodic Hypoxia Model

Hypoxia is a serious threat to mammals because it jeopardizes organ metabolism and function. Acute hypoxia leads to stimulation of the peripheral chemoreceptors, which, in turn, directly increases sympathetic outflow. It has long been known that epinephrine is excreted into adrenal venous blood during asphyxia, stimulating sympathoadrenal-renal discharge to counter the stress of oxygen lack (12,13). Norepinephrine is a ganglionic neurotransmitter of the peripheral sympathetic nervous system (SNS) and adrenal medulla. The adrenal medulla and the peripheral SNS act together during hypoxia to preserve homeostasis by increasing cardiac output, modifying blood flow distribution, and altering metabolism to improve oxygen delivery to vital tissues. With this background, we developed a method of providing recurrent short periods of hypoxia to rats for 35 days, episodically stimulating the chemoreceptors and the SNS to examine the cardiovascular response of this animal to recurrent EH.

From 1990–1992 we designed and constructed 25 chambers where small animals could be exposed to rapid swings in ambient oxygen concentration (FI_{O_2}) which induced changes in oxygen saturation (Sa_{O_2}) similar to that seen in humans with sleep apnea (Figs. 1 and 2). The animals are housed in identical cylindrical Plexiglas chambers (length 28 cm, diameter 10 cm, volume 2.4 L) with snug-fitting lids. Using a timed solenoid valve, nitrogen (100%) is distributed to each chamber for 12 sec at a flow that is adjusted to reduce the F_{IO_2} to 3–5% for approximately 3–6 sec. This is followed by infusion of compressed air, allowing gradual return (over 15–18 sec) to an F_{IO_2} of 20.9%. The cycle is repeated twice per minute during the day for 6 to 8 hr on consecutive days. Multiple serial arterial blood samples as well as continuous arterial catheter oximetry monitoring during episodic hypoxia have shown the average nadir level of Sa_{O_2} in this system to be 70% (range 60 to 80%) (Fig. 2).

At the same time nitrogen is being distributed to hypoxic chambers, compressed air at approximately the same liter flow is distributed to sham cages simulating the same noise and air disturbance. A dampening device at the intake end of the chamber is used to dissipate the airstream so that no direct gas jets

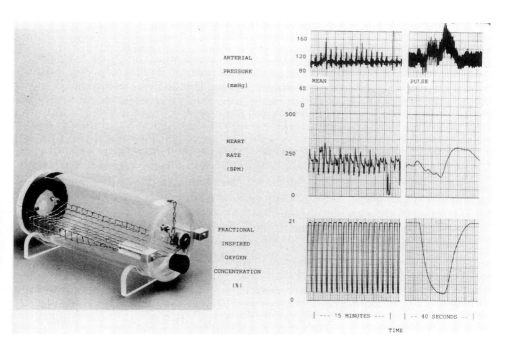

Figure 1 Normobaric chamber where infusion of N_2 and CO_2 lowers F_{IO_2} or raises F_{ICO_2}, creating transient hypoxia or asphyxia. Infusion of gases lasts about 12 sec (with a range of 6–14 sec), followed by compressed air for the balance of each 30-sec cycle. Tracing at the right shows a hypertensive response to acute hypoxia at slow-and high-speed traces. The rat is conscious and unrestrained during these studies. (From Ref. 57.)

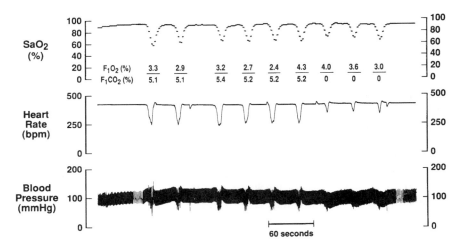

Figure 2 Example of continuous oxyhemoglobin saturation change (Sa_{O_2}) (top channel), continuous heart rate (middle channel), and blood pressure (bottom channel) in a single rat undergoing acute episodic hypoxia challenge (FI_{O_2} (%) is indicated in the numerator) with and without added CO_2 (FI_{CO_2} (%) is indicated in the denominator). At the end of the sixth desaturation, the added CO_2 is cut off, with rapid return to hypocapnic hypoxia, reducing the bradycardia and blood pressure response. The continuous Sa_{O_2} was measured with an indwelling fiberoptic catheter placed in the carotid artery of the rat.

disturb the animal. The tubing to the system can be manipulated to combine nitrogen with varying concentrations of CO_2 such that both eucapnia and hypercapnia can be induced along with the hypoxia, creating asphyxia (Fig. 2). Thus, any blood gas change associated with apnea can be simulated in this model and administered chronically.

It is important to note that the rat is nocturnal and sleeps during the day. Thus, the 8-hr EH exposure period is during the usual sleep cycle of the rat. Behaviorally, the rats do continue to sleep during the day (albeit with disturbed sleep) throughout the 35-day cycle.

The first publication describing the EHR model demonstrated that repetitive EH patterned after that seen in sleep apnea can contribute to persistent mean arterial pressure (MAP) elevation (14). Six Sprague-Dawley rats were subjected to intermittent hypoxia, 8 hr per day for 35 days, while 6 controls were placed in similar chambers for the same time period but exposed only to exchanges of compressed air. Measuring BP by the tail cuff method revealed a 21-mmHg increase in diurnal (nonhypoxic) systolic BP ($p < 0.05$), while the sham controls and four unhandled controls showed no change from baseline measurements. A similar study was performed using Wistar Thomae rats in which BP was measured intra-arterially. This time, some rats were removed from EH at 20, 30, and 35 days. There was a progressive increase in MAP among the three groups, with the 35-day Wistar EHR showing a 13.7-mmHg increase in MAP (Fig. 3). Sham (compressed air) and unhandled controls showed no MAP change (14).

III.   The Sympathetic Nervous System and BP in Chronic Episodic Hypoxia

Since we hypothesized that EH stimulated carotid chemoreceptors and thereby induced increased sympathetic activity, our next two studies examined the role of chemoreceptors and the peripheral sympathetic nervous system (SNS) in producing the diurnal BP increase in the EHR (15,16). Carotid-body denervation was performed on two groups of male Wistar rats by severing both carotid sinus nerves (15). A sham-operated, nondenervated group exposed to EH displayed a 13-mmHg increase in MAP while carotid body–denervated rats exposed to EH showed no change. Unhandled sham-operated rats and unhandled carotid body–denervated rats showed no significant change in BP from baseline (Fig. 4). This study showed that intact peripheral chemoreceptors were necessary for the BP to increase in response to chronic EH.

A similar study examined the role of the peripheral SNS in the EHR (16). Chemical sympathectomy was performed using a drug (6-OH dopamine) that accumulates only at norepinephrine uptake sites, destroying nerve synapses of the peripheral SNS. Intrinsically, the adrenals are not affected, but any sympathetic innervation to the adrenals would be damaged. Two intraperitoneal injections of 6-OH dopamine were given 20 days apart in two groups of male Wistar Thomae rats, one subjected to EH and one remaining unhandled (16). A third group received only vehicle but was subjected to EH. Rats injected with vehicle and exposed to EH showed a 7.7-mmHg increase (post 40 days) in MAP above baseline while the 6-OH dopamine injected, EH and unhandled controls showed no change in MAP. Measurement of catecholamines in cardiac muscle homogenate confirmed sympathetic denervation in 6-OH dopamine animals. The results showed that the SNS plays a major role in the diurnal BP increase in the EHR.

From the above study, it appeared certain that the SNS is greatly involved in the *chronic* BP response to EH. We performed a series of acute studies to confirm this by direct measurement of sympathetic nerve activity and blockade of the peripheral sympathetic receptors (17). This study examined whether episodic eucapnic hypoxia was a more potent stimulus to *acute* BP elevation than episodic hypocapnic hypoxia, as well as the role of the sympathetic and parasympathetic nervous systems in the heart rate and BP response. The techniques of invasive BP measurement describe above were used. Prazosin (an α_1-adrenergic blocker), yohimbine (α_2-adrenergic blocker) and atropine were used to block sympathetic

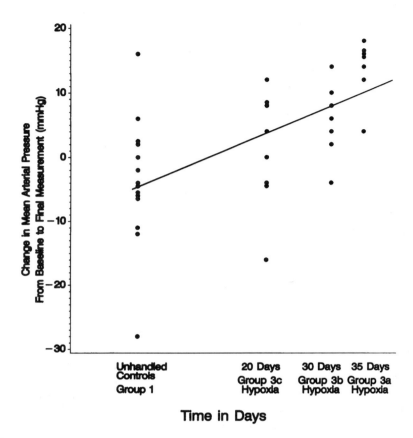

Figure 3 Change in mean arterial pressure from baseline to final measurement in unhandled controls (zero hypoxia exposure) and rats (Wistar Thomae) exposed to 20, 30, and 35 days of episodic hypoxia. The linear slope of 0.42 mmHg/day points to a duration-of-exposure response to episodic hypoxia. (From Ref. 14.)

and parasympathetic responses. Eucapnic hypoxia caused a threefold greater elevation in systolic BP and greater bradycardia than hypocapnic hypoxia (Fig. 5). Prazosin but not yohimbine blunted the BP response and atropine blocked the hypoxia-associated bradycardia (Fig. 5). Direct recording of splanchnic nerve activity in the awake, unrestrained rat confirmed that adding CO_2 to EH caused a profound increase in SNS activity (Fig. 6). This study confirmed that in *acute studies*, eucapnic hypoxia is a more potent stimulus to BP elevation than hypocapnic hypoxia.

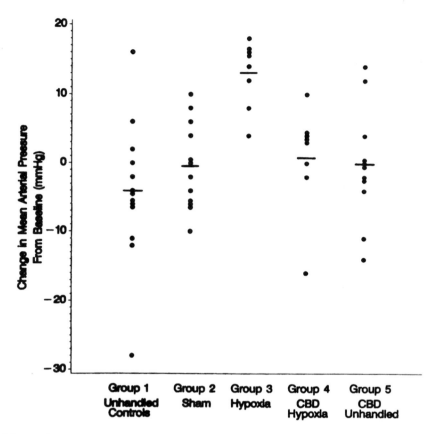

Figure 4 Change in mean arterial pressure (MAP) from baseline in five groups of rats. Group 3 (non-CBD receiving episodic hypoxia) showed a significant increase in MAP (13 mmHg) compared to unhandled controls. No other group showed any significant blood pressure (BP) changes from baseline to day 35 treatment. All non-CBD rats received ''sham'' neck surgery at the beginning of the study. CBD, carotid body–denervated; sham refers to daily episodic compressed air instead of episodic hypoxia. (From Ref. 15.)

Since the usual blood gas change of apnea is mildly increased CO_2 and the BP change of *acute* apnea is markedly enhanced by hypercapnia (17), we hypothesized that chronic EH ranging from eucapnia to hypercapnia might cause a greater *chronic* increase in BP than the usual hypocapnic hypoxia (18). Arterial blood gases were drawn in 33 rats to establish blood gas changes occurring under varying conditions of Fi_{CO_2}, using the same chambers and gas intake time (Fig.

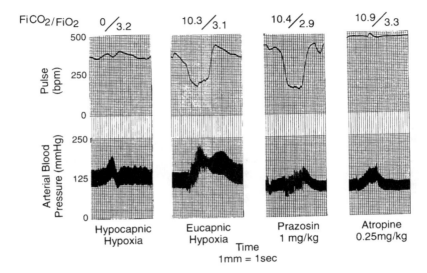

Figure 5 Continuous pulse (upper channel) and blood pressure (lower channel) from a single F1 rat exposed to hypocapnic hypoxia, eucapnic hypoxia, prazosin and eucapnic hypoxia, and prazosin + atropine + eucapnic hypoxia. Eucapnic hypoxia produced a greater pressor response than hypocapnic hypoxia, with more profound bradycardia. Prazosin blocks much of the pressor response, doing little to the bradycardia. Atropine completely eliminated the bradycardia, doing little to the pressor response. F_{ICO_2} (%) for each eucapnic hypoxia (EH) episode appears in the numerator (top) and F_{IO_2} appears in the denominator. (From Ref. 37.)

7). Five groups of male Sprague-Dawley rats were used in the *chronic* experiment. These included unhandled and sham-air controls, hypocapnic hypoxia (no added CO_2—ie., the usual EH), eucapnic hypoxia (7–10% F_{ICO_2}), and hypercarbic hypoxia (11–14% F_{ICO_2}). MAP was measured as in previous studies in conscious animals at baseline and after 35 days under their respective study conditions. Neither episodic eucapnic nor hypercarbic hypoxia had any additional effect upon changes in chronic diurnal BP compared to hypocapnic hypoxia (Fig. 8). These results suggest that the SNS or other neurohumoral systems contributing to *chronic* diurnal BP elevation may already be maximally stimulated by hypoxia or there may be some protective mechanism limiting the BP response to eucapnic or hypercapnic hypoxia in the EHR.

Another controversy has emerged in the process of studying the acute hemodynamic response to OSA. This is the role of arousal itself in eliciting acute cardiovascular changes. It is well known that arousal from sleep or startle in the awake animal or human causes a sympathetic discharge and other cardiovascular

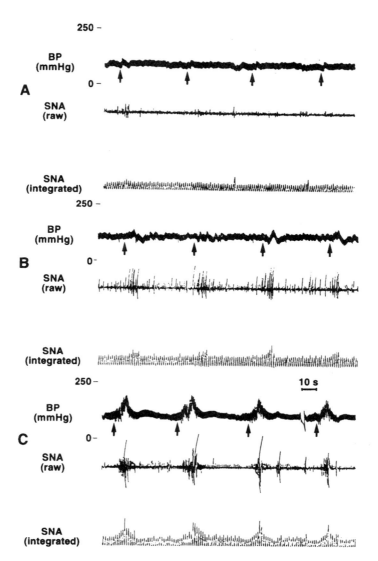

Figure 6 Tracing showing blood pressure (BP) and sympathetic nerve activity (SNA) in a single rat. (A) At baseline during episodes (arrows) of compressed air; (B) four episodes of hypocapnic hypoxia ($FI_{O_2} = 10\%$, $FI_{CO_2} = 0$); (C) four episodes of hypoxia plus CO_2 ($FI_{O_2} = 10\%$, $FI_{CO_2} = 5\%$). Heart rate is not shown. (From Ref. 17.)

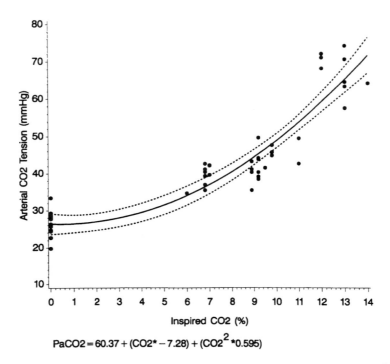

$$PaCO2 = 60.37 + (CO2* - 7.28) + (CO2^2 *0.595)$$

Figure 7   The quadratic relationship between FI_{CO_2} and arterial PCO_2 under conditions of transient hypoxia and supplemented CO_2 ranging from an FI_{CO_2} of 6–14% with FI_{O_2} of around 2–3%. Insufflations of N_2 and CO_2 cycled on for 12 sec followed by a compressed air flush, total cycle 30 sec. $N = 50$ samples drawn from 33 conscious, unrestrained rats. The amount of supplemental CO_2 required to return the hyperventilating rat to eucarbia was about 8–9% and for hypercarbia about 13%. Some points are superimposed. The dashed lines indicate the 95% confidence interval for the estimated regression function. (From Ref. 18.)

changes seen with hypoxia (19,20). Ringler et al. examined 11 obstructive apnea patients during sleep and found that apneas recorded during oxygen supplementation were associated with equivalent postapneic mean arterial blood pressure elevations compared to apneas without oxygen supplementation. Furthermore, when hypoxemia down to arterial saturation of 80% was induced with nitrogen, elevation of blood pressure was not seen if respiratory and sleep disruption were avoided (19). A subsequent study by the same authors supported these findings, suggesting that arousal and sleep disruption could be important factors in acute and chronic BP changes with apnea (20).

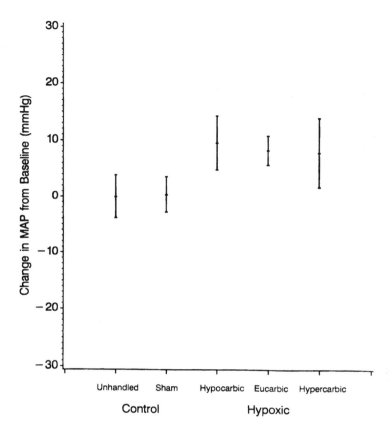

Figure 8 Change in mean blood pressure from baseline to follow-up after 35 days of no handling (unhandled), sham (compressed air), episodic hypocarbic hypoxia, or episodic hypoxia with 9% (eucarbic) or 13% $F_{I_{CO_2}}$ (hypercarbic). Shown are the means $\pm$ 2 SE. (From Ref. 18.)

For these reasons we were interested in testing the chronic effect of repetitive arousal. We exposed 12-week-old ($N = 10$) Sprague-Dawley rats in individual chambers to recurrent buzzer noise (500 Hz, 100 dB) 6 out of every 30 sec for 8 hr per day for 35 days. Nine sham rats housed in identical cages were not exposed to noise (21). An infrared beam with detector was positioned at the end of each cage, quantifying motion by registering the number of times the rat broke the beam per 8-hr "sleep" period. MAP was invasively measured in unrestrained conscious animals at baseline and at the end of 35 days of their respective conditions. All animals showed a significant *acute* BP response to noise, which diminished after 30–60 min of noise exposure. Acoustic-stimulated rats showed higher movement activity throughout the day than did the nonstimulated rats, but there was no difference in MAP in either group before or after the respective 35-day experimental conditions.

Establishing that the SNS plays a direct role in the chronic BP response to EH, we undertook a study to further dissect how the various components of the SNS interacted (22). We were interested in the specific roles of the renal artery sympathetics and the adrenal medulla in the chronic BP increase. Male Sprague-Dawley rats had either adrenal medullectomy or bilateral renal artery denervation or an abdominal incision only (sham surgery). Demedullated rats, sham-operated rats, and renal denervated rats were subjected to EH, as described above, for 35 days. Control groups were subjected either to compressed air or

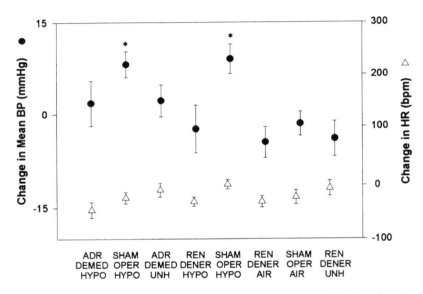

Figure 9 Change in mean arterial pressure (MAP) and heart rate (HR) from baseline in eight groups of rats exposed to control or study conditions. Closed circles represent change in MAP and open triangles represent change in HR. The first five data points (left side of figure) represent the five groups of rats exposed to control or study conditions described in the text for renal artery denervation study. The last three data points (right side of figure) represent the three groups of rats exposed to control or study conditions described in the text for adrenal demedullation study. See text for further explanation of groups. *A significant change from baseline at $p < 0.05$ or greater. SHAM OPER, sham operations (abdominal incision); HYPO, hypoxia; ADR, adrenal; DEMED, demedullated; UNH, unhandled; REN, renal; DENER, denervated. Brackets indicate ± 1 SE. (From Ref. 22.)

were left unhandled. Intra-arterial BP was measured at baseline and after cessation of EH or control conditions. Both adrenal demedullation and, separately, renal artery denervation (Fig. 9) eliminated the chronic diurnal BP response to EH, while sham-operated controls continued to show elevation of systemic BP. Plasma and renal tissue catecholamines at the end the experiment confirmed successful adrenal demedullation or renal denervation in the respective groups. In the sham-operated, hypoxia-exposed rats, plasma norepinephrine was elevated five times above baseline at the end of the hypoxia period (see discussion below). The findings of this study indicate that the chronic EH-mediated increase in diurnal BP require *both* intact renal artery nerves as well as an intact adrenal medulla.

One possible mechanism for renal sympathetic involvement in chronic BP elevation in the EHR is through stimulation of the renin-angiotensin system, discussed below. However, if renal sympathetic overactivity were the only mechanism modulating BP in EH, it would be difficult, in the above study, to explain why adrenal medullectomy eliminated the rise in BP after EH exposure. The results of the study suggest that adrenal-secreted, circulating epinephrine may also be an important regulator of BP in the setting of chronic EH (22). There are at least two possible ways that combined action of adrenal epinephrine and renal artery sympathetic nerves may both bring about diurnal BP elevations in this model. One is that circulating epinephrine binds to presynaptic SNS receptors and enhances norepinephrine release across the neural junction, facilitating neurogenic vasoconstriction, as described by Floras et al. (23,24). The other is that the renin-angiotensin system may participate in the diurnal BP increase, its release stimulated by renal artery sympathetics (25). It is known however, that the secretion of renin may persist in the face of renal artery denervation, and the existence of an extrarenal site that is stimulated by circulating adrenal epinephrine is postulated (26,27). (For further details see 22).

IV. Plasma Catecholamines and Renin in the EHR

Plasma catecholamines can be measured in the resting, nonstimulated human or animal, suggesting relationships between sympathetic and cardiovascular activity. However, absolute levels of catecholamines may not reflect true body and organ turnover or activity when release and clearance of the catecholamines are unknown. For example, in humans, it has been shown that hypoxia causes increased SNS activity (measured by muscle sympathetic nerve signals) with minimal change in plasma norepinephrine (28). This is explained by a significant increase in both release and clearance of norepinephrine. Also, catecholamine values are somewhat labile, as judged by a wide standard error, since they are rapidly changed by movement or activity of the animal. Thus, if catecholamine turnover is unknown, a low or normal plasma catecholamine level does not rule out increased SNS activity. A high plasma level, if drawn under ideal conditions, may indicated increased SNS activity but could also reflect artifact if the animal arouses. The major reason for measuring catecholamine levels in some of our previous studies was to confirm successful organ (adrenal demedullation) or nervous system ablation (peripheral SNS or renal denervation). However, a review of the plasma and tissue catecholamine levels yields some information suggestive of increased sympathetic activity in the EHR.

The technique for drawing and measuring plasma catecholamines was the same for all studies. Between 0.4 and 0.6 mL of whole blood was rapidly withdrawn from an indwelling arterial catheter connected to tubing extended outside of individual bedded cages. The levels were always measured at midmorning in a quiet room, with the rats unrestrained, resting, or behaviorally asleep. Plasma catecholamines were measured using high-performance liquid chromatography with electrochemical detection (29). As proof of successful chemical denervation (16) and renal artery denervation (22), animals were sacrificed at the end of the study and the heart or kidneys harvested and flash-frozen in liquid nitrogen. Tissue was stored at $-70°C$ until assay. Later, 100 mg of kidney tissue was sonicated in 0.5 mL of buffer (pH 4.0) containing 0.17 M citrate acetate and 10% methanol. The sonicated tissue was centrifuged and the clear aspirate subjected to microfiltration (Amicon, W. R. Grace, Beverly, MA) and high-performance liquid chromatography with electrochemical detection. Low levels of tissue norepinephrine indicated successful sympathetic denervation.

Our first attempt at measuring plasma catecholamines in the EHR was in the carotid-body denervation study (15). We found no significant differences in resting catecholamine levels between the various groups (Table 1).

In order to confirm successful chemical denervation with 6-OH dopamine (16), we measured plasma catecholamines within 2 days following cessation of EH in all groups (Table 2). The vehicle-treated EH group showed a significantly higher norepinephrine level after chronic EH than the unhandled controls. This suggested that elevated plasma norepinephrine in the EH group might reflect increased peripheral SNS activity. These results were also supported by the adrenal demedullation and renal artery denervation studies (22). Pre- and post-EH plasma epinephrine and norepinephrine were drawn in the adrenal demedullated and sham groups at baseline and within 4 days of the end of chronic EH. The sham-operated, EH-exposed animals showed plasma epinephrine 2.5 times that of their own baseline values (Fig. 10). The two demedullated groups both showed very low epinephrine levels pre- and post-35 days, which is compatible with successful demedullation. Norepinephrine, on the other hand, was elevated in both groups exposed to EH (sham-operated and adrenal demedullated) compared to baseline. However, the adrenal demedullated unhandled rats also showed elevated norepinephrine at day 37. The latter finding could represent normal aging or faulty blood-drawing technique or perhaps could be related to SNS compensa-

Table 1 Resting Plasma Catecholamines, Carotid Body Denervation Study[a]

	Group 1 unhandled (N = 13)	Group 2 Sham Controls (N = 9)	Group 3 Hypoxia (N = 8)	Group 4 CBD-Hypoxia (N = 5)	Group 5 CBD-Unhandled (N = 6)	p
Epinephrine (nmol/L)	0.87 (0.29)	0.24 (0.05)	0.41 (0.13)	0.34 (0.14)	0.24 (0.04)	N.S.
Norepinephrine (nmol/L)	0.43 (0.10)	1.37 (0.31)	0.60 (0.07)	0.83 (0.19)	0.91 (0.18)	N.S.
Dopamine (nmol/L)	0.45 (0.18)	0.78 (0.09)	0.97 (0.24)	0.56 (0.22)	0.34 (0.08)	N.S.

[a] Values are means $\pm$ two standard errors in μmol/L; N is the number of rats per study.
Source: From Ref. 15.

Table 2 Resting Plasma Catecholamines—Chemical SNS Denervation Study

	Vehicle Unhandled (n = 13)	Vehicle Hypoxia (n = 8)	6-OH Dopamine Hypoxia (n = 8)	6-OH Dopamine Unhandled (n = 11)	p^a
Epinephrine (nmol/L)	0.41 (0.10)	0.41 (0.12)	0.25 (0.11)	0.25 (0.10)	ns
Norepinephrine (nmol/L)	0.60 (0.05)	*1.14 (0.12)	0.78 (0.12)	0.72 (0.11)	<0.05
Dopamine (nmol/L)	0.93 (0.20)	1.32 (0.17)	1.14 (0.17)	1.17 (0.14)	ns

[a] Statistical differences between group means (*) using Tukey's multiple-comparison tests. The norepinephrine value for vehicle/hypoxia varied significantly from group 1 unhandled controls.
Source: From Ref. 16.

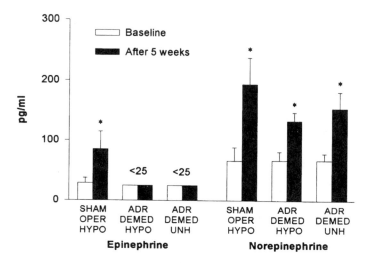

Figure 10 Mean levels of catecholamines for adrenal demedulated and sham operated hypoxia-exposed rats before (open bars) and after 35 days exposure to episodic hypoxia (closed bars). Same abbreviations as in Figure 9. Catecholamine levels are expressed in picograms per milliliter. Brackets indicate ± 1 SE. *Change at $p < 0.05$ or greater. (From Ref. 22.)

tion for the adrenal ablation. Again, the implication of changes in plasma norepinephrine levels related to peripheral SNS activity must be interpreted with caution.

For similar reasons (to confirm effective and sustained sympathetic renal artery denervation), tissue catecholamines were measured in excised kidneys of EH and control rats at the end of the renal denervation experiment (about 4 days after the last EH day) (22). Based upon these results, successful renal artery denervation was achieved in the renal-denervated rats, since renal tissue norepinephrine was low in all denervated animals at 35 days compared to sham-operated, compressed-air controls (Fig. 11). The sham-operated EH animals showed renal tissue norepinephrine levels that were twofold higher than those of sham-operated compressed-air rats. This suggests that EH may have caused increased renal SNS activity in the kidneys of these animals. Tissue epinephrine levels were borderline elevated in the renal denervated rats, but this difference was probably not physiologically relevant.

To assure successful chemical sympathectomy in the 6-OH dopamine study, we measured myocardial tissue catecholamines (16). Control values for norepinephrine levels in the cardiac ventricles have been reported at 500–950

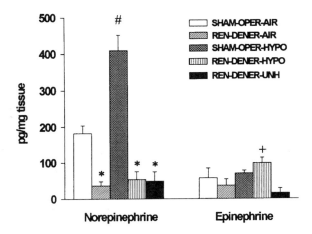

Figure 11 Mean levels of renal tissue catecholamines for renal-denervated and sham-operated hypoxia-exposed (HE) or control rats described in text, after 35 days exposure to various study conditions. # = Sham-operated EH values varied from all other groups at $p < 0.05$ level. *Groups differed from other groups at $p < 0.05$ or greater. + = Variation from renal-denervated by $p < 0.05$. Brackets indicate $\pm$ 1 SE. Same abbreviations as in Figure 9. (From Ref. 22.)

pg/mg (30,31), which were consistent with the value of 965 pg/mg in our unhandled controls (Table 3). The right ventricular epinephrine and norepinephrine values in our vehicle-treated, EH-exposed animals were 1.5–2.0 times that of unhandled controls respectively, while the levels in the left ventricle were not statistically different. Since the methods of analysis were identical and the samples were run concurrently, these results should be valid. Chronically administered intermittent hypoxia (4 continuous hr per day, 24–75 exposures) has been shown to be a potent stimulus to pulmonary artery vasoconstriction, right ventricular stress, and hypertrophy (32–35). One could speculate that sympathetic activity to the right heart might be differentially increased over that of the left in the present model. Kinetic studies of catecholamine turnover are more accurate for determining myocardial sympathetic activity and would be needed for definitive proof.

Although not classified as a catecholamine, plasma renin activity (PRA) may be regulated by sympathetic activity and may affect chronic BP through the renin-angiotensin system. Based upon the results of the renal denervation experiment, it was logical to question the role of the renin-angiotensin system in the chronic EHR preparation. To that end, we examined PRA in 24 Sprague-Dawley rats after 35 days of EH. Half of the group was treated with losartan [an angiotensin 1 (AT_1) receptor blocker] 15 mg/kg per day by gastric gavage and

Table 3 Myocardial Catecholamine Levels[a]

Parameter	Group 1, Vehicle Unhandled (n = 8)	Group 2, Vehicle and Hypoxia (n = 9)	Group 3, 6OH-DOP and Hypoxia (n = 7)	Group 4, 6OH-DOP Unhandled (n = 10)	p
Epinephrine					
Right Ventricle pg/mg	15.8 (2.7)	+*30.1 (3.3)	8.2 (1.6)	12.1 (2.3)	<0.05
Left Ventricle pg/mg	*18.1 (3.1)	*24.0 (3.2)	5.7 (1.1)	9.3 (2.7)	<0.05
Norepinephrine					
Right Ventricle pg/mg	*965 (104)	+*1535 (89)	226 (38)	140 (26)	<0.05
Left Ventricle pg/mg	*1004 (73)	*988 (62)	174 (30)	141 (17)	<0.05

[a] Asterisk (*) indicates that the epinephrine or norepinephrine values in the myocardium of the vehicle injected animals differed significantly from those in the 6-OH-dopamine–injected animals using Tukey's multiple-comparison tests. Plus sign (+) indicates group 2 values also varied from group 1 by $p <$ 0.05. Catecholamine values are expressed in terms of picograms per gram of actual muscle weight.

Source: From Ref. 15.

Table 4 Resting Plasma Renin Levels, Losartan Study

BP	DAY 0 BP (mmHg)	DAY 0 PRA (pg/mL)	DAY 14 BP (mmHg)	DAY 28 BP (mmHg)	DAY 36 BP (mmHg)	DAY 36 PRA (pg/mL)
HYPO	92.3	1.7	*101.5	*105.1	*102.3	*6.6
HYPO+LO	98.2	2.1	88.0	87.8	85.9	*16.7
UNH	94.0	1.8	—	—	94.5	1.9
UNH+LO	95.2	1.7	—	—	82.3	*18.7

Plasma renin activity (PRA) at baseline (day 0) and after cessation of hypoxia (day 36) along with baseline, day 14, day 28, and day 36 blood pressure (BP) in four groups of rats. There are no 14- or 28-day BP values for the unhandled and unhandled losartan-treated animals, since their BP was measured by indwelling catheters at the beginning and end of the study. The other rats' BP could be monitored continuously throughout the 35-day period by telemetry transducers. Methods for drawing and running PRA levels are described in the text. The asterisk (*) indicates that values differ from day-0 levels at $p <$ 0.05 level or greater. BP, blood pressure; HYPO = episodic hypocapnic hypoxia, LO = losartan treated, UNH = unhandled.
Source: From Ref. 36.

half were treated with vehicle only (36). The groups were divided as follows: 5 rats remained unhandled to establish PRA normals for our methods and another 5 unhandled rats received losartan; 7 rats were exposed to EH without losartan and 7 were exposed to EH with losartan. Both at the beginning and at the end of the experiment, in a manner similar to those described for catecholamine blood collection, 2 mL of arterial blood was rapidly withdrawn from quiet, resting rats, yielding 1 mL of plasma. Blood volume was simultaneously replaced by 2 mL of normal saline via venous catheter. Plasma was stored at 70°C for later measurement of angiotensin I and PRA. In the EH and EH-losartan rats, BP was monitored at room air rest (unrestrained) using implanted telemetry sensors (Data Sciences, St. Paul, MN) at baseline and every seventh day throughout a 35-day period. In the remaining rats, BP was measured at baseline and on day 36 by indwelling arterial catheter.

EH was associated with a 10-mmHg increase in MAP and a threefold rise in PRA as compared to no increase in BP or PRA in the unhandled controls (Table 4). Unhandled losartan-treated animals showed a fall in MAP over 35 days. Losartan effectively blocked the BP response to EH. The results show that PRA increases in response to EH and that the AT_1 antagonist prevents the rise in BP. As would be expected in any study with AT_1 blockade, losartan caused a small fall in MAP in the unhandled and EH rats along with a large increase in PRA in all treated animals. We concluded that chronic BP elevation from EH is in part implemented through the renin angiotensin system.

V. Ventricular Hypertrophy in the EHR

With the development of elevated BP, either in the pulmonary or systemic circuit, one might expect hypertrophy of the respective ventricular muscle. We nearly always examined right and left ventricular weights at the end of each EH experiment. The following technique was uniformly used in each study. The rats were anesthetized and rapidly exsanguinated; then the heart was removed. The atria and great vessels were dissected away, the right ventricle was separated from the left ventricle and septum, and the two muscles were weighed separately. This favors higher accuracy in the left ventricular segment, since it includes the septal wall which could be subject to hypertrophy of either ventricle.

Since we did not measure pulmonary artery pressure in any of the animal preparations, we cannot address the issue of possible elevated pulmonary artery pressure in the EHR. Examination of the right ventricular free wall to body-weight ratio (RV/TBW) helps very little in this regard (Table 5). The RV/TBW was significantly higher in EH rats than in sham (compressed air) or unhandled rats in the Sprague-Dawley rats of the first experiment (14), the Wistar Thomae EH rats with carotid-body denervation (hypoxic on room air when denervated)

Table 5   Right Ventricular/Total-Body-Weight Ratios from All Chronic Studies

	Episodic Hypoxia, mean	Compressed air, mean	Unhandled, mean
First study (14)			
Sprague-Dawley	0.62*	0.54	0.56
Wistar Thomae	0.52	0.48	0.48
Carotid Body–denervated (15)			
Sham operated	0.52		
Carotid body–denervated	0.60 *	0.46	0.46
Chemical sympathectomy (16)			
Sympathectomy	0.48		0.47
Vehicle-treated	0.48		0.47
Effect of CO_2 (18)			
Hypocapnic	0.59	0.50	0.52
Eucapnic	0.58		
Asphyxia	0.69*		
Renal denervation (22)			
Renal-denervated	0.52	0.56	0.56
Sham-operated	0.53		
Denervated—compressed air	0.53		
Adrenal (22)			
Demedullation	0.54	0.52	0.45*
F1 generation (37)			
Eucapnic hypoxia—8.4%	0.57	0.56	0.57
Eucapnic hypoxia—10.5%	0.67		
Hypocapnic hypoxia—0%	0.66		

Asterisk (*) indicates variation from other groups < 0.05 or less, one-way ANOVA, Bonferroni test. Standard errors omitted because of space constraints.

(15), and the Sprague-Dawley rats given episodic asphyxia for 35 days (18). In all other studies, the difference between RV/TBW in EH and controls was not statistically significant.

The data on left ventricular weights paint a more convincing picture. Examining Table 6, the left ventricle/total body weight (LV/TBW) of EH rats significantly exceeds the compressed air and unhandled rat LV/TBW in nearly every study except the renal denervation study. One might at first assume that this is hypertrophy secondary to the observed BP increase associated with EH. This is not the case, as LV/TBW increased in relation to EH but not to BP change. All animals in column one (EH) were exposed to episodic hypoxia, but because of various blocking manipulations, some did not develop elevated BP. For example, the carotid body–denervated rats exposed to EH did not elevate BP at 35 days

Table 6 Left Ventricular/Total-Body-Weight Ratios from All Chronic Studies[a]

	Episodic Hypoxia, mean	Compressed air, mean	Unhandled, mean
First study (14)			
Sprague-Dawley	2.39* ↑ BP	2.19	2.28
Wistar Thomae	2.00 ↑ BP	1.80	1.75
Carotid body-denervated (15)			
Sham-operated	1.98* ↑ BP		
Carotid body–denervated	2.05* ↔ BP	1.80	1.70
Chemical sympathectomy (16)			
Sympathectomy	1.90* ↔ BP		1.75
Vehicle-treated	1.90* ↑ BP		1.75
Effect of chronic episodic hypoxia (EH) with CO_2 (18)			
Hypocapnic EH	2.49* ↑ BP	2.33	2.10
Eucapnic	2.51* ↑ BP		
Asphyxia	2.40* ↑ BP		
Renal denervation (22)			
Renal denervation	1.83 ↔ BP	1.94	1.98
Sham-operated	1.83 ↑ BP		
Denervated—compressed air	1.92 ↔ BP		
Adrenal demedullation (22)			
Demedullation	1.81* ↔ BP		1.67
Sham-operated	1.83* ↑ BP		
F1 generation (37)			
Eucapnic hypoxia—8.4%	2.41* ↓ BP	2.30	2.26
Eucapnic hypoxia—10.5%	2.44* ↓ BP		
Hypocapnic hypoxia—0%	2.20 ↑ BP		

[a] Asterisk (*) indicates variation from other groups < 0.05 or less, one-way ANOVA, Bonferroni test. Standard errors are omitted because of space but can be found in original publications. The numbers in parentheses refer to the original study from which the table values are taken.

but did have higher, LV/TBW (nearly the same as the sham-operated EH) compared to compressed air–treated and unhandled controls (15). Chemical-sympathectomy rats exposed to EH had no BP change, but the LV/TBW was as high as in the vehicle-treated rats exposed to EH, which did show BP elevation (16). The same is true with the adrenal-demedullated EH and sham-operated EH rats (22). Both had increased LV/TBW over unhandled controls, yet only one group (sham-operated) had increased BP. All Sprague-Dawley rats exposed to EH with added CO_2 had increased LV/TBW compared to sham and unhandled controls (18). Of note is the fact that despite a *lowering* of 35-day BP in F1-generation rats exposed to eucapnic EH (see below), the LV/TBW weights were higher than those in the controls, in which the BP remained at baseline at 35 days (37). This again confirms the independent effect of EH on LV/TBW as opposed to a chronic change in BP. We cannot explain why the F1 hypocapnic EH rats did not show a higher LV/TBW, nor can we explain why none of the renal-denervated EH or sham-operated EH rats in the renal denervation study showed an elevated LV/TBW (22).

It is difficult to find data on the isolated effect of hypoxia on left ventricular hypertrophy. However, an increase in left ventricular weight in response to hypoxia but without elevation in systemic blood pressure has been reported previously (38,39). One possible cause of this could be pulmonary hypertension–induced right ventricular *septal* hypertrophy contributing to the increased left ventricular weight. Since we did not weigh the septa separately, we cannot rule this out as one factor, but we view is as unlikely, since all studies showed minimal differences between RV weights. Ou and Smith (39) have demonstrated increased LV/TBW exclusive of septal hypertrophy in hypoxia-exposed rats without "systemic hypertension" (specific blood pressure data were not given). They exposed two strains of Sprague-Dawley rats, one "altitude sensitive" and one "altitude resistant," to a simulated altitude of 18,000 ft for 35 days. Both groups developed marked right ventricular hypertrophy, but the altitude-sensitive rats showed a LV/TBW (septa removed) of 1.98 mg/g compared to 1.49 mg/g for sea-level controls and 1.43 mg/g for hypoxia-exposed altitude-resistant rats. It could be speculated that hypoxia induces blood or endothelial factors such as platelet activating factor, tissue renin, thromboxanes, prostaglandins, cytokines, endothelin, or other factors that could induce vascular smooth muscle contraction and growth or myocardial cell growth in direct response to hypoxia (40).

VI. Genetic Factors in the EHR

The "Folkow hypothesis" proposes that repeated episodes of sympathetic overactivity resulting from stimulation of the CNS "defense area" (for example, environmental stress) may trigger a series of events resulting in chronically elevated arterial BP (41,42). This presumes that some humans or animals have a genetic predisposition allowing the development of systemic hypertension when challenged while others do not. Such may be the case in hypertension associated with OSA; not all patients with OSA develop systemic hypertension. For example, the stress of chronic, recurrent episodic hypoxia may induce a secondary form of systemic hypertension in OSA, but only in genetically predisposed individuals. Correction of the apnea with removal of EH early in the disease might allow return of BP to normal. If the apnea is not corrected, the blood pressure elevation may be perpetuated by vascular remodeling or a secondary renal response to chronic preglomerular vasoconstriction and altered renal perfusion. Later correction of the apnea might then be unsuccessful in correcting the hypertension. The best nonhuman example of such "genetic predisposition" and increased end-organ susceptibility to systemic hypertension is the spontaneously hypertensive rat (SHR) (43).

In searching for the maximal BP response to chronic EH, we investigated several different rat strains. We chose to examine a rat strain that became hypertensive only when subjected to stress rather than the SHR that develops increased BP with age. The first-generation cross (F1 generation or borderline hypertensive

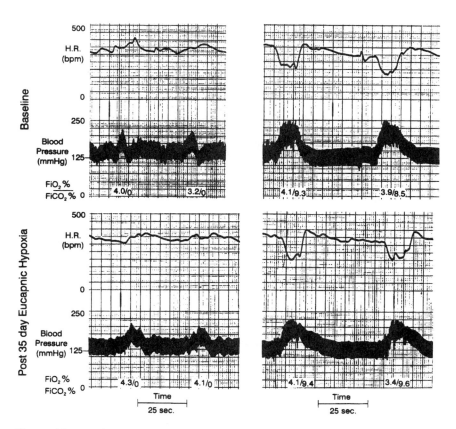

Figure 12 Continuous pulse (upper channel) and blood pressure (lower channel) from a single F1 rat exposed to episodic hypocapnic hypoxia (upper left panel) and eucapnic hypoxia (upper right panel) at baseline and after 35 days (7 hr/day) of exposure to chronic eucapnic hypoxia (lower panels respectively). Eucapnic hypoxia, as evidenced in the middle two panels, frequently induced transient bradycardia. (From Ref. 37.)

rat) between the SHR and the normotensive Wistar Kyoto rat (WKY) provides an excellent genetic model of BP which develops in response to environmental stress (44,45). Hemodynamic measurements in conscious F1 rats exposed to *behavioral stress* show increased mean BP, systemic vascular resistance, and cardiac index, which appear mediated by increased SNS activity (46).

We examined both acute and chronic BP response to episodic hypocapnic hypoxia and eucapnic hypoxia in borderline hypertensive rats (F1 generation) (37). Five groups of male F1 rats were studied after 35-day exposure to the following conditions: UNHANDLED ($N=8$) received no treatment; SHAM ($N=10$) received episodic compressed air only; HYPOHYPO ($N=14$) received daily EH to mean F_{IO_2} of levels 2.7% without added CO_2; EUHYPO$_1$ ($N=12$) received EH to mean F_{IO_2} levels of 2.9% along with CO_2 to mean F_{ICO_2} levels of 8.4%, which caused an arterial Pa_{CO_2} of approximately 40 mmHg (Fig. 7); and EUHYPO$_2$ ($N=11$) received EH to F_{IO_2} levels of 2.8% and CO_2 to mean F_{ICO_2} levels of 10.5%, which caused an arterial Pa_{CO_2} of approximately 45 mmHg. Under *acute condi-*

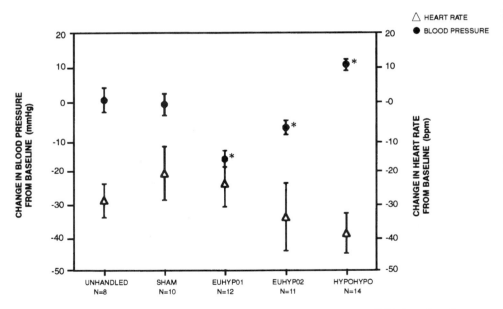

Figure 13 Change in mean arterial pressure (MAP) and heart rate (HR) from baseline in five groups of F1 hybrid rats exposed to various control or study conditions. Closed circles represent change in MAP; open triangles represent change in HR. See text for further explanation of groups. *Significant change from baseline. EUHYPO1, eucapnic hypoxia with added CO_2 of 8.4%; EUHYPO1, eucapnic hypoxia with added CO_2 of 10.5%; HYPOHYPO, hypocapnic hypoxia (without added CO_2). (From Ref. 37.)

tions, HYPOHYPO caused a 34.2-mmHg and EUHYPO a 77.9-mmHg increase in group mean BP (Fig. 12). Under chronic conditions, HYPOHYPO caused a 10.3-mmHg increase in daytime MAP, while EUHYPO caused a *fall* in MAP of −16.6 and −9.3 mmHg in the two separately studied groups (Fig. 13). In the hypertension-prone F1 rat, *acute* EUHYPO caused an accentuated elevation of BP, but *chronic* EUHYPO caused a fall. The acute response to EUHYPO is not predictive of what occurs after chronic exposure in the hypertension-prone F1 rat. Polygenetic factors control the BP response to chronic EH, with a specific difference between eucapnic versus hypocapnic hypoxia.

Because of differences in the BP response to 35 days of EH between several strains of rats, we examined the chronic BP response to EH in two additional strains, one known to be sensitive to high altitude (Sprague-Dawley Hilltop) and one morbidly obese strain (Zucker) (unpublished). BP was also measured in unhandled controls. The increase in diurnal BP was minimal (4 mmHg) (Hilltop) and there was no change in response to EH in the Zucker rats.

VII. Summary

Summarizing the studies from this laboratory to date, our data create the following scenerio regarding chronic recurrent EH and diurnal BP in the EHR. Acute and chronic hypoxia stimulate the peripheral chemoreceptors (15,37), which then elevate BP, probably through increased α-adrenergic sympathetic receptor activity (17). This is verified by observations of acutely increased splanchnic nerve sympathetic activity and BP and heart rate change in response to EH, which is then blocked by prazosin but not yohimbine (17). Diurnal (chronic, nonstimulated) increased BP changes are blocked by chemical sympathectomy (16). Increased plasma norepinephrine (16) as well as right ventricular myocardial catecholamines also support this. It appears that both the adrenal gland, via circulating epinephrine, as well as renal sympathetics participate in the chronic diurnal BP elevation (22). Common links between these two end organs of sympathetic activity may be 1) potentiation of SNS transmission by the binding of circulating (adrenal) epinephrine to peripheral SNS synapses, increasing peripheral neural transmission, and/or 2) by facilitation of the release of renin through α-adrenergic receptors in the kidney as well as circulating epinephrine-stimulated release of renin from nonrenal sites (22). The renin angiotensin system is activated in EHR, and the BP response to EH is blocked by AT-1 receptor blockers (36). Finally, genetics appears to play a role in the predisposition for the diurnal BP increase to occur (37).

Overactivity of the SNS is postulated to be critical in the pathogenesis of several forms of hypertension, but evidence remains indirect. Several forms of hypertension in experimental models have associated SNS overactivity with lesions believed to be related to an increased adrenergic state. These include the renovascular hypertensive rat (47), genetic hypertension in the SHR (44,48), and the spontaneously hypertensive turkey (49). Neurogenic tone is reported to be greater in the small arterioles in the cremaster muscle of SHR as assessed by neural blockade with tetrodotoxin (50). It is suggested that an increased responsiveness to SNS stimulation could be due to an altered presynaptic and/or postsynaptic receptor mechanism (51). An increase in the presynaptic release of norepinephrine (perhaps because of presynaptic circulating epinephrine binding) has been proposed as a mechanism for the increased reactivity of peripheral resistance vessels during hypertension. Norepinephrine release during SNS stimulation has been shown to be increased in the SHR. Common to these models is increased vessel contractility, increased smooth muscle cells resulting in medial hypertrophy, greater wall stress than in control animals, and intimal proliferative lesions that lead to a hypertension-associated type of atherosclerosis (52).

Enhanced adrenergic drive could lead to vascular damage through alterations of arterial flow and cellular and metabolic changes in the arterial wall. Enhanced adrenergic drive results in increased BP, heart rate, and blood velocity, possibly leading to arterial flow turbulence (53). The increase in BP may lead to changes in arterioles (typical target-organ damage seen in hypertension, retinopathy, etc.) and alteration of flow pattern in large arteries, resulting in typical intimal thickening, atherosclerotic plaques, and aneurysms, etc. Increased BP and flow turbulence have been shown to play a role in increased endothelial permeability by causing denudation or functional endothelial alterations and cell turnover, perhaps through shear stress (54). Could it be that change in shear stress and turbulent flow with endothelial cell damage/permeability are worse in cyclic constriction-relaxation (versus continuous), such as that seen in recurrent hypoxemia? Norepinephrine is known to be atherogenic in some animals on normal diets (55), including the SHR (56). Hypertension and high catecholamines appear to be risk factors for atherosclerosis in the spontaneously hypertensive turkey (57). In vitro work demonstrates that catecholamines produce an increase in growth rate of smooth muscle cells in secondary cultures of rat aorta (58). Thus, there appear to be many possibilities for an etiological relationship between recurrent EH, hypertension, and atherosclerosis.

Evidence for a link between systemic hypertension and sleep apnea and possibly atherosclerotic events (acute myocardial occlusion, stroke) in middle-aged and older males is strong, but a cause-and-effect relationship remains unproven. The slow time course and delayed diagnosis of sleep apnea and hypertension clearly limit our ability to examine such possibilities in humans until specific mechanisms of diurnal hypertension are worked out. For this reason, it is extremely important to develop animal preparations that can mimic some manifestations of OSA over a reasonable time period, allowing study of likely scenarios in the relationship between OSA and hypertension, stroke, myocardial infarction, and early cardiovascular death. The flexibility of the EHR allows manipulation of stress factors (noise, CO_2 and nadir O_2 levels), and control of exposure periods. It also allows many invasive functional and anatomical studies not possible in humans, producing a better understanding of endocrine, neural, and renal mechanisms operating to elevate BP. This model responds quickly (30–35 days), so that multiple risk factors (e.g., genetics, age, body weight, etc.) and mechanisms can be studied. Similar mechanisms of BP control and analogous diurnal and sleeping BP patterns between human and rat lend further validity to the EHR preparation. Such knowledge may enhance management of hypertension in patients with sleep-disordered breathing.

REFERENCES

1. Guilleminault C, Tilkian A, Dement WC. The sleep apnea syndromes. Annu Rev Med 1976; 27:465–484.
2. Tilkian AG, Guilleminault C, Schroeder JS, Lehrman KL, Simmons FB, Dement WC. Hemodynamics in sleep-induced apnea: studies during wakefulness and sleep. Ann Intern Med 1976; 85:714–719.
3. Lugaresi E, Coccagna G, Cirignotta F, et al. Breathing during sleep in man in normal and pathological conditions. Adv Exp Med Biol 1978; 99:35–45.
4. Lavie P, Ben-Yosef R, Rubin AE. Prevalence of sleep apnea syndrome among patients with essential hypertension. Am J Cardiol 1985; 55:1019–1022.
5. Kales A, Cadieux RJ, Shaw LC, Vela-Bueno A, Bixler EO, Schneck DW, Locke TW, Soldatos CR. Sleep apnoea in a hypertensive population. Lancet 1984; 2:1005–1008.
6. Fletcher EC, DeBehnke RD, Lovoi MS, Gorin AB. Undiagnosed sleep apnea in patients with essential hypertension. Ann Intern Med 1985; 103:190–195.
7. Williams AJ, Houston D, Finberg S, Lam C, Kinney JL, Santiago S. Sleep apnoea syndromes and essential hypertension. Am J Cardiol 1985; 55:1019–1022.
8. O'Donnell, CP, Ayuse T, King ED, Schwartz AR, Smith PL, Robotham JL. Airway obstruction during sleep increases blood pressure without arousal. J Appl Physiol 1996; 80:773–781.
9. Shepard JW Jr. Gas exchange and hemodynamics during sleep. Med Clin North Am 1985; 69:1243–1263.
10. Kimoff RJ, Makino H, Horner RL, Kozar LF, Lue F, Slutsky AS, Phillipson EA. Canine model of obstructive sleep apnea: model description and preliminary application. J Appl Physiol 1994; 76:1810–1817.
11. Brooks D, Horner RL, Kozar LG, Render-Teixeir CL, Phillipson EA. Obstructive sleep apnea as a cause of systemic hypertension: evidence from a canine model. J Clin Invest 1997; 99:106–109.
12. Korner PI, White, SW. Circulatory control in hypoxia by the sympathetic nerves and adrenal medulla. J Physiol 1966; 184:272–290.
13. Johnson TS, Young JB, Landsberg L. Sympathoadrenal response to acute and chronic hypoxia in the rat. J Clin Invest 1983; 71:1263–1272.

14. Fletcher EC, Lesske J, Qian W, Miller CC, Unger T. Repetitive, episodic hypoxia causes diurnal elevation of systemic blood pressure in rats. Hypertension 1992; 19: 555–561.
15. Fletcher EC, Lesske J, Behm R, Miller CC, Unger T. Carotid chemoreceptors, systemic blood pressure, and chronic episodic hypoxia mimicking sleep apnea. J Appl Physiol 1992; 72:1978–1984.
16. Fletcher EC, Lesske J, Culman J, Miller CC, Unger T. Sympathetic denervation blocks blood pressure elevation episodic hypoxia. Hypertension 1992; 20:612–619.
17. Bao G, Fletcher EC. Mechanism of acute blood pressure elevation during episodic hypercapnic hypoxia in rats simulating sleep apnea. J Appl Physiol 1997; 82:1071–1078.
18. Fletcher EC, Bao G, Miller CC. Effect of recurrent episodic hypocapnic, eucapnic, and hypercapnic hypoxia on systemic blood pressure. J Appl Physiol 1995; 78:1516–1521.
19. Ringler J, Basner RC, Shannon R, Schwartzstein R, Manning H, Weinberger SE, Weiss JW. Hypoxemia alone does not explain blood pressure elevations after obstructive apneas. J Appl Physiol 1990; 69:2143–2148.
20. Ringler JE, Garpestad RC, Basner RC, Weiss JW. Systemic blood pressure elevation after airway occlusion during NREM sleep. Am J Respir Crit Care Med 1994; 150: 1062–1066.
21. Bao G, Metreveli N, Fletcher EC. Acute and chronic blood pressure response to recurrent acoustic arousal in rats. Am J Hypertens 1999; 12:504–510.
22. Bao G, Metreveli N, Li R, Taylor A, Fletcher EC. Blood pressure response to chronic episodic hypoxia: role of the sympathetic nervous system. J Appl Physiol 1997; 83: 95–101.
23. Floras JS, Aylward PE, Victor RG, Mark AL, Abboud FM. Epinephrine facilitates neurogenic vasoconstriction in humans. J Clin Invest 1988; 81:1265–1274.
24. Floras JS. Aylward PE. Mark AL, Abboud FM. Adrenalin facilitates neurogenic vasoconstriction in borderline hypertensive subjects. J Hypertens 1990; 8:443–448.
25. Loeffler JR, Stockigt JR, Ganong WF. Effect of alpha and beta adrenergic blocking agents on the increase in renin secretion produced by stimulation of renal nerves. Neuroendocrinology 1972; 10:129–138.
26. Blair ML, Hisa H, Sladek, CD, Radke KJ, Gengo FM. Dual adrenergic control of renin during non-hypotensive hemorrhage in conscious dogs. Am J Physiol 1991; 260:E910–E919.
27. Blair ML, Gengo FM. β-adrenergic control of renin in sodium-deprived conscious dogs: renal versus extrarrenal location. Can J Physiol Pharmacol 1995; 73:1198–1202.
28. Leuenberger U, Gleeson K, Wroblewski K, Prophet S, Zelis R, Zwillich C, Sinoway L. Norepinephrine clearance is increased during acute hypoxemia in humans. Am J Physiol 1991; 261:H1659–H1664.
29. Goldstein DS, Feuerstein G, Izzo JL Jr. Liquid chromatography for measuring norepinephrine and epinephrine in man. Life Sci 1981; 28:467–475.
30. Torda T, Culman J, Petrikova M. Distribution of phenylethanolamine-N-methyltransferase in the rat heart: effect of 6-hydroxydopamine. Eur J Pharmacol 1987; 141:305–308.
31. Fluharty SJ, Vollmer RR, Meyers SA, McCann MJ, Zigmond MJ, Stricker EM.

Recovery of chronotropic responsiveness after systemic 6-hydroxydopamine treatment: Studies in the pithed rat. J Pharm Exp Ther 1987; 243:415–423.

32. Nattie EE, D Bartlett Jr, Johnson K. Pulmonary hypertension and right ventricular hypertrophy caused by intermittent hypoxia and hypercapnia in the rat. Am Rev Respir Dis 1978; 118:653–658.

33. Ressl J, Urbanova D, Widimsky J. Reversibility of pulmonary hypertension and right ventricular hypertrophy induced by intermittent high altitude hypoxia in rats. Respiration 1974; 31:38–46.

34. Widimsky J, Urbanova D, Ressl J. Effect of intermittent altitude hypoxia on the myocardium and lesser circulation in the rat. Cardiovasc Res 1973; 7:798–808.

35. McGrath JJ, Prochazka J, Pelouch B, Ostadal B. Physiological response of rats to intermittent high altitude stress: effects of age. J Appl Physiol 1973; 34:289–293.

36. Fletcher EC, Li R, Bao G. Renin activity and blood pressure in chronic episodic hypoxia (abstr). Hypertension 1999; 34:309–314.

37. Fletcher EC, Bao G. The effect of recurrent episodic eucapnic and hypocapnic hypoxia on systemic blood pressure in hypertension prone rats. J Appl Physiol 1996; 81:2088–2094.

38. Fregly MJ. Effect of chronic exposure to hypoxia on development and maintenance of renal hypertension in rats. Proc Soc Exp Biol Med 1970; 134:78–82.

39. Ou LC, Smith RP. Probable strain differences of rats in susceptibilities and cardiopulmonary responses to chronic hypoxia. Respir Physiol 1983; 53:367–377.

40. Luscher TF, Boulanger CM, Dohi Y, Yang Z. Endothelium-Derived contracting factors. Hypertension 1992; 19:117–130.

41. Folkow B. Physiological aspects of primary hypertension. Physiol Rev 1982; 62:347–504.

42. Folkow B. Psychosocial and central nervous influences in primary hypertension. Circulation 1987; 76(suppl i):i10–i19.

43. Yamori Y, Ikeda K, Kulakowski EC, McCarty R, Lovenberg W. Enhanced sympathetic-adrenal medullary response to cold exposure in spontaneously hypertensive rats. J Hypertens 1985; 3:63–67.

44. Lawler JE, Barker GF, Hubbard JW, Allen MT. Conflict and tonic levels of BP in the genetically borderline hypertensive rat. Psychophysiology 1980; 17:363–370.

45. Lawler JE, Sanders BJ, Chen Y, Nagahama S, Oparil S. Hypertension from a high sodium diet in borderline hypertensive rat. Clin Exp Hypertens 1987; A9:1713–1731.

46. Hubbard JW, Cox RH, Sanders BJ, Lawler JE. Changes in cardiac output and vascular resistance during behavioral stress in the rat. Am J Physiol 1986; 251:R82–R90.

47. Wolinsky H. Response of the rat aortic media to hypertension. Circ Res 1976; 26:507–512.

48. Mulvany JJ, Halpern W. Contractile properties of small arterial resistance vessels in spontaneously hypertensive and normotensive rats. Circ Res 1977; 41:19–26.

49. Pagnan A, Thiene G, Pessina AC, Dal Palu C. Serum lipoproteins and atherosclerosis in hypertensive broad breasted white turkeys. Artery 1980; 6:320–327.

50. Lombard J, Chenoweth JL, Stekiel WJ. Nonneural vascular smooth muscle tone in arterioles of the hamster. Hypertension 1984; 6:540–535.

51. Lokhandwala MF and Eikenburg DC. Presynaptic receptors and alteration in norepinephrine release in spontaneously hypertensive rat. Life Sci 1983; 33:1527–1542.

52. Pauletto P, Scannapieco G, Pessina AC. Sympathetic drive and vascular damage in hypertension and atherosclerosis. Hypertension 1991; 17(suppl III):III 75–III 81.

53. Spence JD. Effects of antihypertensive drugs on blood velocity: implications for prevention of cerebral vascular disease. Can J Neurol Sci 1977; 4:93–97.

54. Davies PF, Remuzzi A, Gordon EJ, Forbes DC, Gimbrone MA. Turbulent fluent shear stress induced vascular endothelial cell turnover in vitro. Cell Biol 1986; 83:2114–2117.

55. Helin P, Lorenzen I, Garbarsch C, Matthiessen E. Arteriosclerosis in rabbit aorta induced by noradrenalin. Atherosclerosis 1970; 12:125–132.

56. Yamori Y, Tarazi RC, Oshima O. Effect of beta-receptor blocking agents on cardiovascular structural changes in spontaneous and noradrenaline-induced hypertension in rats. Clin Sci 1980; 59:457s–460s.

57. El Halawani ME, Weibel PE, Appel JR, Good AL. Catecholamine and monoamine-oxidase activity in turkeys with high or low blood pressure. Trans NY Acad Sci 1973; 35:463–470.

58. Blaes N, Bloissel JP. Growth-stimulating effect of catecholamines on rat aortic smooth muscle cells in culture. J Cell Physiol 1983; 116:167–171.

9

The Acute Hemodynamic Response to Upper Airway Obstruction During Sleep

J. WOODROW WEISS, SANDRINE H. LAUNOIS, and AMIT ANAND

Beth Israel Deaconess Medical Center
and Harvard Medical School
Boston, Massachusetts

I. Introduction

The repetitive pauses in airflow that define obstructive sleep apnea are each punctuated by abrupt increases in heart rate and arterial pressure and by a sudden decrease in ventricular stroke volume. Considerable research has been devoted in recent years to defining the factors that contribute to these hemodynamic oscillations. Among the factors that have been considered are chemostimulation, changes in lung volume, and arousal—the abrupt change in sleep state. While evidence exists supporting a hemodynamic contribution from each of these factors, the relative impact of these and other factors to the hemodynamic events that characterize sleep apnea remain controversial. In this review we describe in detail the hemodynamic events that characterize upper airway obstruction during sleep and detail some of the controversies regarding the nature of the acute response to obstructive apneas, focusing on the effects of arousal and chemostimulation. This chapter does not address, except indirectly, the contribution of these acute events to the chronic hemodynamic consequences of sleep apnea, such as hypertension. These chronic changes are covered in other chapters in this volume.

213

II. The Acute Response to Upper Airway Obstruction During Sleep

The highest heart rate and the peak arterial pressure of the apnea-recovery cycle occur 5–7 sec following apnea termination (1,2). Conversely, the lowest heart rate and pressure occur at the beginning of the apnea, at the onset of obstruction (Fig. 1). Rate and pressure build during the apnea, but there is a sudden increase as the apnea ends, coincident with arousal from sleep, resumption of respiration, and the lowest oxygen saturation (Sa_{O_2}) of the apnea-recovery cycle. Several lines of evidence indicate that stroke volume decreases following apnea termination (3–6), but the magnitude of the decrease is uncertain; thus it is not yet clear whether the increase in heart rate completely buffers the decrease in stroke volume to maintain cardiac output constant or whether cardiac output declines following resumption of ventilation. Some human studies suggest that cardiac output falls after apnea termination, but other human and animal studies suggest that there is an increase in output following resumption of ventilation.

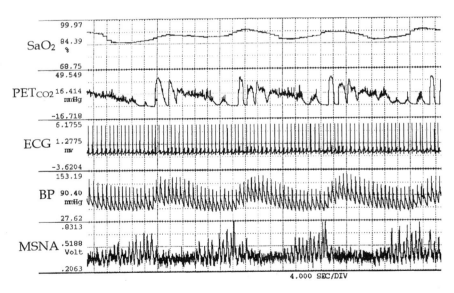

Figure 1 Recording of oxygen saturation (SaO_2), end-tidal carbon dioxide (PET_{CO2}), heart rate on electrocardiogram (ECG), arterial pressure (BP), and muscle sympathetic nerve activity (MSNA) in a patient experiencing repetitive obstructive apneas during sleep. Note the oscillations in arterial pressure, measured noninvasively through digital photoplethysmography. The peaks of arterial pressure occur after the resumption of airflow as measured by end-tidal carbon dioxide.

Whether the increase in heart rate is sufficient to increase cardiac output is uncertain, but other evidence suggests the heart rate oscillation is crucial to the typical oscillations in arterial pressure. One such piece of evidence is the finding that atropine abolishes the increase in arterial pressure following release of obstruction (7). Another piece of evidence is the finding, in a recent preliminary report, that heart transplant recipients with sleep apnea do not have typical oscillations in arterial pressure during sleep (8). This suggests that heart rate must increase for arterial pressure to rise after release of obstruction.

Whether the increase in heart rate is sufficient to maintain cardiac output postapnea is difficult to resolve, but pharmacological studies suggest that the increase in arterial pressure at apnea termination is at least in part due to systemic vasoconstriction. First, O'Donnell and co-workers have administered hexamethonium to dogs subjected to tracheal occlusion during sleep (9). In these animals, the ganglionic blocker prevented the increase in arterial pressure previously demonstrated in intact animals. Morgan and co-workers also used hexamethonium in normal human volunteers performing voluntary breath-holds (10). Again, the ganglionic blocker prevented the previously demonstrated increase in end-apnea arterial pressure. Finally, preliminary reports from Remsburg et al. (11) and from Leuenberger's laboratory (12) documented limb vasoconstriction in the postapnea period using venous plethysmography (Remsburg) and Doppler ultrasound (Leuenberger).

A. Heart Rate Changes During the Apnea-Recovery Cycle

Several studies have noted an association between sleep apnea and oscillations in heart rate (13,14). In fact, some early investigators suggested that regular reductions in heart rate during the sleep period might serve as a diagnostic marker for obstructive sleep apnea (15). While heart rate analysis has not proven sufficiently sensitive or specific to serve as a routine screening test for sleep apnea, there continues to be interest regarding the nature of the alternating tachycardia and bradycardia.

Zwillich and colleagues (16) were among the first to examine the changes in heart rate in association with sleep apnea. These investigators observed heart rate slowing during the latter portion of the apnea and pursued the nature of this slowing by examining the heart rate changes in normal subjects during a breath-hold. In an elegant series of studies in dogs, Daly and colleagues (17,18) had previously determined that when increases in respiration are constrained, hypoxia causes a decrease in heart rate. In contrast, when ventilation is allowed to increase with hypoxic exposure, heart rate also increases. Similarly, in normal humans, Zwillich and co-workers established that apneic hypoxia is associated with bradycardia, and these authors speculated that bradycardia occurs during obstructive apneas as a consequence of the apneic asphyxia. Tolle et al. (19) also examined the heart rate changes in patients experiencing obstructive apneas during sleep. They described an 11% decrease in rate during the apnea compared to the baseline heart rate during wake before sleep.

Although Zwillich et al. (16) and Tolle et al. (19) described decreases in heart rate during progressive apnea, more recent investigators have described progressive tachycardia during the apnea, followed by further increases in heart rate following apnea termination (1,3,20). Garpestad and co-workers (3) divided the apneic period in half, into early apnea and late apnea, and compared heart rate during these periods to heart rate following resumption of respiration (recovery). These authors found a progressive increase in heart rate from early to late apnea, with a further sharp increase at recovery. Interestingly, this pattern of heart rate change was not altered by administration of supplementary oxygen at sufficient flows to ameliorate but not abolish apnea-related desaturation (minimum Sa_{O_2} 93%). Similar progressive increases in heart rate during the apnea have been described by Stoohs and Guilleminault (20), who, like Garpestad et al., studied patients with severe sleep apnea.

The discrepancy between the findings of Zwillich and co-workers (16) and those of Garpestad et al. (3) are difficult to reconcile but may be related to technique as well as to patient selection. Zwillich, for example, compared heart rate in the final seconds of the apnea to the heart rate in the seconds immediately preceding the apnea. Thus, heart rate at the end of the apnea was compared to heart rate during a period that may include the period of recovery analyzed by Garpestad et al. (3)—a time when most authors describe substantial tachycardia (1,20). Similarly, Tolle et al. compared heart rate at end-apnea to heart rate during waking, a comparison that may be misleading, since numerous reports document a consistent decrease in heart rate during non–rapid-eye-movement (NREM) sleep (21,22) in normal humans. These methodological techniques may not entirely account for the different results, however. There may also be differences among patients in the heart rate response to obstructive apneas during sleep. Although Garpestad et al. described progressive tachycardia in their patients, approximately 10% of sleep apnea patients develop severe bradycardia in association with obstructive episodes (23). Furthermore, case reports document episodes of sinus pauses and heart block at end-apnea in specific patients (24). Thus, there may be differences among patients in terms of the changes in heart rate observed. It remains uncertain whether these differences can be accounted for by other factors, such as degree of desaturation or stage of sleep.

B.   Fluctuations in Systemic Arterial Pressure During the Apnea-Recovery Cycle

In normal human subjects, arterial pressure consistently decreases from waking to stable NREM sleep (21,22). This decrease in pressure is primarily attributable to a decrease in cardiac output that occurs as a consequence of a decrease in heart rate (21). In healthy young volunteers, systemic vascular resistance changes little with sleep onset (25).

Numerous clinical studies have established that the normal decrease in arterial pressure is lacking in patients with obstructive sleep apnea (26,27). Instead, patients with sleep apnea experience repetitive surges in arterial pressure, with the peak arterial pressure occurring 5–7 sec after apnea termination (1,2). These oscillations in pressure may be extreme, with patients who are apparently normotensive during the day displaying peak systolic pressures greater that 280 mmHg after obstructive apneas. In general, the oscillations in arterial pressure are greater in REM than in NREM sleep even when matching for degree of oxygen desaturation (28).

C. Changes in Ventricular Stroke Volume During and After Obstructive Apneas

The oscillations in arterial pressure that occur during and after upper airway obstruction during sleep are easily characterized using standard invasive and noninvasive techniques available for both human and animal investigations. In contrast, the techniques available to characterize changes in ventricular stroke volume are technically difficult and all are poorly validated for the measurement of stroke volume during the complex physiological events that occur with airway collapse and recovery.

Early investigators attempted to resolve the changes in ventricular function during and after obstructive events using the thermodilution technique to measure cardiac output. Tilkian and colleagues (6) and Podzus and colleagues (27) performed thermodilution measurements in patients with spontaneous apneas and failed to find consistent changes. However, Guilleminault and co-workers, using the same technique, noted a 30–35% fall in cardiac index during the apnea followed by a 15% increase in output during the immediate postapnea period (30). But by definition, the thermodilution technique requires a steady state for accurate measurement. In addition, the technique consumes several seconds and is unable to resolve rapid transients in cardiac function.

Unlike thermodilution, impedance cardiac output measurements are capable of resolving more rapid changes in ventricular function. This technique uses continuous measurement of thoracic impedance to assess changes in thoracic blood volume that are assumed to reflect changes in ventricular volume (30). Tolle et al. (19) were the first to apply this technique to patients with sleep apnea. However, they confined their analysis to the period of obstruction, because of concern that changes in lung volume at apnea termination might alter the results. Their results indicated that left ventricular stroke volume (LVSV) decreased 18% during the obstruction relative to the waking baseline. Again comparing their results to the waking baseline, they determined that cardiac output decreased during the apnea as heart rate fell (see above) and stroke volume decreased. Simultaneous measurement of esophageal pressure allowed them to relate the changes in stroke volume to changes in thoracic pressure. Because stroke volume decreased with more negative intrapleural pressure, these authors postulated that the changes in stroke volume were attributable to decreases in left ventricular filling.

This impedance technique was also used by Stoohs and Guilleminault (20) to study patients with obstructive apneas. These authors did compare the period of obstruction to the period between apneas. During apneas occurring in NREM sleep, these authors described a decrease in stroke volume from the beginning of the obstruction to the end of the apnea. Stroke volume did not decrease further during the period between apneas. In findings similar to those of Tolle and colleagues (19), Stoohs and Guilleminault (20) reported that progressively more intense respiratory efforts, resulting in more negative pleural pressure, accounted for the change in stroke volume during the apnea.

Garpestad and colleagues used a different technique to resolve the changes in stroke volume associated with apnea and resumption of ventilation. In two studies (3,31), these authors used a nuclear technique to monitor left ventricular function. After technetium labeling in vitro of autologous red blood cells, a non-imaging scintillation probe was placed over the left ventricular blood pool using a lead target. The probe provided a continuous output of the left ventricular blood pool, which approximates left ventricular volume (32). As noted above, these authors divided the apnea into early and late and compared those periods to recovery, defined as the time from the resumption of ventilation to the peak of arterial pressure. Like Stoohs and Guilleminault (20), these authors described a progressive decrease in LVSV during the apnea, but unlike the other authors, Garpestad and colleagues found a further decrease in LVSV immediately after apnea termination. Of note, Garpestad et al. compared cardiac function to the first seconds of the interapnea period, while Stoohs considered all cardiac cycles from the end of one apnea to the beginning of the next. This difference in data analysis is important, because in the study of Garpestad et al., patients' LVSV was least immediately upon resumption of ventilation and increased progressively over the subsequent seconds, suggesting that further data collection might have obscured the magnitude of the early change in stroke volume.

Two other monitoring techniques have now been used to monitor ventricular function in patients with sleep apnea. These also suggest that stroke volume decreases during the period immediately after apnea termination. Bonsignore et al. (4) placed flow probes in the pulmonary arteries of patients with obstructive sleep apnea (OSA) and then allowed the subjects to sleep, recording oscillations in flow in association with the obstructive events. These investigators reported that right ventricular stroke volume, as measured by the catheters, decreased immediately after apnea termination. By relating the changes in flow to simultaneous measurements of pleural pressure, these authors could account for the flow change through the effects of negative pleural pressure on cardiac performance. Escourrou and colleagues used pulse contour analysis to assess the changes in stroke volume during spontaneous apneas in sleeping OSA patients (5). This technique also indicated that stroke volume decreases after apnea termination. In this study, however, the change in stroke volume was compensated for by the increase in heart rate, so that cardiac output increased after release of obstruction.

III. The Role of Chemostimulation in the Acute Hemodynamic Response to Obstructive Apneas

Because obstructive apneas are accompanied by oscillations in Sa_{O_2} that occur in association with the hemodynamic fluctuations, there is obvious reason to invoke chemostimulation as an explanation for the changes in heart rate and arterial pressure. A number of lines of investigation support the view that hypoxemia is the stimulus that primarily accounts for the hemodynamic changes described above.

One line of evidence that supports a primary role for hypoxemia comes from studies of normal volunteers simulating apneas during wakefulness. Aardweg and Karemaker (33) simulated sleep apnea by having normal volunteers perform breath-holds after breathing from a spirometer filled either with air or 100% oxygen. In these subjects, apneas during hypoxia consistently resulted in increases in arterial pressure, while those performed after breathing oxygen had no effect on pressure. Furthermore, in these subjects, the increase in pressure was proportional to the degree of desaturation. Leuenberger and colleagues (34) also compared voluntary apneas in subjects exposed to hypoxia and hyperoxia. In addition to heart rate and arterial pressure, these investigators also monitored muscle sympathetic nerve activity (MSNA). During room-air apneas, MSNA increased 94% and mean arterial pressure rose 6.5 mmHg. During hypoxic apneas (after breathing 10.5% oxygen), MSNA rose 616% and arterial pressure rose 10.8 mmHg. Thus, hypoxemia augmented both MSNA and arterial pressure responses to voluntary apneas. In another study, Morgan and co-workers (35) studied the effects of voluntary apnea during both room air and oxygen breathing, comparing the effects of breath-holds and sustained Mueller maneuvers in normal volunteers. These investigators also monitored MSNA as well as arterial pressure and heart rate. Although the subjects breathed room air immediately prior to the voluntary apneas at baseline, so that desaturation was mild, nevertheless, the increases in both arterial pressure and MSNA that were observed with room-air maneuvers were markedly attenuated by supplementary oxygen.

Studies in sleep apnea patients also suggest that chemostimulation may contribute to the complex hemodynamic changes in patients with sleep apnea. Leuenberger and colleagues (36) measured arterial pressure and MSNA in patients with spontaneous apneas before and after oxygen supplementation. One hundred percent oxygen was administered to prevent any decrease in oxygen saturation during obstructive episodes. Spontaneous apneas were characterized by surges in sympathetic activity during the apnea. Bursts diminished in amplitude and frequency following apnea termination, but arterial pressure continued to rise, peaking approximately 7 sec following resumption of respiration. Oxygen supplementation markedly attenuated the rise in sympathetic activity during the apnea. Interestingly, the peak arterial pressure after apnea termination was not altered by oxygen. Because the arterial pressure nadir during the apnea did not fall as low during oxygen therapy, however, the magnitude of the oscillation was damped by oxygen.

Smith and colleagues also studied sleep apnea patients during spontaneous apneas, apneas with oxygen supplementation, simulated apneas awake, and induced hypoxemia (37). These investigators induced hypoxemia with one to four breaths of nitrogen in patients breathing from a mouthpiece. Arterial pressure and sympathetic nerve activity were monitored under the different conditions. Sympathoexcitation during spontaneous apneas was twice that observed during induced hypoxemia. Oxygen supplementation ameliorated the increase in SNA. The authors concluded that hypoxemia contributed but did not account for all the sympathoexcitation observed during obstructive apneas.

IV. The Role of Arousal in the Acute Hemodynamic Response to Obstructive Apneas

The major other possible contributor to the acute arterial pressure surge at end-apnea is arousal, the abrupt change in sleep state. Ringler et al. (1) monitored arterial pressure in patients with sleep apnea to examine the relative contribution of hypoxemia and arousal to the postapnea pressure surge. These investigators compared the arterial pressure at termination of apneas with oxygen saturation (Sa_{O_2}) nadirs of 78–82% to the pressure following apneas in which supplementary oxygen ameliorated the desaturation ($Sa_{O_2} > 90\%$, mean 93%). In this group of patients, oxygen supplementation did not alter the peak arterial pressure obtained after release of obstruction. Then, by placing the same patients on nasal continuous positive airway pressure (CPAP) sufficient to abolish the obstructive events, the authors examined the effects of sleep disruption without desaturation on arterial pressure. Using acoustic arousals induced by an audiometer, these investigators found that arousal without desaturation was sufficient to reproduce the arterial pressure peak observed after naturally occurring apneas. Their conclusion was that hypoxemia was not *necessary* for the increase in arterial pressure that follows relief of obstruction.

Since this study, others have specifically examined the hemodynamic effects of sleep disruption. Davies and co-workers studied five normal volunteers during sleep, monitoring sleep stage, electrocardiogram, and beat-to-beat arterial pressure with a noninvasive cuff (38). Non-respiratory arousals were created with a tactile stimulus, and arousals were graded by intensity and duration. Arousal stimuli resulted in increases in arterial pressure, with an average increase in systolic pressure of 10 mmHg. During NREM sleep, there was a tendency for arousals of greater intensity to result in greater increases in arterial pressure. The increase in arterial pressure was estimated to be 75% of that occurring after episodes of obstructive apnea. Morgan et al. (39) expanded on these observations by monitoring muscle sympathetic nerve activity and arterial pressure during arousals produced in normal volunteers using an auditory stimulus. Heart rate and stroke volume (impedance cardiography) were also monitored. Stimuli that evoked electroencephalographic (EEG) evidence of arousal also evoked one to two large bursts of sympathetic activity. Stimuli that did not produce visible evidence of EEG arousal resulted in lesser increases in arterial pressure, but sympathetic activation was not evident.

Animal studies have added substantially to our understanding of the hemodynamic consequences of arousal. O'Donnell and colleagues have used a canine model of sleep apnea in which occlusions are created by inflation of a balloon in a tracheostomy tube (8,40). By matching occlusions for duration, these investigators were able to create ''apneas'' of similar length that did and did not result in EEG arousal (9). Apneas that were terminated before arousal resulted in an increase in arterial pressure of 13.8 mmHg. When arousal occurred at end-apnea, there was a further 11.8-mmHg increase in pressure. When autonomic blockade was induced in the animals using hexamethonium, arterial pressure fell in the immediate postobstruction period whether or not arousal occurred. Brooks and co-workers (41) created a chronic dog model of sleep apnea, with occlusions created by solenoid occlusion of a tracheotomy in animals remotely monitored for sleep by telemetry. These investigators compared the hemodynamic effects of repetitive airway occlusions to those of repetitive auditory arousals. Although auditory arousals mimicked the acute changes in arterial pressure of airway occlusion, only repetitive occlusions resulted in sustained increases in waking arterial pressure.

These studies suggest that arousal does contribute to the surge in arterial pressure that follows termination of apnea in patients with OSA. They further suggest, however, that arousal alone likely does not account for the complex nocturnal hemodynamic changes that occur in apnea patients.

V. The Role of Lung Volume and Intrathoracic Pressure Changes in the Acute Hemodynamic Response to Obstructive Apneas

Although most studies of hemodynamics in sleep apnea patients have focused on the influences of chemostimulation and arousal on arterial pressure, these patients also experience marked fluctuations in lung volume and intrathoracic pressure during the apnea-recovery cycle. The extensive literature examining influences of lung volume and thoracic pressure on cardiovascular function and hemodynamics has been well reviewed (42,43) and is not summarized here. However, some studies have focused specifically on the hemodynamic effects of respiratory effort patients with obstructive sleep apnea.

The effects of respiratory effort on ventricular stroke volume are well documented (44,45). Tolle et al., however, were among the first to look at the effect of pleural pressure on left ventricular stroke volume during an obstructive apnea (19). These authors related changes in stroke volume to changes in pleural pressure during the period of apnea and concluded that at pleural pressures less than 10 cmH$_2$O below the resting end-expiratory level, pleural pressure changes accounted for much of the variance in stroke volume observed. More recently, Stoohs and Guilleminault (20) have used methods similar to those of Tolle and were also able to relate changes in ventricular stroke volume to the degree of respiratory effort. Garpestad and co-workers (31) examined the effects of oxygen supplementation on cardiac function in patients with sleep apnea. These authors found that oxygen at sufficient flow rates to ameliorate the nadir of desaturation did not alter the changes in stroke volume that were observed during the apnea-recovery cycle. Although these authors previously showed that acoustic arousal reproduced the arterial pressure peak that occurs after apnea termination (1), they found that arousal alone was not sufficient to recreate the decrease in ventricular stroke volume that occurs during recovery from the obstructive event (31). In a subsequent study, these same investigators had sleep apnea patients recreate spontaneous apneas awake by copying the pleural pressure and airflow pattern recorded during sleep (44). When apneas were recreated during wakefulness, stroke volume decreased in the same pattern as observed during spontaneous apneas asleep, suggesting that the mechanical events of intrathoracic pressure change and chest wall inflation might account for the changes in stroke volume.

Morgan and co-workers have examined the impact of changes in intrathoracic pressure on arterial pressure and MSNA in normal volunteers (35). During the Mueller maneuvers, subjects maintained pleural pressure at -40 cmH$_2$O for the full period. During the sustained Mueller maneuvers, arterial pressure initially fell but then rose progressively. Similarly, sympathetic nerve activity (SNA) was initially suppressed by the maneuver but rose as the apnea progressed. During breath holds, arterial pressure and SNA rose progressively through the apnea, with no initial decrease. As noted above, oxygen supplementation ameliorated the MSNA and changes in arterial pressure during both Mueller maneuvers and breath-holds.

VI. Conclusion

Obstructive apneas during sleep are associated with marked oscillations in arterial pressure, heart rate, and ventricular function. The hemodynamic events occur in association with changes in sleep state, chemostimulation, and lung volume as well as intrathoracic pressure. From the studies summarized here, it seems likely that all these factors contribute to the complex hemodynamic pattern that characterizes the apnea-recovery cycle. We are still some distance, however, from defining the precise contribution of each of these variables to the dramatic oscillations that may occur in sleep apnea patients experiencing upper airway obstructions. If, as seems likely, these oscillations contribute to cardiovascular morbidity and even mortality in these patients, then we need to better our understanding of these events to help prevent the peaks and valleys of arterial pressure that cause such extreme oscillations in cardiac workload during sleep.

Acknowledgments

This work was supported in part by HL 46951 and by MO1-RR01032 to the Beth Israel Deaconess Medical Center General Clinical Research Center from the National Institutes of Health.

References

1. Ringler J, Basner RC, Shannon R, Schwartzstein RM, Manning H, Weinberger SE, Weiss JW. Hypoxemia alone does not explain blood pressure elevations after obstructive apneas. J Appl Physiol 1990; 69:2143–2148.
2. Tilkian AG, Guilleminault C, Schroeder JS, Lehrman KL, Simmons FB, Dement WC. Hemodynamics in sleep induced apnea. Ann Intern Med 1976; 85:714–719.
3. Garpestad E, Katayama H, Parker TA, Ringler J, Lilly J, Yasuda T, Moore RH, Strauss HW, Weiss JW. Stroke volume and cardiac output decrease at termination of obstructive apneas. J Appl Physiol 1992; 73:1743–1748.
4. Bonsignore MR, Marrone O, Romano S, Piero D. Time course of right ventricular stroke volume and output in obstructive sleep apnea. Am J Respir Crit Care Med 1994; 149:155–159.
5. Escourrou P, Tessier O, Bourgin P. Non-invasive hemodynamics during snoring and sleep apnea. Presented at the 3rd International Marburg Symposium on Cardiocirculatory Function During Sleep. Marburg, Germany, 1994.

6. Schneider H, Schaub CD, Andreoni KA, Schwartz AR, Smith PL, Robothom JL, O'Donnell CP. Systemic and pulmonary hemodynamic responses to normal and obstructed breathing during sleep. J Appl Physiol 1997; 83:1671–1680.

7. Tilkian AG, Guilleminault C, Schroeder JS, Lehrman KL, Simmons FB, Dement WC. Hemodynamics in sleep induced apnea. Ann Intern Med 1976; 85:714–719.

8. Edwards N, Wilcox I, Keogh A, Sullivan CE. Hemodynamic responses to obstructive apneas during sleep are attenuated in heart transplant recipients. Am J Respir Crit Care Med 1997; 155:A678.

9. O'Donnell CP, Ayuse T, King ED, Schwartz AR, Smith PL, Robothom JL. Airway obstruction during sleep increases blood pressure without arousal. J Appl Physiol 1996; 80:773–781.

10. Katragadda S, Xie A, Puleo D, Skatrud JB, Morgan BJ. Neural mechanism of the pressor response to obstructive and nonobstructive apnea. J Appl Physiol 1997; 83: 2048–2054.

11. Remsburg S, Lantin M, Weiss JW. Forearm vascular resistance and MAP increase following apnea termination in patients with OSA. Am J Respir Crit Care Med 1996; 153:A198.

12. Imadojemu VA, Leuenberger U, Sinoway L. Transient arterial hypertension in obstructive sleep apnea during sleep is accompanied by peripheral vasoconstriction. Am J Respir Crit Care Med 1998; 155:A777.

13. Guilleminault C, Tilkian A, Dement WC. The sleep apnea syndromes. Annu Rev Med 1976; 27:465–484.

14. Guilleminault C, Connolly SJ, Winkle RA. Cardiac arrhythmia and conduction disturbances during sleep in 400 patients with sleep apnea syndrome. Am J Cardiol 1983; 52:490–494.

15. Guilleminault C, Connolly S, Winkle R, Melvin K, Tilkian A. Cyclical variations of the heart rate in sleep apnea syndrome: mechanisms and usefulness of 24h electrocardiography as a screening technique. Lancet 1984; 1:126–131.

16. Zwillich C, Devlin T, White D, Douglas N, Weil J, Martin R. Bradycardia during sleep apnea: characteristics and mechanism. J Clin Invest 1982; 69:1286–1292.

17. Daly MD, Hazzeldine JL. The effects of artificially induced hyperventilation on the primary cardiac reflex response to stimulation of the carotid bodies in the dog. J Physiol (Lond) 1963; 168:872–879.

18. Angell James JE, Daly MD. Cardiovascular responses in apneic asphyxia: role of arterial chemoreceptors and the modification of their effects by a pulmonary vagal inflation reflex. J Physiol (Lond) 1969; 201:87–104.

19. Tolle FA, Judy WV, Yu P, Markand ON. Reduced stroke volume related to pleural pressure in obstructive sleep apnea. J Appl Physiol 1983; 55:1718–1724.

20. Stoohs R, Guilleminault C. Cardiovascular changes associated with the obstructive sleep apnea syndrome. J Appl Physiol 1992; 72:582–589.

21. Khatri IM, Freis ED. Hemodynamic changes during sleep. J Appl Physiol 1967; 22: 867–873.

22. Somers VK, Dyken ME, Mark AL, Abboud FM. Sympathetic-nerve activity during sleep in normal subjects. N Engl J Med 1993; 328:303–307.

23. Miller WP. Cardiac arrhythmias and conduction disturbances in the sleep apnea syndrome: prevalence and significance. Am J Med 1982; 73:317.

24. Grimm W, Hoffmann J, Menz V, et al. Electrophysiologic evaluation of sinus node function and atrioventricular conduction in patients with prolonged ventricular asystole during obstructive sleep apnea. Am J Cardiol 1996; 77:1310.
25. Minimasawa K, Tochikubo O, Ishii M. Systemic hemodynamics during sleep in young or middle-aged and elderly patients with essential hypertension. Hypertension 1994; 23:167–173.
26. Podzus T, Mayer J, Penzel T, et al. Nocturnal hemodynamics in patients with obstructive sleep apnea. Eur J Respir Dis 1986; 69:435.
27. Guilleminault C, Tilkian A, Dement WC. The sleep apnea syndromes. Annu Rev Med 1976; 27:465–484.
28. Garpestad E, Ringler J, Parker JA, Remsburg S, Eiss JW. Sleep stage influences the hemodynamic response to obstructive apneas. Am J Respir Crit Care Med 1995; 152:199–203.
29. Guilleminault C, Motta J, Mihm F, Melvin K. Obstructive sleep apnea and cardiac index. Chest 1986; 74:331–334.
30. Kubicek WG, Karnegis JN, Patterson RP, Witsoe DA, Mattson RH. Development and evaluation of an impedance cardiac output system. Aerosp Med 1976; 47:1046–1051.
31. Garpestad E, Parker JA, Katayama H, Lilly J, Yasuda T, Ringler J, Strauss HW, Weiss JW. Decrease in ventricular stroke volume at apnea termination is independent of oxygen saturation. J Appl Physiol 1994; 77:1602–1608.
32. Wilson RA, Sullivan PJ, Moore RH, Zielonla JS, Alpert NM, Boucher CA, McKusick KA, Strauss HW. An ambulatory function monitor: validation and preliminary clinical results. Am J Cardiol 1983; 52:601–606.
33. Aardweg JG van den, Karemaker JM. Repetitive apneas induce periodic hypertension in normal subjects through hypoxia. J Appl Physiol 1992; 72:821–827.
34. Hardy JC, Gray K, Whisler S, Leuenberger U. Sympathetic and blood pressure responses to voluntary apnea are augmented by hypoxia. J Appl Physiol 1994; 77:2360–2365.
35. Morgan BJ, Denahan T, Ebert TJ. Neurocirculatory consequences of negative intrathoracic pressure vs. asphyxia during voluntary apnea. J Appl Physiol 1993; 74:2969–2975.
36. Leuenberger U, Jacob E, Sweer L, Waravdekar N, Zwillich C, Sinoway L. Surges of muscle sympathetic nerve activity during obstructive apnea are linked to hypoxemia. J Appl Physiol 1995; 79:581–588.
37. Smith ML, Niedermaier ON, Hardy SM, Decker MJ, Strohl KP. Role of hypoxemia in sleep-induced sympathoexcitation. J Auton Nerv Syst 1996; 56:184–190.
38. Davies RJ, Belt PJ, Roberts SJ, Ali NJ, Stradling JR. Arterial blood pressure responses to graded transient arousal from sleep in normal humans. J Appl Physiol 1993; 74:1123–1130.
39. Morgan BJ, Crabtree DC, Puleo DS, Badr MS, Toiber F, Skatrud JB. Neurocirculatory consequences of abrupt change in sleep state in humans. J Appl Physiol 1996; 80:1627–1636.
40. O'Donnell CP, King ED, Schwartz AR, Robothom JL, Smith PL. Relationship between blood pressure and airway obstruction during sleep in the dog. J Appl Physiol 1994; 77:1819–1828.

41. Brooks D, Horner RL, Kozar LF, Render-Teixeira CLB, Phillipson EA. Obstructive sleep apnea as a cause of systemic hypertension: evidence from a canine model. J Clin Invest 1997; 99:106–119.

42. Kaufman MP, Cassidy SS. Reflex effects of lung inflation and other stimuli on the heart and circulation. In: Scharf SM, Cassidy SS, eds. Heart-Lung Interactions in Health and Disease. New York: Marcel Dekker, 1989:339–363.

43. Robotham JL, Peters J. How changes in alveolar pressure cause changes in afterload and preload. In: Scharf SM, Cassidy SS, eds. Heart-Lung Interactions in Health and Disease. New York: Marcel Decker, 1989:251–283.

44. Condos W, Latham R, Hoadley S, Pasipoularides A. Hemodynamics of the Mueller maneuver in man: right and left heart micromanometry and Doppler echocardiography. Circulation 1987; 76:1020–1028.

45. Buda AJ, Pinsky MR, Ingels NB Jr., Daughters GT 2nd, Stinson EB, Alderman EL. Effect of intrathoracic pressure on left ventricular performance. N Engl J Med 1979; 301:453–459.

10

Nocturnal Myocardial Ischemia and Cardiac Arrhythmias

Importance of Cardiorespiratory Homeostasis

RICHARD L. VERRIER

Harvard Medical School
and Beth Israel Deaconess Medical Center
Boston, Massachusetts

I. Introduction

The periodic reexcitation the brain experiences during normal cycling from non–rapid-eye-movement (NREM) to REM sleep results in significant perturbations in cardiac autonomic tone (1). In individuals with heart disease, these sleep state–dependent fluctuations in autonomic pattern may compromise coronary artery blood flow and trigger life-threatening arrhythmias (2). Impairment of ventilation during sleep by central or obstructive sleep apnea can produce significant reductions in oxygen supply to the heart. Obstructive sleep apnea afflicts 5–10 million Americans, or 2–4% of the population (3), and has been strongly implicated in the development of hypertension, ischemia, arrhythmias, myocardial infarction, and sudden death in individuals with coexisting ischemic heart disease. Cardiac function in patients with heart failure further deteriorates when respiration is disturbed. Atrial fibrillation may be precipitated by autonomic or respiratory disturbances during sleep in certain patient populations.

 The goal of this chapter will be to discuss the pathophysiological mechanisms responsible for sleep-related cardiac morbidity and mortality, particularly in the context of disturbed nighttime breathing.

II. Cardiorespiratory Homeostasis During Sleep

Maintaining homeostasis during sleep requires coordinating control over two different types of systems: the respiratory, necessary for oxygen exchange, and the cardiovascular, for blood transport (4). The difficult balancing act of regulating two systems, one supplying somatic musculature (i.e., diaphragmatic, intercostal, abdominal, and upper airway musculature) and the other involving control of autonomic pathways to the heart and vasculature is a daunting task. This challenge is particularly difficult in individuals who have diseased respiratory or cardiovascular systems.

NREM sleep is associated with relative stability of autonomic regulation (1). Respiratory sinus arrhythmia is marked, indicating a high degree of parasympathetic tone (1,4,5). NREM sleep is accompanied by hypotension, bradycardia, and reductions in cardiac output and systemic vascular resistance (1,5). The bradycardias appear to be due mainly to an increase in vagal activation, whereas the hypotension is primarily the result of a reduction in sympathetic vasomotor tone (6). During transitions from slow-wave to REM sleep, bursts of vagus nerve firing may culminate in pauses in heart rhythm and frank asystole (7).

REM sleep, in serving brain neurochemical functions and behavioral adaptations, can disturb cardiorespiratory homeostasis (1,4,5). The brain's increased excitability during REM sleep can result in major surges in cardiac sympathetic activity to the coronary and skeletal muscular vessels. Cardiac efferent vagal tone is usually suppressed during REM, and breathing patterns are irregular (4,8,9). Such changes can significantly affect cardiovascular functioning, as is evident in alterations in heart rate and arterial blood pressure in normal subjects and in the occurrence of arrhythmias and ischemia in patients whose myocardium is compromised.

III. Central and Peripheral Mechanisms Responsible for Surges in Heart Rhythm

Distinct mechanisms associated with specific brain sites contribute to discrete sleep state–dependent perturbations in cardiac rhythm. Several investigators have documented REM-induced sinus tachycardia in experimental animals (6,10–16). One distinct heart rate response that has recently been characterized involves an abrupt though transitory 35–37% increase in rate that occurs mainly during phasic REM and is followed by a baroreceptor-mediated deceleration; it is eliminated by surgical ablation of sympathetic neural input to the heart (Fig. 1) (13–15). The phenomenon, observed in dogs, differs from that observed by Baust and Bohnert (11) in felines in that the increase in heart rate observed is more pronounced and is not contingent on withdrawal of parasympathetic nerve activity.

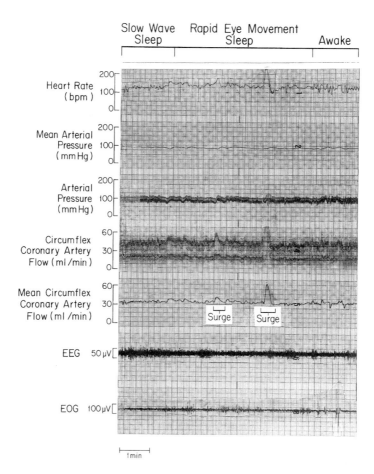

Figure 1 Effects of NREM sleep, REM sleep, and quiet wakefulness on heart rate, phasic and mean arterial blood pressure, phasic and mean left circumflex coronary flow, electroencephalogram (EEG), and electro-oculogram (EOG) in the dog. Sleep spindles are evident during NREM sleep, eye movements during REM, and grosser eye movements on awakening. Surges in heart rate and coronary flow occur during REM sleep. (From Ref. 13.)

An enhanced frequency of heart rate surges was observed during periods of REM marked by phasic eye movements (10,11,15).

A second, distinct REM sleep state–dependent surge in heart rate appears to be due to the primary involvement of central nervous system (CNS) activation, as it is accompanied by a concomitant increase in hippocampal theta frequency, pontogeniculo-occipital (PGO) activity, and eye movements (16). This increase in frequency was observed in felines, a species in which the appearance of theta waves is characteristic of arousal, orienting activity, alertness, and REM sleep, when they are typically closely associated with PGO activity and eye movements (17–20). The finding that cardioselective β-adrenergic blockade with atenolol markedly reduced the phenomenon suggests that these REM-induced heart rate surges are primarily mediated by bursts of cardiac sympathetic efferent fiber activity that affect heart rate directly.

IV. Mechanisms Mediating Heart Rhythm Pauses

An abrupt deceleration in heart rhythm that occurs predominantly during tonic REM sleep and is not associated with any preceding or subsequent change in

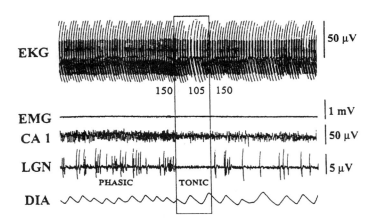

Figure 2 Representative polygraphic recording of a primary heart rate deceleration during tonic REM sleep in a cat. During this deceleration, heart rate decreased from 150 to 105 beats per minute, or 30%. The deceleration occurred during a period devoid of pontogeniculo-occipital (PGO) spikes in the lateral geniculate nucleus (LGN) or theta rhythm in the hippocampal (CA1) leads. The deceleration is not a respiratory arrhythmia, as it is independent of diaphragmatic movement. The abrupt decreases in amplitude of hippocampal theta (CA1), PGO waves (LGN), and respiratory amplitude and rate (DIA) are typical of transitions from phasic to tonic REM. EKG, electrocardiogram; EMG, electromyogram, LGN, lateral geniculate nucleus; CA1, hippocampus CA1 region; DIA, diaphragm. (From Ref. 21.)

heart rate or arterial blood pressure has recently been observed in felines (Fig. 2) (21). Vagus nerve discharge appears to be directly initiated by central influences, as there is no antecedent or subsequent change in resting heart rate or arterial blood pressure. The primary involvement of central nervous system activation is suggested by the consistent antecedent abrupt termination of PGO activity and concomitant interruption of hippocampal theta rhythm.

The likely basis for the abrupt deceleration in heart rate during tonic REM sleep is an alteration in the centrally induced pattern of autonomic activity to the heart. This may be the result of a reduction in sympathetic nerve activity or increased vagal tone, either alone or in combination. Muscarinic blockade with glycopyrrolate completely abolished the phenomenon, suggesting that the tonic REM-induced decelerations may be primarily mediated by bursting of cardiac

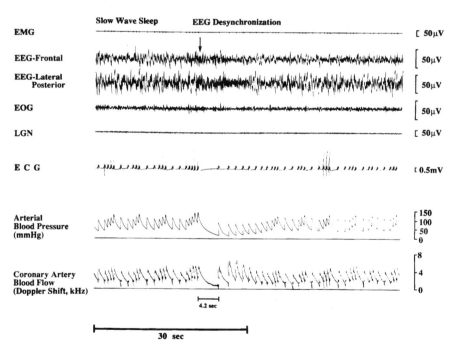

Figure 3 Coronary blood flow (CBF) surge during deep NREM sleep interrupted by electroencephalographic (EEG) desynchronization in a dog. This response pattern is common and appears to represent a brief, low-grade arousal. The 4.2-sec pause in heart rhythm was followed by a brief increase of 46% in average peak CBF and a decrease of 49% in the rate pressure (HR × SBP) product. EMG, electromyogram; EEG, electroencephalogram; EOG, electro-oculogram; LGN, lateral geniculate nucleus field potential recordings; ECG, electrocardiogram. (From Ref. 7.)

vagal efferent fiber activity. This finding is consonant with the established observation that enhanced vagal activity can abruptly and significantly affect sinus node firing rate (22). Withdrawal of cardiac sympathetic tone does not appear to be integral to the changes in heart rate, as cardioselective β_1-adrenergic blockade with atenolol did not affect the incidence or magnitude of decelerations. Respiratory interactions do not appear to be essential to the deceleration, as the phenomenon often occurred without any temporal association with inspiratory effort.

This primary pause phenomenon differs from the baroreceptor-mediated reductions in heart rate, in which heart rhythm pauses almost invariably followed accelerations in rate and increases in arterial blood pressure (Fig. 3) (7). This second group of heart rhythm pauses was observed in canines and occurs mainly during transition from slow-wave sleep (SWS) to desynchronized sleep and more frequently during phasic REM than tonic REM sleep. They persist from 1 to 8 sec and are followed by dramatic increases in coronary blood flow, averaging 30% and ranging up to 84%, which are not linked to metabolic activity of the heart, as indicated by the heart rate–blood pressure product. A strong burst of vagus nerve activity is likely to produce the phenomenon, since the decelerations appear against a background of pronounced respiratory sinus arrhythmia, varying degrees of heart block with nonconducted P waves, and low heart rate. Guilleminault and colleagues reported similar pauses in young adults (23).

V. Experimental Models Defining Effects of Obstructive Sleep Apnea on Systemic Circulatory Function

Notwithstanding the established importance of obstructive sleep apnea in the development of important cardiac disease conditions—including hypertension, myocardial infarction, arrhythmias, and sudden cardiac death—there has been a paucity of experimental studies directed to define the relationship between disturbed nocturnal breathing and cardiovascular function. This has been due in part to the absence of natural models and also to difficulty in implementing suitable techniques to emulate obstructive sleep apnea. To date, only one natural large land mammal model of sleep apnea has been described. Hendricks and coworkers (24) found that the English bulldog, because of its unusual upper airway anatomy with enlargement of the soft palate and narrow oropharynx, exhibits spontaneous sleep-disordered breathing. These animals experience significant oxygen desaturation to <90% during REM sleep. However, they do not experience apnea during NREM sleep. During wakefulness, the animals are hypersomnolent, as evidenced by shortened sleep latency. Although several studies of CNS and respiratory physiology have been explored with this model, it has not been employed in cardiovascular studies.

The main sleep apnea models employed in the cardiac physiology literature have involved endotracheal obstruction with a balloon occluder (25–29) or laryn-

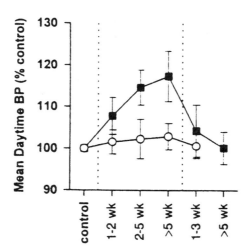

Figure 4 Mean daytime arterial blood pressure in four dogs during obstructive sleep apnea (OSA) (filled squares) and sleep fragmentation (open circles). The dashed lines indicate the beginning and end, respectively, of the OSA or sleep fragmentation phase. The post-OSA or post-sleep fragmentation values represent the first recovery night. Values = means ± SEM. The duration of the OSA and sleep fragmentation phases ranged from 5–14 weeks and 5–7.5 weeks, respectively. Data points are joined for ease of interpretation; note, however that the time periods between points on the X axis are unequal. (From Ref. 28.)

geal stimulation (30). Significant state-dependent alterations in heart rhythm and systemic hemodynamic function have been reported in association with airway obstruction. Among the most clinically relevant studies is that of Brooks and co-workers (28), who demonstrated that intermittent airway occlusion during sleep over the course of a 1- to 3-month period could induce systemic hypertension in a canine model. Mean arterial blood pressure was raised by 16 ± 4 mmHg, a highly significant result (Fig. 4). The development of hypertension could not be attributed to recurrent arousals from sleep but was probably due to changes in neurohumoral control of the heart. The underlying mechanisms deserve intense investigation, especially given the high prevalence of both hypertension and obstructive sleep apnea in the general population and the central role of these pathologies in the genesis of cardiorespiratory disease.

VI. Coronary Hemodynamic Function During Sleep

Marked changes in coronary blood flow occur during REM and sleep-state transitions (13–15,31). Vatner and co-workers (31) observed baboons during the nocturnal period and determined that coronary artery blood flow fluctuated by as much as twofold when the animals were judged to be asleep by behavioral indicators. The periodic fluctuations in blood flow were not associated with changes in heart rate or arterial blood pressure and occurred while the animals remained motionless with eyes closed. No data were obtained regarding sleep stage, nor was the mechanism for the coronary blood flow surge defined.

Concomitant with heart rate surges of REM sleep observed in dogs (13–15) described above were sizable episodic surges in coronary blood flow with

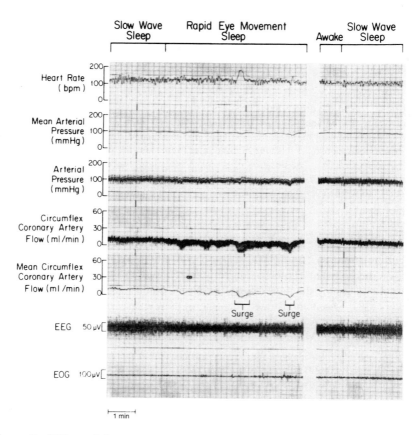

Figure 5 Effects of sleep stage on heart rate, mean and phasic arterial blood pressures, and mean and phasic left circumflex coronary artery blood flow in a typical dog during stenosis. Note phasic decreases in coronary flow occurring during heart rate surges while the dog is in REM sleep. EEG, electroencephalogram; EOG, electro-oculogram. (From Ref. 14.)

corresponding decreases in coronary vascular resistance (Fig. 1). These phenomena occurred mainly during periods of REM sleep characterized by intense phasic activity, as defined by the frequency of eye movements (15). There were no appreciable changes in mean arterial blood pressure. Heart rate was elevated during the flow surges, indicating an increase in cardiac metabolic activity as the cause of the coronary vasodilation. In fact, the close coupling between rate-pressure product—an index of metabolic demand—and the magnitude of the flow surge suggests that the surges do not represent a state of myocardial hyperperfusion. These increases in coronary blood flow appeared to result from increased adrenergic discharge, since they were abolished by bilateral stellectomy. They did not appear to be due to nonspecific effects of somatic activity or respiratory fluctuations.

During coronary artery stenosis, with baseline flow reduced by 60%, phasic reductions in coronary arterial blood flow rather than increases were found during REM sleep coincident with these heart rate surges (14) (Fig. 5). The increase in adrenergic activity could lead to a decrement in coronary blood flow by at least two possible mechanisms: stimulation of α-adrenergic receptors on the coronary vascular smooth muscle or a decrease in diastolic coronary perfusion time due to the surges in heart rate. The accuracy of the latter explanation is supported by the strong correlation ($r^2 = 0.96$) between the magnitude of the increase in heart rate and the decrease in coronary blood flow (14). The association between REM-induced changes in heart rate and the occurrence of coronary insufficiency in patients with advanced coronary artery disease is in accord with the clinical experience of Nowlin and co-workers (32).

VII. Consequences of Airway Obstruction on Coronary Artery Blood Flow

A few studies have been performed on the effects of mechanical obstruction of the airway on coronary and myocardial hemodynamic function during sleep. Pinto and co-workers (25) determined in a porcine model that endotracheal obstruction lasting ~10 sec during REM or NREM sleep was not associated with any significant effects on heart rate, mean arterial blood pressure, coronary artery blood flow, or coronary vascular resistance. However, arousal from sleep during airway obstruction was associated with significant increases in all variables, especially in coronary vascular resistance. α-adrenergic receptor blockade eliminated the associated increases in both arterial pressure and coronary vascular resistance. Follow-up studies by the same group indicated that β-adrenergic blockade eliminated the heart rate and coronary blood flow responses (26) and that intracerebroventricular β-blockade prevented the increases in coronary vascular resistance in this model (27). Caution should be exercised in extrapolating these receptor blocking studies to the clinical arena because of the established differences in porcine and human responses to β-adrenergic blockade (33). The increases in coronary blood pressure and vascular resistance could prove especially important in individuals with coronary artery disease, who may experience excessive coronary artery reactivity and have a compromised coronary vascular reserve, conditions that can lead to impaired myocardial perfusion, ischemia, and even arrhythmias.

A similar model of upper airway obstruction during sleep was employed in canines (29), allowing investigators to document marked oscillation in ventricular output throughout the apnea cycle and to determine that heart rate, and not stroke volume, is the dominant factor moderating ventricular output in response to apnea. A second canine model of apnea involved laryngeal stimulation, produced either by inflating a small balloon positioned in the rostral portion of the trachea or by squirting water on the larynx through a catheter inserted through a tracheos-

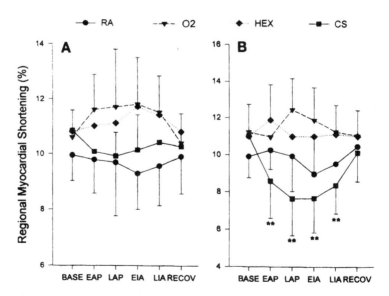

Figure 6 Effects of periodic obstructive apneas on LV regional myocardial segmental shortening, indicating regional myocardial ischemia. (A), Area perfused by left circumflex (LCX) coronary artery. (B), Area perfused by LAD coronary artery. RA, room-air breathing; O2, breathing O_2; CS, breathing room air after critical coronary stenosis; Hex, breathing room air after hexamethonium; Base, baseline; EAP, early apnea; LAP, late apnea; EIA, early interapnea; LIA, late interapnea; Recov, recovery. Values = means ± SEM; each data point represents 5 sec of data. **Significance compared with baseline, $p < 0.01$. (From Ref. 34.)

tomy (30). Subarousal stimuli during NREM produced apnea and bradycardia. During REM, the apnea was prolonged (>10 sec) and bradycardia was marked.

Chen and Sharf (34) examined the effects of periodic obstructive apneas in sedated pigs with coronary artery stenosis. They determined that obstructive apneas led to regional myocardial ischemia, as indicated by segmental shortening of the territory supplied by the stenosed vessels (Fig. 6) and a corresponding decrease in intramyocardial pH, indicative of impaired metabolic activity with propensity to regional metabolic acidosis.

The important gap in knowledge regarding the involvement of apnea in myocardial ischemia and infarction could be addressed if the techniques of airway obstruction were combined with coronary artery stenosis in a large animal model during natural sleep. Such a model would be extremely useful in elucidating mechanisms responsible for the clinical findings of heightened risk for myocardial infarction and sudden cardiac death in individuals with advanced coronary artery disease and sleep apnea and perhaps in providing opportunities for exploring therapeutic interventions.

VIII. Arrhythmogenesis During Sleep

The concept that NREM sleep is generally protective with respect to ventricular arrhythmogenesis is consonant with studies of neurocardiac interactions and clinical experience (2). Profound activation of the vagus nerve as occurs during the NREM state decreases heart rate, blood pressure, and coronary vascular resistance (35), increases cardiac electrical stability, and reduces the rate-pressure product, an index of cardiac metabolic activity. These characteristics can lead to an improved supply–demand relationship in stenotic coronary artery segments. However, in the setting of severe coronary disease or acute myocardial infarction, hypotension can conduce to myocardial ischemia because of inadequate coronary perfusion pressure, and this set of circumstances, consequently, can also provoke arrhythmias and myocardial infarction (5,36,37). Nocturnal surges in vagus nerve activity could precipitate myocardial ischemia and arrhythmias as a result of vasoconstriction rather than dilation in atherosclerotic coronary artery segments due to impaired release of endothelium-derived relaxing factor (38). Finally, the abrupt enhancement in vagal tone that can occur during periods of REM or sleep-state transitions can produce significant pauses in heart rhythm, bradyarrhythmias (7), and, potentially, triggered activity, a mechanism of the lethal cardiac arrhythmia torsades de pointes. Patients with long-QT syndrome who have the type 3 phenotype are prone to experience torsades de pointes at night rather than in the more typical settings of stress or exercise (39).

Because of the attendant surges in autonomic activity and in heart rate, REM sleep also has the potential for triggering ventricular and supraventricular arrhythmias because of the arrhythmogenic influence of neurally released cate-cholamines (40,41). The striking respiratory variability can also significantly affect cardiovascular functioning. The few clinical studies in which sleep staging has been employed have identified REM as the state in which arrhythmias occurred (5,42–44).

REM sleep is also capable of inducing ischemia (32), with potential for increasing sympathetic nerve activity and, in turn, cardiac vulnerability by complex mechanisms. Experimental studies of ischemia-induced arrhythmogenesis have determined that the direct profibrillatory mechanisms are derangements in impulse formation, conduction, or both (41). Increased levels of catecholamines activate β-adrenergic receptors, which, in turn, alter adenylate cyclase activity and intracellular calcium flux. These actions are probably mediated by the cyclic nucleotide and protein kinase regulatory cascade, which can alter spatial heterogeneity of calcium transients and consequently increase dispersion of repolarization. The major indirect mechanisms include impaired oxygen supply–demand ratio due to increased cardiac metabolic activity and coronary vasoconstriction, particularly in vessels with injured endothelium and in the context of altered preload and afterload (45).

Experimental findings on sleep state–dependent cardiac function during myocardial infarction are extremely limited. Ventricular ectopic activity but not ventricular fibrillation has been observed during NREM sleep in pigs following myocardial infarction (46). This pattern may be attributable to slowing of heart rate and increased vagus nerve activity during NREM sleep, conditions that can remove the normal overdrive suppression of ventricular rhythms by sinoatrial node pacemaker activity and result in firing of latent ventricular pacemakers and triggered activity. Snisarenko (47) observed significant elevations in heart rate following myocardial infarction in a feline model but did not discuss heart rhythm.

IX. Summary and Conclusions

Sleep states have a significant effect on cardiorespiratory homeostasis. This is a consequence of the changing brain activity during the normal cycling between NREM and REM sleep. Because of the close neurohumoral coupling between central structures and the cardiorespiratory system, sleep state–dependent fluctuations occur in heart rhythm, arterial blood pressure, coronary artery blood flow, and ventilation. NREM sleep is associated with relative autonomic stability and coordination between respiration, pumping action of the heart, and maintenance of arterial blood pressure. During REM sleep, there are sizable alterations in the pattern of both sympathetic and parasympathetic nerve activity, resulting in significant surges and pauses in heart rhythm. Whereas the perturbations in autonomic nervous system activity are well tolerated in normal individuals, those with heart disease and/or sleep apnea may be at particular risk during REM sleep, as the stress on the system has the potential for triggering atrial and ventricular arrhythmias and myocardial infarction. During NREM sleep, a potential for hypotension exists in the diseased circulatory system that can, in turn, impair delivery to stenotic cerebral and coronary vessels. Despite the evidence that autonomic factors have the potential for significantly altering susceptibility to arrhythmias, the observation that the heart rate surges of REM sleep conduce to myocardial ischemia, and the epidemiological data on the extent of sleep-induced cardiac events (48), there is a dearth of information regarding the effects of sleep states on susceptibility to arrhythmias during myocardial ischemia and infarction in experimental animals. Given the overwhelming evidence that the coexistence of heart disease and sleep apnea is associated with heightened risk and that the affected population is sizable, there is a need for intensified research of this major public health problem.

Acknowledgments

Supported by grant HL50078 from the National Heart, Lung, and Blood Institute and ES 08129 from National Institutes of Environmental Health, National Institutes of Health, Bethesda, Maryland.

References

1. Verrier RL, Harper RM, Hobson AJ. Central and autonomic mechanisms regulating cardiovascular function during sleep. In: Kryger MH, Roth T, Dement WC, eds. Principles and Practice of Sleep Medicine, 3d ed. Philadelphia: WB Saunders, 2000.
2. Verrier RL, Mittleman MA. Sleep-related cardiac risk. In: Kryger MH, Roth T, Dement WC, eds. Principles and Practice of Sleep Medicine, 3d ed. Philadelphia: WB Saunders, 2000.
3. Young T, Palta M, Dempsey J, Skatrud J, Weber S, Badr S. The occurrence of sleep-disordered breathing among middle-aged adults. N Engl J Med 1993; 328:1230–1235.
4. Harper RM, Frysinger RC, Zhang J, Trelease RB, Terreberry RR. Cardiac and respiratory interactions maintaining homeostasis during sleep. In: Lydic R, Biebuyck JF, eds. Clinical Physiology of Sleep. Bethesda, MD: American Physiological Society, 1988.
5. Mancia G. Autonomic modulation of the cardiovascular system during sleep. N Engl J Med 1993; 328:347–349.
6. Baccelli G, Guazzi M, Mancia G, Zanchetti A. Neural and non-neural mechanisms influencing circulation during sleep. Nature 1969; 223:184–185.
7. Dickerson LW, Huang AH, Nearing BD, Verrier RL. Primary coronary vasodilation

associated with pauses in heart rhythm during sleep. Am J Physiol. 1993; 264:R186–R196.

8. Phillipson EA, Bowes G. Control of breathing during sleep. In: Cherniack NS, Widdicombe JG, eds. Handbook of Physiology: Section III. The Respiratory System. Bethesda, MD: American Physiological Society, 1986.

9. Snyder F, Hobson JA, Morrison DF, Goldfrank F. Changes in respiration, heart rate, and systolic blood pressure in human sleep. J Appl Physiol 1964; 19:417–422.

10. Gassel MM, Ghelarducci B, Marchiafava PL, Pompeiano O. Phasic changes in blood pressure and heart rate during the rapid eye movement episodes of desynchronized sleep in unrestrained cats. Arch Ital Biol 1964; 102:530–544.

11. Baust W, Bohnert B. The regulation of heart rate during sleep. Exp Brain Res 1969; 7:169–180.

12. Baust W, Holzbach E, Zechlin O. Phasic changes in heart rate and respiration correlated with PGO-spike activity during REM sleep. Pflugers Arch 1972; 331:113–123.

13. Kirby DA, Verrier RL. Differential effects of sleep stage on coronary hemodynamic function. Am J Physiol 1989; 256:H1378–H1383.

14. Kirby DA, Verrier RL. Differential effects of sleep stage on coronary hemodynamic function during stenosis. Physiol Behav 1989; 45:1017–1020.

15. Dickerson LW, Huang AH, Thurnher MM, Nearing BD, Verrier RL. Relationship between coronary hemodynamic changes and the phasic events of rapid eye movement sleep. Sleep 1993; 16:550–557.

16. Rowe K, et al. Heart rate surges during REM sleep are associated with theta rhythm and PGO activity in cats. Am J Physiol 1999; 277:R843–R849.

17. Sakai K, Sano K, Iwahara S. Eye movements and hippocampal theta activity in cats. Electroencephalogr Clin Neurophysiol 1973; 34:547–549.

18. Kemp IR, Kaada BR. The relation of hippocampal theta activity to arousal, attentive behaviour and somato-motor movements in unrestrained cats. Brain Res 1975; 95: 323–342.

19. Lerma J, Garcia-Austt E. Hippocampal theta rhythm during paradoxical sleep: effects of afferent stimuli and phase relationships with phasic events. Electroencephalogr Clin Neurophysiol 1985; 60:46–54.

20. Sei H, Morita Y. Acceleration of EEG theta wave precedes the phasic surge of arterial pressure during REM sleep in the rat. Neuroreport 1996; 7:3059–3062.

21. Verrier RL, Lau RT, Wallooppillai U, Quattrochi J, Nearing BD, Moreno R, Hobson JA. Primary vagally mediated decelerations in heart rate during tonic rapid eye movement sleep in cats. Am J Physiol 1998; 43:R1136–R1141.

22. Pappano AJ. Modulation of the heartbeat by the vagus nerve. In: Zipes DP, Jalife J, eds. Cardiac Electrophysiology: From Cell to Bedside. Philadelphia: WB Saunders, 1995.

23. Guilleminault CP, Pool P, Motta J, Gillis AM. Sinus arrest during REM sleep in young adults. N Engl J Med 1984; 311:1006–1010.

24. Hendricks JC, Kline LR, Kovalski RJ, O'Brien JA, Morrison AR, Pack AI. The English bulldog: a natural model of sleep-disordered breathing. J Appl Physiol 1987; 63:1344–1350.

25. Pinto JMB, Garpestad E, Weiss JW, Bergau DM, Kirby DA. Hemodynamic changes

associated with obstructive sleep apnea followed by arousal in a porcine model. J Appl Physiol 1993; 75:1439–1443.

26. Kirby DA, Pinto JM, Weiss JW, Garpestad E, Zinkovska S. Effects of beta-adrenergic receptor blockade on hemodynamic changes associated with obstructive sleep apnea. Physiol Behav 1995; 58:919–923.

27. Zinkovska S, Kirby DA. Intracerebroventricular propranolol prevented vascular resistance increases on arousal from sleep apnea. J Appl Physiol 1997; 82:1637–1643.

28. Brooks D, Horner RL, Kozar LF, Render-Teixeira CL, Phillipson EA. Obstructive sleep apnea as a cause of systemic hypertension: evidence from a canine model. J Clin Invest 1997; 99:106–109.

29. Schneider H, Schaub CD, Andreoni KA, Schwartz AR, Smith PL, Robotham JL, O'Donnell CP. Systemic and pulmonary hemodynamic responses to normal and obstructed breathing during sleep. J Appl Physiol 1997; 83:1671–1680.

30. Sullivan CE, Murphy E, Kozar LF, Phillipson EA. Waking and ventilatory responses to laryngeal stimulation in sleeping dogs. J Appl Physiol Respir Environ Exerc Physiol 1978; 45:681–689.

31. Vatner SF, Franklin D, Higgins CB, Patrick T, White S, Van Citters RL. Coronary dynamics in unrestrained conscious baboons. Am J Physiol 1971; 221:1396–1401.

32. Nowlin JB, Troyer WG Jr, Collins WS, Silverman G, Nichols CR, McIntosh HD, Estes EH Jr, Bogdonoff MD. The association of nocturnal angina pectoris with dreaming. Ann Intern Med 1965; 63:1040–1046.

33. Benfey BG, Elfellah MS, Ogilvie RI, Varma DR. Anti-arrhythmic effects of prazosin and propranolol during coronary artery occlusion and re-perfusion in dogs and pigs. Br J Pharmacol 1984; 82:717–725.

34. Chen L, Scharf SM. Systemic and myocardial hemodynamics during periodic obstructive apneas in sedated pigs. J Appl Physiol 1998; 84:1289–1298.

35. Kovach JA, Gottdiener JS, Verrier RL. Vagal modulation of epicardial coronary artery size in dogs: a two-dimensional intravascular ultrasound study. Circulation 1995; 92:2291–2298.

36. Broughton R, Baron R. Sleep patterns in the intensive care unit and on the ward after acute myocardial infarction. Electroencephalogr Clin Neurophysiol 1978; 45:348–360.

37. Deedwania PC. Increased demand versus reduced supply and the circadian variations in ambulatory myocardial ischemia: therapeutic implications (editorial). Circulation 1993; 88:328–331.

38. Ludmer PL, Selwyn AP, Shook TL, Wayne RR, Mudge GH, Alexander RW, Ganz P. Paradoxical vasoconstriction induced by acetylcholine in atherosclerotic arteries. N Engl J Med 1986; 315:1046–1051.

39. Schwartz PJ, Priori SG, Locati EH, Napolitano C, Cantú F, Towbin AJ, Keating MT, Hammoude H, Brown AM, Chen LK, Colatsky TJ. Long QT syndrome patients with mutations of the SCN5A and HERG genes have differential responses to Na+ channel blockade and to increases in heart rate. Implications for gene-specific therapy. Circulation 1995; 92:3381–3386.

40. Lown B, Verrier RL. Neural activity and ventricular fibrillation. N Engl J Med 1976; 294:1165–1170.

41. Janse MJ, Wit AL. Electrophysiological mechanism of ventricular arrhythmias resulting from myocardial ischemia and infarction. Physiol Rev 1989; 69:1049–1169.
42. Smith R, Johnson L, Rothfeld D, Zir L, Tharp B. Sleep and cardiac arrhythmias. Arch Intern Med 1972; 130:751–753.
43. Rosenblatt G, Hartman E, Zwilling GR. Cardiac irritability during sleep and dreaming. J Psychosom 1973; 17:129–134.
44. Otsuka K, Yanaga T, Ichimaru Y, Seto K. Sleep and night-type arrhythmias. Jpn Heart J 1982; 23:479–486.
45. Verrier RL. Autonomic modulation of arrhythmias in animal models. In: Rosen MR, Wit AL, Janse MJ, eds. Cardiac Electrophysiology: A Textbook in Honor of Brian Hoffman. New York: Futura Press, 1990.
46. Skinner JE, Mohr DN, Kellaway P. Sleep-stage regulation of ventricular arrhythmias in the unanesthetized pig. Circ Res 1975; 37:342–349.
47. Snisarenko AA. Cardiac rhythm in cats during physiological sleep in experimental myocardial infarction and beta-adrenergic receptor blockade. Cor Vasa 1986; 38: 306–314.
48. Lavery CE, Mittleman MA, Cohen MC, Muller JE, Verrier RL. Nonuniform nighttime distribution of acute cardiac events: a possible effect of sleep states. Circulation 1997; 96:3321–3327.

11

Obstructive Sleep Apnea and Cardiac Ischemia in Humans

PATRICK J. HANLY

University of Toronto
and St. Michael's Hospital
Toronto, Ontario, Canada

I. Introduction

There are a number of factors that promote the coexistence of obstructive sleep apnea (OSA) and coronary artery disease (CAD) in a single patient. First, both are common conditions. The prevalence of OSA, defined as an apnea-hypopnea index (AHI) greater than 5/hr, in a population-based study of middle- aged adults was found to be 9% in women and 24% in men (1). The prevalence of CAD is also high in both men and women. By the age of 60 years, 6% of women and 20% of men in the United States have had a coronary event (2). Second, OSA and CAD share many risk factors such as male gender (1,2), obesity (1,3), advancing age (1,4), and diabetes mellitus (5,6), which predispose an individual patient to develop both conditions. Third, it has been suggested that OSA is associated with the pathogenesis of CAD (7,8), possibly by promoting the development of coronary atherosclerosis secondary to hypoxemia during sleep (9).

Many of the physiological changes that accompany OSA can also provoke myocardial ischemia. OSA is characteristically associated with recurrent hypoxemia, which occurs during each obstructive apnea or hypopnea. Chierchia et al. (10) continuously monitored oxygen saturation in the coronary sinus (CSO_2S) in six males with CAD who had frequent angina at rest. It was found that a sharp drop in CSO₂S consistently preceded the onset of myocardial ischemia, reflected by electrocardiographic and hemodynamic changes (Fig. 1). Interestingly, only 10 of 137 ischemic episodes were associated with anginal pain, which typically occurred 50–120 sec after the onset of ST-segment and T-wave changes. Ironically, patients with OSA are repetitively exposed to reduced myocardial oxygen supply at a time when their myocardial oxygen demand is increasing. Repeated attempts to inspire against an occluded upper airway are accompanied by more negative pressure around the heart, thereby increasing left ventricular afterload (11,12) and heart rate, both of which increase myocardial oxygen demand. Changes in heart rate before and throughout episodes of myocardial ischemia, reflected by ST-segment depression, were recorded in 11 patients with nocturnal and daytime angina by Quyyumi et al. (13). In 94% of nocturnal episodes and 100% of daytime episodes, the heart rate increased before the onset of ST segment depression; in all but one episode, the heart rate returned to baseline before the ST segment (Fig. 2). These changes were observed regardless of whether the episodes of segment depression were accompanied by anginal pain. This imbalance between myocardial oxygen demand and supply during obstructive apneas predisposes these patients to myocardial ischemia, and this imbalance is amplified during rapid-eye-movement (REM) sleep, when apneas are characteristically

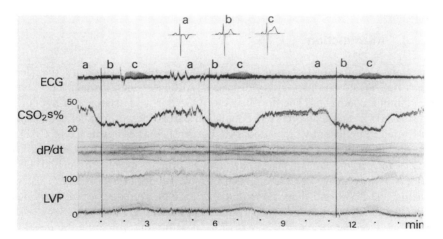

Figure 1   Low-speed playback (paper speed 0.3 mm/sec) of ECG, coronary sinus O_2 saturation (CSO₂S), left ventricular pressure (LVP), and dp/dt during three successive asymptomatic ischemic episodes in a single patient over a period of about 15 min. At the top are electrocardiographic patterns (lead V_2) in resting conditions (a), at the onset (b), and at the peak (c) of the ischemic episode. Vertical lines correspond to the onset of the ST-T–wave changes. A sharp drop of CSO₂S consistently precedes the onset of ECG and hemodynamic changes (From Ref. 10.)

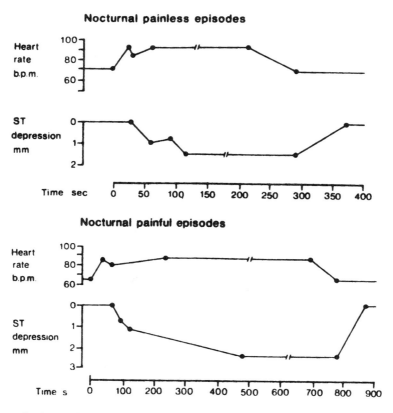

Figure 2 Mean changes in heart rate during episodes of painless and painful nocturnal ST-segment depression in five patients (From Ref. 13.)

longer and the severity of hypoxemia is greater. Furthermore, REM sleep itself has been associated with nocturnal angina (14), possibly through associated changes in autonomic tone.

Thus, there is a good theoretical basis for the development of myocardial ischemia during obstructive apnea, *particularly* in patients with CAD, which is quite likely to coexist with OSA. What evidence is there that myocardial ischemia develops during obstructive apnea in patients with and without CAD?

II. OSA in Patients with CAD (Table 1)

Wei and Bradley selected 10 subjects with angiographically proven CAD who had stable exertional angina and episodic nocturnal angina (15). Following over-

Table 1 Myocardial Ischemia in OSA Patients with CAD

Ref.	Demographics		OSA		Evidence CAD				Evid. MI		CPAP	
	n (m/f)	Age	AHI	Min SaO$_2$	AP	Ex ECG	Angio	Thallium	AP	ST	AP	ST
Wei, 1992 (15)	8(7/1)	69 ± 4	36 ± 11	76 ± 3	+		+		+		+	
DeOlazabal, 1982 (16)	17	36–63	20	~80	+		+		−	−		
Goldman, 1993 (17)	34(33/1)	69 ± 6	?	?	+				−	+		
Koehler, 1991 (20)	20	47–68	33 ± 13	75	+	+	+		−	+		
Franklin, 1995 (22)	10(10/0)	63 ± 7	40 ± 19	?	+		+		+	+	+	+
Philip, 1993 (23)	34(32/2)	53 ± 10		<50%	+	+		+	+	+	+	+

n(m/f), number of subjects (male/female ratio); OSA, obstructive sleep apnea; AHI, apnea-hypopnea index; min Sa$_{O_2}$, minimum oxygen saturation during sleep; Evidence CAD, evidence of coronary artery disease based on a history of angina pectoris (AP), electrocardiographic changes on exercise (Ex ECG), coronary angiography (Angio), or thallium perfusion scan (Thallium); Evid. MI, evidence of myocardial ischemia based on a history of angina pectoris (AP) or ST-segment changes during continuous electrocardiographic monitoring (ST); CPAP, effect of nasal continuous positive airway pressure (CPAP) on AP and ST during sleep; +, present; −, absent.

night polysomnography, 8 patients were found to have significant OSA with a mean AHI of 36 ± 11 hr, which was associated with significant hypoxemia (lowest oxygen saturation 76.1 ± 3.3%). Six patients were treated with nasal CPAP, which corrected their OSA and associated nocturnal hypoxemia. During a follow-up period of 10.3 ± 1.4 months, none of these patients had any further episodes of nocturnal angina, although they continued to experience exertional daytime angina. In contrast, the two patients who did not receive treatment with nasal CPAP continued to experience episodes of nocturnal angina. Although this descriptive study is limited by the lack of objective monitoring of cardiac ischemia during sleep, these observations suggest that OSA can exacerbate myocardial ischemia in patients with coexisting CAD.

De Olazabal et al. recruited 17 male patients with angiographically proven CAD for overnight polysomnography (16). All patients had "symptoms of coronary insufficiency" and 7 "occasionally complained" of nocturnal chest pain. Significant CAD was defined as more than 50% occlusion of a coronary vessel. The extent of coronary artery involvement varied from one vessel (29% of patients) to two vessels (29% of patients) to triple vessel disease (41% of patients). In addition to standard overnight polysomnography, all patients had continuous electrocardiographic (ECG) monitoring, which was reviewed for evidence of ST-segment depression. Thirteen of the 17 patients recruited for the study were found to have sleep-disordered breathing: 11 had OSA and 2 had Cheyne-Stokes respiration. The average AHI was 20/hr, and there was a modest fall in oxygen saturation during apnea ranging from 6 to 15%. In addition, 11 patients continued to take propranolol for control of angina pectoris throughout the study. In contrast to the findings of Wei and Bradley, these investigators found no objective evidence of myocardial ischemia during sleep in patients with either OSA or Cheyne-Stokes respiration. These findings may be explained by the fact that the patients had less severe sleep apnea with milder hypoxemia during sleep, which was less likely to provoke myocardial ischemia, particularly in those who continued to take beta blockers.

Goldman et al. investigated an older group of patients (59 to 82 years of age) referred for elective abdominal or carotid reconstructive vascular surgery (17). Eighteen of these 34 patients had cardiac anesthetic risk factors (defined as previous myocardial infarction, exertional angina pectoris, or diastolic pressure greater than 100 mmHg). All patients had noninvasive monitoring, which included ECG monitoring for 18–21 hr and overnight oximetry. The ECG was reviewed for ST-segment depression, which was defined as greater than 1 mm of depression below baseline persisting for more than 60 msec after the J point and appearing in consecutive beats lasting for more than 60 sec. The overnight oximetry recordings were reviewed for evidence of repetitive oscillation in oxygen saturation and heart rate, which is characteristically seen in patients with OSA. Significant oscillation was defined as a 4% or greater fall in oxygen saturation followed by a 3% increase associated with a cyclic tachycardia in excess of 10% of the baseline heart rate. Individuals who manifested 50 or more such respiratory events during an overnight oximetry recording were described as having "nocturnal respiratory abnormality" (NRA). These investigators found ST-segment depression in 59% of patients, and all of these episodes were clinically silent. This reflects the high prevalence of occult myocardial disease in this patient population. However, the timing of ST-segment depression was different between patients who had NRA and those who did not (Fig. 3). In patients without NRA, ST-segment depression occurred between 6:00 and 7:00 A.M., which has been reported as the peak time for myocardial ischemia in previous studies (18,19). In contrast, in patients with evidence of NRA, maximum ST-segment depression occurred between midnight and 5:00 A.M. In addition, five patients who had NRA but no evidence of CAD did not exhibit ST-segment depression. Assuming that NRA reflects the presence of OSA, these findings support the concept that OSA provokes myocardial ischemia in patients who have coexisting CAD but does not cause myocardial ischemia in patients without CAD.

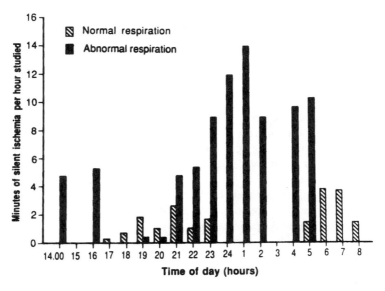

Figure 3 Diurnal variation in ischemia for 10 patients with ECG evidence of silent myocardial ischemia. Each bar represents the hourly duration of silent ischemia. Hatched bars are the average of eight patients with normal nocturnal respiratory patterns. Solid bars are the average of two patients with abnormal nocturnal respiratory patterns. Patients with significantly abnormal nocturnal respiration developed more ischemia during the night (From Ref. 17.)

Koehler et al. investigated 30 patients with OSA, 20 with evidence of CAD and 10 without (20). CAD was confirmed by coronary angiography (15 patients) or a positive stress test (5 patients). Of the 10 patients without CAD, 7 had normal coronary angiography and 3 had a normal stress test. All patients had overnight polysomnography, which revealed an AHI of 33 ± 13/hr; simultaneous six-lead ECG monitoring was analyzed for ST-segment depression and T-wave changes. ST-segment depression greater than 0.1 mV below the baseline and T-wave inversion were considered pathological. ST-segment depression was documented only if it lasted for at least 10 sec. All cardiac medications were discontinued at least 48 hr prior to overnight monitoring. ST-segment depression was found almost exclusively in patients with CAD, specifically in 5 of the 20 patients with CAD and 1 of the remaining 10 patients without evidence of CAD. In fact, the single patient in the non-CAD group who had ST-segment depression also had an abnormal coronary angiogram reflected by "diffuse wall defects without significant stenosis." The duration of ST-segment depression ranged from 12 to 96 sec. Moreover, ST-segment depression was temporally associated with apnea and hypoxemia (Figs. 4 and 5) and 84% of such events occurred during REM sleep.

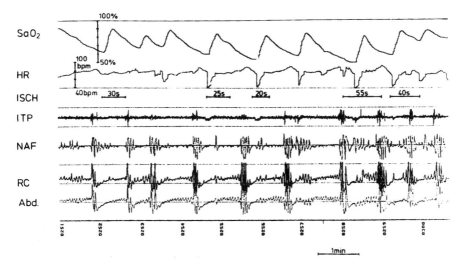

Figure 4   Polysomnography obtained in a patient with single coronary vessel disease, severe sleep apnea, and nocturnal oxygen desaturations below 60%. Episodes of myocardial ischemia (ISCH), reflected by ST-segment and T-wave changes, are represented by horizontal bars and are coincidental with termination of obstructive apneas. SaO₂, oxygen saturation; HR, heart rate. ITP, intrathoracic pressure; NAF, nasal airflow; RC and ABD, thoracic and abdominal respiration. (From Ref. 20.)

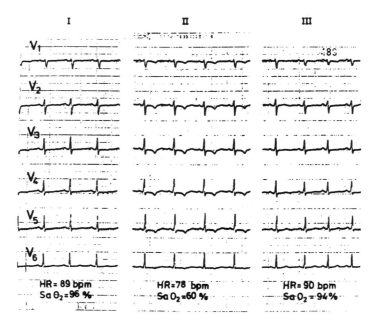

Figure 5 ST-segment and T-wave morphology in a single patient before (I), during (II), and following (III) termination of an obstructive apnea. Note ST-segment depression and T-wave inversion during apnea (II), which normalizes when apnea is terminated (III). (From Ref. 20.)

A follow-up report from the same investigators reiterated these findings with two additional observations (21). First, sustained-release nitrates did not reduce the frequency of ischemic ECG changes; second, ischemic episodes, which were asymptomatic, were associated with more arousals, which led these authors to suggest that asymptomatic myocardial ischemia can cause sleep disruption.

Franklin et al. selected 10 men with severe angina occurring both during wakefulness and sleep (22). All patients had angiographically proven CAD with greater than 50% stenosis in at least one vessel. Eight patients had triple-vessel disease. Investigations, completed in 9 patients, included overnight polysomnography and continuous ECG monitoring for "ST segment deviation," which was measured at 20 msec after the J point. A reversible increase for at least 40 sec in the magnitude of the ST-change vector by over 0.05 mV was defined as myocardial ischemia. All patients were found to have evidence of sleep apnea with a mean apnea-hypopnea index of 40 ± 19/hr. The type of apnea was predominantly obstructive, although 1 patient had exclusively central sleep apnea and 2 patients had evidence of both obstructive and central sleep apnea. Unfortunately, the authors did not report the severity of associated hypoxemia. Nevertheless, 4 patients experienced nocturnal angina reflected by typical chest pain associated with ST-segment changes (Fig. 6). In 3 patients, angina was preceded by apnea, and in 1 patient angina was preceded by an increase in heart rate during REM sleep. There were 32 episodes of ST-segment changes in 6 patients and 18 episodes were associated with apnea or hypopnea occurring during the preceding 90 sec. The authors reported that the ST-segment changes were equally distributed between REM and non-REM (NREM) sleep in all but one patient.

These authors evaluated the impact of nasal CPAP therapy on myocardial ischemia during sleep. Nasal CPAP successfully corrected sleep apnea, as reflected by a reduction in the mean AHI from 44 ± 19 to 12 ± 15/hr. This was associated with resolution of nocturnal angina and a significant reduction in the frequency of ST-segment changes, which persisted in 5 patients for a total of 9 separate episodes. Following discharge from the sleep laboratory to their home environment, 8 of the 9 patients continued to be free of nocturnal angina while on nasal CPAP therapy.

Finally, Philip and Guilleminault reviewed a database of 4000 patients with OSA and identified 34 subjects (32 men, 2 women) with a positive history of exertional and nocturnal angina (23). CAD was confirmed in all patients by a

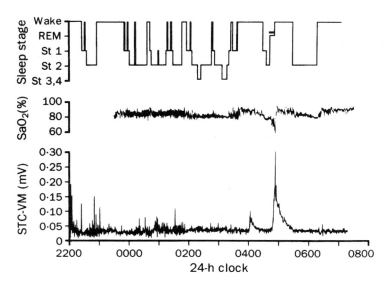

Figure 6 Sleep stage, oxygen saturation (SaO$_2$), and ST-segment change (STC-VM) in a patient who was awakened by an attack of angina at 0446 hr that was preceded by apnoea and hypoxemia. (From Ref. 22.)

positive exercise test and an abnormal thallium scan. All patients underwent overnight polysomnography and simultaneous eight-lead ECG monitoring. ST-segment depression of greater than 0.1 mV below baseline for greater than 10 sec was found in all 34 patients during sleep. Thirty-one patients awoke from sleep complaining of chest pain during these ECG changes. In the remaining 3 patients, ST-segment depression occurred without arousal from sleep or a history of chest pain. The authors reported that both complaints of nocturnal chest pain and ST-segment depression were associated with severe hypoxemia, defined as a fall in oxygen saturation to 50% or below. In addition, the authors found that most patients had significant comorbid disease. Specifically, 25 patients had evidence of previous myocardial infraction, 12 had non-insulin-dependent diabetes mellitus, and 19 had hypertension. As in the case of previous reports, the authors found that treatment with either nasal CPAP or nasal BiPAP corrected both complaints of nocturnal angina and associated ST-segment depression. Recruitment of only 34 patients from such a large database suggests that the prevalence of myocardial ischemia in patients with OSA is low. However, this may reflect the sensitivity of their methods to identify myocardial ischemia and most likely underestimates the true prevalence of symptomatic CAD in this patient population.

In summary, there is reasonable evidence that the development of significant hypoxemia during sleep in patients who have coexisting OSA and CAD can provoke myocardial ischemia, reflected by either nocturnal angina or ST-segment depression on ECG monitoring. Furthermore, it appears that treatment of OSA with nasal CPAP not only corrects their OSA and associated symptoms but also significantly reduces the prevalence of accompanying myocardial ischemia during sleep.

III. OSA and Myocardial Ischemia in Patients Without CAD (Table 2)

There are only three published reports on the interaction between OSA and myocardial ischemia in patients without CAD. In the previously mentioned report by Koehler et al. (20), there were no episodes of myocardial ischemia, as reflected by ST-segment changes on the ECG, during sleep in 10 patients who had OSA without evidence of CAD. An additional study by Andreas et al. (24) investigated 15 patients with OSA who had no evidence of CAD, either from clinical history or exercise testing. The mean apnea index was 45 ± 28/hr and the minimum oxygen saturation during sleep was $71 \pm 14\%$. In addition to overnight polysomnography, all patients had continuous Holter monitoring for ST-segment and T-wave changes. The authors found no evidence of ST-segment depression on the

Table 2 Myocardial Ischemia in OSA Patients Without CAD

Ref.	Demographics		OSA		Evidence CAD				Evid. MI		CPAP	
	n (m/f)	Age	AHI	Min SaO$_2$	AP	Ex ECG	Angio	Thallium	AP	ST	AP	ST
Koehler, 1991 (20)	10	47–68	33 ± 13	75	—	—	—		—	1		
Andreas, 1991 (23)	15	53 ± 8	45 ± 28	71 ± 14	—	—			—	—		
Hanly, 1993 (24)	23 (21/2)	48 ± 12	64 ± 22	<90%	—	1		1	—	+		+

n(m/f), number of subjects (male/female ratio); OSA, obstructive sleep apnea; AHI, apnea-hypopnea index; min Sa$_{O_2}$, minimum oxygen saturation during sleep; Evidence CAD, evidence of coronary artery disease based on a history of angina pectoris (AP), electrocardiographic changes on exercise (Ex ECG), coronary angiography (Angio), or thallium perfusion scan (Thallium); Evid. MI, evidence of myocardial ischemia based on a history of angina pectoris (AP) or ST-segment changes during continuous electrocardiographic monitoring (ST); CPAP, effect of nasal continuous positive airway pressure (CPAP) on AP and ST during sleep; +, present; −, absent.

ECG during sleep and concluded that OSA does not cause myocardial ischemia in the absence of coexisting CAD.

These findings contrast markedly with those of Hanly et al. (25), who recruited 23 consecutive patients with significant OSA prior to treatment with nasal CPAP. Twenty-two patients had no evidence of CAD either by clinical history, baseline ECG, or exercise testing (done in 17 patients). A single patient had asymptomatic myocardial ischemia reflected by typical ischemic ST-segment depression of 2 to 3 mm during exercise. A follow-up exercise thallium scan demonstrated reversible myocardial ischemia. All patients returned to the sleep laboratory for a CPAP titration study, during which overnight polysomnography was repeated in addition to a simultaneous three-channel Holter monitor. An episode of myocardial ischemia was defined as ST-segment depression greater than 1 mm from baseline for more than 0.08 sec after the J point, lasting for at least 1 min and separated from the next episode by at least 1 min. Each patient was randomly assigned to receive nasal CPAP for the first or second half of the night. This study design enabled the investigators to assess their patients for episodes of ST-segment depression, to determine the relationship of such episodes to the severity of OSA, and also to evaluate the effect of nasal CPAP therapy.

Without nasal CPAP, these patients had severe OSA with a mean AHI of 65 ± 35/hr and oxygen saturation less than 90% for 44 ± 27% of the total sleep time. In addition, 7 patients (30%), including the single patient with evidence of CAD, had ST-segment depression during sleep. The duration of ST-segment depression ranged from 4 to 57 min/hr of sleep, and this occurred predominantly during stages 1 and 2 NREM sleep ($77 + 22$% of the total sleep time). In contrast to the report by Koehler et al. (20), who found that ST-segment depression in patients with CAD occurred predominantly during REM sleep (84%), Hanly et

ST SEGMENT TREND (ENTIRE STUDY)

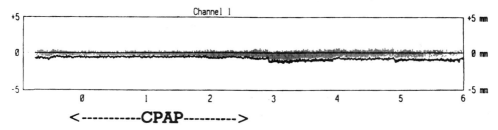

Figure 7a ST-segment trend in lead V_5 for the entire sleep study in a single patient, with the dark lines indicating significant ST-segment depression. Note that almost all ST-segment depression occurred with the subject off nasal continuous positive airway pressure (CPAP). (From Ref. 25.)

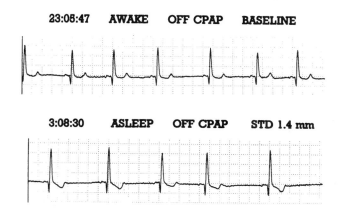

Figure 7b Examples of electrocardiographic tracings while the subject was awake and asleep (off continuous positive airway pressure), indicating different ST- and T-wave morphology. (From Ref. 25.)

al. found that ST-segment depression occurred infrequently during REM sleep (20 ± 19% of total duration of ST-segment depression). Nasal CPAP significantly reduced the duration of ST-segment depression in all patients (Fig. 7). Overall, the duration of ST-segment depression fell from 30 ± 17 min/hr of sleep off nasal CPAP to 11 + 13 min/hr of sleep on nasal CPAP. It was concluded that ST-segment depression is relatively common in patients with OSA even in the absence of coexisting CAD and that the duration of ST-segment depression is significantly reduced by nasal CPAP therapy. It was acknowledged that although ST-segment depression may reflect true myocardial ischemia, it is also possible that these ECG changes may be caused either by nonspecific changes unrelated to OSA or nonischemic changes associated with OSA (discussed below).

In summary, there is conflicting evidence as to whether patients with severe OSA who do not have coexisting CAD experience myocardial ischemia during sleep.

IV. Limitations of ST Segment Monitoring

It can be seen from the preceding literature review that objective monitoring of myocardial ischemia has relied heavily on ECG monitoring to detect ST-segment depression. Although ST-segment depression can reflect myocardial ischemia, these ECG changes are not specific for myocardial ischemia. In fact, the pathogenesis of ST-segment depression in this patient population can be due to nonspecific changes unrelated to OSA, myocardial ischemia caused by OSA, and nonischemic changes associated with OSA.

A. Nonspecific Changes Unrelated to OSA

There are a variety of factors unrelated to OSA that can cause nonspecific ST- and T-wave changes on continuous ECG monitoring. First, it is critical that electrodes be located appropriately on the chest for accurate interpretation of changes in ST segments. The resting ECG should be reviewed for baseline ST- and T-wave changes, preexisting left ventricular hypertrophy or preexcitation syndromes. In addition, certain medications can affect ST segments and T waves as well as electrolyte abnormalities. Valvular heart disease, such as aortic stenosis or mitral valve prolapse, can confound interpretation of ST-segment depression on Holter monitoring. Finally, changes in body position during sleep have been reported to cause changes in the ST segment during ECG monitoring (26).

B. Myocardial Ischemia Caused by OSA

ST-segment depression has been shown in previous human studies to reflect true myocardial ischemia (27,28). Inspiration against an occluded upper airway reduces intrathoracic pressure, resulting in increased left ventricular preload and afterload and thereby enhancing left ventricular wall stress and myocardial oxygen demand (29). Previous animal experiments have shown that these mechanical changes alone, in the absence of hypoxemia, may cause myocardial ischemia in dogs, with partial occlusion of the left anterior descending artery (11). However, most obstructive apneas are also accompanied by hypoxemia, which is known to cause myocardial ischemia in patients with CAD (28). The concurrent decrease in myocardial oxygen supply at a time of increased oxygen demand substantially enhances the risk that myocardial ischemia will develop in patients with significant CAD.

C. Nonischemic Changes Associated with OSA

A number of physiological changes occur during repetitive obstructive apneas that may cause changes on ECG monitoring. For example, obstructive apneas are typically terminated by an arousal from sleep. Such arousals are usually accompanied by relative hyperventilation, which has been shown to cause both ST-segment depression and T-wave abnormalities on the ECG (30–32). In addition, patients with OSA have increased sympathetic nervous system activity, which is further increased by arousal from sleep. This may explain why Hanly et al. found that some patients without CAD developed ST-segment depression during sleep, which was corrected by nasal CPAP therapy. These investigators evaluated the temporal relationship between ST-segment changes and alteration in sleep and respiration and found that the apnea and arousal indexes were significantly higher when ST segments were depressed compared to when ST segments were isoelectric; this raises the possibility that ST-segment changes were due to sleep disruption rather than myocardial ischemia.

Alteration of intrathoracic pressure during obstructive apnea may render the gastroesophageal sphincter less competent, leading to esophageal reflux and possibly esophageal spasm (33). These changes, which may be subclinical, have been reported to cause ST- and T-wave changes (34). Nasal CPAP reduces esophageal reflux and thereby associated ST-segment depression (33). Obstructive sleep apnea has also been reported to increase intracranial pressure (35) and reduce cerebral perfusion (36), both of which are corrected by nasal CPAP. Once again, ST- and T-wave changes may accompany these neurological events (37) and mimic the electrocardiographic changes of myocardial ischemia.

V. Conclusion

There is reasonably strong evidence that OSA can cause myocardial ischemia in patients with coexisting CAD. This evidence is based predominantly on a history of typical chest pain with or without ECG changes, such as ST-segment depression, and their resolution with nasal CPAP therapy. However, the prevalence of myocardial ischemia in patients with OSA is not known. Furthermore, it remains to be clarified whether OSA alters the natural history of CAD and how the development of myocardial ischemia during sleep affects mortality associated with OSA.

It is not clear whether myocardial ischemia develops during sleep in patients who have OSA without coexisting CAD. There has been very limited research on this question in human subjects. The use of continuous electrocardiographic monitoring as the only objective monitor of myocardial ischemia has significant limitations, and better investigative tools to monitor myocardial perfusion are required to progress further in this area of clinical research.

References

1. Young T, Palta M, Dempsey J, et al. The occurrence of sleep-disordered breathing among middle aged adults. N Engl J Med 1993; 328:1230–1235.
2. National Center for Health Statistics. Vital Statistics of the United States, 1989. Vol. II. Mortality. Part A. DHH publication no. (PHS) 93-1101. Washington DC: U.S. Government Printing Office, 1993.
3. Manson JE, Colditz GA, Stampfer MJ, et al. A prospective study of obesity and risk of coronary heart disease in women. N Engl J Med 1990; 322:882–889.

4. Rich-Edwards JW, Manson JE, Hennekens CH, Buring JE. The primary prevention of coronary heart disease in women. N Engl J Med 1995; 332:1758–1758.

5. Katsumata K, Okada T, Miyao M, Katsumata Y. High incidence of sleep apnea syndrome in a male diabetic population. Diabetes Res Clin Pract 1991; 13:45–51.

6. Kannel WB, McGee DL. Diabetes and cardiovascular disease: the Framingham study. JAMA 1979; 241:2035–2038.

7. Hung J, Whitford EG, Parsons RW, Hillman DR. Association of sleep apnea with myocardial infarction in men. Lancet 1990; 336:261–264.

8. Saitor T, Yoshikawa T, Sakamoto Y, Tanaka K, Inoue T, Ogawa R. Sleep apnea in patients with acute myocardial infarction. Crit Care Med 1991; 19:938–941.

9. Strohl KP, Boehm KD, Denko CW, Novak RD, Decker MJ. Biochemical morbidity in sleep apnea. Ear, Nose Throat J 1993; 72(1):34, 39–41.

10. Chierchia S, Brunelli C, Simonetti I, Lazzari M, Maseri A. Sequence of events in angina at rest: primary reduction in coronary flow. Circulation 1980; 61:759–768.

11. Scharf S, Graver M, Balaban K. Cardiovascular effects of periodic occlusions of the upper airways in dogs. Am Rev Respir Dis 1992; 146:321–329.

12. Marrone O, Bellia V, Ferrara G, Milone F, Romano L, Salvaggio A, et al. Transmural pressure measurements: importance in the assessment of pulmonary hypertension in obstructive sleep apneas. Chest 1989; 95:338–342.

13. Quyyumi A, Wright C, Mockus L, Fox K. Mechanisms of nocturnal angina pectoris: importance of increased myocardial oxygen demand in patients with severe coronary heart disease. Lancet 1984; i:1207–1209.

14. Nowlin J, Troyer W, Collins W, Silverman G, Nichols C, McIntosh H, Estes E, Boddonoff M. The association of nocturnal angina pectoris with dreaming. Ann Intern Med 1965; 63:1040–1046.

15. Wei K, Bradley T. Association of obstructive sleep apnea and nocturnal angina. Am Rev Respir Dis 1992; 145:A443.

16. De Olazabal J, Miller M, Cook W, Mithoefer J. Disordered breathing and hypoxia during sleep in coronary artery disease. Chest 1982; 82:548–552.

17. Goldman M, Reeder M, Muir A, Loh L, Young J, Gitlin D, Casey K, Smart D, Fry J. Repetitive nocturnal arterial oxygen desaturation and silent myocardial ischemia in patients presenting for vascular surgery. J Am Geriatr Soc 1993; 41:703–709.

18. Mulcahy D, Keegan J, Cunningham D, et al. Circadian variation of total ischemic burden and its alteration with anti-anginal agents. Lancet 1988; ii:755–759.

19. Muller JE, Stone PH, Turi ZG, et al. Circadian variation in the frequency of acute myocardial infarction. N Engl J Med 1985; 313:1315–1322.

20. Koehler U, Dubler H, Glaremin T, Junkermann H, Lubbers C, Ploch T, Peter J, Pomykaj T, von Wichert P. Nocturnal myocardial ischemia and cardiac arrhythmia in patients with sleep apnea with and without coronary heart disease. Klin Wochenschr 1991; 69:474–482.

21. Schaffer H, Koehler U, Ploch T. Sleep-related myocardial ischemia and sleep structure in patients with obstructive sleep apnea and coronary heart disease. Chest 1997; 111:387–393.

22. Franklin K, Nilsson J, Sahlin C, Naslund U. Sleep apnoea and nocturnal angina. Lancet 1995; 345:1085–1087.

23. Philip P, Guilleminault C. ST segment abnormality, angina during sleep and obstructive sleep apnea. Sleep 1993; 16:558–559.
24. Andreas S, Hajak G, Natt P, Auge D, Ruther E, Kreuzer H. ST Strecken Veranderungen and Rhythmusstorungen bei obstruktiver Schlafapnoe. Pneumologie 1991; 45:720–724.
25. Hanly P, Sasson Z, Zuberi N, Lunn K. ST-segment depression during sleep in obstructive sleep apnea. Am J Cardiol 1993; 71:1341–1345.
26. Noble RJ, Zipes DP. Long-term continuous electrocardiographic recording. In: Hurst JW, Schlant RC, Rackley CE, Sannenblick EH, Wenger NK, eds. The Heart, 7th ed. New York: McGraw-Hill, 1990:1834–1841.
27. Gottlieb SO. Asymptomatic or silent myocardial ischemia in angina pectoris: pathophysiology and clinical implications. Cardiol Clin 1991; 9:49–61.
28. Barach AL, Steinder A, Eckman M, Molomut N. The physiologic action of oxygen and carbon dioxide on the coronary circulation, as shown by blood gas and electrocardiographic studies. Am Heart J 1941; 22:13–34.
29. Parish JM, Shepard JW. Cardiovascular effects of sleep disorders. Chest 1990; 97:1220–1226.
30. McHenry PL, Cogan OJ, Elliott WC, Knoebel SB. False positive ECG response to exercise secondary to hyperventilation: cineangiographic correlation. Am Heart J 1970; 79:683–687.
31. Goldschlager L. Electrocardiographic changes during hyperventilation resembling myocardial ischemia in patients with normal coronary arteriograms. Am Heart J 1974; 87:383–390.
32. Biberman L, Sarma RN, Surawicz B. T-Wave abnormalities during hyperventilation and isoproterenol infusion. Am Heart J 1971; 81:166–174.
33. Kerr P, Shoenur JP, Millar T, Buckle P, Kryger MH. Nasal CPAP reduces gastroesophageal reflux in obstructive sleep apnea syndrome. Chest 1982; 101:1539–1544.
34. Hick DG, Morrison JFB, Casey JF, Al-Ashhab W, Williams GJ, Davies GA. Oesophageal motility, luminal pH and electrocardiographic-ST segment analysis during spontaneous episodes of angina like chest pain. GUT 1992; 33:79–86.
35. Jennum P, Borgesen SE. Intracranial pressure and obstructive sleep apnea. Chest 1989; 95:279–283.
36. Meyer JS, Sakai F, Karacan I, Derman S, Yamamoto M. Sleep apnea, narcolepsy and dreaming: regional cerebral hemodynamics. Ann Neurol 1980; 7:479–485.
37. Davies KR, Gelb AW, Manninen PH, Boughner DR, Bisnaire D. Cardiac function in aneurysmal subarachnoid haemorrhage: a study of electrocardiographic and echocardiographic abnormalities. Br J Anaesth 1991; 67:58–63.

12

Epidemiological Evidence for an Association of Sleep-Disordered Breathing with Hypertension and Cardiovascular Disease

TERRY YOUNG and PAUL E. PEPPARD

University of Wisconsin—Madison
Madison, Wisconsin

I. Introduction

The causal link between the abnormal breathing events of sleep-disordered breathing (SDB) and immediate cardiovascular perturbations is well established, but the extent of cardiovascular *disease* (CVD) that may result from nightly exposure to SDB is largely unknown. Epidemiological studies are uniquely able to address relationships between outcomes and exposures as they naturally occur in populations and to estimate the overall population impact of that exposure. Additionally, epidemiological studies are often the only means to investigate causes and consequences of diseases with natural histories spanning decades. For example, the role of low-level, chronic SDB throughout adulthood in the development of CVD in later life cannot be determined from experiments on nonhumans. Population-based prospective epidemiological investigations in which people with and without SDB are followed to compare incidence of CVD are best suited to answer the pressing questions of how much, if any, CVD can be attributed directly to SDB, what level of SDB severity makes a significant contribution to CVD outcomes, and what factors (e.g., age, gender, other CVD risk factors) modify the associations identified.

Prospective studies are usually not initiated until sufficient evidence warrants the large investment of resources, including large samples and observations spanning several years, that are almost always required. Typically, findings from other types of observational studies—including cross-sectional analyses and case-control studies—as well as clinical observations and biological plausibility, provide the rationale for prospective cohort studies. Over the past 15 years, several epidemiological studies employing cross-sectional or case-control designs of SDB and CVD have been completed. In addition, reports from two populations-based prospective studies of snoring and CVD and a few mortality follow-up studies have been published. Although tallies of positive and negative findings on SDB and CVD or hypertension from "all" past studies suggest a lack of agreement, positive evidence from the methodologically stronger studies have stimulated the initiation of population-based prospective studies. A limited number of prospective studies specifically designed to test the hypothesis that objectively measured SDB has a causal role in the development of hypertension and CVD are under way, and results should be available within a few years.

II. Methodological Issues in Observational Studies of SDB and CVD

In an attempt to gather the soundest epidemiological evidence regarding SDB and CVD, a major emphasis in this chapter is on population-based studies. Epidemiological studies can be based on patient populations, but only when there is a high probability that medically recognized cases of the condition of interest are representative of all cases. At present, only a fraction of people with SDB ever enter the medical care system. In an area with minimal health care barriers and an established sleep laboratory, it was estimated that less than 7% of women and 18% of men with SDB meeting clinical guidelines for treatment were actually diagnosed (1). Accordingly, existing sleep apnea patient populations are the product of various known and unknown referral and selection biases, and this can result in a distorted picture of the epidemiology of SDB. For example, based on clinic populations, SDB was thought to be rare in women, but population-based studies have shown that relative to women with sleep apnea, men have been overrepresented in patient populations (2–5). Furthermore, the factors that bring patients into evaluation may vary greatly from laboratory to laboratory. In some places, a higher level of knowledge of sleep apnea in primary care may cast a wider net, while in other areas, most referrals may come from hospitalized patients observed to have severe sleep apnea.

In general, patients evaluated for a specific chronic condition have a higher prevalence of other types of morbidity as compared to the general population. A major reason for this is that people with medically recognized morbidity (e.g.,

CVD), by having more frequent contact with health care providers, have more opportunity for underlying conditions (e.g., SDB) to be uncovered. As a result, comorbidity will be disproportionately higher in sleep clinic populations, and this undermines the ability to use the patients in observational study designs. Furthermore, the comorbidity bias is most likely to operate on those with the least severe SDB. People with the most severe SDB may be referred to a sleep clinic primarily on the basis of their obvious nighttime apneic activity; but among people with only mild indications of SDB—e.g., asymptomatic snoring—another problem such as CVD may be needed to warrant a referral for evaluation of SDB. This bias would tend to reduce any difference in comorbidity between those with little or no SDB and severe SDB, making cross-sectional studies within sleep clinic samples invalid.

With increased awareness of sleep disorders in health care, a high proportion of significant cases of SDB may be evaluated and diagnosed in the future. Under such conditions, the validity of using patient samples would improve. At the present, however, research questions regarding SDB and CVD cannot be addressed confidently with observational studies based on existing patient populations.

Other methodological problems in both population- and clinic-based studies of SDB and CVD can also limit interpretation of results. In the earliest reviews, positive findings from clinical comparisons were appropriately questioned because obesity, a strong correlate of both SDB and cardiovascular disorders, had not been accounted for in the analyses (6,7). In studies that followed, steps were taken to control for obesity and other potential confounding factors of age and gender, either by matching, multiple regression modeling, or stratification. When the measured association of SDB and blood pressure became reduced in magnitude or lost statistical significance after accounting for confounding factors, conclusions were too hastily drawn that the widely reported relationship between SDB and CVD was spurious and due primarily to obesity acting as a confounding factor (8,9). Overestimation of an association due to confounding is always a concern in epidemiological analyses, but this is not the only serious methodological problem that must be attended to. Many study flaws, in fact, result in *underestimation* of associations, such that true relationships are missed (10). Indeed, attenuation of findings toward no relationship has undoubtedly occurred in most studies to date, undermining the validity of the negative results every bit as much as the lack of controlling for obesity would invalidate positive results. Important methodological problems that lead to inaccurate estimates of associations (in either direction) include 1) inappropriate study populations (see above discussion of clinic-based samples); 2) measurement error; and 3) confounding factors. Measurement error and confounding are briefly discussed below.

Error in measuring SDB or CVD and hypertension can seriously bias estimates of their association. The validity of subjective measures (e.g., snoring) of

SDB is poor or unknown, and even polysomnographically determined apneas and hypopneas are likely to be measured with error. Summary measures, such as event frequency, may not capture the pathophysiological aspect of SDB relevant to the outcome (e.g., oxygen desaturation versus arousals) and are also subject to intraperson night-to-night variation. The resulting extraneous variability, or noise, in the measurement of SDB will diminish the ability to detect meaningful associations. Similar issues apply to the measurement of CVD and hypertension. The use of antihypertensive medication poses additional problems in the measurement of blood pressure. If SDB is causally linked to hypertension, those persons with SDB will be more likely to be using antihypertensives and their unmedicated blood pressure will be obscured. Clearly, this can affect the outcome of interest, possibly leading to underestimates of the relationship of SDB and blood pressure. Although exclusion from analysis of people using antihypertensive medication is a common approach used to circumvent this problem, this too can result in an underestimate by leaving out those people who demonstrate the strongest relationship between SDB and blood pressure.

Uncontrolled confounding and improper modeling of confounding variables yield biased estimates of associations (10). A pertinent example for SDB and CVD/hypertension is body habitus. The use of crude summary measures (e.g., obese vs. not obese) is likely to produce overestimates of the relationship between SDB and CVD by incompletely controlling for the confounding influence of body habitus (11). In addition, failing to account for all relevant aspects of body habitus will bias estimates of associations between SDB and CVD. Some researchers have suggested that large neck circumference or central body fat distribution are the important etiological aspects of obesity with respect to SDB (12–18). Thus, in examining the relationship between SDB and CVD, it may be necessary to consider measures of body habitus other than the typically used body-mass index (BMI).

It is important to properly control for confounding variables, but it is possible to "over-control" in an analysis. For example, in some studies examining the relationship between SDB and mortality, history of CVD has been used as a control variable (19,20). Since one of the major hypothesized pathways by which SDB could affect mortality is via CVD, controlling for CVD could obscure a possible connection. That is, it may be difficult to find a connection between SDB and mortality independent of CVD. Adjusting for a variable intermediate in a putative causal pathway between the independent variable and outcome of interest can reduce the apparent effect of the independent variable (10).

Finally, statistical analyses must be careful and thorough. An expensive and well-designed study can be entirely wasted if analyses are inappropriate. With regard to statistical analyses, we offer the following cautions and suggestions:

1. The distribution of SDB, as measured on a continuum of event frequency is strongly "right-tailed" in the general population. That is, many individuals have no or little SDB, but a few have severe SDB. Failure to account for this (e.g., with transformation functions, distribution-free methods, or grouping) may lead to invalid inference in many common statistical models by allowing the few individuals with severe SDB to have inordinate influence on estimated associations.

2. Automated analysis approaches to regression modeling (e.g., stepwise regression) are poorly suited to properly assess confounding and interactions or to deal with violation of modeling assumptions (e.g., influential outliers, nonlinearity) and multicollinearity (e.g., among several measures of body habitus). Many studies in this field seem to have used automated approaches as their primary statistical tool, thus weakening confidence in their findings.

3. Several authors have argued that measures of body habitus other than BMI—such as central obesity, neck obesity or body composition—are more important to control for when examining SDB and CVD (12–18). It may be premature to declare that there are one or two most important measures of body habitus because different measures may be more important among subgroups (21). Furthermore, measures of body habitus are typically highly correlated, so that controlling for one measure may not lead to estimates of association markedly different than those obtained by controlling for another measure. Pending further research in this area, it is reasonable to examine multiple measures of body habitus as potential confounders.

4. For studies examining SDB and blood pressure that include people using antihypertensive medications, grouping individuals over a certain blood pressure cutpoint (e.g., 140/90 mmHg) with individuals using antihypertensives (regardless of measured blood pressure) in logistic regression analyses is often done to avoid the problem of bias (underestimation of associations) discussed earlier, but not without the cost of statistical power and interpretability. Another approach is using statistical models for censored data in which the blood pressures of subjects using antihypertensives are treated as censored at some value, such as 140/90 mmHg. This approach has the advantage of using actual measured blood pressures from unmedicated subjects. However, the censored data models may make somewhat unrealistic assumptions about the blood pressures of medicated subjects (22). Still, we expect the censored data approach to be an improvement over multiple linear regression models when there are a substantial number of subjects using antihypertensive medications. Simply "controlling" for antihyperten-

sive medication use in multiple linear regression analyses does not eliminate and may even exacerbate bias.

5. If the true association is small, as is often the case for outcomes with multifactorial etiology, large sample sizes are needed in order to detect the association with statistical significance. And, equally important, in the case where there is no true association, power must be sufficient to have confidence in a null finding.

In summary, in epidemiological studies that lack proper attention to the methodological issues inherent in the topic of SDB and CVD, underestimation as well as overestimation of a true effect is a major concern. Concern is amplified if the effect to be detected is small, as small associations are easily biased toward no association by study flaws that lead to underestimation and are easily influenced by confounding factors that may lead to overestimation. It is with these methodological issues in mind that findings from the current literature are summarized in this chapter. Section III.A addresses the association of SDB and blood pressure, for which findings are most abundant, and Section III.B examines findings on SDB and CVD morbidity and mortality.

III. Observational Studies of SDB and CVD

A. Studies of SDB and Blood Pressure

Although hypertension is not considered to be a cardiovascular disease, elevated blood pressure is a well-established CVD risk factor and may be considered an intermediate outcome for CVD. Chronically elevated blood pressure and hypertension have been widely examined as intermediate outcomes of SDB. Some reviewers, however, have advocated focusing primarily on CVD rather than hypertension as the disease outcome of interest (23). We agree on the importance of keeping in mind that one ultimate goal of studying the relationship between SDB and blood pressure is an understanding of the causal role of SDB in known clinical sequelae of hypertension. However, there are strong pragmatic reasons to examine blood pressure directly as an intermediate outcome of SDB. First, in prospective studies, use of an intermediate outcome allows a shorter follow-up period. In cross-sectional studies, use of intermediate outcomes reduces the potential for the disease outcome of interest to alter the exposure under study. For example, the measurement of SDB in someone who has had a myocardial infarction may not be a valid indicator of SDB status prior to the myocardial infarction. Second, hypertension per se has substantial health care costs (e.g., physician visits and antihypertensive medication). Third, elucidation of mechanisms by which SDB affects CVD—whether by nighttime cardiovascular disturbance, elevated daytime blood pressure, or both—could lead to strategies to break a causal chain. That is, if SDB affects CVD only through nocturnal cardiovascular disturbance, then treatment of SDB would be the most direct way to stem future CVD due to SDB. If SDB affects CVD primarily through chronically elevated blood pressure, then CVD sequelae of SDB could be reduced by treatment of either SDB or hypertension. For reasons such as these, intermediate outcomes, such as elevated blood pressure, are commonly used in epidemiological studies (24). Thus, even though hypertension is not the endpoint of ultimate interest, studies of SDB and blood pressure are particularly useful in addressing the role of SDB in CVD.

Population-Based Studies of Objectively Measured SDB and Blood Pressure

Studies with Full Polysomnography

Recent findings from two methodologically strong studies have indicated that SDB as measured by polysomnography is significantly associated with blood pressure, independent of age, sex, smoking, alcohol, education, use of antihypertensive medication, and body habitus (including BMI and indications of body fat distribution). Results from these studies, discussed below, represent cross-sectional analyses of baseline data from prospective population-based studies.

Wisconsin Sleep Cohort Study. The Wisconsin Sleep Cohort Study is a prospective study of the natural history and outcomes of medically unrecognized SDB. The cohort comprises middle-aged men and women who were employed by the state of Wisconsin in 1989 (for study design, see 25). At 4-year intervals, participants in the cohort undergo in-laboratory overnight polysomnography and other tests, including several measurements of blood pressure: standard seated and supine blood pressure, 24-h ambulatory blood pressure, and Doppler-assisted arm and ankle blood pressure. Several other measurements are taken, including weight, height, neck, waist, and hip circumferences. Extensive self-reported data on health history, demographics, and lifestyle are collected.

A summary of results from the Sleep Cohort Study relating SDB to blood pressure and hypertension (26) is given in Table 1. SDB is indicated by the number of polysomnographically determined apneas and hypopneas per hour of sleep (AHI), with an apneic event defined as 10 sec or more of no oral and nasal airflow and a hypopneic event defined as a reduction in breathing amplitude measured by calibrated Respitrace and accompanied by a 4% arterial blood oxygen desaturation. The table presents estimated increases in mean systolic and diastolic blood pressure and odds of hypertension ($>140/90$ mmHg or using antihypertensives) for comparison of a given level of SDB versus no SDB. Estimates are adjusted for age and sex for an individual with a BMI $= 28$. Adjustment for other factors (e.g., alcohol, smoking, physical activity, central and neck obesity) did not appreciably alter the estimates. All estimates are statistically significant at $p < 0.05$. Of note, SDB appears to be more strongly related to systolic than diastolic blood

Table 1 Linear Regression Coefficients for Apnea-Hypopnea Index (AHI) Predicting Blood Pressure (mmHg) and Odds Ratios for AHI and Hypertension Adjusted for Age, Sex, and Body-Mass Index in the Wisconsin Sleep Cohort Study ($n = 1069$)

AHI (Events per Hour) Comparison	β-Coefficient (s.e.) Systolic BP	β-Coefficient (s.e.) Diastolic BP	Odds Ratio (95% C.I.) Hypertension
5 vs. <1	1.2 (0.4)	0.6 (0.3)	1.2 (1.1, 1.3)
15 vs. <1	3.6 (1.2)	1.8 (0.8)	1.8 (1.3, 2.4)
30 vs. <1	7.2 (2.4)	3.6 (1.5)	3.1 (1.7, 5.7)

Source: Adapted from Ref. 26.

pressure. As shown in Table 1, the associations are modest: holding confounders constant, persons with AHI = 15, compared to those with AHI <1, are expected to have 3.6 and 1.8 mmHg higher systolic and diastolic blood pressures, respectively. Similarly, persons with AHI = 15 have a 1.8-fold greater chance of being hypertensive.

Corroborating data from ambulatory blood pressure monitoring on a sample of 554 participants in the Sleep Cohort Study is demonstrated in Figure 1 for

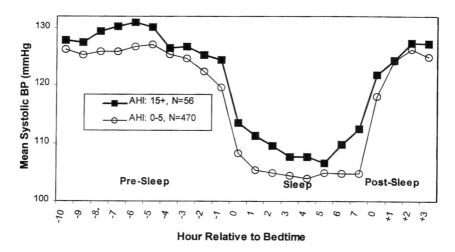

Figure 1 Estimated mean hourly systolic blood pressure from ambulatory monitoring during sleep and wake in the Wisconsin Sleep Cohort Study for subjects ($n = 554$) with SDB (AHI = 15 or more, heavy line) and without SDB (AHI <5, light line). Estimates are adjusted for age, sex, and BMI.

systolic blood pressure and in Figure 2 for diastolic blood pressure. The figures contrast hourly blood pressure patterns for people with SDB (AHI >15) and people without (AHI <5). Again, the effects are small, statistically significant, and stronger for systolic than for diastolic blood pressure. A line indicating the pattern in people with AHI between 5 and 15 has been omitted for visual clarity; that line, if displayed, would lie almost entirely above the AHI <5 line. There is no evidence from the plots that people with SDB as a group fail to show a substantial nighttime dip in blood pressure.

Sleep Heart Health Study. The Sleep Heart Health Study is a prospective multicenter study designed specifically to investigate the role of SDB in cardiovascular disease occurrence, progression, and mortality. The design is based on the addition of overnight in-home polysomnography and other measures relevant to sleep disorders to samples of participants from several established cohort studies. The study design and methods have been described in detail (27). Reports on the association of AHI and hypertension have not yet been published, but preliminary findings presented by Nieto et al. (28) have shown an association of SDB and hypertension independent of age, gender, race, BMI, and neck circumference (Table 2). Prevalence of hypertension, adjusted for confounders, increased with AHI category level. The odds ratio [95% confidence interval (C.I.)] for AHI >30 versus <5 was 1.5 (1.1,2.1). The odds ratios for the two less severe

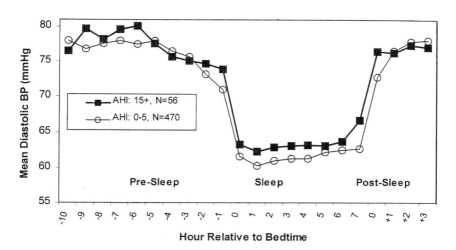

Figure 2 Estimated mean hourly diastolic blood pressure from ambulatory monitoring during sleep and wake in the Wisconsin Sleep Cohort Study for subjects ($n = 554$) with SDB (AHI = 15 or more, heavy line) and without SDB (AHI <5, light line). Estimates are adjusted for age, sex, and BMI.

Table 2 Odds Ratios for Apnea-Hypopnea Index (AHI) and
Hypertension Adjusted for Age, Sex, Race, Smoking, Body-Mass
Index, and Neck Circumference in the Sleep Heart Health Study
($n = 2840$)

AHI Category	Percent with Hypertension	Odds Ratio (95% C.I.) for Hypertension
<5	39	1 (reference category)
5–15	47	1.2 (1.0, 1.5)
15–30	46	1.1 (0.9, 1.5)
>30	59	1.5 (1.2, 2.1)

Source: Adapted from Ref. 28.

AHI categories versus AHI <5 were low and of borderline statistical significance, but the upper bound of both 95% confidence intervals was 1.5.

The rigorous design of both of these studies with similar results increases confidence that the findings are not driven by sample bias and are not due to confounding from any of the known correlates of both SDB and CVD. It is possible that there are uncontrolled confounding factors that cause the association. However, given the enormous amount of research into risk factors for hypertension, it is unlikely that there is an unknown strong risk factor for elevated blood pressure that is also strongly related to SDB. The major drawback to these findings is the uncertainty of the temporal order: some or all of the association may be due to the effect of high blood pressure on increased SDB. Assuming that the more biologically plausible direction of SDB causing elevated blood pressure accounts for most of the association, these studies 1) provide strong evidence for a true association between SDB and blood pressure; 2) indicate that the magnitude of the association is not large; and 3) suggest that the association is graded, with even mild SDB related to some increased risk of elevated blood pressure.

Studies with Some Physiological Measure of SDB Other Than Full Polysomnography

In one of the earliest community studies, Stradling and Crosby (29,30) used overnight home oximetry to detect SDB in a random sample of 748 British men. Blood pressure was measured in the men's homes in the early evening and a flexible oximetry probe was left for self-application. The authors reported almost no correlation between >4% desaturation events per hour of sleep and mean blood pressure after adjustment for several confounders. Results of the statistical analyses, however, were not fully presented. The authors generally noted *p* values; the only estimates from multivariate analysis given to express the magnitude of the association of SDB and blood pressure was that <1% of the variation in mean blood pressure was explained by the dip rate. No estimates were given for the dip rate and systolic blood pressure, diastolic blood pressure, or hypertension.

Olson et al. (31,32) studied a sample of 441 Australian men and women drawn from various sources. SDB in this study was measured by breathing sounds and chest and abdominal movement sounds, all detected by microphones that subjects applied themselves before bed. The adjusted odds ratio (95% C.I.) for $\geq$ 15 events per hour and self-reported hypertension was 1.5 (0.7, 3.3) but lacked statistical significance.

Schmidt-Nowara (33) investigated SDB using end-tidal CO_2 monitoring and hypertension based on blood pressure measurement and medication history in a probability sample of 275 Hispanic adults in New Mexico. SDB status was indicated by three apnea-per-hour categories: <10, 10–19, and >20. The odds ratio (95% C.I.) for AHI >10 versus <10, adjusted for confounders, was of borderline significance: 2.6 (1.0, 6.8). The odds ratio for AHI >20 versus AHI <10 was 1.8 (0.5, 6.0). Thus, there was no evidence for a dose-response relationship.

Jennum et al. (34) recorded 748 Danish men and women enrolled in the Copenhagen sample of the MONICA study, a multicenter study of cardiovascular risk factors. Measurements of blood pressure and other CVD risk factors were described in detail, but the measurement of SDB was described only as the number of apneas and hypopneas per hour of sleep detected by inductive plethysmography. Neither the equipment, the monitoring procedure, nor the scoring was described. The authors concluded that their index of abnormal events per hour was not statistically associated with blood pressure (p >0.6), but no supporting data were shown. Although hypertension was discussed as an endpoint for analysis, no finding for SDB and hypertension was given.

Little insight can be gleaned from the studies in which actual estimates of the strength of the associations were missing or incompletely presented. The two studies with some documentation of findings showed a statistically insignificant estimate in the range of that reported in the Sleep Cohort Study and the Sleep Heart Health Study. In view of the greater SDB measurement error in these studies using unattended monitoring with unconventional parameters, underestimation and loss of study power was likely to occur. Overall, findings from the Schmidt-Nowara et al. study and the Olson et al. study were not inconsistent with those of the Sleep Cohort Study and Sleep Heart Health Study, and findings from the other studies are not clear enough to provide evidence to the contrary.

Large Population-Based Studies with SDB Indicated by Habitual Snoring

Mailed Surveys of Self-Reported Snoring and Hypertension

Prospective and cross-sectional survey data provided by Nurses' Health Study participants were analyzed for associations between self-reported snoring (non-snoring, occasional snoring, regular snoring) and self-reported blood pressure and physician-diagnosed hypertension (35). The cross-sectional analysis represented 73,231 U.S. female nurses, ages 40–65 years, in 1986. Prevalence of reported physician-diagnosed hypertension in 1986 was 24% (n = 17,511). After adjustment for age, BMI, waist girth, cigarette smoking, alcohol use, and physical activity, the prevalence of hypertension was statistically significantly higher in occasional and regular snorers than in nonsnorers. The adjusted odds ratio (95% C.I.) for occasional snoring versus no snoring was 1.22 (1.16, 1.27) and for regular snoring versus no snoring was 1.43 (1.33, 1.53). Similar associations were found among incident cases of hypertension in an analysis of 8-year follow-up data obtained from nurses who were normotensive in 1986 (incidence rate ≈ 2 hypertension cases per 100 person-years). The adjusted relative risk for hypertension for occasional versus no snoring was 1.29 (1.22, 1.37) and for regular versus no snoring, 1.55 (1.42, 1.70).

As part of the Sleep Cohort Study, a baseline and 4-year follow-up survey that included identical questions on snoring (five semiquantitative response categories plus "do not know") and hypertension (taking antihypertensive drugs or diagnosed hypertension) were conducted. Snoring and hypertension data for baseline and follow-up were available for 3723 men and women. Using logistic regression to adjust for several confounders, we estimated the odds ratios for hypertension based on the initial and follow-up surveys separately. The robustness of the association was impressive: an odds ratio of 1.4 and 95% C.I. of (1.1, 1.8) for habitual snorers versus slight or nonsnorers resulted from both the initial and follow-up surveys.

Gislason et al. (36), using a survey, examined habitual snoring and hypertension (defined by being under medical care for hypertension) in 3201 Icelandic men 30–69 years of age and found a significant association only in men aged 40–49. An identical study (37) on 1505 women 40–59 years of age conducted several years later showed an association not restricted to any age subgroup (relative risk of hypertension in habitual snorers = 1.7, 95% C.I. = 1.5–2.4).

Koskenvuo et al. (38) studied snoring and self-reported hypertension in men and women enrolled in the Finnish Twin Cohort Study. The cohort comprises twin pairs born in Finland before 1958; various data are collected longitudinally on these twins. A survey of the participants aged 40–69 was conducted in 1981 and a well-constructed question on snoring (semiquantitative response categories including "do not know") was included, along with questions on history of hypertension, angina pectoris, and myocardial infarction. The response rate was 84%, yielding a sample size of 7511. The authors found that habitual snoring (always or almost always) was significantly related to hypertension, independent of age and BMI, for both men (odds ratio = 1.5, $p < 0.05$) and women (odds ratio = 2.77, $p < 0.001$). In addition, male habitual snorers compared to those who were not snorers were twice as likely to report a history of angina pectoris.

Self-Reported Snoring in Conjunction with Laboratory or Field Measures of Blood Pressure

The relationship between snoring and blood pressure has been investigated in the Sleep Cohort Study. A preliminary report on 147 participants who underwent ambulatory monitoring showed that habitual snorers with AHI <5 (simple snorers) had blood pressure values slightly higher than those of nonsnorers throughout the course of the recording (approximately 5 P.M. to 9 A.M.) (39). After adjustment for confounding factors, however, most differences between the snorers and nonsnorers were not statistically significant. The analysis was repeated after a larger sample accrued, and the pattern of a small increase in blood pressure persisted (40). Using data on standard blood pressure measures in the early evening (seated) and the next morning (supine), the morning and evening systolic and evening diastolic mean blood pressures were statistically significantly higher (p <0.05) in simple snorers (126 and 82 mmHg) compared to nonsnorers (122 and 80 mmHg).

Schmidt-Nowara et al. (41) investigated snoring and measured blood in a sample of 1206 Hispanic Americans in New Mexico. Loud snoring (often or always) was not related to hypertension, defined as systolic blood pressure ≥140 mmHg or diastolic blood pressure ≥90 mmHg or using antihypertensive medications (odds ratio = 1.0, adjusted for confounders). However, an odds ratio of 1.8 (95% C.I.= 0.9, 3.6) for loud snoring and myocardial infarction of borderline statistical significance was reported.

By adding snoring questions to the Male Copenhagen Study, Jennum et al. (42) were able to study self-reported snoring and measured blood pressure on a sample of 3323 employed men aged 54–74 years. There was only a slight univariate association between snoring and blood pressure; the authors stated that the association was not statistically significant after controlling for confounders.

Grunstein et al. (43) studied a sample of 3034 obese participants in a weight-loss study (Swedish Obesity Study) in Sweden. Data on self-reported loud snoring and breathing pauses were used to identify participants who had a high likelihood of SDB (frequent loud snoring and breathing pauses) and a low likelihood of SDB (never or rare loud snoring and no observed breathing pauses). Multiple regression, controlling for several confounders, showed that the SDB variable was a strong predictor of diastolic blood pressure in men and systolic blood pressure in women. It is not clear whether the gender difference was significant because a test for a difference was not reported. The study is unique in demonstrating than even among very obese people, a slight SDB association with blood pressure can be detected.

A major issue in interpreting the above study findings on snoring and blood pressure is an insufficient understanding of the pathophysiological state reflected in the self-report of loud, disruptive, or heavy snoring. Although most people with frequent apneas and hypopneas (i.e., AHI >5) do snore, most snorers in unselected populations do not have severe SDB (25,44). Assuming, then, that most people in the category of heavy or habitual snoring have SDB at the milder end of the severity spectrum, the weak associations found in most of the above studies could indicate that even very mild SDB is related to increased blood pressure, or that an association with more severe SDB and blood pressure is strong enough to surface even when a crude surrogate for SDB is used.

The assessment of findings from studies using snoring for SDB status is made even more difficult by misclassification based on self-reported snoring (45). Self-reported snoring is not only subjective but often also secondary information. Although snoring is self-perceived by some people, many must rely on information from others—e.g., bed partners. When asked about their snoring, people must integrate past information from others and then draw their own conclusion regarding their snoring status. Consequently, it is highly likely that the accuracy and reliability of self-reported snoring will vary not only by factors such as age and gender but also by unmeasured characteristics such as the vigilance level of household members, candidness of informants, and acceptance by the snorer of informants' accounts. The validity of self-reported snoring has not been adequately tested: monitoring over several nights would be needed to assess any responses except "always" and "never." In view of the underestimation that would occur with the substantial misclassification inherent in self-reported snoring, it is remarkable that significant associations with hypertension and blood pressure have been found and that the associations appear to be reliable, as shown in the baseline and 4-year follow-up analyses of the Sleep Cohort Study and cross-sectional and prospective analyses of the Nurses' Health Study.

Clinic Studies of SDB and Blood Pressure

Of the studies based on sleep clinic populations, statistically significant associations of SDB and blood pressure have been found in some (15,46–49). Most clinic-based studies have failed to detect a significant independent association (50–55). As discussed above, intractable design problems in clinic-based studies seriously limit interpretation of findings based on sleep clinic samples. Although the validity of some studies may indeed be better than others, there is no way to assess the amount and probable direction of bias in each study. However, provocative hypotheses that warrant investigation have been generated by the clinic-based studies. In particular, there is considerable interest in whether the diurnal pattern of blood pressure is affected by SDB. The following two hypotheses are based on observations of evening and morning blood pressures in sleep apnea patients: 1) the effect of SDB on blood pressure may be fairly acute, i.e., the morning blood pressure reflects the effect of the events the night before, and the effect diminishes as the day progresses (52) and 2) SDB may abolish or diminish the normal dip in blood pressure during sleep (48,51,52,56–58).

B. Studies of SDB and CVD

SDB has been examined in relation to the following CVD endpoints: myocardial infarction, angina, coronary artery disease, mortality due to ischemic heart disease, and overall mortality.

Population-Based Studies of SDB and CVD Morbidity and Mortality

Ancoli-Israel et al. (19) conducted an 8- to 10-year follow-up on a probability sample of 426 community-dwelling persons 65 years of age or older at study entry. The sample had been studied at baseline by in-home recording of thoracic and abdominal breathing excursions; an activity monitor was used to estimate sleep. The researchers were able to follow up all but 4 persons from the original cohort. There was a higher proportion of cardiovascular deaths in people with a respiratory distress index (RDI) of 15 or greater: 35, 59, and 54% for groups with RDI <15, 15–30, and >30 respectively. Survival analysis showed a significant difference in survival time ($p = 0.003$), with an average survival of 7.9 years for those with an RDI >30 and 9.4 years for those with RDI <15. However, using a Cox proportional hazards regression model that included terms for age, gender, BMI, and history of CVD, RDI was not a significant predictor of mortality. Since CVD should be intermediate in the causal pathway of SDB and CVD death, it is not surprising that RDI was no longer significant.

Lindberg and colleagues (59) followed 3100 men for 10 years for mortality outcomes. The men, aged 30–69 at study entry, were randomly selected from a population register in Uppsala, Sweden. Based on answers to mailed questionnaires, the men were partitioned into four categories: snorers with and without excessive daytime sleepiness and nonsnorers with and without excessive daytime sleepiness. Over the 10-year follow-up, 213 deaths were ascertained by accessing a national death registry. After adjustment for self-reported BMI, age, hypertension, diabetes, and heart disease in a Cox proportional hazards regression model, younger men (<60 years) with both snoring and excessive daytime sleepiness were more likely to die over the follow-up period than men with neither snoring nor sleepiness. The adjusted relative risk (95% C.I.) for overall mortality was 2.2 (1.3, 3.8) and for cardiovascular mortality was 2.0 (0.8, 4.7). There was no significant elevation in mortality (cardiovascular or overall) for older (>60 years) sleepy snoring men or for snoring or sleepiness in isolation, regardless of age. That is, snoring only imparted an excess risk of mortality in younger men with excessive daytime sleepiness.

Koskenvuo et al. (60) surveyed 4388 male participants 40–69 years of age in the Finnish twin cohort on snoring status in 1981 and then ascertained CVD status with hospital discharge data and mortality records up to 1984. Among the men free of ischemic heart disease at the time of the survey (i.e., no history of angina or myocardial infarction), the odds ratio (95% C.I.) for new ischemic heart disease was 1.4 (1.15, 1.71) for habitual and frequent snorers versus occasional and nonsnorers, independent of BMI, age, smoking, alcohol and hypertension.

Jennum et al. (61) conducted a similar large prospective study ($n = 2937$), the Copenhagen Male Study. Participants aged 54–74 were surveyed on snoring and then followed for ischemic heart disease outcomes through hospital and mortality records for up to 6 years. In this study, however, snoring was not related to ischemic heart disease (relative risk = 1.0, adjusted for confounding factors).

The disparity in results from the two Scandinavian studies with similar study methods and large, well-constructed samples is puzzling. Jennum et al. (61) suggested that an association may be present only younger men, below the age range of the Copenhagen study. The findings of Lindberg et al. (59) support this explanation. Additionally a recent survey of sleep disorders in older adults, Enright et al. (62) found no correlation between snoring and outcomes often associated with SDB (including hypertension) in middle-aged adults. It is also possible that other factors, such as genetics, may modify the effect of SDB on CVD development and that these factors differ in the two Scandinavian samples. Also, if simple snoring or snoring without significant apneic events does not itself carry a CVD risk, it is possible that the prevalence of more serious sleep apnea was higher in the Finnish sample.

CVD Morbidity and Mortality in Sleep Apnea Patients

Treated Versus Untreated Sleep Apnea Patients

A few studies have been conducted in which incident CVD or CVD mortality in sleep clinic patients was ascertained some years after diagnosis. The problem in assessing morbidity associated with sleep apnea lies in selection of the proper comparison group. Because of the overall selection bias that ensures more comorbidity among patients, comparison of patients' mortality with that of the general population is not useful. Three studies attempted to circumvent this problem by comparing morbidity and mortality in untreated patients with sleep apnea with patients who had been treated by tracheostomy.

In a widely cited early study, He et al. (63) attempted to ascertain the vital status of 706 sleep apnea patients. The mortality experiences of treated versus untreated, mild versus severe, and younger versus older apnea patients were compared in 385 patients who were successfully tracked. Conservatively treated patients (e.g., weight loss was advised) were found to have a significantly higher death rate than patients treated by tracheotomy. In addition to a lack of randomization to treatment group, a serious limitation of the study was the large proportion of patients whose vital status was not found. Even a small tendency for lower ascertainment of untreated people who survived versus treated people who survived could account for the association.

Using a similar study design, Partinen et al. conducted a 5-year mortality follow-up (64) and a 7-year morbidity follow-up (65) on 200 sleep apnea patients. Extensive tracking was used and the status of 198 of the patients was ascertained, increasing confidence in the findings. In the mortality follow-up study, the conservatively treated patients, compared to those treated by tracheostomy, had nearly five times the risk of cardiovascular or stroke-related death. In the morbidity follow-up study, the relative risk (95% C.I.) of new vascular disease for the untreated compared to treated group was 2.3 (1.5, 3.6).

These clinic-based studies, with the power of prospective analyses, indicate that people with untreated SDB are at greater risk of CVD and mortality. However, as discussed above, the use of clinic samples for addressing the role of SDB in CVD is fraught with problems. If it had been possible to randomize patients in these two studies to treatment or no treatment, concern would be diminished. Without randomization, it is possible that observed differences at follow-up merely reflect the different baseline health of the groups. However, for sleep apnea patients in the era in which these studies were based, the expected bias would be that the sickest patients would be treated aggressively (tracheostomy); indeed, the comparisons of AHI, weight, and other factors in the He et al. (63) and Partinen et al. (64,65) studies support this. Consequently, these studies do provide support for a causal role of SDB in CVD. An important caveat, however, is that these studies were conducted on patients with quite severe SDB, so the findings may not be applicable to mild or moderate SDB.

Case-Control Studies Linking SDB with CVD

Hung et al. (66) performed overnight polysomnography on 101 Australian patients who had survived myocardial infarction and 53 volunteers from community clubs who served as heart disease–free controls. These men were screened by medical history and by a treadmill stress test to ascertain their control status. Both apnea index and snoring history were significantly associated with myocardial infarction independent of BMI and other potential confounding factors. Men with an apnea index over 5 were 23 times more likely to have had a myocardial infarction. The confidence interval for this very high odds ratio is wide (95% C.I. = 4, 140) but even the low boundary indicates a substantial risk. Being a current snorer carried nearly as high a risk (odds ratio = 11, 95% C.I. = 3, 40). Concerns regarding estimation of past SDB with current status have been raised. The possibility that the myocardial infarction preceded the SDB cannot be ruled out. Perhaps the most serious concern is that the control group was healthier than the general population and that an abnormally low level of SDB and snoring in this group was responsible for the relationship.

A more conservative approach to construction of the control group was taken by D'Alessandro et al. (67) in a case-control study of myocardial infarction and snoring history conducted in Italy. For each case recruited from new hospital admissions for myocardial infarction ($n = 50$), both a hospital control (the next acute illness hospital admission after each case's admission for myocardial infarction) and a community control randomly selected from the community census listing were used (matched on age and sex). Using both control groups together, the odds ratio (adjusted for confounders) for snoring and myocardial infarction was 4.4 (95% C.I. = 1.1, 17.8). Again, the authors controlled for hypertension, which may have resulted in an underestimation of snoring and myocardial infarction if hypertension is intermediate in a causal pathway.

More recently, Mooe et al. studied coronary artery disease and SDB in 192 Swedish men (68) and in 152 women (69) using a case-control design. For both studies, cases were identified based on coronary angiographic evidence of coronary artery disease and controls were randomly selected from the population registry. All participants had an in-hospital sleep study; apneas were defined by a 10-sec airflow cessation detected by thermistry and hypopneas were defined by a decrease in airflow accompanied by a 4% or more oxygen desaturation detected by oximetry. The results showed that men and women with AHI in the upper quartile (≥ 5 events per hour for women, ≥ 14 events per hour for men) versus those with lesser AHI were 4.5 and 4.1 times more likely to have coronary artery disease, respectively. Odds ratios, adjusted for BMI, hypertension, smoking and diabetes, were statistically significant at $p < 0.05$. The response rates for the comparison groups in both studies were excellent, reducing concern for an overly healthy control group. A weakness of these studies as well as the earlier case-control studies is that the past SDB status (prior to the development of CVD) is estimated by the current status. Findings in the earlier studies have been questioned because myocardial infarction may affect breathing during sleep (70). Although the Mooe et al. studies (68,69) suffer from the same limitation, concern is lessened because the cases had newly diagnosed coronary artery disease and consequently less severe pathology that might otherwise affect breathing during sleep. In spite of the limitations of the case-control studies, the magnitude of the association was large and independent of potential confounding factors and of hypertension.

IV. Summary

The relationships between SDB (variously defined) and CVD, hypertension, or mortality have been examined in several epidemiological studies: a substantial number of studies have found a small to modest statistically significant relationship; a substantial number of studies have demonstrated a small to modest but not statistically significant relationship; a small number of studies have found a large relationship; and a small number of studies have found no relationship whatsoever.

All the findings discussed or referred to in this review are likely to be biased to some degree. Bias can be both toward underestimation (e.g., from mismeasurment of SDB) and overestimation (e.g., from inadequate control of confounders), and the net magnitude of competing biases undoubtedly varies from study to study. Because those studies designed to detect small to modest relationships (the Sleep Cohort Study and Sleep Heart Health Study) *have* found modest relationships with hypertension, we conclude that the data are most consistent with a small to modest independent relationship between SDB and CVD/hypertension. This conclusion is bolstered by the observation that even those studies that have found no significant relationship do have confidence limits for their estimates that include small but important positive associations. However, we cannot yet rule out the possibility that there is no relationship, and temporal precedence has not yet been established. Since SDB is quite prevalent and CVD and hypertension are major causes of poor quality of life, disability, and death, it is imperative that 1) well-designed studies continue in this area and, for policy purposes, 2) we assume that SDB and CVD/hypertension *are* modestly linked until it is conclusively demonstrated that their association is negligible.

References

1. Young T, Evans L, Finn L, Palta M. Estimation of the clinically diagnosed proportion of sleep apnea syndrome in middle-aged men and women. Sleep 1997; 20:705–706.
2. Redline S, Kump K, Tishler PV, Browner I, Ferrette V. Gender differences in sleep disordered breathing in a community-based sample. Am J Respir Crit Care Med 1994; 149:722–726.
3. Young T. Analytic epidemiology studies of sleep disordered breathing—what explains the gender difference in sleep disordered breathing? Sleep 1993; 16(suppl): S1–S2.
4. Young T, Hutton R, Finn L, Badr S, Palta M. The gender bias in sleep apnea diagnosis: are women missed because they have different symptoms? Arch Intern Med 1996; 156:2445–2451.
5. Bearpark H, Elliott L, Grunstein R, et al. Occurrence and correlates of sleep disordered breathing in the Australian town of Busselton: a preliminary analysis. Sleep 1993; 16(suppl):S3–S5.
6. Jeong DU, Dimsdale JE. Sleep apnea and essential hypertension: a critical review of the epidemiological evidence for co-morbidity. Clin Exp Hypertens Theory Pract 1989; 11:1301–1323.

7. Waller PC, Bhopal RS. Is snoring a cause of vascular disease? An epidemiological review. Lancet 1989; 1:143–146.

8. Hoffstein V. Is snoring dangerous to your health? Sleep 1996; 19:506–516.

9. Wright J, Johns R, Watt I, Melville A, Sheldon T. Health effects of obstructive sleep apnoea and the effectiveness of continuous positive airways pressure: a systematic review of the research evidence. BMJ 1997; 314:851–860.

10. Rothman KJ, Greenland S. Modern Epidemiology. Philadelphia: Lippincott-Raven, 1998.

11. Marshall JR, Hastrup JL. Mismeasurement and the resonance of strong confounders: uncorrelated errors. Am J Epidemiology 1996; 143:1069–1078.

12. Katz I, Stradling J, Slutsky AS, Hoffstein V. Do patients with obstructive sleep apnea have thick necks? Am Rev Respir Dis 1990; 141:1228–1231.

13. Levinson PD, McGarvey ST, Carlisle CC, Eveloff SE, Herbert PN, Millman RP. Adiposity and cardiovascular risk factors in men with obstructive sleep apnea. Chest 1993; 103:1336–1342.

14. Millman RP, Carlisle CC, McGarvey ST, Eveloff SE, Levinson PD. Body fat distribution and sleep apnea severity in women. Chest 1995; 107:362–366.

15. Grunstein R, Wilcox I, Yang TS, Gould Y, Hedner J. Snoring and sleep apnoea in men: association with central obesity and hypertension. Int J Obes Rel Metab Disord 1993; 17:533–540.

16. Hoffstein V, Mateika S. Differences in abdominal and neck circumferences in patients with and without obstructive sleep apnoea. Eur Respir J 1992; 5:377–381.

17. Davies RJ, Ali NJ, Stradling JR. Neck circumference and other clinical features in the diagnosis of the obstructive sleep apnoea syndrome. Thorax 1992; 47:101–105.

18. Horner RL, Mohiaddin RH, Lowell DG, et al. Sites and sizes of fat deposits around the pharynx in obese patients with obstructive sleep apnoea and weight matched controls. Eur Respir J 1989; 2:613–622.

19. Ancoli-Israel S, Kripke DF, Klauber MR, et al. Morbidity, mortality and sleep-disordered breathing in community dwelling elderly. Sleep 1996; 19:277–282.

20. Lavie P, Herer P, Peled R, et al. Mortality in sleep apnea patients: a multivariate analysis of risk factors. Sleep 1995; 18:149–157.

21. Peppard PE, Young T, Palta M, Skatrud J. Sex-differences in the relationship between obesity and sleep-disordered breathing. Am J Respir Crit Care Med 1998; 157:A60.

22. White IR, Chaturvedi N, McKeigue PM. Median analysis of blood pressure for a sample including treated hypertensives. Stat Med 1994; 13:1635–1641.

23. Stradling J, Davies RJO. Sleep apnea and hypertension—what a mess! Sleep 1997; 20:789–793.

24. Munoz A, Gange SJ. Methodological issues for biomarkers and intermediate outcomes in cohort studies. Epidemiol Rev 1998; 20:29–42.

25. Young T, Palta M, Dempsey J, Skatrud J, Weber S, Badr S. The occurrence of sleep-disordered breathing among middle-aged adults. N Engl J Med 1993; 328:1230–1235.

26. Young T, Peppard P, Palta M, et al. Population-based study of sleep-disordered breathing as a risk factor for hypertension. Arch Intern Med 1997; 157:1746–1752.

27. Quan SF, Howard BV, Iber C, et al. The Sleep Heart Health Study: design, rationale, and methods. Sleep 1997; 20:1077–1085.

28. Nieto JF, Young T, Samet J, et al. Sleep apnea and systemic hypertension: the Sleep Heart Health Study. Circulation 1998; 97:828.

29. Stradling JR, Crosby JH. Relation between systemic hypertension and sleep hypoxaemia or snoring: analysis in 748 men drawn from general practice. BMJ 1990; 300:75–78.

30. Stradling JR, Crosby JH. Predictors and prevalence of obstructive sleep apnoea and snoring in 1001 middle aged men. Thorax 1991; 46:85–90.

31. Olson LG, King MT, Hensley MJ, Saunders NA. A community study of snoring and sleep-disordered breathing: health outcomes. Am J Respir Crit Care Med 1995; 152:717–720.

32. Olson LG, King MT, Hensley MJ, Saunders NA. A community study of snoring and sleep-disordered breathing: prevalence. Am J Respir Crit Care Med 1995; 152: 711–716.

33. Schmidt-Nowara WW. Cardiovascular consequences of sleep apnea. Progr Clin Biol Res 1990; 345:377–385.

34. Jennum P, Sjol A. Snoring, sleep apnoea and cardiovascular risk factors: the MONICA II Study. Int J Epidemiol 1993; 22:439–444.

35. Hu FB, Willett WC, Colditz GA, et al. Prospective study of snoring and risk of hypertension in women. Am J Epidemiol 1999; 150:806–816.

36. Gislason T, Aberg H, Taube A. Snoring and systemic hypertension—an epidemiological study. Acta Med Scand 1987; 222:415–421.

37. Gislason T, Benediktsdottir B, Bjornsson JK, Kjartansson G, Kjeld M, Kristbjarnarson H. Snoring, hypertension, and the sleep apnea syndrome: an epidemiologic survey of middle-aged women. Chest 1993; 103:1147–1151.

38. Koskenvuo M, Kaprio J, Partinen M, Langinvainio H, Sarna S, Heikkila K. Snoring as a risk factor for hypertension and angina pectoris. Lancet 1985; 1:893–896.

39. Hla KM, Young TB, Bidwell T, Palta M, Skatrud JB, Dempsey J. Sleep apnea and hypertension: a population-based study. Ann Intern Med 1994; 120:382–388.

40. Young T, Finn L, Hla KM, Morgan B, Palta M. Hypertension in sleep disordered breathing: snoring as part of a dose-response relationship between sleep-disordered breathing and blood pressure. Sleep 1996; 19(suppl):S202–S205.

41. Schmidt-Nowara WW, Coultas DB, Wiggins C, Skipper BE, Samet JM. Snoring in a Hispanic-American population: risk factors and association with hypertension and other morbidity. Arch Intern Med 1990; 150:597–601.

42. Jennum P, Hein HO, Suadicani P, Gyntelberg F. Cardiovascular risk factors in snorers: a cross-sectional study of 3,323 men aged 54 to 74 years: the Copenhagen male study. Chest 1992; 102:1371–1376.

43. Grunstein RR, Stenlof K, Hedner J, Sjostrom L. Impact of obstructive sleep apnea and sleepiness on metabolic and cardiovascular risk factors in the Swedish Obese Subjects (SOS) Study. Int J Obes Rel Metab Disord 1995; 19:410–418.

44. Bearpark H, Elliott L, Grunstein R, et al. Snoring and sleep apnea: a population study in Australian men. Am J Respir Crit Care Med 1995;151:1459–1465.

45. Young TB. Some methodologic and practical issues of reported snoring validity. Chest 1991; 99:531–532.

46. Carlson JT, Hedner JA, Ejnell H, Peterson LE. High prevalence of hypertension in sleep apnea patients independent of obesity. Am J Respir Crit Care Med 1994; 150: 72–77.

47. Millman RP, Redline S, Carlisle CC, Assaf AR, Levinson PD. Daytime hypertension in obstructive sleep apnea: prevalence and contributing risk factors. Chest 1991; 99: 861–866.

48. Pankow W, Nabe B, Lies A, Becker H, Lohmann FW. Influence of sleep apnea on 24-hour blood pressure. Chest 1997; 112:1253–1258.

49. Strohl KP, Novak RD, Singer W, et al. Insulin levels, blood pressure and sleep apnea. Sleep 1994; 17:614–618.

50. Davies RJO, Crosby J, Prothero O, Stradling JR. Ambulatory blood pressure and left ventricular hypertrophy in subjects with untreated obstructive sleep apnea and snoring, compared with matched control subjects and their response to treatment. Clin Sci 1994; 86:417–424.

51. Nabe B, Lies A, Pankow W, Kohl FV, Lohmann FW. Determinants of circadian blood pressure rhythm and blood pressure variability in obstructive sleep apnea. J Sleep Res 1995; 4:97–101.

52. Hoffstein V, Mateika J. Evening-to-morning blood pressure variations in snoring patients with and without obstructive sleep apnea. Chest 1992; 101:379–384.

53. Rauscher H, Popp W, Zwick H. Systemic hypertension in snorers with and without sleep apnea. Chest 1992; 102:367–371.

54. Mendelson W. The relationship of sleepiness and blood pressure to respiratory variables in obstructive sleep apnea. Chest 1995; 108:966–972.

55. Escourrou P, Jirani A, Nedelcoux H, Duroux P, Gaultier C. Systemic hypertension in sleep apnea syndrome. Chest 1990; 98:1362–1365.

56. Noda A, Okada T, Hayashi H, Yasuma F, Yokota M. 24-hour ambulatory blood pressure variability in obstructive sleep apnea syndrome. Chest 1993; 103:1343–1347.

57. Wilcox I, Grunstein RR, Collins FL, Doyle JM, Kelly DT, Sullivan CE. Circadian rhythm of blood pressure in patients with obstructive sleep apnea. Blood Pressure 1992; 1:219–222.

58. Suzuki M, Guilleminault C, Otsuka K, Shiomi T. Blood pressure "dipping" and "non-dipping" in obstructive sleep apnea syndrome patients. Sleep 1996; 19:382–387.

59. Lindberg E, Janson C, Svardsudd K, Gislason T, Hetta J, Boman G. Increased mortality among sleepy snorers: a prospective population based study. Thorax 1998; 53: 631–637.

60. Koskenvuo M, Kaprio J, Telakivi T, Partinen M, Heikkila K, Sarna S. Snoring as a risk factor for ischaemic heart disease and stroke in men. BMJ 1987; 294:16–19.

61. Jennum P, Hein HO, Suadicani P, Gyntelberg F. Risk of ischemic heart disease in self-reported snorers. Chest 1995; 108:138–142.

62. Enright PL, Newman AB, Wahl PW, Manolio TA, Haponik EF, Boyle PJR. Prevalence and correlates of snoring and observed apneas in 5,201 older adults. Sleep 1996; 19:531–538.

63. He J, Kryger MH, Zorick FJ, Conway W, Roth T. Mortality and apnea index in obstructive sleep apnea: experience in 385 male patients. Chest 1988; 94:9–14.

64. Partinen M, Jamieson A, Guilleminault C. Long-term outcome for obstructive sleep apnea syndrome patients. Mortality. Chest 1988; 94:1200–1204.
65. Partinen M, Guilleminault C. Daytime sleepiness and vascular morbidity at seven-year follow-up in obstructive sleep apnea patients. Chest 1990; 97:27–32.
66. Hung J, Whitford EG, Parsons RW, Hillman DR. Association of sleep apnoea with myocardial infarction in men. Lancet 1990; 336:261–264.
67. D'Alessandro R, Magelli C, Gamberini G, et al. Snoring every night as a risk factor for myocardial infarction: a case-control study. BMJ 1990; 300:1557–1558.
68. Mooe T, Rabben T, Wiklund U, Franklin KA, Eriksson P. Sleep-disordered breathing in men with coronary artery disease. Chest 1996; 109:659–663.
69. Mooe T, Rabben T, Wiklund U, Franklin KA, Eriksson P. Sleep-disordered breathing in women: occurrence and association with coronary artery disease. Am J Med 1996; 101:251–256.
70. Saito T, Yoshikawa T, Sakamoto Y, Tanaka K, Inoue T, Ogawa R. Sleep apnea in patients with acute myocardial infarction. Crit Care Med 1991; 19:938–941.

13

Cerebrovascular Disease and Sleep Apnea

MARK ERIC DYKEN

University of Iowa College of Medicine
Iowa City, Iowa

I. Introduction

Stroke and obstructive sleep apnea are common. In the United States, stroke is responsible for greater than half of all acute neurological hospital admissions, is the third leading cause of death, and is the leading cause of serious long-term disability (1). In a random sample of 602 people, between 30 and 60 years of age, the prevalence of obstructive apnea in the general population ranged between 4 and 9% for women and between 9 and 24% for men (2).

Stroke and obstructive sleep apnea are also associated with many of the same health problems, including hypertension and cardiovascular disease (3,4). Risk factors for both include age, gender, diabetes mellitus, and cigarette smoking. Although obstructive sleep apnea has not been proven to be a risk factor for stroke, the literature suggests that a cause-and-effect relationship can occur (3).

II. Snoring

Snoring is common in obstructive sleep apnea (OSA). A continuum appears to exist between snoring and obesity and the obstructive sleep apnea syndrome

(OSAS) (5,6). Snoring is a loud, inspiratory noise produced by vibrations of a compliant oropharynx (7). Without polysomnography, clinical impression and a snoring history can suggest the diagnosis of OSA.

Even after adjusting for gender, age, smoking, and obesity, frequent snoring has been associated with angina (8), hypertension (8–12), and heart disease (11,13,14). A controlled study showed snoring to be an independent risk factor for myocardial infarction (14). Habitual snoring has also been associated with a greater relative risk of Alzheimer's disease and multi-infarct dementia (15), combined ischemic heart disease and stroke (16), and stroke (17–21).

In a study of 167 men with stroke, 36% suffered stroke in sleep (18). Stepwise multiple logistic regression analysis showed that among potential stroke risk factors (obesity, age, smoking, alcohol, and diabetes mellitus), only snoring was significantly related to stroke in sleep. A similar study reported that the odds ratio of snoring as a risk factor for stroke was increased if there was an association with classic signs and symptoms for OSA (obesity and sleepiness) (20).

Snoring studies have many limitations (21). People who sleep alone may not be able to knowingly report snoring. The histories of patients with significant cerebrovascular disease may be limited due to aphasia, confusion, stupor or coma, or as a result of impaired cognition due to a multitude of concomitant health problems and medication effects.

The severity of OSA and snoring may not progress in parallel. If OSA worsens in regard to duration and frequency, the severity of snoring may decrease, as snoring should not occur during a full obstruction.

Isolated snoring without apnea is common. Occasional snoring occurs more frequently than OSA, with an estimated prevalence of 42.0% in the general adult population (11). Habitual snoring has been reported in approximately 14% of women and 24% of men (8–10). In addition, some individuals with OSA have been shown not to snore during polysomnography (22). False-positive and false-negative diagnoses are likely when one is attempting to diagnose OSA on the basis of snoring.

III. Polysomnography

A number of sleep laboratories have analyzed stroke patients polysomnographically (see Table 1) (22–36). Abnormal sleep-related respiratory events have been defined as hypopneas and apneas (37). Hypopneas are associated with significantly reduced airflow when compared to the normal waking, resting respiratory patterns. Airflow is absent during apneas (38).

Hypopneas and apneas are classified as obstructive, central, or mixed. During central apnea, there is no respiratory effort. During an obstructive apnea, respiratory effort continues. A mixed apnea starts with a central component and is followed by an obstruction. In practice, a mixed apnea is considered an obstruction.

In adults, a significant apnea or hypopnea persists for at least 10 sec and/ or occurs with an arousal and/or an oxygen saturation drop of 3% or more. A diagnosis of apnea has traditionally been associated with an apnea/hypopnea index (the average number of events per hour of sleep) greater than or equal to 10 and/or any events associated with oxygen desaturations to or below 86% (when the baseline is greater than 86%) (38–42).

IV. Unselected, Retrospectively Studied Populations and Case Reports

In a retrospective study of 55 unselected patients with mild to moderate OSA, 19% (10 subjects) had a history of stroke (23). Each patient had a total of two polysomnograms performed at a mean interval of 77 weeks. The initial and follow-up studies showed respective mean apnea/hypopnea indices of 21.8 and 33.4 events per hour. The specific apnea/hypopnea and oxygen-saturation low indices were not given for the stroke patients.

Some cases reports are limited in clinical and laboratory description. Although an abstract from 1987 reported polygraphic evidence of obstructive sleep apnea in a patient with stroke and transient ischemic attacks, oxygen saturation and apnea/hypopnea indices were not provided (26).

Brainstem stroke and OSA were addressed polysomnographically in a 1982 case report, where a 46-year-old hypertensive male required intubation within 3 months of a right lateral medullary infarction (24). A sleep study showed an oxygen saturation low of 60% and an apnea index of 18.0 events per hour. The patient was successfully treated with tracheostomy. It was hypothesized that injury to the nucleus ambiguus (a brainstem area that provides upper motor neuron innervation to the upper airways) resulted in OSA. Nevertheless, apnea would have been expected acutely, and reports of progressive weight gain, sleepiness, and snoring suggest that OSA was not a primary result of stroke.

In 1988, OSA was polysomnographically diagnosed in a patient with a unilateral lateral medullary brainstem infarction (27). A 2-night study revealed an oxygen saturation low value of 80% and a mean apnea/hypopnea index of 25.0 events per hour. This individual had 51 central apneas (a finding often associated with brainstem stroke) and 99 obstructive apneas. Nevertheless, this patient may have been predisposed to OSA due to anatomic considerations (long uvula, septal deviation, and nasal occlusion).

A potential relationship between ischemic hemispheric stroke and OSA was suggested polysomnographically in 1985 (25). During the early morning hours, an obese 34-year-old man (with a history of hypertension, diabetes, snor-

Table 1 Studies of Stroke Patients Analyzed Polysomnographically

Study Type/Authors/Year	Number of Stroke/Controls	% OSA[a]	A/H[b]	Sa_{O_2} (LS) (%)[c]	Location	Type (No. pts)
Unselected retrospectively studied populations and case reports						
Pendlebury et al., 1997 (23)	Stroke = 19	100.0	NG	NG	NG	NG
Chaudhary et al., 1982 (24)	Stroke = 1	100.0	18.0	60.0	Brainstem	I
Tilkare et al., 1985 (25)	Stroke = 1	100.0	78.0	70.0	Hemispheric	I
Rivest/Reiher, 1987 (26)	Stroke = 1	100.0	NG	NG	Brainstem	I
Askenasy/Goldhammer, 1988 (27)	Stroke = 1	100.0	25.0	80.0	Brainstem	I
Dyken et al., 1991 (28,29)	Stroke = 1	100.0	36.0	60.0	Subcortical	H
Pressman et al., 1995 (30)	Stroke = 1	100.0	22.0	<50.0	Hemispheric	I
Selected populations						
Kapen et al., 1991 (31)	Stroke 47[d] (31)	72.0	28.0	NG	Hemispheric	I
Hudgel et al., 1993 (32)	Stroke = 8	NG	44.0	82.0	NG	I/H
	Control = 8	NG	12.0	90.0	—	—
Mohsenin/Valor, 1995 (33)	Stroke = 10	80.0 (OSA) 10.0 (CSA)	52.0	NG	Hemispheric (9) Subcortical (1)	I (9) H (1)
	Control = 10	—	3.0	NG	—	—
Good et al., 1996 (34)	Stroke = 19	95.0	36.0	NG	Hemispheric (16) Brainstem (3)	I

Unselected consecutively studied populations

Population	Group				Location	
Bassetti et al., 1996 (35)	Stroke = 23	70.0	32.0	82.0	"Anterior circ."[e] (74%)	I
					"Posterior circ." (26%)	—
	Control = 19	16.0	6.0	89.0		
Dyken et al., 1996 (22)	Stroke = 24	71.0	26.0	85.0	Hemispheric (12)	I (20)
					Subcortical (8)	H (4)
					Cerebellar (2)	
					Brainstem (2)	
	Control = 27	19.0	4.0	91.0		
Bassetti et al., 1997 (36)	Stroke = 39	54.0 (OSA)	26.0 (NREM)	82.0 (ST)	Hemispheric (28)	I
		10.0 (CSB)	30.0 (REM)	83.0 (IT)	Brainstem (9)	
					Pontocerebellar (1)	
					Cerebellum (1)	

[a] Percentage of patients diagnosed polysomnographically with obstructive sleep apnea.
[b] Apnea/hypopnea index.
[c] Lowest value during sleep.
[d] Only 31 of 47 patients in data pool had full polysomnograms.
[e] Data pool was mixed with transient ischemic attack patients.
I, ischemic; H, hemorrhagic; circ., circulation; CSB, Cheyne-like breathing; ST, supratentorial; IT, infratentorial.

ing, and sleepiness) suffered an acute right hemiplegia. A computed tomographic (CT) scan of the head performed within 1 to 2 days of the event revealed a paraventricular area of low attenuation. He was noted to have a stertorous breathing pattern when lying supine. Subsequent polysomnography showed an oxygen saturation low of 70% and an apnea/hypopnea index of 78 events per hour. The authors acknowledged that other medical problems (such as hypertension) may have been responsible for this stroke. Nevertheless, they suggested that hypoxia and cardiac arrhythmia, commonly observed in OSA, might have contributed.

In 1991 a case report concerning the possible relationship between hemorrhagic stroke and polysomnographically documented OSA was published. A 34-year-old man, after a hemorrhagic stroke in sleep, had a sleep study showing oxygen desaturations to 60% and an apnea/hypopnea index of 36 events per hour (28). The history was remarkable for snoring, sleepiness, and obesity without hypertension, cardiac disease, or previous stroke. A hypertensive event was suggested by the location of the patient's stroke. A noncontrast CT of the brain showed a hemorrhage involving the putamen and the proximal portion of the posterior limb of the right internal capsule (see Fig. 1).

Previous studies with arm cuff and intra-arterial monitoring techniques documented elevated blood pressures after nocturnal obstructive respiratory events

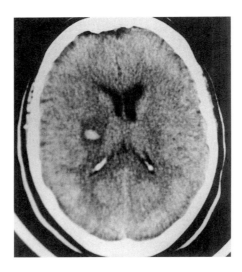

Figure 1 A brain CT without contrast reveals a hemorrhage, with a surrounding area, greater than 1-cm in diameter, of low density, consistent with edema, involving the putamen and the proximal posterior limb of the right internal capsule.

(43–45). These findings led to the hypothesis that stroke may result from apnea-induced hypertensive bleeding (28,29).

In 1995, a 59-year-old obese, hypertensive woman awoke with right hemiparesis (30). She had a history of weight gain, snoring, and gasping arousals associated with palpitations and diaphoresis, morning headaches, and hypersomnolence. The family history was suggestive of OSA with sudden unexplained death in sleep. Polysomnography revealed an oxygen saturation low value less than 50% and an apnea/hypopnea index of 22.0 events per hour. The patient was successfully treated with continuous positive airway pressure (CPAP) therapy.

V. Selected, Prospectively Studied Populations

In 1991, a total of 31 subjects with ischemic hemispheric stroke were selected for polysomnography (31). The findings were added to those of an unpublished study where an additional 16 patients had incomplete polysomnograms, without monitoring of oxygen saturation or respiratory effort (46). The overall mean apnea/hypopnea index was 28 events per hour. For the 72% (34 of 47 patients) diagnosed with OSA, the mean apnea/hypopnea index was 37.9 events per hour. The apneics tended to be heavier, older, and sleepier than nonapneics (the mean sleep latency was 9 min for apneics and 12 min for nonapneics).

In 1993, a total of 8 elderly patients with finger-pulse oximetry studies suggestive of apnea were selected for polysomnography at least 1 month after unilateral ischemic or hemorrhagic stroke (32). Controls were similar in gender, age, weight, and height. The respective mean oxygen saturation low indices in the control and stroke groups were 90 and 82%. The respective mean apnea/hypopnea indices in the control and stroke groups were 12 and 44 events per hour. The number of apneics was not reported in either group.

Wider tidal volume oscillations and greater hypopharyngeal pressures were found in the stroke group. Referencing previous studies, it was suggested that hypoxemia and oscillations in intracranial pressures and blood flow predisposed obstructive sleep apneics to ischemic stroke (47–49).

In 1995, a total of 10 subjects from a rehabilitation facility with stroke within the year were selected for polysomnography (33). Previous to stroke, no patient had significant snoring, apnea, obesity, hypersomnolence, or neurological problems. A control group was matched for obesity, age, smoking, and hypertension. The respective mean apnea/hypopnea indices for the control and stroke groups were 3 and 52 events per hour. Of the 10 patients with stroke, 8 had significant sleep apnea. Predominately obstructive events were found in 7 patients, and primarily central apneas occurred in 1 individual. Graphically, control subjects and stroke patients were shown to have respective oxygen desaturations below 80 and 70% (mean oxygen saturation low values were not provided).

The authors intended to provide stronger evidence for a cause-and-effect relationship between hemispheric stroke and sleep apnea by selecting out hypertension. They concluded that sleep-associated breathing disorders might be a sequela of stroke. Nevertheless, there was a bias against finding OSA as a cause of stroke, as patients with previous obesity, snoring, and apnea were also selected out.

In 1996, a highly selective study polysomnographically analyzed only 19 of 47 stroke patients after overnight oximetry screens (34). Of the 19 individuals, 18 were diagnosed with OSA, with a mean apnea/hypopnea index of 36 events per hour. In the 16 patients with hemispheric strokes, 93% of all apneas were obstructive, while only 7% were central. In the 3 subjects with brainstem stroke, 42% of the apneas were central. The polysomnographic mean oxygen saturation low values could not be determined owing to the combination of data.

VI. Unselected, Prospective, Consecutively Studied Populations

In 1996, a total of 23 consecutively encountered patients with acute stroke were evaluated polysomnographically (35). The mean oxygen saturation low value was 82% and the mean apnea/hypopnea index was 32 events per hour. Seventy percent of the subjects were diagnosed with OSA. Nineteen control subjects, with histories of limited alcohol use, without known apnea or significant snoring, had a mean oxygen saturation low value of 89% and a mean apnea/hypopnea index of 6 events per hour.

In 1996, another prospective study compared polysomnograms of 27 healthy age- and gender-matched control individuals without stroke to 24 consecutively studied, nonselected inpatients with recent stroke (22). Information regarding many of the known risk factors for OSA [excessive daytime sleepiness (50), snoring (5), obesity (2,51), hypertension (52,53), and cardiac disease (54)] and stroke [smoking, diabetes mellitus, hypertension, and cardiac disease (3)] was gathered.

OSA was diagnosed in 19% of the controls, 71% of the stroke patients, 64% of the women with stroke (14% of female controls), and 77% of the men with stroke (23% of male controls). The mean lowest oxygen saturation was 91% in the control group and 85% in the stroke group. Overall, the mean apnea/hypopnea index was 4 events per hour for controls and 26 events per hour for stroke patients. For women, the mean apnea/hypopnea index was 3.0 events per hour for controls and 32 events per hour for stroke patients. For men, the mean apnea/hypopnea index for controls was 5 events per hour and for stroke patients was 22 events per hour. No patient had primarily central sleep apnea or Cheyne-Stokes respirations.

In females, the mean body-mass index was less in the controls (with or without apnea). In males, there was no significant difference in the mean body-mass index. In addition, in the stroke group, 15 individuals smoked and 7 had diabetes mellitus.

A total of 82% of women and 69% of men with stroke had previous systemic hypertension. Cardiac disease was reported in 55% and 31% of the respective females and males with stroke. Eighty percent (4 out of 5) nonhypertensive/noncardiac disease stroke patients had OSA, with a mean apnea/hypopnea index of 35.6 events per hour. No significant difference was found between the mean body-mass index of the nonhypertensive/noncardiac disease subgroup of stroke patients and the nonhypertensive/noncardiac disease subgroup of controls.

Fifty-four percent of the patients (13 of 24) suffered their strokes during sleep (12 ischemic and 1 hemorrhagic). A 4-year follow-up revealed that of the 5 patients with OSA, who had subsequently died, 4 had their strokes in sleep. These findings led to the speculation that the hypoxemia and previously documented autonomic responses (28,29,55–60) associated with obstructive apnea might produce acute and chronic changes predisposing to stroke. When cardiac disease and hypertension were selected out, OSA still had a relatively high prevalence in the stroke population. In these selected subgroups, there was no significant difference between the mean body-mass indices of the nonstroke subjects and those of stroke patients.

In 1997, polysomnography was performed on 39 (24 men and 15 women) noncomatose adult stroke patients (mean age 57 years) within a mean of 10 days from their first stroke (36). Twenty-one patients (54%; 14 men and 7 women) had OSA (7 with Cheyne-Stokes–like breathing patterns in sleep), while 4 individuals had Cheyne-Stokes breathing in sleep (without OSA). Obstructive apnea was more frequent in subjects with bulbar or pseudobulbar palsy. The overall apnea/hypopnea indices were categorized by stroke location and major sleep stage. For supratentorial strokes, the mean apnea/hypopnea indices in NREM and REM sleep, respectively, were 22.0 and 27.7 events per hour. For infratentorial strokes, the mean apnea/hypopnea indices for NREM and REM sleep, respectively, were 37.4 and 35.9 events per hour.

VII. Studies of Transient Ischemic Attack

People with transient ischemic attacks are at high risk for stroke. A 1987 study reported that a 64-year-old man (with recent embolic vertebrobasilar stroke) had recurrent transient left hemiparesis, ophthalmoplegia, and Babinski signs precipitated by sleep (26). All attacks captured polysomnographically were immediately preceded by obstructive apneas. In this case, it was hypothesized that apnea produced temporary hemodynamic instability, which precipitated transient nocturnal attacks as a result of ischemia to a previously injured brainstem.

In 1995, a 64-year-old woman without major stroke risk factors awoke with a motor aphasia that resolved within 3 hr (30). Her blood pressure was 154/82 mmHg; with the exception of aphasia, her examination was normal. A brain CT, magnetic resonance imaging (MRI) angiogram, and carotid and transcranial Doppler sonograms were unremarkable.

During overnight oximetry the patient was hypersomnolent and snored loudly. The study showed oxygen desaturations below 50%. Subsequently, overnight polysomnography revealed an apnea/hypopnea index of 83.4 events per hour. Obstructive apnea was successfully treated with nasal CPAP therapy. Subsequently, there were dramatic improvements in sleep quality and daytime alertness as well as a resolution of transient ischemic attacks. These findings suggested that, in some cases, treatment of transient ischemic attacks (stroke prevention) could be equated with treating apnea.

In 1996, a controlled, polysomnographic study of 13 consecutive subjects with transient ischemic attacks was performed (35). Obstructive sleep apnea was diagnosed in 16% of controls and in 69% of patients with transient ischemic attacks. Patients with transient ischemic attacks had a mean oxygen saturation low value of 79% and a mean apnea/hypopnea index of 19 events per hour. The high frequency of OSA in patients with transient ischemic attacks suggested that apnea may precipitate stroke.

VIII. Central Respiratory Abnormalities

Stroke can precipitate apnea (61). There is a well-established temporal relationship between abnormal respiration and damage high in brainstem (62–66) and cervical spinal cord centers (67–70) for automatic respiration. Furthermore, in stupor and coma from uncal or central transtentorial brain herniation, there is a classic progression from eupneic to Cheyne-Stokes to hyperventilation and ataxic respiratory patterns (71). Waking respiratory abnormalities can also occur with bilateral dysfunction of the cervical spinal cord, pons, diencephalon, or cerebrum (70–72).

Animal studies have identified two neuronal centers for automatic respiration in the medulla oblongata of the brainstem. These include a ventrolateral group (associated with the retroambiguus and ambiguus nuclei) and a dorsal group (associated with the solitary tract nucleus) (65,73,74). Associated neuronal tracts in the paramedian reticular formation of the brainstem tegmentum descend toward the ventrolateral portions of the high cervical spinal cord near the spino-thalamic tract (62,68,70,75).

Lesions in these areas, rostral to the upper portions of the cervical spinal cord and caudal to the fifth cranial nerve, can result in "Ondine's curse" (failure of automatic respiration) (76,77). In addition, there are areas rostral to the pons— in the mesencephalic and diencephalic nuclei and fronto-orbital, cingulate, insular, anterior temporal, and sensorimotor cortices—that are also associated with the control of respiration (78,79).

Central apneas and Cheyne-Stokes respirations have been associated with brainstem stroke. In 1976, a total of 23 patients with acute brainstem strokes were evaluated for respiratory abnormalities (80). All subjects with prominent Cheyne-Stokes respirations had bilateral pontine lesions; however, not all patients with large pontine infarctions had Cheyne-Stokes respirations. Sleeping Cheyne-Stokes respiratory patterns were only rarely found in 10 of the patients with normal waking respirations. Otherwise, no clear distinctions were made between respiratory abnormalities in the sleeping and waking states. Owing to technical limitations, obstructive sleep apnea could not be addressed.

Supratentorial and infratentorial lesions have been associated with Cheyne-Stokes respirations in waking and sleeping states (36,79). By Fourier transformed respiratory frequency analysis, 17 of 32 subjects (4 of 10 infratentorial and 13 of 22 supratentorial stroke patients) were found to have Cheyne-Stokes respiratory patterns during waking periods.

In 1993 a polysomnographic study of subjects with unilateral cerebral stroke (selected for periodic breathing in sleep) showed no difference when compared to controls in regard to respiratory periodicity (32). Nevertheless, stroke patients had more obstructive sleep apneic events and larger fluctuations in tidal volume and upper airway resistance.

It has been assumed that all respiratory abnormalities that follow injury to the brainstem medulla should be central in nature, as associated injury to the solitary nucleus can produce diaphragmatic dysfunction (24,76,81,82). Nevertheless, a report from 1982 suggested that obstructive sleep apnea can occur after brainstem stroke due to associated injury of the nucleus ambiguus (a location of upper motor neurons for the upper airways) (24,26,27).

In 1977, there was a case report of central sleep apnea with a unilateral medullary infarction (76). However, in this patient, obesity and cardiomegaly, respectively, could have predisposed to and resulted from chronic underlying OSA. As the patient had a tracheostomy, underlying obstructive apneas, if they existed, could not have been appreciated.

There are other studies where OSA was believed to be the result of unilateral medullary brainstem stroke (24,27). Nevertheless, preexisting signs and symptoms—such as progressive weight gain, nasal occlusion and septal deviation, a long uvula, underlying cardiac disease and hypertension, and loud snoring—occasionally suggest that apnea preceded stroke.

IX. Circadian Rhythms

Sleep and the early morning hours are associated with a relatively high frequency of ischemic stroke and myocardial infarction (22,83–89). If stroke had an equal probability of occurring anytime over a 24-hr period, a full 33% should occur during an 8-hr sleep period. In a study of 24 patients with recent stroke of whom 71% had OSA, a higher than expected percentage of individuals suffered stroke in sleep (54%; $p = 0.0304$) (22).

The most prolonged rapid-eye-movement (REM) sleep period occurs in temporal proximity to the circadian preference for ischemic stroke (the early morning hours). During REM sleep, healthy subjects without OSA have been shown to experience significant autonomic nervous system instability, with sympathetic activation (90) and blood pressures that reach normal waking levels (91). In addition, surges in blood pressure have been associated with muscle twitches that normally occur during active REM periods.

The early morning hours are associated with the highest levels of catecholamines, blood viscosity and platelet activity and aggregability, and the lowest fibrinolytic activity (92–94). It has been suggested that elevated catecholamine levels associated with obstructive sleep apnea (95) may increase thrombus formation—and the risk of stroke—in the otherwise normal morning hematological milieu (86).

During REM sleep, cerebral blood flow increases throughout the brain (96,97). An increase in intracranial pressure with reduced cerebral perfusion pressure has been reported to occur during obstructive apneas (48). This may predispose obstructive sleep apneics to ischemic stroke at a time when there normally is an increased demand of the brain for oxygen.

The oropharyngeal effects of the paresis that is normally associated with REM sleep may precipitate obstructive apnea (98). This phenomenon, along with the previously mentioned circadian, hematological, autonomic, and metabolic concomitants, may increase the risk of stroke during REM sleep.

X. Autonomic Studies

Excessive sympathetic and parasympathetic activation, with subsequent profound blood pressure fluctuations and cardiac arrhythmias, can occur as the result of obstructive sleep apneic events (see Figs. 2 and 3) (56,57,59,60,99,100). Microneurography allows direct measurement of efferent sympathetic nervous activity from postganglionic unmyelinated C fibers through the introduction of a tungsten

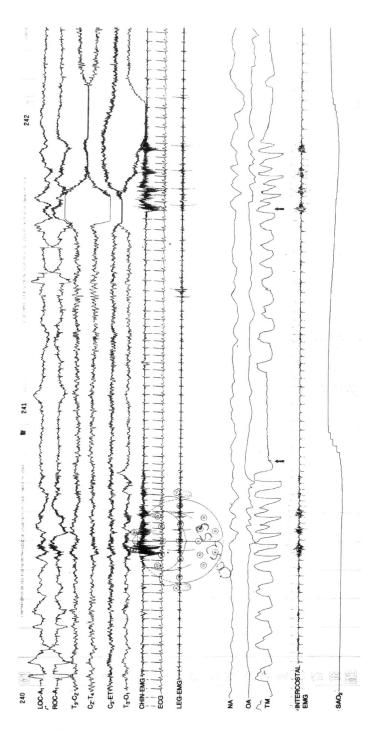

Figure 2 A polysomnographic tracing (paper speed 10 mm/sec) has been reduced to correspond to a temporally related microneurographic tracing (Fig. 3; paper speed 5 mm/sec). Arrows indicate a prolonged mixed apnea of approximately 26-sec duration occurring during REM sleep, associated with severe oxygen desaturation. LOC, left outer canthus; ROC, right outer canthus; T, temporal; C, central; ET, ears tied; O, occipital; EMG, electromyogram; ECG, electrocardiogram; N, nasal airflow; OA, oral airflow; TM, thoracic movement.

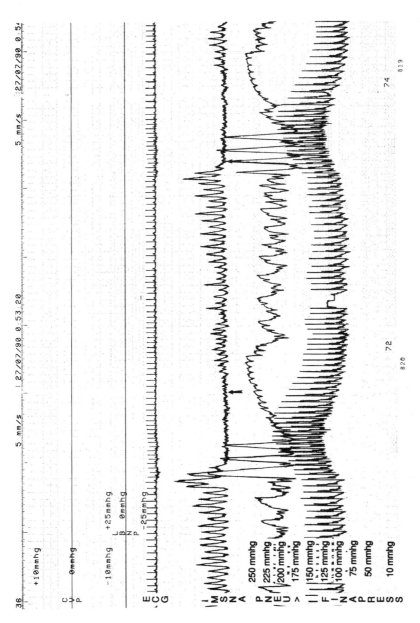

Figure 3 The arrows in this microneurographic tracing recorded from the peroneal nerve indicate a gradual elevation of efferent sympathetic nerve activity during a mixed apnea. The activity peak is immediately followed by cessation of the apnea, with a subsequent marked elevation of arterial blood pressure to 215/130 mmHg from a baseline of 135/80 mmHg. MSNA, muscle sympathetic nerve activity; Pneu, chest excursion; Finapress; fingertip blood pressure.

needle into the peroneal nerve (99). The reflex effects of the hypoxia, hypercap-nia, and decreased input from thoracic stretch receptors—which result from ob-structive apneas—are believed to cause this increase in sympathetic activity (55).

In 1992, microneurographic comparisons were made between patients with OSA and subjects with simulated apneas (59). A mildly hypertensive, 23-year-old nonapneic demonstrated elevated sympathetic and parasympathetic (bradycardia, sinus pause, and complete heart block) activity during voluntary end-expiratory apneas. Similar findings were found in a 43-year-old hypertensive apneic during nocturnal obstructive events. He experienced falls in blood pressure from approx-imately 180/100 mmHg (prior to apneas) to less than 50 mmHg during apneas. Sinus arrest, lasting up to 10 sec, was noted during some obstructions.

In 1993, nine volunteers were studied microneurographically during Mueller maneuvers (inspiring against a closed glottis; simulating obstructive sleep apnea) (60). During the initial 10 sec of the maneuver, there was a drop in sympathetic activity and mean blood pressure (from 95 to 81 mmHg). In the 5-sec interval preceding the release of the maneuver, there was a dramatic in-crease in sympathetic activity. Upon release of the maneuver, the mean blood pressure surged to 104 mmHg.

In 1995, ten patients with obstructive sleep apnea had simultaneous blood pressure, sympathetic nerve activity, and polysomnographic monitoring (100). In four of the subjects these evaluations were performed before and after continuous positive airway pressure therapy (CPAP) was introduced. The mean blood pres-sure increased from 92 mmHg in the waking state to 127 mmHg in REM sleep. The peak sympathetic activity, as measured over the last 10 sec of each apnea, increased by 246% during REM sleep. Decreases in blood pressure and sympa-thetic activity occurred with CPAP.

Autonomic studies indicate that during obstructive sleep apneic events, ele-vated sympathetic activity can lead to blood pressure instability. These marked blood pressure changes have been associated with a significant reduction in intra-cerebral perfusion (48,56,101,102). In addition, microneurographic studies show that persons with OSA have increased sympathetic tone even when awake (100). These findings suggest that OSA, through an autonomic mechanism, may induce acute and chronic changes that predispose to stroke.

XI. Morbidity and Mortality

There is evidence that undertreated OSA has negative health consequences and can contribute to stroke (103,104). In 1988, a total of 198 patients with OSA were treated with either tracheostomy (71 subjects) or weight loss (127 subjects). After 7 years, only 1 and 2% respectively in the tracheostomy group, suffered a new stroke or myocardial infarction, while 3% died (1% from a vascular etiology). In the weight-loss group 9 and 5% respectively experienced a new stroke or myocardial infarction, while 17.3% died (11% from a vascular etiology). These results (independent of obesity, age, and apnea/hypopnea index) suggest that undertreated OSA can lead to higher morbidity and mortality.

In 1996, a 4-year reassessment of 24 subjects (originally studied polysom-nographically after recent stroke) showed that all patients who died had OSA (22). Only one of these subjects used CPAP; her death was due to urosepsis. Retrospective analysis of the polysomnographic data revealed respective mean apnea/hypopnea indices of 22.1 events per hour and 41.3 events per hour, respectively, for patients found to be alive and dead, at follow-up. The findings suggest that the diagnosis and severity of OSA in stroke may be associated with greater mortality.

In 1996, the functional abilities were determined for 19 patients with recent stroke who had been selected for polysomnography (34). Outcome variables included ability to return home at discharge; continued residence at home at 3 and 12 months poststroke; the Barthel Index at discharge, 3 months, and 12 months; and death within 12 months. Obstructive sleep apnea was diagnosed in 95% of the subjects. Oximetry measurements correlated with return home after discharge. Patients with abnormal oximetry readings, histories of snoring, and hemispheric strokes tended to have the worst functional outcomes. The authors concluded that sleep-related respiratory disorders in individuals with stroke may independently predict worse functional outcome.

XII. Conclusions

Sleep apnea can result from cerebrovascular disease. Whether obstructive sleep apnea can lead to stroke is not clear. In a recent review of 54 epidemiological studies that examined the association between sleep apnea and health-related outcomes, most were found to be poorly designed, with only weak or contradictory evidence for an association between apnea and cardiovascular disease and stroke (105).

To date, there are no published, large, well-run, prospective, double-blind, controlled experiments where polysomnographic evaluations have been performed prior to and after stroke that compare treated and untreated obstructive sleep apneics. Logistic and ethical constraints may not permit such experiments. Nevertheless, the literature suggests that obstructive sleep apnea can contribute to stroke. Health care professionals should consider obstructive sleep apnea when treating stroke.

References

1. The American Heart Association Heart and Stroke Statistical Update. Dallas: AHA, 1998.

2. Young T, Palta M, Dempsey J, Skatrud J, Weber S, Safwan B. The occurrence of sleep-disordered breathing among middle-aged adults. N Engl J Med 1993; 328: 1230–1235.

3. Wolf PA, D'Agostino RB, Belanger AJ, Kannel WB. Probability of stroke: a risk profile from the Framingham study. Stroke 1991; 22:312–318.

4. Dyken ME, Somers V, Yamada T, Yeh M, Ren Z, Zimmerman MB. The effect hypertension, cardiac disease and stroke has on clinically suspected obstructive sleep apnea (abstr). Sleep Res 1995; 24:388.

5. Berry DTR, Webb WB, Block AJ, Switzer DA. Sleep-disordered breathing in a subclinical population. Sleep 1986; 9:478–483.

6. Bliwise DL, Feldman DE, Bliwise NG, Carskadon MA, Kraemer HC, North CS, Petta DE, Seidel WF, Dement WC. Risk factors for sleep disordered breathing in heterogeneous geriatric populations. Am Geriatr Soc 1987; 35:132–141.

7. Lugaresi E, Cirignotta F, Montagna P, Sforza E. Snoring: pathogenic, clinical, and therapeutic aspects. In: Kryger MH, Roth T, Dement WC, eds. Principles and Practice of Sleep Medicine, 2d ed. Philadelphia: Saunders, 1994:621–629.

8. Koskenvuo M, Kaprio J, Partinen M, Langinvainio H, Sarna Seppo, Heikkila K. Snoring as a risk for hypertension and angina pectoris. Lancet 1985; 1:893–895.

9. Gislason T, Aberg H, Taube A. Snoring and systemic hypertension—an epidemiological study. Acta Med Scand 1987; 222:415–421.

10. Lugaresi E, Cirignotta F, Coccagna G, Piana C. Some epidemiological data on snoring and cardiocirculatory disturbances. Sleep 1980; 3:221–224.

11. Norton PG, Dunn EV. Snoring as a risk factor for disease: an epidemiological survey. BMJ 1985; 291:630–632.

12. Mondini S, Zucconi M, Cirignotta F, Aguglia U, Lenzi PL, Zauli C, Lugaresi E. Snoring as a risk factor for cardiac and circulatory problems: an epidemiological study. In: Guilleminault C, Lugaresi E, eds. Sleep/Wake Disorders: Natural History, Epidemiology and Long-Term Evolution. New York: Raven Press, 1983:99–105.

13. Partinen M, Alihanka J, Lang H, Kalliomaki L. Myocardial infarction in relation to sleep apneas (abstr). Sleep Res 1983; 12:272.

14. D'Alessandro R, Magelli C, Gamberini G, Bacchelli S, Cristina E, Magnani B, Lugaresi E. Snoring every night as a risk factor for myocardial infarction: a case-control study. BMJ 1990; 300:1557–1558.

15. Erkinjuntti T, Partinen M, Sulkava R, Palomaki H, Tilvis R. Snoring and dementia. Age Ageing 1987; 16:305–310.

16. Koskenvuo M, Kaprio J, Telakivi T, Partinen M, Heikkila K, Sarna S. Snoring as a risk factor for ischaemic heart disease and stroke in men. BMJ 1987; 294:16–19.

17. Partinen M, Palomaki H. Snoring and cerebral infarction. Lancet 1985; 2:1325–1326.

18. Palomake H, Partinen M, Juvela S, Kaste M. Snoring as a risk factor for sleep-related brain infarction. Stroke 1989; 10:1311–1315.

19. Spriggs D, French JM, Murdy JM, Bates D, James OFW. Historical risk factors for stroke: a case control study. Age Ageing 1990; 19:280–287.

20. Palomake H. Snoring and the risk of ischemic brain infarction. Stroke 1991; 22: 1021–1025.

21. Palomaki H, Partinen M, Erkinjuntti T, Kaste M. Snoring, sleep apnea syndrome, and stroke. Neurology 1992; 42(suppl 16):75–81.

22. Dyken ME, Somers VK, Yamada T, Ren Z-Y, Zimmerman MB. Investigating the relationship between stroke and obstructive sleep apnea. Stroke 1996; 27:401–407.

23. Pendlebury ST, Pepin JL, Veale D, Levy P. Natural evolution of moderate sleep apnoea syndrome: significant progression over a mean of 17 months. Thorax 1997; 52:872–878.

24. Chaudhary BA, Elguindi AS, King DW. Obstructive sleep apnea after lateral medullary syndrome. South Med J 1982; 75:65–67.

25. Tikare SK, Chaudhary BA, Bandisode MS. Hypertension and stroke in a young man with obstructive sleep apnea syndrome. Postgrad Med 1985; 78:59–66.

26. Rivest J, Reiher J. Transient ischemic attacks triggered by symptomatic sleep apneas (abstr). Stroke 1987; 18:293.

27. Askenasy JJM, Goldhammer I. Sleep apnea as a feature of bulbar stroke. Stroke 1988; 19:637–639.

28. Dyken ME, Somers VK, Yamada T. Hemorrhagic stroke; part of the natural history of severe obstructive sleep apnea? (abstr) Sleep Res 1991; 20:371.

29. Dyken ME, Somers VK, Yamada T. Stroke, sleep apnea and autonomic instability. In: Togawa K, Katayama S, Hishikawa Y, Ohta Y, Horie T, eds. Sleep Apnea and Rhonchopathy. Basel: Karger, 1993:166–168.

30. Pressman MR, Schetman WR, Figueroa WG, Van Uitert B, Caplan HJ, Peterson DD. Transient ischemic attacks and minor stroke during sleep. Stroke 1995; 26: 2361–2365.

31. Kapen S, Park A, Goldberg J, Wynter J. The incidence and severity of obstructive sleep apnea in ischemic cerebrovascular disease (abstr). Neurology 1991; 41(suppl 1):125.

32. Hudgel DW, Devadatta P, Quadri M, Sioson ER, Hamilton H. Mechanism of sleep-induced periodic breathing in convalescing stroke patients and healthy elderly subjects. Chest 1993; 104:1503–1510.

33. Mohsenin V, Valor R. Sleep apnea in patients with hemispheric stroke. Arch Phys Med Rehabil 1995; 76:71–76.

34. Good DC, Henkle JQ, Gelber D, Welsh J, Verhulst S. Sleep-disordered breathing and poor functional outcome after stroke. Stroke 1996; 27:252–258.

35. Bassetti C, Aldrich MS, Chervin RD, Quint D. Sleep apnea in patients with transient ischemic attack and stroke: a prospective study of 59 patients. Neurology 1996; 47:1167–1173.

36. Bassetti C, Aldrich MS, Quint D. Sleep-disordered breathing in patients with acute supra- and infratentorial strokes: a prospective study of 39 patients. Stroke 1997; 28:1765–1772.

37. Rechtschaffen A, Kales A, eds. A manual of standardized terminology, techniques and scoring system for sleep stages of human subjects. Natl Inst Health 1968; 204: 1–13.

38. Thorpy MJ and the Diagnostic Classification Steering Committee. The International Classification of Sleep Disorders: Diagnostic and Coding Manual. Rochester, MN: American Sleep Disorders Association, 1990:52–58.

39. He J, Kryger MH, Zorich FJ, Conway W, Roth T. Mortality and apnea index in obstructive sleep apnea: experience in 385 male patients. Chest 1988; 94:9–14.

40. Guilleminault C, Connolly SJ, Winkle RA. Cardiac arrhythmia and conduction disturbances during sleep in 400 patients with sleep apnea syndrome. Am J Cardiol 1983; 52:490–494.

41. Shepard JW, Garrison MW, Grither DA, Dolan GF. Relationship of ventricular ectopy to oxyhemoglobin desaturation in patients with obstructive sleep apnea. Chest 1988; 88:335–340.

42. Zwillich C, Devlin T, White D, Douglas N, Weil J, Martin R. Bradycardia during sleep apnea: characteristics and mechanism. J Clin Invest 1982; 69:1286–1292.

43. Tilkian AG, Guilleminault C, Schroeder JS, Lehrman KL, Simmons FB, Dement WC. Hemodynamics in sleep-induced apnea: studies during wakefulness and sleep. Ann Intern Med 1976; 85:714–719.

44. Coccagna G, Mantovani M, Brignani F, Parchi C, Lugaresi E. Continuous recording of the pulmonary and systemic arterial pressure during sleep in syndromes of hypersomnia with periodic breathing. Bull Physiol Pathol 1972; 8:1159–1172.

45. Lugaresi E, Coccagna G, Mantovani M, Brignani F. Effects of tracheostomy in two cases of hypersomnia with periodic breathing. J Neurosurg Psychiatry 1973; 36:15–26.

46. Personal communication with Dr. Kapen (5/97).

47. Sugita Y, Iijima S, Teshima T, Shimizu N, Nishimura T, Tsutsomi H, Hayashi H, Kaneda H, Hishikawa Y. Marked episodic elevation of cerebrospinal fluid pressure during nocturnal sleep in patients with sleep apnea hypersomnia syndrome. Electroencephalogr Clin Neurophysiol 1985; 60:214–219.

48. Jennum P, Borgesen SE. Intracranial pressure and obstructive sleep apnea. Chest 1989; 95:279–283.

49. Daly JA, Giombetti R, Miller B, Garrett K. Impaired awake cerebral perfusion in sleep apnea. Am Rev Respir Dis 1990; 141(4):A376.

50. Guilleminault C. Clinical features and evaluation of obstructive sleep apnea. In: Kryger MH, Roth T, Dement WC, eds. Principles and Practice of Sleep Medicine, 2d ed. Philadelphia: Saunders, 1994:667–677.

51. Stradling JR, Crosby JH. Predictors and prevalence of obstructive sleep apnoea and snoring in 1001 middle aged men. Thorax 1991; 46:85–90.

52. Kales A, Bixler EO, Cadieux RJ, Shaw LC, Vela-Bueno A, Bixler EO, Schneck DW, Locke TW, Soldatos CR. Sleep apnea in a hypertensive population. Lancet 1984; 2:1005–1008.

53. Fletcher EC, DeBehnke RD, Lavoi MS, Gorin AB. Undiagnosed sleep apnea in patients with essential hypertension. Ann Intern Med 1985; 103:190–194.

54. Hung J, Whitford EG, Parsons RW, Hillman DR. Association of sleep apnoea with myocardial infarction in men. Lancet 1990; 336:261–264.

55. Somer VK, Mark AL, Abboud FM. Sympathetic activation by hypoxia and hypercapnia: implications for sleep apnea. Clin Exp Hypertens 1988; A10(suppl 1):413–422.

56. Hedner J, Ejnell H, Sellgren J, Hedner T, Wallin G. Is high and fluctuating muscle nerve sympathetic activity in sleep apnoea syndrome of pathogenetic importance for the development of hypertension? J Hypertens 1988; (6 suppl 4):529–531.

57. Somers VK, Dyken ME, Mark AL, Abboud FM. Autonomic and hemodynamic responses during sleep in normal and sleep apneic humans (abstr). Clin Res 1991; 39:735.

58. Dyken ME, Somers VK, Yamada T, Adams HP, Zimmerman MB. Investigating the relationship between sleep apnea and stroke (abstr). Sleep Res 1992; 21:30.

59. Somers VK, Dyken ME, Mark AL, Abboud FM. Parasympathetic hyperresponsiveness and bradyarrhythmias during apnea in hypertension. Clin Auton Res 1992; 2: 171–176.

60. Somers VK, Dyken ME, Skinner JL. Autonomic and hemodynamic responses and interactions during the Mueller maneuver in humans. J Auton Nerv Syst 1993; 44: 253–259.

61. Simon RP. Respiration. In: Asbury AK, McKhann GM, McDonald WI, eds. Diseases of the Nervous System: Clinical Neurobiology. Vol I. Philadelphia: Saunders, 1986: 651–664.

62. Adelman S, Dinner DS, Goren H, Little J, Nickerson P. Obstructive sleep apnea in association with posterior fossa neurologic disease. Arch Neurol 1984; 41:509–510.

63. Haponik EF, Givens D, Angelo J. Syringobulbia-myelia with obstructive sleep apnea. Neurology 1983: 33:1046–1049.

64. Chokroverty S, Sachdeo R, Masdeu J. Autonomic dysfunction and sleep apnea in olivopontocerebellar degeneration. Arch Neurol 1984; 41:926–931.

65. Beal MF, Richardson EP, Brandstetter R, Hedley-Whyte ET, Hochberg FH. Localized brainstem ischemic damage and Ondine's curse after near-drowning. Neurology 1983; 33:717–721.

66. Boor JW, Johnson RJ, Canales L, Dunn DP. Reversible paralysis of automatic respiration in multiple sclerosis. Arch Neurol 1977; 34:686–689.

67. Belmusto L, Brown E, Owens G. Clinical observations on respiratory and vasomotor disturbances as related to cervical cordotomies. J Neurosurg 1963; 20:224–232.

68. Mullan S, Hosobuchi Y. Respiratory hazards of high cervical cord percutaneous cordotomy. J Neurosurg 1968; 28:291–297.

69. Tenicela R, Rosomoff HL, Feist J, Safar P. Pulmonary function following percutaneous cordotomy. Anesthesiology 1968; 29:7–16.

70. Krieger AJ, Rosomoff HL. Sleep-induced apnea: A respiratory and autonomic dysfunction syndrome following bilateral percutaneous cervical cordotomy. J Neurosurg 1974; 39:168–180.

71. Plum F, Posner JB. The Diagnosis of Stupor and Coma, 3d ed. Philadelphia: Davis, 1980.

72. Lee MC, Klassen AC, Resch JA. Respiratory pattern disturbances in ischemic cerebral vascular disease. Stroke 1974; 5:612–616.

73. Merrill EG. The lateral respiratory neurones of the medulla: their associations with nucleus ambiguus, nucleus retroambigualis, the spinal accessory nucleus and the spinal cord. Brain Res 1970; 24:11–28.

74. Berger AJ, Mitchell RA, Severinghaus JW. Regulation of respiration. N Engl J Med 1977; 297:92–97, 138–142, 194–201.

75. Pitts R. The respiratory center and its descending pathways. J Comp Neurol 1940; 72:605–625.

76. Levin BE, Margolis G. Acute failure of automatic respirations secondary to a unilateral brainstem infarct. Ann Neurol 1977; 1:583–586.
77. Severinghaus JW, Mitchell RA: Ondine's curse-failure of respiratory center automaticity while awake(abstr). Clin Res 1962; 10:122.
78. Hugelin A. Forebrain and midbrain influence on respiration. In: Fishman AP, Cheniak NS, Widdicombe JG, Geige SR, eds. Handbook of Physiology. Sec. 3: The Respiratory System. Vol. II. Control of Breathing: Part 1. Bethesda, MD: American Physiological Society 1986:69–91.
79. Nachtmann A, Siebler M, Rose G, Sitzer M, Steinmetz H. Cheyne-Stokes respiration in ischemic stroke. Neurology 1995; 45:820–821.
80. Lee MC, Klassen AC, Heaney LM, Resch JA. Respiratory rate and pattern disturbances in acute brain stem infarction. Stroke 1976; 7:382–385.
81. Devereaux MW, Keane JR, Davis RL. Automatic respiratory failure associated with infarction of the medulla: report of two cases with pathologic study of one. Arch Neurol 1973; 29:46–52.
82. Guilleminault C, Dement W, eds. Sleep Apnea Syndromes. New York: Liss 1978: 11.
83. Muller JE, Stone BH, Turi ZG, Rutherford JD, Czeiler CA, Parker C, Poole K, Passamani E, Roberts R, Robertson T, Sobel BE, Willerson JT, Braunwald E, MILIS Study Group. Circadian variation in the frequency of onset of acute myocardial infarction. N Engl J Med 1985; 313:1315–1322.
84. Muller JE, Ludmer PL, Willich SN, Tofler GH, Aylmer G, Klangos I, Stone PH. Circadian variation in the frequency of sudden cardiac death. Circulation 1987; 75: 131–138.
85. Muller JE, Tofler GH, Stone PH. Circadian variation and triggers of onset of acute cardiovascular disease. Circulation 1989; 79:733–743.
86. Marsh E, Biller J, Adams H, Marler JR, Hulbert JR, Love BB, Gordon DL. Circadian variation in onset of acute ischemic stroke. Arch Neurol 1990; 47:1178–1180.
87. Marshall J. Diurnal variation in occurrence of strokes. Stroke 1977; 8:230–231.
88. Tsementzis SA, Gill JS, Hitchcock ER, Gill SK, Beevers DG. Diurnal variation of and activity during the onset of stroke. Neurosurgery 1985; 17:901–904.
89. Marler JR, Price TR, Clark GL, Muller JE, Robertson T, Mohr JP, Hier DB, Wolf PA, Caplan LR, Foulkes MA. Morning increase in onset of ischemic stroke. Stroke 1989; 20:473–476.
90. Hornyak M, Cejnar M, Elam M, Matousek M, Wallin G. Sympathetic muscle nerve activity during sleep in man. Brain 1991; 114:1281–1295.
91. Somers VK, Dyken ME, Mark AL, Abboud FM. Sympathetic nerve activity during sleep in normal humans. N Engl J Med 1993; 328:303–307.
92. Andreotti F, Davies GJ, Hackett DR, Khan MI, De Bart ACW, Aber VR, Maseri A, Kluft C. Major circadian fluctuations in fibrinolytic factors and possible relevance to time of onset of myocardial infarction, sudden cardiac death and stroke. Am J Cardiol 1988; 62:635–637.
93. Tofler GH, Brezinski D, Schafer AI, Czeisler CA, Rutherford JD, Willich SN, Gleason RE, Williams GH, Muller JE. Concurrent morning increase in platelet aggregability and the risk of myocardial infarction and sudden cardiac death. N Engl J Med 1987; 316:1514–1518.

94. Musumeci V, Rosa S, Caruso A, Zuppi C, Zappacosta B, Tutinelli F. Abnormal diurnal changes in in vivo platelet activation in patients with atherosclerotic diseases. Atherosclerosis 1986; 60:231–236.

95. Fletcher EC, Miller J, Schaaf JW, Fletcher JG. Urinary catecholamines before and after tracheostomy in patients with obstructive sleep apnea and hypertension. Sleep 1987; 10:35–44.

96. Greenberg JH. Sleep and the cerebral circulation. In: Orem J, Barnes CD, eds. Physiology in Sleep. New York: Academic Press, 1980:57–95.

97. Klingelhofer J, Hajak G, Sander D, Schulz-Varszegi M, Ruther E, Conrad B. Assessment of intracranial hemodynamics in sleep apnea syndrome. Stroke 1992; 23:1427–1433.

98. Issa FG, Sullivan CE. Upper airway closing pressures in obstructive sleep apnea. J Appl Physiol 1984; 57:520–527.

99. Valbo AB, Hagbarth KE, Torebjork HE, Wallin BG. Somatosensory, proprioceptive, and sympathetic activity in human peripheral nerves. Physiol Rev 1979; 59:919–957.

100. Somers VK, Dyken ME, Clary MP, Abboud FM. Sympathetic neural mechanisms in obstructive sleep apnea. J Clin Invest 1995; 96:1897–1904.

101. Podszus T, Kohler U, Mayer J, Penzel T, Peter JH, Von Wichert P. Systemic arterial pressure decreases during obstructive sleep apnea (abstr). Sleep Res 1986; 15:155.

102. McGinty D, Beahm E, Stern N, Littner M, Sowers J, Reige W. Nocturnal hypotension in older men with sleep-related breathing disorders. Chest 1988; 94:305–311.

103. Partinen M, Jamieson A, Guilleminault C. Long-term outcome for obstructive sleep apnea syndrome patients: mortality. Chest 1988; 94:1200–1204.

104. Partinen M, Guilleminault C. Daytime sleepiness and vascular morbidity at seven-year follow-up in obstructive sleep apnea patients. Chest 1990; 97:27–32.

105. Wright J, Johns R, Watt I, Melville A, Sheldon T. Health effects of obstructive sleep apnoea and the effectiveness of continuous positive airways pressure: a systematic review of the research evidence. Br Med J 1997; 314:851–860.

14

Circadian Variation in the Incidence of Cardiovascular and Cerebrovascular Ischemic Events

CRAIG A. CHASEN and JAMES E. MULLER*

University of Kentucky Medical Center
Lexington, Kentucky

I. Cardiovascular Disease

A. Introduction

Despite recent advances in therapy, cardiovascular disease continues to be our nation's number one health problem. Each year, approximately 1.5 million acute myocardial infarctions and 500,000 cardiac deaths occur in the United States alone. Randomized, controlled, clinical trials regarding acute myocardial infarction (MI) and its treatment, have generated knowledge that may contribute to prevention. Data provided by these trials suggest that acute cardiac events occur in a nonrandom fashion. Circadian and seasonal variations in the incidence of onset of acute MI, myocardial ischemia, sudden cardiac death, and ventricular arrhythmias suggest that activities and the environment may trigger these disorders.

In 1910 Obraztsov and Strazhesko (1) wrote that activities such as climbing stairs, unpleasant conversation, and emotional distress during a game of cards could trigger a myocardial infarction. From the 1930's to the early 1980's, the prevailing belief was that activities are of little importance in causing disease onset. Objective evidence accumulated over the past decade reinforces the importance of triggering of acute coronary syndromes.

---

* *Current affiliation*: Massachusetts General Hospital, Boston, Massachusetts.

B. Myocardial Infarction

It is now well established that onset of myocardial infarction has a distinct daily pattern with a peak incidence in the hours after awakening and arising (2). The Multicenter Investigation of Limitation of Infarct Size (MILIS) (3) and the Intravenous Streptokinase in Acute Myocardial Infarction Study (ISAM) (4) (Figure 1) utilized serial creatine kinase measurements to document a morning increase in the time of onset of MI. In 849 patients with confirmed MI in the MILIS (3) trial, a marked variation in time of onset of infarction was noted by Muller et al (1985). A maximum of 45 infarcts occurred between 9AM and 10AM, and a minimum of 15 occurred between 11PM and midnight. In the ISAM (4) study, myocardial infarction occurred 3.8 times more frequently between 8 AM and 9 AM (hour of maximum incidence) than between 12:00 midnight and 1:00 AM (hour of minimum incidence). The morning was found to be a risk period both for patients with mild as well as severe coronary artery disease. Goldberg et al (5) noted that approximately 23% of patients reported onset of initial symptoms of MI within one hour after awakening. Willich et al (6) supported this finding with the observation that the increased incidence of MI occurs within the first 3 to 4 hours after awakening and onset of activity. Subsequently, in the Thrombolysis in Myocardial Infarction (7) (TIMI II) Trial, 34.4% of episodes of MI occurred between 6AM and noon vs. 15.4% between midnight and 6AM. Recently, Cannon and asso-

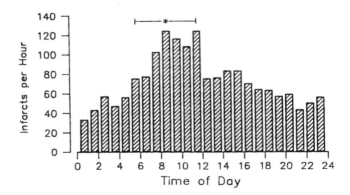

Figure 1 Bar graph of incidence of myocardial infarction of 1741 patients of the ISAM (Intravenous Streptokinase in Acute Myocardial Infarction) study. There is a marked circadian variation ($p < 0.001$) with a peak during the morning hours. Myocardial infarction occurred 1.8 times more frequently between 6:00 and 12:00 A.M. compared with the average of other quarters of day. The risk of myocardial infarction in the afternoon and evening was approximately equally distributed, whereas during the night, a trough period occurred in the incidence of myocardial infarction. (From Ref. 4.)

ciates (8) documented a morning increase in the onset of unstable angina and non-Q-wave MI in patients enrolled in the Thrombolysis in Myocardial Ischemia (TIMI) III Registry and Trial.

Hjalmarson et al (9) reviewed a total of 4800 cases of acute myocardial infarction and noted that the morning increase was blunted or abolished in subgroups of patients with advanced age, cigarette use, diabetes mellitus and previous infarction. Ridker et al (10) noted that physicians treated with aspirin experienced a selective 59% reduction in MI during the morning hours. In the ISAM (4) trial the group of patients receiving beta-adrenergic blocking therapy before the event did not show an increased morning incidence of myocardial infarction.

Hjalmarson et al (9) and others (11,12) have suggested that in the evening hours (between 6 PM and 12 MN), a second but lower peak of onset of myocardial infarction is present. This may relate to the evening meal or other triggers concentrated in those hours.

C. Sudden Cardiac Death

Most studies of the timing of onset of sudden cardiac death have revealed a prominent midmorning peak, thought to be related to a surge in catecholamines associated with arising and assuming the upright posture, that is blunted or eliminated by the administration of beta blockers. Data from the Framingham Heart Study (13) revealed a significant circadian variation in the occurrence of sudden cardiac death, with a peak incidence from 7 to 9 AM and a decreased incidence from 9 AM to 1 PM. The risk of sudden cardiac death was at least 70% higher during the peak period than was the average risk during the other times of the day. In another study, death certificates of 2203 individuals dying out of the hospital in Massachusetts in 1983 were reviewed and revealed a prominent circadian variation of sudden cardiac death with a low incidence during the night and an increased incidence from 7 to 11 AM (14). Levine and coworkers (15) identified a morning peak of sudden cardiac death in out-of-hospital cardiac arrests in the City of Houston Emergency Medical Services. The multicenter trial Veterans Affairs Congestive Heart Failure–Survival Trial of Antiarrhythmic Therapy (CHF-STAT) documented a morning increase of sudden cardiac death in patients with CHF (16). The Cardiac Arrhythmia Suppression Trial (CAST) revealed that patients randomized to flecainide, encainide and moricizine experienced a significant increase in the morning peak of sudden cardiac death, as compared to placebo (17).

Out of hospital sudden cardiac death in the Beta-blocker Heart Attack Trial also demonstrated a marked morning increase in the placebo group. However, patients randomized to beta blocker therapy received a major protective effect during morning hours (18). One reason for this benefit may be that beta blockers blunt the morning peak of ventricular tachyarrhythmias (19). A recent analysis of the Danish Verapamil Infarction Trials (DAVIT I and II) suggest that verapamil is associated with a preferential reduction in morning sudden cardiac deaths (20). The study of the patterns of sudden cardiac death may yield important clues to the pathophysiology of the disease process (21).

D. Arrhythmias/Implantable Defibrillators

Malignant tachyarrhythmias are the most common cause of sudden cardiac death. Canada et al (22) noted that ventricular ectopy reveals a prominent peak during the daytime hours and a trough at night. Twidale et al (23) observed that the peak incidence of sustained symptomatic ventricular tachycardia in 68 patients occurred between 10AM and noon. Arntz et al (24) identified a primary peak of frequency of ventricular fibrillation between 6AM and noon.

Tofler et al (25) in an analysis of 483 patients who had an implantable cardioverter-defibrillator (ICD) implanted between 1990 and 1993, showed that almost 22% of the ventricular tachyarrhythmias occurred between the hours of 9AM and noon. Venditti et al (26) analyzed defibrillation thresholds (DFTs) at different times of day in 134 patients with an ICD. The morning DFT (8 AM to noon) was fifteen joules versus thirteen joules in the mid (noon to 4 PM) and late (4 PM to 8 PM) afternoon, (*p <.02). In a separate group of 930 patients implanted with an ICD system with date and time stamps for each therapy, Venditti and colleagues reviewed 1,238 episodes of ventricular tachyarrhythmias treated with shock therapy. There was a significant peak in failed first shocks in the morning compared with other time intervals, supporting the concept that greater amounts of energy are required for termination of morning tachyarrhythmias. These findings may have important implications for appropriate ICD function.

Not all arrhythmias demonstrate a morning increase. Yamashita and associates (27) studied 150 patients with paroxysmal atrial fibrillation in a drug-free state identified from among 25,500 consecutive Holter recordings. Analysis of the onset, maintenance, and termination of this arrhythmia as hourly data and probabilities revealed the following results: onset of arrhythmia had no circadian variation, maintenance of arrhythmia showed a trough and termination of arrhythmia peaked at 11 AM. Parasympathetic as well as sympathetic activity may be of importance in occurrence of atrial fibrillation.

E. Transient Myocardial Ischemia

Nademanee et al (28) studied 68 patients with chronic stable angina and 9 patients with Prinzmetal angina for circadian periodicity. Among the patients with chronic stable angina, both silent and painful episodes had a peak occurrence in the morning and early afternoon hours (8 AM and 3 PM); the fewest episodes occurred between 1 AM and 5 AM. In the case of Prinzmetal's angina, no clear periodicity in the distribution of the ischemic episodes was noted. Rocco et al (29) recruited

32 patients with chronic stable symptoms of coronary artery disease to undergo one or more days of ambulatory monitoring during routine activities. A significant circadian variation in ischemic ST segment depression was noted and 39% of episodes and 46% of total ischemic time occurred between 6 AM and 12 PM. The peak increase in ischemia occurred within the first 2 hours after rising.

Parker and colleagues (30) enrolled 20 patients with stable CAD to assess the role of activity in causing the morning increase of myocardial ischemia. The ability of nadolol to block the morning peak was also studied. Ambulatory ECG monitoring was performed during regular activity and delayed activity days. The investigators noted that the morning increase in ambulatory ischemic episodes was due to physical activity patterns. The majority of ischemic episodes were found to be preceded by a heart rate increase of 5 beats per minute or more and it was those episodes that were primarily responsible for the morning increase in ischemia. Delaying the time of arising and onset of morning activity deferred the time of peak ischemia. Therapy with nadolol caused a 50% reduction in the total number of ischemic episodes and the elimination of the circadian peak in ischemic episodes. Unfortunately, nadolol caused a significant increase in ST segment depression not associated with a heart rate increase. The clinical significance of this finding is not known. Not all cardiac agents are efficacious in treating this disorder. Short-acting calcium channel blockade has been shown to have no appreciable affect on the morning increase in silent ischemia (31).

F. Other Cardiovascular Disorders

Gallerani and associates (32) reported on 70 cases of spontaneous acute dissection of the thoracic aorta that were treated at St. Anna Hospital of Ferrara, Italy from January 1985 to December 1994. The authors demonstrated that spontaneous acute thoracic rupture occurs with a circadian pattern, with a peak of onset in the morning hours (~10 AM) and a secondary peak in the evening (~8 PM). A circadian distribution with a morning peak has also been noted for fatal pulmonary thromboembolism (33).

G. Mechanisms of Action

A variety of mechanisms (arterial blood pressure surge (34), increase in coronary tone (35) and shear stress (36), and hemostatic factors) alone or in combination could account for the morning augmentation in cardiovascular disease onset. A growing body of evidence supports a role for hemostatic factors in triggering cardiovascular events. Ehrly and Jung (37) noted a morning increase in blood viscosity. Higher levels of fibrinogen and factor VII activity have been documented in patients with CAD (38). Factor VII activity and plasminogen activator inhibitor-1 (PAI-1) levels follow a circadian pattern that favors morning hypercoagulability and hypofibrinolysis (39). Decousus et al (40) identified a circadian variation in the efficacy of a constant intravenous infusion of heparin by noting a nadir in activated PTT levels in the morning hours. Kurnik (41) noted that efficacy of thrombolytic therapy is reduced in the morning hours.

Tofler and associates (42) measured platelet activity at 3-hour intervals for 24 hours in 15 healthy men. The period from 6 to 9 AM was the only interval in the 24-hour period during which platelet aggregability increased significantly. The morning increase in platelet aggregability was not observed when the subjects remained supine and inactive. Subsequently, Brezinski et al (43) demonstrated that in vitro platelet responsiveness to adenosine diphosphate and epinephrine increased only after assumption of the upright posture. During that same interval, plasma levels of epinephrine and norepinephrine increased significantly. Epinephrine-stimulated release of platelets from the spleen into the circulation may also be a contributor to the increased platelet activity.

Recently, Murakami et al (44) noted an association between coronary artery endothelial dysfunction and a circadian increase in coronary sinus serotonin levels. Since serotonin is contained inside dense granules of platelets, the early morning increase in coronary sinus plasma serotonin suggests that secretion by platelets in the cardiac circulation increased during that time period.

H. Cardiovascular Triggers

The primary significance of the recognition of circadian variation of MI onset is the evidence it provides supporting the concept that activities of the patient can trigger the onset of MI at any time of the day. The Myocardial Infarction Onset Study, supported by the NHLBI, has identified four triggers of onset of infarction: start of activity in the morning, anger, heavy physical exertion and sexual activity (45–47). Together these triggers account for approximately 16% of all infarctions or more than 250,000 events annually in the United States. The evidence supporting these triggers is given below.

Anger

A study of anger as a trigger was conducted in 1623 patients from the Determinants of Myocardial Infarction Onset Study who were interviewed an average of four days after myocardial infarction. Anger was assessed by the onset anger scale (a single-item, seven-level, self-report scale) and the state anger subscale of the State-Trait Personality Inventory. The onset anger scale identified 2.4% (39 patients) with episodes of anger in the two hours before the onset of myocardial infarction. Using a newly developed case-crossover study design (48) the relative risk of MI in the two hours after an episode of anger was 2.3. The state anger subscale corroborated these findings with a relative risk of 1.9. Regular users of aspirin had a significantly lower relative risk that anger would trigger MI (relative risk = 1.4) than nonusers. (47) Reich et al (49) noted that anger was the probable trigger for 15% of the life-threatening arrhythmias identified in 117 patients.

Heavy Exertion

Exercise can both prevent and cause acute myocardial infarction and sudden cardiac death. A sedentary lifestyle has been identified as a risk factor of equal importance to hypertension, hypercholesterolemia, or cigarette smoking (50).

In the TIMI-2 trial, moderate or marked physical activity was reported to occur at onset of MI in 18.7% of patients (7). Almost half (48%) of the 849 patients from the Multicenter Investigation of Limitation of Infarct Size (MILIS) indicated exposure to one or more possible triggers including moderate physical activity (14%) and heavy physical activity (9%) (51). In the Determinants of Onset of Myocardial Infarction Study, 4.4% of subjects reported heavy exertion within an hour of onset of myocardial infarction. Heavy exertion was classified as 6 METS or more, and was regarded as at least vigorous with panting and sweating. The range of activities included jogging, speed walking, shoveling snow, heavy gardening, and overhead work. The overall relative risk of MI in the hour after heavy physical exertion was 5.9. However, increasing levels of habitual physical activity were associated with progressively lower relative risks. Sedentary individuals (those exercising less than once per week) experienced a relative risk of 107 for myocardial infarction onset to occur within one hour after heavy physical exertion. Among people who usually exercised one to two, three to four, or five or more times per week, the respective relative risks were 19.4, 8.6 and 2.4 (45).

Heavy physical exertion is also associated with sudden cardiac death. Vuori (52) reported that the risk of SCD during cross-country skiing was 4.5 fold higher than the risk during sedentary activities. Siscovick and colleagues (53) have demonstrated that sudden cardiac death in men is more likely to occur following heavy physical exertion than during sedentary behavior. However, among habitually vigorous men, the overall risk of cardiac arrest—i.e., during and not during vigorous activity—was only 40% that of the sedentary men. Although the risk of primary cardiac arrest is transiently increased during vigorous exercise, habitual vigorous exercise is associated with an overall decreased risk of primary cardiac arrest.

Sexual Activity

Although sexual activity is associated with an average energy expenditure of 3–4 METS, a lower level than that associated with triggering the onset of myocardial infarction, data from the Myocardial Infarction Onset Study indicates that sexual activity may trigger infarction. Nine percent of patients reported sexual activity within 24 hours of MI and three percent engaged in sexual relations within 2 hours of symptom onset. Case-crossover analysis yielded a relative risk of 2.5 (95% CI 1.7–3.7) for infarction within two hours after sexual activity (46). Although baseline risk is increased, there was no increased relative risk for patients with prior cardiac disease—a finding that should be used to reassure patients during cardiac rehabilitation.

Physical exertion may trigger infarction in several ways. First, hemodynamic stress may trigger the disruption of a vulnerable atherosclerotic plaque. Second, in the presence of endothelial dysfunction, vasoconstriction rather than dilatation may occur with physical as well as emotional stress. Narrowing of stenotic segments may lead to increased shear forces and platelet deposition. Third, in patients with CAD, exercise may induce a prothrombotic state characterized by platelet activation and a reduced fibrinolytic response and reduced prostacyclin release (54). It is not known if physical exertion leads directly to plaque rupture, or whether the exertion merely adds a thrombotic or vasoconstrictive element to the causal pathway.

Recommendations for Patients

While certain external stressors have been identified as triggers of onset of MI, the absolute risk of infarction with each trigger is low, because baseline risk is low. For example, the risk of MI may double in the two hours after sexual activity, but since the baseline risk of MI for a healthy 50 year-old male in any given hour is 1/1,000,000, the absolute risk increases only to 2/1,000,000. Similarly, the baseline risk of sudden cardiac death (SCD) in people engaging in vigorous exercise is 10 times higher in cardiac patients than in apparently healthy people. Since the baseline risk is very low in the healthy individual, the absolute risk of SCD is also low (1:60,000 vs. 1:565,000 person-hours) (55). Physical activity favorably influences several risk factors including total cholesterol, HDL cholesterol, and triglycerides. In addition, physical activity is associated with reduced blood pressure, improved glucose tolerance, increased insulin sensitivity and reduced blood coagulability (56).

The finding that more infarcts occur in the morning raises questions about the desirability of exercise in the morning; however, Murray and colleagues (57) found no difference in risk between individuals who attended cardiac rehabilitation programs in the morning and those who attended in the afternoon.

Other Considerations

Seasonal and Weekly Variations of Acute MI

The seasonal distribution of acute myocardial infarction in the second national registry of myocardial infarction (NRMI-2) was examined by Spencer et al (58) (Figure 2). Participating hospitals reported 259,891 cases of acute MI to the

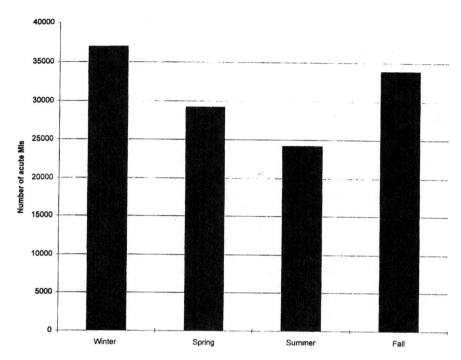

Figure 2 Cases of acute myocardial infarction reported each season to the NRMI-2. Counts were normalized to a 90-day season length. (From Ref. 58.)

NRMI-2 during the 25-month period beginning June 1994. There were 53% more cases of AMI noted during the winter months than in summer, with a peak incidence in January. A marked nadir in July was also appreciated. Nine of 10 distinct geographic areas in the U.S. followed this pattern. Colder weather has been shown to alter hemodynamic (BP, sympathetic tone) and hematologic (platelet count, fibrinogen) factors favoring arterial thrombosis (59–62).

A seasonal variation in cardiac mortality with an increased incidence during the winter months has been noted by several investigators (63–66).

Many authors have reported a hebdomadal (weekly) variation of MI with a peak incidence on Monday (67–71). The transition to work from the weekend may be responsible for this increase.

Mental Stress

Mental stress is considered by some to be a risk factor for the development of CAD (72) and a trigger for the onset of acute cardiovascular events. Within the first week of missile attacks on Israel during the 1991 Iraqi war, 20 people developed an acute myocardial infarction at one hospital compared to eight MIs during a control period (73). Frasure-Smith et al (74) found that MI survivors with high levels of psychological stress had three times the cardiac mortality of post-MI patients with low levels of stress. In patients with long QT syndrome, mental stress can precipitate ventricular arrhythmia and sudden death (75). Barry et al (76) noted that transient ischemia was more likely to occur as the intensity level of mental activity increased.

Frimerman and colleagues (77) examined 27 healthy accountants in Tel Aviv, Israel and demonstrated that long-term mental stress caused by increased workload induces a state of hypercoagulability through an increase in thrombocyte number and activity, as well as an elevation in coagulation factors (fibrinogen, factors VII and VIII). Patients with known coronary artery disease and echocardiographic evidence of ischemia during mental stress testing demonstrate significant ischemic episodes on ambulatory ECG monitoring during sedentary activities. This finding may reflect greater functional severity of CAD or a propensity toward coronary vasoconstriction while sedentary (78).

Trichopoulos et al (79) found an excess of cardiac deaths in the days following the Athens earthquake of 1981 and proposed that this was due to the excess mental stress acting as a trigger. The 1994 earthquake that occurred in the Los Angeles area provided an unusual opportunity to clarify the relationship between stress and the triggering of acute cardiac events. Leor and Kloner (80) found a significant rise in the number of sudden cardiac deaths on the day of the earthquake. A 35% increase in the number of hospital admissions for acute myocardial infarction in Southern California occurred during the week following the earthquake (81). Additionally, Kloner's group detected an increase in the incidence of ventricular tachycardia or fibrillation among patients with implantable cardioverter-defibrillators during the two weeks following the earthquake (82).

II. General Theory of Thrombosis

The new information on circadian variation and triggering has provided the basis for a general theory of onset of coronary thrombosis (83) (Fig. 3). This general theory adds the concept of triggering activities to the general scheme of the role of thrombosis in the acute coronary syndromes advanced by Falk (84), Davies (85), Fuster (86), and Willerson (87). The important new concepts included are: vulnerable plaques, triggers, and acute risk factors. It is proposed that the initial step in the process is the development of an atherosclerotic plaque vulnerable to disruption. This process is presumably a dynamic, potentially reversible disorder caused by several factors including a lipid-rich plaque, a thin fibrous cap and increased macrophage activity with elaboration of metaloproteinases (88,89). The fibrous cap is often thinnest and weakest at its junction with the nearby intima

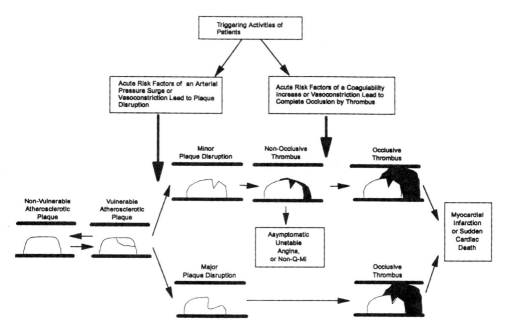

Figure 3 Hypothetical method by which daily activities may trigger coronary thrombosis. Three triggering mechanisms are presented: 1) physical or mental stress producing hemodynamic changes leading to plaque rupture, 2) activities causing an increase in coagulability, and 3) stimuli leading to vasoconstriction. The scheme depicting the role of coronary thrombosis in unstable angina, myocardial infarction, and sudden cardiac death has been well described by numerous investigators. The novel portion of this figure is the additional of triggers. Non-Q-MI, non-Q-wave myocardial infarction. (From Ref. 83.)

(90). Recently, Lodder and associates (91) from the University of Kentucky have been able to demonstrate lipoprotein distribution in arterial plaques in vivo using near-infrared imaging and spectroscopy.

The onset of myocardial infarction might be triggered by a stress (physical or mental) that produces a hemodynamic change which is sufficient to disrupt the vulnerable plaque. A synergistic combination of triggering activities may account for thrombosis in a setting in which each activity alone may not exceed the threshold for causation of infarction. For example, heavy physical exertion (producing a minor plaque disruption) in a sedentary cigarette smoker (producing an increase in coronary artery vasoconstriction and a relatively hypercoagulable state (92)) may be needed to cause occlusive thrombosis and disease onset. However, in a patient with an extremely vulnerable plaque, even the nonstrenuous activities of daily living may be sufficient to trigger the cascade leading to the cardiovascular event. The acute risk factor is defined as the pathophysiological change (vasoconstrictive, hemodynamic, or hemostatic) potentially leading to occlusive coronary thrombosis. It results from a combination of an external stress (physical or mental) and the individual's reactivity to that stress. If plaque disruption is major, with extensive exposure of collagen and atheromatous core contents to the lumen, it may lead immediately to occlusive thrombosis with infarction or sudden cardiac death. Far more commonly, a minor disruption occurs and the resulting non-occlusive thrombus causes no symptoms, unstable angina or non-Q-wave infarction.

Given the current state of knowledge of circadian variation of disease onset, and in view of the potentially harmful physiological processes involved, it seems reasonable that pharmacological protection should be provided during the morning hours for patients already being administered anti-ischemic and antihypertensive therapy. Therapies should include anti-platelets (aspirin, glycoprotein IIb/IIIa inhibitors), beta blockers, and regular aerobic exercise. Lipid lowering therapy with HMG-CoA reductase inhibitors have had early favorable effects in reducing cardiac events, presumably through plaque stabilization (93).

With further epidemiological, clinical, and basic science research, we may achieve a better understanding of the mechanisms that provoke the onset of acute cardiovascular disease. This knowledge would help investigators design effective preventive therapies for these disorders.

III. Cerebrovascular Disease

A. Introduction

Cerebrovascular disease is the 3rd leading cause of death and an important cause of hospital admission and long-term disability in the United States. Every year there are approximately 500,000 cerebrovascular accidents (CVA) and 175,000 fatalities. Chronic diseases such as allergic rhinitis, angina, rheumatoid and osteoarthritis, asthma, epilepsy, hypertension and ulcer disease commonly exhibit daily, menstrual cycle (in women) and seasonal patterns (94). The identification of circadian (daily), hebdomadal (weekly), and circannual (seasonal) variations in the incidence of onset of stroke and its subtypes may help to define better strategies to treat and prevent this disorder.

B. Ischemic Infarcts

Cerebral infarction is the most common type of stroke seen in the middle-aged and elderly population and is often due to atherothrombosis. The atheromatous process in brain arteries is identical to that in the aorta and coronary circulation and has a tendency to form at branching and curves of the cerebral arteries. As expected, hypertension, hyperlipidemia, diabetes mellitus and cigarette smoking are risk factors that are associated with ischemic stroke (95). Younger patients (ages 15–44) with cerebral arterial infarction have fewer atherosclerotic risk factors and a different spectrum of potential etiologies (i.e. pregnancy (96), illicit drug use, hematologic disorders, vasculopathies) (97). Very recently, Wagner et al (98) reported that the presence of phospholipase A2 polymorphism of platelet glycoprotein IIb/IIIa (a membrane receptor for fibrinogen and von Willebrand factor and implicated in the pathogenesis of acute coronary syndromes) appears to be associated with increased ischemic stroke risk in young caucasian females.

An overall male preponderance of stroke is noted in most age groups (99) with the exception of young adults (<40 years) and subjects greater than age 70 (95). In addition to gender differences in stroke, racial variations have also been reported. Most recently, Sacco et al (100) found that in the urban community of northern Manhattan, African Americans had a 2.4-fold increase and Hispanics a 2-fold increase in strokes compared to Caucasians.

Numerous investigators have identified a circadian variation of cerebral infarction with a peak incidence of onset during the morning hours between 6 AM and noon (101–110). Marler et al (102) noted that more strokes occurred in awake patients from 10 AM to noon than during any other 2-hour interval. Marsh et al (111) noted that 24% of all infarctions occurred within the first hour after awakening. In contrast, Marshall (112) and Moulin (95) noted an increased incidence of ischemic infarction during sleep and at night. Haapaniemi et al (107) reported an evening peak of cerebral infarction in young adults (ages 16–40).

Pasqualetti et al (104) noted a hebdomadal (weekly) variation of ischemic stroke with an increased incidence of onset during the weekend. Haapaniemi (107) reported a weekend and holiday peak occurrence of cerebral infarction in young adults, possibly associated with alcohol ingestion or other lifestyle-related issues.

Seasonal variation in onset of cerebral infarction has been studied but no clear consensus has emerged. Multiple investigators noted an increased incidence of onset during the winter months (104,105,113–115). Sobel et al (116) reported an increase in onset of ischemic stroke during the months of February through April. Gallerani et al (109) noted a peak occurrence of cerebral infarction during the month of October. In contrast, several investigators found no significant seasonal variation for this disorder (95,117,118). Woo et al (119) recorded an association between the occurrence of cerebral infarcts and maximum temperature on the day of onset in patients aged 70 years or above. Biller et al (120) noted an increase in referrals for ischemic stroke during the warmer months.

Independent risk factors for death after first cerebral infarction include: severity of the clinical deficits (121), atrial fibrillation (122,123) age, congestive heart failure, recurrent stroke, ischemic heart disease (124). Recently, Tanne et al (125) studied 8586 Israeli men over a 21-year period and noted an inverse relationship between serum HDL-C levels and ischemic stroke mortality. A long-term prospective study of cerebrovascular and cardiovascular mortality conducted in Ohasama, Japan, found that those subjects with the lowest and highest quintiles of home systemic blood pressure levels demonstrated a significantly high all cause mortality (126). Mortality from cerebral infarction and its relationship to ambient temperature has also been studied. Haberman et al (127) described a high fatality rate in winter and spring and low mortality in late summer. More recently, Pan et al (113) noted a U-shaped mortality curve for cerebral infarction in elderly Chinese. In their study, the death rate was 66% higher at 32°C than at 27–29° C. In addition, the death rate increased by 3% for every degree the ambient temperature fell below 27–29° C. Kunst et al (128) reported that total mortality increased in the Netherlands when the outdoor temperature rose above or fell below 20–25° C. Temperature-related swings on serum coagulation factors and cholesterol may be playing a role. Woodhouse (61,129) noted that plasma fibrinogen, factor VII, and serum lipids are higher during the winter. Keatinge (130) reported that exposure to high temperatures result in increased platelet count, blood viscosity, and serum cholesterol measurements.

Recent data by Macko et al (131) suggest that both febrile and nonfebrile infectious/inflammatory syndromes may be a common predisposing risk factor for brain infarction and the period of increased risk is confined within a brief temporal window of less than 1 week. Kubota et al (132) reported that hot-spring bathing may precipitate cerebral infarction or acute myocardial infarction.

C. Transient Ischemic Attacks (TIAs)

A circadian variation in onset of transient ischemic attacks has been noted with a peak incidence in the morning hours (108,109,133). A seasonal variation in onset of TIAs has been studied by several authors with varying results. Giroud et al (134) and Sobel et al (116) noted a peak occurrence during the warm summer months. Alternatively, Butchart et al (133) reported a peak incidence in winter. Biller et al (120) found that TIA was not influenced by seasonal climatic variables.

D. Subarachnoid Hemorrhage

Circadian, hebdomadal, and seasonal variations in the onset of subarachnoid hemorrhage (SAH) have been considered by numerous investigators but with variable results. Pasqualetti et al (104) and Wroe et al (106) reported no significant circadian distribution whereas Johansson and colleagues (135) found a single peak of occurrence in the afternoon. Ricci et al (105), Lejeune et al (136), and Fogelholm et al (137) found an increased incidence of onset of subarachnoid hemorrhage in the morning hours. Sloan and colleagues (138) and Kleinpeter et al (139) also identified a significant morning increase in onset but only in patients with systemic hypertension. Several other investigators have reported a bimodal distribution of SAH with increased incidence of onset in the morning and evening (110,140,141). More recently, Vermeer et al noted that the risk of SAH "remained high throughout the day and evening with a small nadir around noon" (142). The circadian fluctuation of SAH parallels that of blood pressure and plasma concentrations of noradrenaline (143–145). This may explain why strenuous physical exercise (146) sexual intercourse (147,148), micturition/defecation (110), sporting (140) and emotional strain (149) are often associated with the onset of aneurysmal subarachnoid hemorrhage.

Kelly-Hayes et al (150), Haapaniemi et al (107) Hillbom and Kaste (151) and Juvela et al (152) reported an increase incidence of SAH on weekends and holidays. Heavy alcohol intake, a known precipitating factor of this disorder (152–154) probably accounts for this hebdomadal variation. This is in contrast to Lejeune et al (136) and Vermeer et al (142) who did not find a preferred day of the week of onset of acute SAH.

Seasonal distribution of SAH has also been examined. Some authors detected a single peak in either autumn (105) or winter (127,155–157) whereas others found no seasonal peak (104,115–117,120,138,158). Chyatte et al (159) found seasonal and gender fluctuations with men peaking in the late fall and women in the spring. At least two investigators have reported a bimodal seasonal distribution with two major peaks in spring and autumn (141,160). The inconsistent seasonal distribution of SAH may be due to variable interactions between environmental and vascular risk factors.

Gordon (161) noted that subarachnoid hemorrhage occurrence showed a distinct latitudinal pattern, with rates decreasing progressively from north to south. Tsementzis reported a positive correlation between subarachnoid hemorrhage occurrence and hours of sunshine, a factor that may be latitudinally dependent (162).

E. Intracerebral Hemorrhage

Approximately 7–30% (95,118,120) of all strokes are due to primary intracerebral hemorrhage (PIH). Risk factors for this disorder include hypertension, abnormal hemostasis, cerebrovascular malformations (163), diabetes mellitus and alcohol ingestion (164).

Circadian, hebdomadal, and seasonal variations in the onset of PIH have been considered by numerous investigators. Several researchers have noted a peak incidence of onset of PIH in the morning hours between 6AM and noon (110,138,150,165,166) and a nadir at night (110,112). In contrast, Deng (167) and Wang (108) noted a peak occurrence of PIH in the afternoon, whereas Pasqualetti (104) and Wroe (106) reported no circadian variation.

Although no circadian variation was appreciated, Pasqualetti (104) identi-fied a hebdomadal variation of PIH with a peak incidence of onset during the weekend. Kelly-Hayes et al (150) noted that one-third of all intracerebral hemor-rhages occurred on Monday.

A seasonal variation in the onset of PIH has been described by many exam-iners. The majority of reports suggest a peak incidence of onset of intracerebral hemorrhage during the cold winter months (104,115,118,155,165). In contrast, Ricci (105) identified a peak occurrence of PIH during autumn and Deng (167) reported a peak incidence of onset in March. Capon et al (156) found that the incidence of PIH was inversely related to temperature, hours of sunshine, and humidity. However, several researchers noted no seasonal distribution of PIH (116,117,119,138,150,158).

F. Cerebral Emboli

Cerebral arterial emboli often originate from the carotid artery, ascending aorta, or the left-sided cardiac chambers. These emboli may be associated with a cardiac arrhythmia (101,168) such as atrial fibrillation (122). A circadian variation with an increased incidence of onset in the morning (6 AM—noon) has been noted by several investigators (110,111,150,169). Marsh et al (111) reported that 62% of all cerebral emboli occurred between 6 AM and noon. Kelly-Hayes also noted a seasonal variation of cerebral emboli with a peak incidence in winter and often while patients are admitted to the hospital.

IV. Acute Cardiovascular Events and Sleep

The first section of this chapter reviewed the data and rationale for the increased incidence of onset of acute cardiac events during the morning hours. It should be noted that in the United States more than 250,00 acute myocardial infarctions and >38,000 sudden cardiac deaths (SCD) occur at night during sleep each year.

Lavery et al (170) reviewed the medical literature on the incidence of acute cardiac episodes between the hours of midnight and 5:59 AM and compiled 19 published studies on acute myocardial infarction, 7 published studies on auto-matic implantable cardioverter-defibrillator (AICD) discharges, and 12 published studies on sudden cardiac death. The distribution of all three cardiac events during this time period was nonrandom; the peak incidence of myocardial infarction and AICD discharge occurred between midnight and 0:59 AM, and the peak incidence of SCD took place between 1:00 and 1:59 AM. The nadir in incidence of MI and AICD discharge occurred between 3:00 and 3:59 AM, and the trough for SCD was between 4:00 and 4:59 AM.

Normal sleep is not a physiologically uniform nor quiescent state. It is a dynamic process involving complex regulation of autonomic nervous system ac-tivity (171). Rapid eye movement (REM) sleep, in particular, is associated with sympathetic nervous system output approaching levels perceived during the awake state. In this catecholamine milieu, the hemodynamic and thrombotic processes activated may cause plaque rupture, coronary vasospasm (172) and ventricular tachyarrhythmias (173) in patients with CAD. During non-REM deep sleep, vagal-mediated decrease in systemic blood pressure (145) may reduce blood flow through stenosed coronary arteries leading to ischemia, thrombi, and possibly evoking emboli either before or after arousal from sleep (174). Therefore, sleep state dependent fluctuations in autonomic nervous system activity may trigger the onset of acute myocardial infarction, ventricular arrhythmias, and sudden cardiac death and provide further impetus for more directly testing this hypothesis at population, individual, and mechanistic levels (170).

Sleep-related disordered breathing (SRDB) is common in patients with coronary artery disease (CAD) (175). Sleep apnea, which occurs in 4% of the adult male population, is associated with increased morbidity (176) and mortality (177) due to cardiovascular disease. Diseases associated with sleep apnea include systemic hypertension, arrhythmias (178) pulmonary hypertension, right heart insufficiency and coronary heart disease. Patients with SRDB and CAD have a high incidence of myocardial dysfunction and cardiac events (179). Electrocardiographic ST segment depression is relatively common in patients with obstructive apnea during sleep and treatment with nasal continuous positive airway pressure significantly reduces the duration of this abnormality (180). This finding suggests that the identification and appropriate therapy of sleep-related disordered breathing may have a beneficial effect on the cardiovascular system.

V. Conclusions

In summary, numerous cardiovascular and cerebrovascular diseases show circadian (daily), hebdomadal (weekly), and circannual (seasonal) variations in incidence and supports the concept of triggering. Hemodynamic, vascular, hematologic and sleep-related processes have been implicated in disease onset. Through further epidemiological, clinical, and basic science research, we may achieve a better understanding of the mechanisms that provoke acute cardiovascular and cerebrovascular disease onset. This knowledge would help devise effective preventive treatments for these disorders. A better understanding of nocturnal triggers may make it possible to reduce acute cardiovascular events during sleep.

References

1. Obraztsov VP, Strazhesko ND. The symptomatology and diagnosis of coronary thrombosis. In: Vorobeva VA, Konchalovaski MP, eds. Works of the First Congress of Russian Therapists: Comradeship Typography of AE Mamontov, 1910:26–43.

2. Muller JE, Tofler GH. Circadian variation and cardiovascular disease (editorial; comment). N Engl J Med 1991; 325:1038–1039.

3. Muller JE, Stone PH, Turi ZG, Rutherford JD, Czeisler CA, Parker C, Poole WK, Passamani E, Roberts R, Robertson T, et al. Circadian variation in the frequency of onset of acute myocardial infarction. N Engl J Med 1985; 313:1315–1322.

4. Willich SN, Linderer T, Wegscheider K, Leizorovicz A, Alamercery I, Schroder R. Increased morning incidence of myocardial infarction in the ISAM Study: absence with prior beta-adrenergic blockade. ISAM Study Group. Circulation 1989; 80:853–858.

5. Goldberg RJ, Brady P, Muller JE, Chen ZY, de Groot M, Zonneveld P, Dalen JE. Time of onset of symptoms of acute myocardial infarction. Am J Cardiol 1990; 66:140–144.

6. Willich SN, Lowel H, Lewis M, Arntz R, Baur R, Winther K, Keil U, Schroder R. Association of wake time and the onset of myocardial infarction. Triggers and mechanisms of myocardial infarction (TRIMM) pilot study: TRIMM Study Group. Circulation 1991; 84:VI62–VI67.

7. Tofler GH, Muller JE, Stone PH, Forman S, Solomon RE, Knatterud GL, Braunwald E. Modifiers of timing and possible triggers of acute myocardial infarction in the Thrombolysis in Myocardial Infarction Phase II (TIMI II) Study Group. J Am Coll Cardiol 1992; 20:1049–1055.

8. Cannon CP, McCabe CH, Stone PH, Schactman M, Thompson B, Theroux P, Gibson RS, Feldman T, Kleiman NS, Tofler GH, Muller JE, Chaitman BR, Braunwald E. Circadian variation in the onset of unstable angina and non-Q-wave acute myocardial infarction (the TIMI III Registry and TIMI IIIB). Am J Cardiol 1997; 79: 253–258.

9. Hjalmarson A, Gilpin EA, Nicod P, Dittrich H, Henning H, Engler R, Blacky AR, Smith SC Jr, Ricou F, Ross J Jr. Differing circadian patterns of symptom onset in subgroups of patients with acute myocardial infarction. Circulation 1989; 80:267–275.

10. Ridker PM, Manson JE, Buring JE, Muller JE, Hennekens CH. Circadian variation of acute myocardial infarction and the effect of low-dose aspirin in a randomized trial of physicians. Circulation 1990; 82:897–902.

11. Thompson DR, Blandford RL, Sutton TW, Marchant PR. Time of onset of chest pain in acute myocardial infarction. Int J Cardiol 1985; 7:139–148.

12. Peters RW, Zoble RG, Liebson PR, Pawitan Y, Brooks MM, Proschan M. Identification of a secondary peak in myocardial infarction onset 11 to 12 hours after awakening: the Cardiac Arrhythmia Suppression Trial (CAST) experience. J Am Coll Cardiol 1993; 22:998–1003.

13. Willich SN, Levy D, Rocco MB, Tofler GH, Stone PH, Muller JE. Circadian variation in the incidence of sudden cardiac death in the Framingham Heart Study population. Am J Cardiol 1987; 60:801–806.

14. Muller JE, Ludmer PL, Willich SN, Tofler GH, Aylmer G, Klangos I, Stone PH. Circadian variation in the frequency of sudden cardiac death (see comments). Circulation 1987; 75:131–138.

15. Levine RL, Pepe PE, Fromm RE, Jr, Curka PA, Clark PA. Prospective evidence

of a circadian rhythm for out-of-hospital cardiac arrests. JAMA 1992; 267:2935–2937.

16. Behrens S, Ney G, Fisher SG, Fletcher RD, Franz MR, Singh SN. Effects of amiodarone on the circadian pattern of sudden cardiac death: Department of Veterans Affairs Congestive Heart Failure-Survival Trial of Antiarrhythmic Therapy). Am J Cardiol 1997; 80:45–48.

17. Peters RW, Mitchell LB, Brooks MM, Echt DS, Barker AH, Capone R, Liebson PR, Greene HL. Circadian pattern of arrhythmic death in patients receiving encainide, flecainide or moricizine in the Cardiac Arrhythmia Suppression Trial (CAST). J Am Coll Cardiol 1994; 23:283–289.

18. Peters RW, Muller JE, Goldstein S, Byington R, Friedman LM. Propranolol and the morning increase in the frequency of sudden cardiac death (BHAT Study). Am J Cardiol 1989; 63:1518–1520.

19. Behrens S, Ehlers C, Bruggemann T, Ziss W, Dissmann R, Galecka M, Willich SN, Andresen D. Modification of the circadian pattern of ventricular tachyarrhythmias by beta-blocker therapy. Clin Cardiol 1997; 20:253–257.

20. Andersen L, Sigurd B, Hansen J. Verapamil and circadian variation of sudden cardiac death. Am Heart J 1996; 131:409–410.

21. Peters RW. Circadian patterns and triggers of sudden cardiac death. Cardiol Clin 1996; 14:185–194.

22. Canada WB, Woodward W, Lee G, DeMaria A, Low R, Mason DT, Laddu A, Shapiro W. Circadian rhythm of hourly ventricular arrhythmia frequency in man. Angiology 1983; 34:274–282.

23. Twidale N, Taylor S, Heddle WF, Ayres BF, Tonkin AM. Morning increase in the time of onset of sustained ventricular tachycardia. Am J Cardiol 1989; 64:1204–1206.

24. Arntz HR, Willich SN, Oeff M, Bruggemann T, Stern R, Heinzmann A, Matenaer B, Schroder R. Circadian variation of sudden cardiac death reflects age-related variability in ventricular fibrillation. Circulation 1993; 88:2284–2289.

25. Tofler GH, Gebara OC, Mittleman MA, Taylor P, Siegel W, Venditti FJ Jr, Rasmussen CA, Muller JE. Morning peak in ventricular tachyarrhythmias detected by time of implantable cardioverter/defibrillator therapy: the CPI Investigators. Circulation 1995; 92:1203–1208.

26. Venditti FJ, Jr, John RM, Hull M, Tofler GH, Shahian DM, Martin DT. Circadian variation in defibrillation energy requirements. Circulation 1996; 94:1607–1612.

27. Yamashita T, Murakawa Y, Sezaki K, Inoue M, Hayami N, Shuzui Y, Omata M. Circadian variation of paroxysmal atrial fibrillation. Circulation 1997; 96:1537–1541.

28. Nademanee K, Intarachot V, Josephson MA, Singh BN. Circadian variation in occurrence of transient overt and silent myocardial ischemia in chronic stable angina and comparison with Prinzmetal angina in men. Am J Cardiol 1987; 60:494–498.

29. Rocco MB, Barry J, Campbell S, Nabel E, Cook EF, Goldman L, Selwyn AP. Circadian variation of transient myocardial ischemia in patients with coronary artery disease. Circulation 1987; 75:395–400.

30. Parker JD, Testa MA, Jimenez AH, Tofler GH, Muller JE, Parker JO, Stone PH.

Morning increase in ambulatory ischemia in patients with stable coronary artery disease: importance of physical activity and increased cardiac demand. Circulation 1994; 89:604–614.

31. Mulcahy D, Keegan J, Cunningham D, Quyyumi A, Crean P, Park A, Wright C, Fox K. Circadian variation of total ischaemic burden and its alteration with anti-anginal agents. Lancet 1988; 2:755–759.

32. Gallerani M, Portaluppi F, Grandi E, Manfredini R. Circadian rhythmicity in the occurrence of spontaneous acute dissection and rupture of thoracic aorta. J Thorac Cardiovasc Surg 1997; 113:603–604.

33. Colantonio D, Casale R, Abruzzo BP, Lorenzetti G, Pasqualetti P. Circadian distribution in fatal pulmonary thromboembolism. Am J Cardiol 1989; 64:403–404.

34. Millar-Craig MW, Bishop CN, Raftery EB. Circadian variation of blood-pressure. Lancet 1978; 1:795–797.

35. Panza JA, Epstein SE, Quyyumi AA. Circadian variation in vascular tone and its relation to alpha-sympathetic vasoconstrictor activity (see comments). N Engl J Med 1991; 325:986–990.

36. Vita JA, Treasure CB, Ganz P, Cox DA, Fish RD, Selwyn AP. Control of shear stress in the epicardial coronary arteries of humans: impairment by atherosclerosis (see comments). J Am Coll Cardiol 1989; 14:1193–1199.

37. Ehrly AM, Jung G. Circadian rhythm of human blood viscosity. Biorheology 1973; 10:577–583.

38. Broadhurst P, Kelleher C, Hughes L, Imeson JD, Raftery EB. Fibrinogen, factor VII clotting activity and coronary artery disease severity. Atherosclerosis 1990; 85: 169–173.

39. Kapiotis S, Jilma B, Quehenberger P, Ruzicka K, Handler S, Speiser W. Morning hypercoagulability and hypofibrinolysis: diurnal variations in circulating activated factor VII, prothrombin fragment F1 + 2, and plasmin-plasmin inhibitor complex. Circulation 1997; 96:19–21.

40. Decousus H, Boissier C, Perpoint B, Page Y, Mismetti P, Laporte S, Tardy B, Queneau P. Circadian dynamics of coagulation and chronopathology of cardiovascular and cerebrovascular events: future therapeutic implications for the treatment of these disorders? Ann NY Acad Sci 1991; 618:159–165.

41. Kurnik PB. Circadian variation in the efficacy of tissue-type plasminogen activator (see comments). Circulation 1995; 91:1341–1346.

42. Tofler GH, Brezinski D, Schafer AI, Czeisler CA, Rutherford JD, Willich SN, Gleason RE, Williams GH, Muller JE. Concurrent morning increase in platelet aggregability and the risk of myocardial infarction and sudden cardiac death. N Engl J Med 1987; 316:1514–1518.

43. Brezinski DA, Tofler GH, Muller JE, Pohjola-Sintonen S, Willich SN, Schafer AI, Czeisler CA, Williams GH. Morning increase in platelet aggregability: association with assumption of the upright posture. Circulation 1988; 78:35–40.

44. Murakami Y, Ishinaga Y, Sano K, Kinoshita Y, Kitamura J, Okada S, Shimada T. Circadian release of serotonin across the coronary bed in patients with endothelial dysfunction. Am J Cardiol 1997; 80:214–216.

45. Mittleman MA, Maclure M, Tofler GH, Sherwood JB, Goldberg RJ, Muller JE. Triggering of acute myocardial infarction by heavy physical exertion: protection

against triggering by regular exertion—Determinants of Myocardial Infarction Onset Study Investigators (see comments). N Engl J Med 1993; 329:1677–1683.

46. Muller JE, Mittleman A, Maclure M, Sherwood JB, Tofler GH. Triggering myocardial infarction by sexual activity. Low absolute risk and prevention by regular physical exertion: Determinants of Myocardial Infarction Onset Study Investigators (see comments). JAMA 1996; 275:1405–1409.

47. Mittleman MA, Maclure M, Sherwood JB, Mulry RP, Tofler GH, Jacobs SC, Friedman R, Benson H, Muller JE. Triggering of acute myocardial infarction onset by episodes of anger: Determinants of Myocardial Infarction Onset Study Investigators (see comments). Circulation 1995; 92:1720–1725.

48. Maclure M. The case-crossover design: a method for studying transient effects on the risk of acute events. Am J Epidemiol 1991; 133:144–153.

49. Reich P, DeSilva RA, Lown B, Murawski BJ. Acute psychological disturbances preceding life-threatening ventricular arrhythmias. Jama 1981; 246:233–235.

50. Fletcher GF, Blair SN, Blumenthal J, Caspersen C, Chaitman B, Epstein S, Falls H, Froelicher ES, Froelicher VF, Pina IL. Statement on exercise: benefits and recommendations for physical activity programs for all Americans—A statement for health professionals by the Committee on Exercise and Cardiac Rehabilitation of the Council on Clinical Cardiology, American Heart Association. Circulation 1992; 86:340–344.

51. Tofler GH, Stone PH, Maclure M, Edelman E, Davis VG, Robertson T, Antman EM, Muller JE. Analysis of possible triggers of acute myocardial infarction: the MILIS study. Am J Cardiol 1990; 66:22–27.

52. Vuori I. The cardiovascular risks of physical activity. Acta Med Scand Suppl 1986; 711:205–214.

53. Siscovick DS, Weiss NS, Fletcher RH, Lasky T. The incidence of primary cardiac arrest during vigorous exercise. N Engl J Med 1984; 311:874–877.

54. Khanna PK, Seth HN, Balasubramanian V, Hoon RS. Effect of submaximal exercise on fibrinolytic activity in ischaemic heart disease. Br Heart J 1975; 37:1273–1276.

55. AHA. Cardiac rehabilitation programs: a statement for healthcare professionals from the American Heart Association. Circulation 1994; 90:1602–1610.

56. Rauramaa R, Salonen JT, Kukkonen-Harjula K, Seppanen K, Seppala E, Vapaatalo H, Huttunen JK. Effects of mild physical exercise on serum lipoproteins and metabolites of arachidonic acid: a controlled randomised trial in middle aged men. Br Med J 1984; 288:603–606.

57. Murray PM, Herrington DM, Pettus CW, Miller HS, Cantwell JD, Little WC. Should patients with heart disease exercise in the morning or afternoon? (see comments). Arch Intern Med 1993; 153:833–836.

58. Spencer FA, Goldberg RJ, Becker RC, Gore JM. Seasonal distribution of acute myocardial infarction in the second National Registry of Myocardial Infarction. J Am Coll Cardiol 1998; 31:1226–1233.

59. Kawahara J, Sano H, Fukuzaki H, Saito K, Hirouchi H. Acute effects of exposure to cold on blood pressure, platelet function and sympathetic nervous activity in humans. Am J Hypertens 1989; 2:724–726.

60. Keatinge WR, Coleshaw SR, Cotter F, Mattock M, Murphy M, Chelliah R. In-

creases in platelet and red cell counts, blood viscosity, and arterial pressure during mild surface cooling: factors in mortality from coronary and cerebral thrombosis in winter. BMJ 1984; 289:1405–1408.

61. Woodhouse PR, Khaw KT, Plummer M, Foley A, Meade TW. Seasonal variations of plasma fibrinogen and factor VII activity in the elderly: winter infections and death from cardiovascular disease (see comments). Lancet 1994; 343:435–439.

62. Bull G, Brozovic M, Chakrabarti R, Mead T, Morton J, North W, Stirling Y. Relationship of air temperature to various chemical, haematological, and haemostatic variables. J Clin Pathol 1979; 32:16–20.

63. Baker-Blocker A. Winter weather and cardiovascular mortality in Minneapolis-St. Paul. Am J Public Health 1982; 72:261–265.

64. Rogers WJ, Bowlby LJ, Chandra NC, French WJ, Gore JM, Lambrew CT, Rubison RM, Tiefenbrunn AJ, Weaver WD. Treatment of myocardial infarction in the United States (1990 to 1993): observations from the National Registry of Myocardial Infarction. Circulation 1994; 90:2103–2114.

65. Marchant B, Ranjadayalan K, Stevenson R, Wilkinson P, Timmis AD. Circadian and seasonal factors in the pathogenesis of acute myocardial infarction: the influence of environmental temperature. Br Heart J 1993; 69:385–387.

66. Beard CM, Fuster V, Elveback LR. Daily and seasonal variation in sudden cardiac death, Rochester, Minnesota, 1950–1975. Mayo Clin Proc 1982; 57:704–706.

67. Spielberg C, Falkenhahn D, Willich SN, Wegscheider K, Voller H. Circadian, day-of-week, and seasonal variability in myocardial infarction: comparison between working and retired patients. Am Heart J 1996; 132:579–585.

68. Gnecchi-Ruscone T, Piccaluga E, Guzzetti S, Contini M, Montano N, Nicolis E. Morning and Monday: critical periods for the onset of acute myocardial infarction: the GISSI 2 Study experience. Eur Heart J 1994; 15:882–887.

69. Massing W, Angermeyer MC. Myocardial infarction on various days of the week. Psychol Med 1985; 15:851–857.

70. Thompson DR, Pohl JE, Sutton TW. Acute myocardial infarction and day of the week. Am J Cardiol 1992; 69:266–267.

71. Willich SN, Lowel H, Lewis M, Hormann A, Arntz HR, Keil U. Weekly variation of acute myocardial infarction: increased Monday risk in the working population. Circulation 1994; 90:87–93.

72. Manuck SB, Kaplan JR, Matthews KA. Behavioral antecedents of coronary heart disease and atherosclerosis. Arteriosclerosis 1986; 6:2–14.

73. Meisel SR, Kutz I, Dayan KI, Pauzner H, Chetboun I, Arbel Y, David D. Effect of Iraqi missile war on incidence of acute myocardial infarction and sudden death in Israeli civilians (see comments). Lancet 1991; 338:660–661.

74. Frasure-Smith N, Lesperance F, Talajic M. Depression following myocardial infarction. Impact on 6-month survival (see comments) [published erratum appears in JAMA 1994 Apr 13; 271(14):1082]. JAMA 1993; 270:1819–1825.

75. Schwartz PJ, Zaza A, Locati E, Moss AJ. Stress and sudden death. The case of the long QT syndrome. Circulation 1991; 83:II71–II80.

76. Barry J, Selwyn AP, Nabel EG, Rocco MB, Mead K, Campbell S, Rebecca G. Frequency of ST-segment depression produced by mental stress in stable angina pectoris from coronary artery disease. Am J Cardiol 1988; 61:989–993.

77. Frimerman A, Miller HI, Laniado S, Keren G. Changes in hemostatic function at times of cyclic variation in occupational stress. Am J Cardiol 1997; 79:72–75.

78. Gottdiener JS, Krantz DS, Howell RH, Hecht GM, Klein J, Falconer JJ, Rozanski A. Induction of silent myocardial ischemia with mental stress testing: relation to the triggers of ischemia during daily life activities and to ischemic functional severity. J Am Coll Cardiol 1994; 24:1645–1651.

79. Trichopoulos D, Katsouyanni K, Zavitsanos X, Tzonou A, Dalla-Vorgia P. Psychological stress and fatal heart attack: the Athens (1981) earthquake natural experiment. Lancet 1983; 1:441–444.

80. Leor J, Poole WK, Kloner RA. Sudden cardiac death triggered by an earthquake (see comments). N Engl J Med 1996; 334:413–419.

81. Leor J, Kloner RA. The Northridge earthquake as a trigger for acute myocardial infarction. Am J Cardiol 1996; 77:1230–1232.

82. Nishimoto Y, Firth BR, Kloner RA. The 1994 Northridge earthquake triggered shocks from implantable cardioverter defibrillators (abstr). Circulation 1995; 92: 606.

83. Muller JE, Abela GS, Nesto RW, Tofler GH. Triggers, acute risk factors and vulnerable plaques: the lexicon of a new frontier. J Am Coll Cardiol 1994; 23:809–813.

84. Falk E. Plaque rupture with severe pre-existing stenosis precipitating coronary thrombosis. Characteristics of coronary atherosclerotic plaques underlying fatal occlusive thrombi. Br Heart J 1983; 50:127–134.

85. Davies MJ, Thomas A. Thrombosis and acute coronary-artery lesions in sudden cardiac ischemic death. N Engl J Med 1984; 310:1137–1140.

86. Fuster V, Badimon L, Badimon JJ, Chesebro JH. The pathogenesis of coronary artery disease and the acute coronary syndromes (2). N Engl J Med 1992; 326: 310–318.

87. Willerson JT, Campbell WB, Winniford MD, Schmitz J, Apprill P, Firth BG, Ashton J, Smitherman T, Bush L, Buja LM. Conversion from chronic to acute coronary artery disease: speculation regarding mechanisms. Am J Cardiol 1984; 54:1349–1354.

88. Davies MJ. The contribution of thrombosis to the clinical expression of coronary atherosclerosis. Thromb Res 1996; 82:1–32.

89. Libby P. Molecular bases of the acute coronary syndromes. Circulation 1995; 91: 2844–2850.

90. Richardson PD, Davies MJ, Born GV. Influence of plaque configuration and stress distribution on fissuring of coronary atherosclerotic plaques (see comments). Lancet 1989; 2:941–944.

91. Dempsey RJ, Cassis LA, Davis DG, Lodder RA. Near-infrared imaging and spectroscopy in stroke research: lipoprotein distribution and disease. Ann NY Acad Sci 1997; 820:149–169.

92. Belch JJ, McArdle BM, Burns P, Lowe GD, Forbes CD. The effects of acute smoking on platelet behaviour, fibrinolysis and haemorheology in habitual smokers. Thromb Haemost 1984; 51:6–8.

93. Brown BG, Zhao XQ, Sacco DE, Albers JJ. Lipid lowering and plaque regression. New insights into prevention of plaque disruption and clinical events in coronary disease. Circulation 1993; 87:1781–1791.

94. Smolensky MH, D'Alonzo GE. Medical chronobiology: concepts and applications. Am Rev Respir Dis 1993; 147:S2–19.

95. Moulin T, Tatu L, Crepin-Leblond T, Chavot D, Berges S, Rumbach T. The Besancon Stroke Registry: an acute stroke registry of 2,500 consecutive patients. Eur Neurol 1997; 38:10–20.

96. Ben Hamouda MRI, Mrabet A, Ben Hamida M. Cerebral venous thrombosis and arterial infarction in pregnancy and puerperium. A series of 60 cases. Rev Neurol (Paris) 1995; 151:563–568.

97. Kittner SJ, Stern BJ, Wozniak M, Buchholz DW, Earley CJ, Feeser BR, Johnson CJ, Macko RF, McCarter RJ, Price TR, Sherwin R, Sloan MA, Wityk RJ. Cerebral infarction in young adults: the Baltimore-Washington Cooperative Young Stroke Study. Neurology 1998; 50:890–894.

98. Wagner KR, Giles WH, Johnson CJ, Ou CY, Bray PF, Goldschmidt-Clermont PJ, Croft JB, Brown VK, Stern BJ, Feeser BR, Buchholz DW, Earley CJ, Macko RF, McCarter RJ, Sloan MA, Stolley PD, Wityk RJ, Wozniak MA, Price TR, Kittner SJ. Platelet glycoprotein receptor IIIa polymorphism P1A2 and ischemic stroke risk: the Stroke Prevention in Young Women Study. Stroke 1998; 29:581–585.

99. Haberman S, Capildeo R, Rose FC. Sex differences in the incidence of cerebrovascular disease. J Epidemiol Commun Health 1981; 35:45–50.

100. Sacco RL, Boden-Albala B, Gan R, Chen X, Kargman DE, Shea S, Paik MC, Hauser WA. Stroke incidence among white, black, and Hispanic residents of an urban community: the Northern Manhattan Stroke Study. Am J Epidemiol 1998; 147:259–268.

101. Agnoli A, Manfredi M, Mossuto L, Piccinelli A. Relationship between circadian rhythms and blood pressure and the pathogenesis of cerebrovascular insufficiency. Rev Neurol 1975; 131:597–606.

102. Marler JR, Price TR, Clark GL, Muller JE, Robertson T, Mohr JP, Hier DB, Wolf PA, Caplan LR, Foulkes MA. Morning increase in onset of ischemic stroke (see comments). Stroke 1989; 20:473–476.

103. Argentino C, Toni D, Rasura M, Violi F, Sacchetti ML, Allegretta A, Balsano F, Fieschi C. Circadian variation in the frequency of ischemic stroke. Stroke 1990; 21:387–389.

104. Pasqualetti P, Natali G, Casale R, Colantonio D. Epidemiological chronorisk of stroke. Acta Neurol Scand 1990; 81:71–74.

105. Ricci S, Celani MG, Vitali R, La Rosa F, Righetti E, Duca E. Diurnal and seasonal variations in the occurrence of stroke: a community-based study. Neuroepidemiology 1992; 11:59–64.

106. Wroe SJ, Sandercock P, Bamford J, Dennis M, Slattery J, Warlow C. Diurnal variation in incidence of stroke: Oxfordshire community stroke project. BMJ 1992; 304:155–157.

107. Haapaniemi H, Hillbom M, Juvela S. Weekend and holiday increase in the onset of ischemic stroke in young women. Stroke 1996; 27:1023–1027.

108. Wang H, Kingsland R, Zhao H, Wang Y, Pan W, Dong X, Guo J, Huang F. Time of symptom onset of eight common medical emergencies (see comments). J Emerg Med 1995; 13:461–469.

109. Gallerani M, Manfredini R, Ricci L, Cocurullo A, Goldoni C, Bigoni M, Fersini C. Chronobiological aspects of acute cerebrovascular diseases. Acta Neurol Scand 1993; 87:482–487.

110. Tsementzis SA, Gill JS, Hitchcock ER, Gill SK, Beevers DG. Diurnal variation of and activity during the onset of stroke. Neurosurgery 1985; 17:901–904.

111. Marsh EEd, Biller J, Adams HP, Jr., Marler JR, Hulbert JR, Love BB, Gordon DL. Circadian variation in onset of acute ischemic stroke (see comments). Arch Neurol 1990; 47:1178–1180.

112. Marshall J. Diurnal variation in occurrence of strokes. Stroke 1977; 8:230–231.

113. Pan W-H, Li L-A, Tsai M-J. Temperature extremes and mortality from coronary heart disease and cerebral infarction in elderly Chinese. Lancet 1995; 345:353–355.

114. Jakovljevic D, Salomaa V, Sivenius J, Tamminen M, Sarti C, Salmi K, Kaarsalo E, Narva V, Immonen-Raiha P, Torppa J, Tuomilehto J. Seasonal variation in the occurrence of stroke in a Finnish adult population: the FINMONICA Stroke Register—finnish monitoring trends and determinants in cardiovascular disease. Stroke 1996; 27:1774–1779.

115. Shinkawa A, Ueda K, Hasuo Y, Kiyohara Y, Fujishima M. Seasonal variation in stroke incidence in Hisayama, Japan. Stroke 1990; 21:1262–1267.

116. Sobel E, Zhang ZX, Alter M, Lai SM, Davanipour Z, Friday G, McCoy R, Isack T, Levitt L. Stroke in the Lehigh Valley: seasonal variation in incidence rates. Stroke 1987; 18:38–42.

117. Rothwell PM, Wroe SJ, Slattery J, Warlow CP. Is stroke incidence related to season or temperature? The Oxfordshire Community Stroke Project. Lancet 1996; 347:934–936.

118. Suzuki K, Kutsuzawa T, Takita K, Ito M, Sakamoto T, Hirayama A, Ito T, Ishida T, Ooishi H, Kawakami K, et al. Clinico-epidemiologic study of stroke in Akita, Japan. Stroke 1987; 18:402–406.

119. Woo J, Kay R, Nicholls MG. Environmental temperature and stroke in a subtropical climate. Neuroepidemiology 1991; 10:260–265.

120. Biller J, Jones MP, Bruno A, Adams HP, Jr., Banwart K. Seasonal variation of stroke—does it exist? (see comments). Neuroepidemiology 1988; 7:89–98.

121. Henon H, Godefroy O, Leys D, Mounier-Vehier F, Lucas C, Rondepierre P, Duhamel A, Pruvo JP. Early predictors of death and disability after acute cerebral ischemic event (see comments). Stroke 1995; 26:392–398.

122. Lin HJ, Wolf PA, Kelly-Hayes M, Beiser AS, Kase CS, Benjamin EJ, D'Agostino RB. Stroke severity in atrial fibrillation. The Framingham Study (see comments). Stroke 1996; 27:1760–1764.

123. European Community Stroke Project F. Ischemic stroke associated with atrial fibrillation: the demographic and clinical characteristics and 30-day mortality in a hospital stroke registry. The European Community Stroke Project, Florence Unit. Ann Ital Med Int 1996; 11:20–26.

124. Petty GW, Brown RD, Jr., Whisnant JP, Sicks JD, O'Fallon WM, Wiebers DO. Survival and recurrence after first cerebral infarction: a population-based study in Rochester, Minnesota, 1975 through 1989. Neurology 1998; 50:208–216.

125. Tanne D, Yaari S, Goldbourt U. High-density lipoprotein cholesterol and risk of

ischemic stroke mortality: a 21-year follow-up of 8586 men from the Israeli Ischemic Heart Disease Study. Stroke 1997; 28:83–87.

126. Imai Y, Tsuji I, Nagai K, Watanabe N, Ohkubo T, Sakuma M, Hashimoto J, Itoh O, Satoh H, Hisamichi S, Abe K. Circadian blood pressure variation related to morbidity and mortality from cerebrovascular and cardiovascular diseases. Ann NY Acad Sci 1996; 783:172–185.

127. Haberman S, Capildeo R, Rose FC. The seasonal variation in mortality from cerebrovascular disease. J Neurol Sci 1981; 52:25–36.

128. Kunst AE, Looman CW, Mackenbach JP. Outdoor air temperature and mortality in The Netherlands: a time-series analysis. Am J Epidemiol 1993; 137:331–341.

129. Woodhouse PR, Khaw KT, Plummer M. Seasonal variation of serum lipids in an elderly population. Age Ageing 1993; 22:273–278.

130. Keatinge WR, Coleshaw SR, Easton JC, Cotter F, Mattock MB, Chelliah R. Increased platelet and red cell counts, blood viscosity, and plasma cholesterol levels during heat stress, and mortality from coronary and cerebral thrombosis. Am J Med 1986; 81:795–800.

131. Macko RF, Ameriso SF, Barndt R, Clough W, Weiner JM, Fisher M. Precipitants of brain infarction: roles of preceding infection/inflammation and recent psychological stress (see comments). Stroke 1996; 27:1999–2004.

132. Kubota K, Tamura K, Take H, Kurabayashi H, Shirakura T. Acute myocardial infarction and cerebral infarction at Kusatsu-spa. Nippon Ronen Igakkai Zasshi 1997; 34:23–29.

133. Butchart EG, Moreno de la Santa P, Rooney SJ, Lewis PA. The role of risk factors and trigger factors in cerebrovascular events after mitral valve replacement: implications for antithrombotic management. J Card Surg 1994; 9:228–236.

134. Giroud M, Beuriat P, Vion P, D'Athis P, Dusserre L, Dumas R. Cerebral vascular complications in the population of Dijon: incidence-breakdown-mortality. Rev Neurol 1989; 145:221–227.

135. Johansson B, Norrving B, Widner H, Wu J, Halberg F. Stroke incidence: circadian and circaseptan (about weekly) variations in onset. Prog Clin Biol Res 1990; 341A: 427–436.

136. Lejeune JP, Vinchon M, Amouyel P, Escartin T, Escartin D, Christiaens JL. Association of occurrence of aneurysmal bleeding with meteorologic variations in the north of France (see comments). Stroke 1994; 25:338–341.

137. Fogelholm RR, Turjanmaa VM, Nuutila MT, Murros KE, Sarna S. Diurnal blood pressure variations and onset of subarachnoid haemorrhage: a population-based study. J Hypertens 1995; 13:495–498.

138. Sloan MA, Price TR, Foulkes MA, Marler JR, Mohr JP, Hier DB, Wolf PA, Caplan LR. Circadian rhythmicity of stroke onset: intracerebral and subarachnoid hemorrhage. Stroke 1992; 23:1420–1426.

139. Kleinpeter G, Schatzer R, Bock F. Is blood pressure really a trigger for the circadian rhythm of subarachnoid hemorrhage? Stroke 1995; 26:1805–1810.

140. Shiokawa K, Takakura K, Kagawa M, Satoh K. Studies on factors influencing the attack of subarachnoid hemorrhage during labor. Sangyo Eiseigaku Zasshi 1995; 37:169–175.

141. Gallerani M, Portaluppi F, Maida G, Chieregato A, Calzolari F, Trapella G, Man-

fredini R. Circadian and circannual rhythmicity in the occurrence of subarachnoid hemorrhage. Stroke 1996; 27:1793–1797.

142. Vermeer SE, Rinkel GJ, Algra A. Circadian fluctuations in onset of subarachnoid hemorrhage. New data on aneurysmal and perimesencephalic hemorrhage and a systematic review. Stroke 1997; 28:805–808.

143. Turton MB, Deegan T. Circadian variations of plasma catecholamine, cortisol and immunoreactive insulin concentrations in supine subjects. Clin Chim Acta 1974; 55:389–397.

144. Mann S, Craig MW, Melville DI, Balasubramanian V, Raftery EB. Physical activity and the circadian rhythm of blood pressure. Clin Sci 1979; 57(suppl 5):291s–294s.

145. Mancia G, Ferrari A, Gregorini L, Parati G, Pomidossi G, Bertinieri G, Grassi G, di Rienzo M, Pedotti A, Zanchetti A. Blood pressure and heart rate variabilities in normotensive and hypertensive human beings. Circ Res 1983; 53:96–104.

146. Lynch P. Ruptured cerebral aneurysm and brawling (letter). BMJ 1979; 1:1793–1794.

147. Locksley HB. Natural history of subarachnoid hemorrhage, intracranial aneurysms and arteriovenous malformations. Based on 6368 cases in the cooperative study. J Neurosurg 1966; 25:219–239.

148. Lundberg PO, Osterman PO. The benign and malignant forms of orgasmic cephalgia. Headache 1974; 14:164–165.

149. Schievink WI, Karemaker JM, Hageman LM, van der Werf DJ. Circumstances surrounding aneurysmal subarachnoid hemorrhage. Surg Neurol 1989; 32:266–272.

150. Kelly-Hayes M, Wolf PA, Kase CS, Brand FN, McGuirk JM, D'Agostino RB. Temporal patterns of stroke onset: The Framingham Study. Stroke 1995; 26:1343–1347.

151. Hillbom M, Kaste M. Alcohol intoxication: a risk factor for primary subarachnoid hemorrhage. Neurology 1982; 32:706–711.

152. Juvela S, Hillbom M, Numminen H, Koskinen P. Cigarette smoking and alcohol consumption as risk factors for aneurysmal subarachnoid hemorrhage. Stroke 1993; 24:639–646.

153. Teunissen L, Rinkel G, Algra A, van Gijn J. Risk factors for subarachnoid hemorrhage: a systematic review. Stroke 1996; 27:544–549.

154. Longstreth WT Jr, Nelson LM, Koepsell TD, van Belle G. Cigarette smoking, alcohol use, and subarachnoid hemorrhage. Stroke 1992; 23:1242–1249.

155. Ramirez-Lassepas M, Haus E, Lakatua DJ, Sackett L, Swoyer J. Seasonal (circannual) periodicity of spontaneous intracerebral hemorrhage in Minnesota. Ann Neurol 1980; 8:539–541.

156. Capon A, Demeurisse G, Zheng L. Seasonal variation of cerebral hemorrhage in 236 consecutive cases in Brussels. Stroke 1992; 23:24–27.

157. Vinall PE, Maislin G, Michele JJ, Deitch C, Simeone FA. Seasonal and latitudinal occurrence of cerebral vasospasm and subarachnoid hemorrhage in the northern hemisphere. Epidemiology 1994; 5:302–308.

158. Giroud M, Beuriat P, Vion P, D'Athis PH, Dusserre L, Dumas R. Stroke in a French prospective population study. Neuroepidemiology 1989; 8:97–104.

159. Chyatte D, Chen TL, Bronstein K, Brass LM. Seasonal fluctuation in the incidence

of intracranial aneurysm rupture and its relationship to changing climatic conditions (see comments). J Neurosurg 1994; 81:525–530.

160. Rosenorn J, Ronde F, Eskesen V, Schmidt K. Seasonal variation of aneurysmal subarachnoid haemorrhage. Acta Neurochir 1988; 93:24–27.

161. Gordon PC. The epidemiology of cerebral vascular disease in Canada: an analysis of mortality data. Can Med Assoc J 1966; 95:1004–1011.

162. Tsementzis SA, Kennet RP, Hitchcock ER, Gill JS, Beevers DG. Seasonal variation of cerebrovascular diseases. Acta Neurochir 1991; 111:80–83.

163. Rosenow F, Hojer C, Meyer-Lohmann C, Hilgers RD, Muhlhofer H, Kleindienst A, Owega A, Koning W, Heiss WD. Spontaneous intracerebral hemorrhage: prognostic factors in 896 cases. Acta Neurol Scand 1997; 96:174–182.

164. Juvela S. Prevalence of risk factors in spontaneous intracerebral hemorrhage and aneurysmal subarachnoid hemorrhage. Arch Neurol 1996; 53:734–740.

165. Gallerani M, Trappella G, Manfredini R, Pasin M, Napolitano M, Migliore A. Acute intracerebral haemorrhage: circadian and circannual patterns of onset. Acta Neurol Scand 1994; 89:280–286.

166. Arboix A, Marti-Vilalta JL. Circadian rhythm and lacunar syndromes. Rev Clin Esp 1997; 197:757–759.

167. Deng JY. Care and analysis of cerebral hemorrhage. Chung Hua Hu Li Tsa Chih 1997; 32:497–498.

168. Lebensztejn W, Jackiewicz H, Klepacki Z, Wisniewska Z, Pryszmont M, Hajdul H. Electrocardiographic changes in acute and past cerebral stroke. Neurol Neurochir Pol 1975; 9:473–479.

169. Yamamoto K, Ikeda U, Fukazawa H, Shimada K. Circadian variation in incidence of cardioembolism. Am J Cardiol 1996; 78:1312–1314.

170. Lavery CE, Mittleman MA, Cohen MC, Muller JE, Verrier RL. Nonuniform nighttime distribution of acute cardiac events: a possible effect of sleep states. Circulation 1997; 96:3321–3327.

171. Verrier RL, Muller JE, Hobson JA. Sleep, dreams, and sudden death: the case for sleep as an autonomic stress test for the heart. Cardiovasc Res 1996; 31:181–211.

172. Somers VK, Dyken ME, Mark AL, Abboud FM. Sympathetic-nerve activity during sleep in normal subjects (see comments). N Engl J Med 1993; 328:303–307.

173. Dickerson LW, Huang AH, Thurnher MM, Nearing BD, Verrier RL. Relationship between coronary hemodynamic changes and the phasic events of rapid eye movement sleep. Sleep 1993; 16:550–557.

174. Mancia G. Autonomic modulation of the cardiovascular system during sleep (editorial; comment). N Engl J Med 1993; 328:347–349.

175. Mooe T, Rabben T, Wiklund U, Franklin KA, Eriksson P. Sleep-disordered breathing in men with coronary artery disease. Chest 1996; 109:659–663.

176. Riess M, Koehler U, Gueldenring D, Fett I, Naumann-Koch C, Peter JH, Ploch T, Stellwaag M, Blanke H, von Wichert P. Results of left heart catheterization study in 64 patients with nocturnal disorders of respiratory control (sleep apnea). Pneumologie 1989; 43(suppl 1):611–615.

177. Peters AJ, Perings C, Schwalen A, Steiner S, Hennersdorf M, Strauer BE, Leschke M. Prognostically relevant parameters in patients with coronary heart disease, arterial hypertension and sleep apnea disorders. Pneumologie 1997; 51(6):580–585.

178. National Heart, Lung, and Blood Institute Working Group on Sleep Apnea. Sleep apnea: is your patient at risk? Am Fam Physician 1996; 53:247–253.

179. Tateishi O, Okamura T, Itou T, Murakami M, Suda T, Nishimuta I, Obata S, Nagata T. Observation of sleep-related breathing disorders in patients with coronary artery disease by ambulatory electrocardiogram-respiration monitoring system. Jpn Circ J 1994; 58:831–835.

180. Hanly P, Sasson Z, Zuberi N, Lunn K. ST-segment depression during sleep in obstructive sleep apnea (see comments). Am J Cardiol 1993; 71:1341–1345.

15

Respiratory and Cardiac Activity During Sleep Onset

JOHN TRINDER

University of Melbourne
Parkville, Victoria, Australia

I. Introduction

This chapter is concerned with the regulatory control exerted by sleep mechanisms over respiratory and cardiac activity and in particular with how that control is manifest during sleep onset. It will be argued that there is emerging evidence to suggest that there are fundamental differences as to how sleep onset affects the respiratory as compared to the cardiac system, such that respiratory activity is markedly altered, with significant changes in regulatory control, while cardiac activity is, by comparison, little affected.

Respiratory and cardiac activity during sleep in general and the effect of non–rapid-eye-movement (NREM) as opposed to REM sleep will not be considered in any detail. This material is covered by other chapters in this volume. However, the effect of NREM sleep on respiratory and cardiac activity are summarized in order to place changes at sleep onset in context. Further, this chapter does not discuss the relationship between presleep levels of physiological functioning and sleep onset—that is, the question of whether high levels of physiological activity delay sleep onset. Rather, the chapter describes the normal changes that occur in respiratory and cardiac activity as one goes to sleep.

II. Respiration and Cardiac Activity During NREM Sleep

Respiration during NREM sleep has been thoroughly investigated and the basic findings are well understood (1). Ventilation is lower than during wakefulness, and while this is partly a consequence of a reduction in the rate of metabolism during sleep, there is a reduction in ventilation over and above the fall in metabolism, as indicated by a rise in Pa_{CO_2}. Sleep is also associated with a rise in airway resistance and the loss of a number of protective reflex mechanisms, such as the reflex compensation for increases in inspiratory load (1,2).

Most authors have interpreted the fall in ventilation as being a consequence of a change in the regulatory control of respiration during sleep, although the precise nature of the change remains uncertain. A widely supported view has been that, during wakefulness, ventilation is augmented by a tonic excitatory component, referred to as the ''wakefulness stimulus,'' but that this component is inactivated during sleep (3). Neurophysiologically the effect has been identified with respiratory-related cells in the reticular formation, which are tonically active in wakefulness but are not respiratory cycle–dependent. It has been shown that during sleep these cells become inactive, suggesting a fall in respiratory drive and thus a reduction in ventilation (4).

The pathway through which sleep affects ventilation has been extensively investigated. One view has been that the withdrawal of the wakefulness stimulus directly reduces ventilatory drive to the respiratory pump muscles (1,3). Alternatively, it has been suggested that ventilation falls as a consequence of poor compensation for an increase in airway resistance (5). It is likely that both components contribute. There are a number of observations indicating that ventilatory drive is lower during sleep. For example, manipulations that have eliminated or minimize the role of the upper airway, as in the case of patients with tracheostomies (6) and normal individuals on CPAP (7), are associated with lower levels of ventilation. Further, the CO_2 threshold at which pump muscle activity is recruited is higher during sleep than wakefulness (8). On the other hand, it is well established that airway resistance is elevated and load compensation reduced during sleep (5).

Cardiac output is also decreased during NREM sleep as compared to wakefulness. This occurs as a consequence of a fall in heart rate (HR). Blood pressure (BP) also falls, in part because of the decrease in HR and in part because of a decrease in peripheral resistance (9,10). However, the complexity of cardiac control makes it difficult to determine whether changes in the pattern of cardiac activity are direct effects of sleep or are the consequence of other sleep related changes, such as the fall in metabolic rate (11) and thermoregulatory changes (12). Similarly, the extent to which these changes are due to sympathetic inhibition or vagal excitation has not yet been clearly resolved.

A variety of studies in both animals and humans have indicated that parasympathetic activity is reduced during NREM sleep. In animals, studies have shown that sympathectomy does not affect the fall in HR from wakefulness to NREM sleep (13), suggesting that the fall in HR is due to increases in parasympathetic activity. Studies in humans using respiratory sinus arrhythmia (RSA) have also shown increases in parasympathetic activity during NREM sleep (14–17). However, a recent study has questioned whether this is a sleep effect (18). Using a constant routine technique, it was shown that there was a rise in parasympathetic activity (RSA) in association with subject's normal sleep onset followed by a reduction in activity in the second half of the sleep period independent of whether subjects were allowed to sleep, raising the possibility that the effect is attributable to the circadian system (Fig. 1).

As indicated above, animal studies suggest that sympathetic inhibition does not contribute to the fall in HR (13). Further, recordings from renal and cervical sympathetic nerves in cats show only small decreases (19) or no change (20,21) in sympathetic activity during NREM sleep. However, consistent with the fall in BP, there does appear to be a reduction in sympathetic vasomotor tone (22) and direct measures of sympathetic nerve activity to skeletal-muscle blood vessels in humans indicates reduced activity during NREM sleep (23–25). These studies provide the strongest evidence yet of a reduction in sympathetic activity during NREM sleep. Nevertheless, it should be noted that microneurographic techniques are intrusive and the observed sleep-wake differences may reflect elevated sympathetic activity during wakefulness as a consequence of the stressful procedures rather than a fall during sleep.

In contrast to the measurement of sympathetic neural activity, studies in humans using the 0.1-Hz peak component obtained from period analyses of heart rate variability suggest that sympathetic activity is unaffected or only slightly reduced during NREM sleep (14–17,26–28). However, these data are difficult to interpret, as recent evidence clearly indicates that the 0.1-Hz peak is not a pure measure of sympathetic activity but rather has a significant parasympathetic input (29). Preejection period (PEP), a variable considered to be a particularly good measure of sympathetic activity (29), has been shown to be elevated (reduced sympathetic activity) during NREM sleep over the sleep period (18,30), an effect specifically associated with sleep (see Fig. 1). Thus, there is strong evidence that sympathetic outflow to vascular beds, particularly to skeletal muscles, is reduced in sleep, leading to vasodilatation and a reduction in BP. However, whether sympathetic activation of the heart is altered remains uncertain.

It should be noted that studies of autonomic functioning during sleep have generally employed a strategy whereby stable periods of wakefulness have been compared to stable periods of NREM or REM sleep under the implicit assumption that the time of measurement within a state is not critical. In assessing NREM

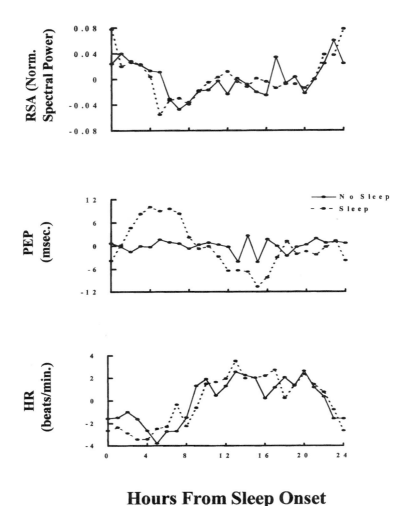

Hours From Sleep Onset

Figure 1 Average RSA (proportion of power spectrum), PEP (msec) and HR (beats per minute) ordered according to time from subject's normal sleep onset. Solid lines, nonsleep routine; dashed lines, sleep routine. Values for each subject standardized to a mean of zero. RSA shows a similar 24-hr variation for sleep and no sleep conditions, suggesting a circadian influence with peak (parasympathetic) activity coinciding with sleep onset. PEP shows a sleep related effect with an increase (decrease in sympathetic activity) during sleep, while HR reflects both sleep and circadian influences. (From Ref. 18.)

sleep, this typically involves comparing presleep wakefulness with the NREM phase of the first sleep cycle. The observations that RSA, PEP, and HR show changes over the sleep period (18,30,31) and that RSA may be under circadian system control (18) indicate that comparisons between sleep and wakefulness are likely to be dependent on when each state is sampled.

III. Sleep Onset

Before describing respiratory activity during sleep onset, it would be of value to comment on the nature of the sleep onset process. Sleep onset does not usually consist of a single transition from wakefulness to sleep but rather involves alternations between transient periods of wakefulness and sleep before stable sleep is obtained. Thus, during sleep onset, there is a period during which the sleep-wake state is unstable. This instability often continues after sleep spindles and K complexes are observed in the electroencephalogram (EEG), with brief arousals interrupting stage 2 sleep. Thus, the occurrence of the first sleep spindle or K complex does not necessarily indicate the attainment of stable sleep. Given the complexity of the sleep onset process, it has been found to be useful to divide it into a number of phases in an attempt to characterize the progression from continuous wakefulness to stable sleep. One such classification, which has been extensively used in the study of respiration during sleep onset, has been suggested by Kay et al. (32). It distinguishes a number of phases based on EEG criteria. Phase 1 is the initial period of wakefulness as defined by alpha or beta activity. Phase 2 consists of alternating periods of predominantly alpha or predominantly theta activity. Phase 3 also contains alternations between wakefulness and sleep, but the periods of theta include sleep spindles and K complexes, while the periods of wakefulness are typically brief. Finally, phases 4 and 5 describe continuous stable stage 2 sleep and slow-wave sleep (SWS), respectively. The classification also allows the distinction between sleep-wake states within phases. Thus, within phases 2 and 3, an individual may be classified as being awake (alpha activity) or asleep (theta activity), while in phase 1 he or she is, by definition, continuously awake and in phases 4 and 5 continuously asleep.

A. Respiratory Activity During Sleep Onset

The study of respiratory activity during sleep onset informs and contributes to the literature on sleep and respiration in three major ways. First, it describes and comments on the nature of sleep onset itself. Second, it provides information as to the timing of regulatory changes, with respect to both sleep and the relationship between variables affected by sleep. Third, changes at sleep onset offer insight into the primary regulatory change relatively independent of subsequent compensatory changes that may mask primary sleep effects in measurements taken during stable sleep. To illustrate this last point, measurements during stable sleep have shown diaphragmatic electromyographic activity (EMG) to be higher than during wakefulness (33–35), indicating that total ventilatory drive is elevated, not reduced, during sleep. However, studies at sleep onset show a reduction in diaphragmatic EMG activity (36). This suggests that a primary reduction in central ventilatory drive occurs immediately upon entry into sleep and is then followed by a compensatory increase in chemical and/or mechanical drive, with the latter components masking the continued absence of the central component.

Investigations of respiration during sleep onset have demonstrated that sleep exerts extraordinarily tight control over respiratory activity. Further, the influence of sleep is manifest very early in sleep onset—indeed, at the first EEG indication of sleep (37,38). As shown in Figure 2, the transition from alpha to theta EEG activity is associated with a rapid (within a breath) fall in ventilation. The fall over the first breath or two of theta activity is not only abrupt but also

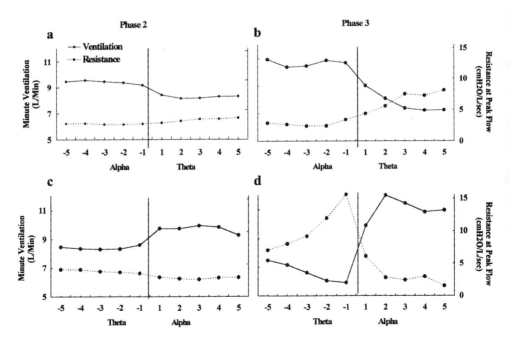

Figure 2 Group transition plots showing mean breath-by-breath changes in minute ventilation (solid lines) and resistance at peak inspiratory flow (dashed lines) over state transitions. a. Phase 2 (early in sleep onset) alpha-(wake) to-theta-(sleep) transitions. b. Phase 3 (late in sleep onset) alpha-to-theta transitions. c. Phase 2 theta-to-alpha transitions. d. Phase 3 theta-to-alpha transitions. (From Ref. 43.)

substantial (approximately 10% of waking ventilation early in sleep onset and over 30% late in sleep onset in normal young individuals) and is larger than the difference between stable wakefulness and stable stage 2 sleep (38). With the return of EEG alpha activity, ventilation immediately increases, overshooting the stable wakefulness level and then returning to this level after several breaths in wakefulness. Further, as indicated in Figure 2, the amplitude of the fluctuation in ventilation increases as sleep onset progresses from phase 2 to phase 3. In phases 1 and 4, when sleep-wake state is stable, ventilation is also stable (37–39).

Thus ventilation is intimately dependent on sleep-wake state (40), such that if sleep-wake state is unstable, as it is during sleep onset, ventilation will also be unstable, fluctuating widely with each transient change in state (38). Further, in accord with Phillipson's model of regulatory control (3), the magnitude of state-dependent fluctuations is augmented by secondary fluctuations in chemical drive. Thus, fluctuations in ventilation during sleep onset are larger in individuals with large ventilatory responses to hypoxia (41) and can be reduced by having subjects breathe a hyperoxic gas mixture (41,42).

Ventilation is not the only respiratory variable to be intimately tied to sleep-wake state. As indicated in Figure 2, airway resistance increases at the state transition from alpha to theta EEG activity and returns to waking levels as soon as there is a return to the waking state (32,43). Further, reflex compensation for loads is also dependent on state during sleep onset. During transient periods of alpha activity, normal waking reflex load compensation is active, such that presentation of a load elicits a reflex response (prolongation of inspiration) and ventilation is maintained. However, during transient periods of theta, the reflex response to a load is, as in established sleep, absent. Indeed, the reflex is lost by the first theta breath and the increase in load that also occurs with the onset of theta is translated into a fall in ventilation (44).

However, the fall in ventilation with the onset of theta activity is not entirely attributable to an increase in resistance. Breath-by-breath analysis of muscle EMG activity during sleep onset indicates that not only do the upper airway muscles—such as the genioglossus and tensor palatini—decrease their activity immediately upon a state transition into theta activity (36,45) but the activity of the diaphragm also decreases (see Fig. 3) (36). This finding offers support to the view that the state-dependent changes in respiratory control affect both direct control of ventilation and airway resistance.

To summarize, the study of respiratory activity during sleep onset indicates a very strong state dependence such that respiratory activity and, by inference, respiratory control are dependent on sleep-wake state such that sleep-regulatory control is instituted within a breath of the onset of dominant theta activity and waking control returns immediately upon the return of alpha activity. The rapidity of the sleep-related changes indicates they are not secondary adaptations to the

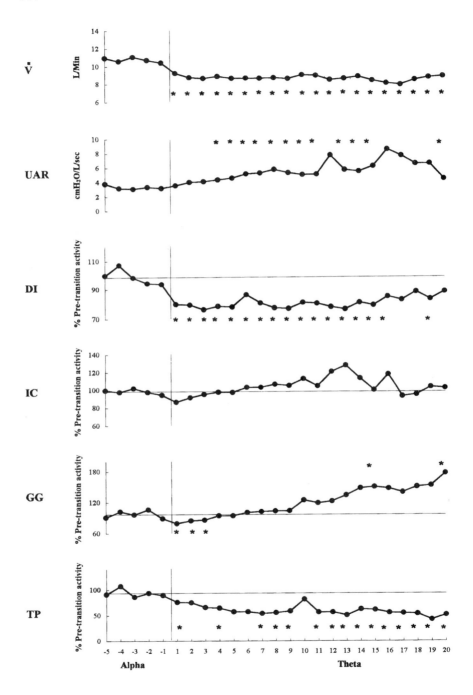

sleep state but rather changes imposed on the respiratory system by sleep mechanisms. Further, the consequences are pervasive, affecting upper airway and pump muscle activity and protective reflex mechanisms.

The relative timing of changes to different components of the respiratory system during sleep onset and in the early sleep period are also of considerable interest. For example, state-dependent changes in ventilation tend to be relatively pronounced early in sleep onset (phase 2) and become larger late in sleep onset (phase 3, see Fig. 2). However, once stable NREM sleep is attained (phase 4), ventilation remains relatively constant as NREM sleep develops (Fig. 4). In contrast, state-dependent changes in airway resistance are very small in phase 2 of sleep onset and then increase markedly in phase 3 (Fig. 2). Further, airway resistance continues to increase during stable sleep as a function of the development of NREM sleep (phases 4 and 5, Fig. 4) (46). The differing time course of ventilation and airway resistance is further evidence that increasing airway resistance is not the only cause of sleep-related hypoventilation. Of considerable interest is the observation that the NREM sleep-related rise in airway resistance is larger in young, healthy, male normal sleepers than in females (Fig. 4) (47).

Measures of muscle EMG activity also show temporally complex changes over the sleep onset period. Respiratory pump muscles, particularly the diaphragm, decrease their activity with a transition from alpha (wakefulness) to theta (sleep) (36); with sustained sleep, however, they tend slowly to recover toward waking levels (Fig. 3). Indeed, as briefly mentioned above, studies during sustained sleep have suggested that activity of the diaphragm is at least as high if not higher during sleep than wakefulness (33–35). The latter observation has contributed to the view that sleep-related hypoventilation is not a function of reduced ventilatory drive, as pump muscles were, if anything, more active during sleep. However, the observation that diaphragmatic EMG activity falls at alpha to theta transitions during sleep onset supports the view that a central drive to ventilation is lost at this time and suggests that, during stable sleep, this effect is masked by increased chemical and/or mechanical drive consequent upon sleep-related hypoventilation and elevated negative airway pressure.

Figure 3 Average breath-by-breath changes in minute ventilation (V), upper airway resistance (UAR), and diaphragm (DI), intercostal (IC), genioglossus (GG) and tensor palatini (TP) EMG activity over transitions from alpha to theta EEG activity extending over 20 posttransition theta breaths. Muscle EMG activity for each data point has been represented as a percentage of the mean of the five pretransition alpha breaths. *Indicates posttransition values that exceed the 95% confidence intervals derived from the five pretransition alpha breaths. The data illustrate the fall in upper airway (GG and TP) and respiratory pump muscle activity (DI and IC) that occurs at sleep onset. (from Ref. 36.)

MALES

FEMALES

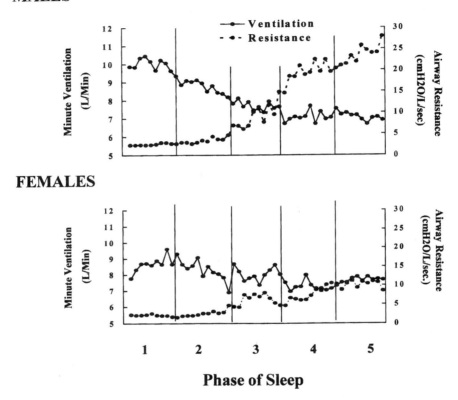

Phase of Sleep

Figure 4 Minute ventilation and airway resistance at peak flow over sleep onset and the NREM phase of the sleep cycle as a function of gender. Subject's progression from wakefulness to SWS was divided into five phases (see text). To average data over subjects, each phase was divided into 10 equal sections comprising equal numbers of breaths, and a mean value for each section was obtained by averaging data for all breaths within the section. Thus each point is a mean value representing a variable number of breaths and a 10% progression through the particular phase. The data indicate that minute ventilation falls over sleep onset (phases 1 to 4), while airway resistance rises most markedly toward the end of sleep onset and during stable sleep (phases 3 to 5). These effects were larger in males than in females. (From Ref. 47.)

White and co-workers (48,49) have suggested that respiratory-related muscles should be distinguished on the basis of whether they are phasic (active in only a portion of the respiratory cycle) or tonic (active throughout the respiratory cycle). Analogous with Orem's view (4), they suggest that muscles which are primarily tonic will decrease more during sleep than muscles which are primarily phasic. The behavior of the upper airway muscles tensor palatini and genioglossus during alpha-to-theta transitions are consistent with this model (36). Thus, as indicated in Figure 3, the level of activity in tensor palatini, a primarily tonic upper airway muscle, abruptly decreases with the loss of alpha activity and then continues to fall and to remain low as long as sleep is maintained. In contrast, genioglossus, a primarily phasic muscle, shows a decrease for several breaths and then rapidly increases its activity above waking levels, presumably under the influence of chemical and/or mechanical drive. It has been suggested that the compensatory activity of the genioglossus is critical in maintaining airway patency during sleep (49,50).

As illustrated in Figure 5, the activity of all muscles dramatically increases on arousal from sleep during sleep onset. The level of activity rebounds well above waking levels, an effect that is partially attributable to the presence of respiratory stimuli have developed during the hypoventilation of the previous sleep period. The behaviour of the tensor palatini is of particular interest in this respect. This muscle does not appear to the responsive to respiratory stimuli, such as elevated chemical stimulation, at least during sleep, yet its activity also overshoots normal waking levels at arousals. This observation is consistent with the possibility that the high level of respiratory activity following an arousal is not entirely due to the presence of sleep-induced respiratory stimuli but also to an arousal-specific effect. This hypothesis is discussed further later in the chapter.

In summary, going to sleep has dramatic effects on the respiratory system. These effects are apparent very early in the sleep onset process—in fact, essentially at the first EEG indication of sleep (39) and well before the traditionally accepted identification of sleep. The pattern of change identified during sleep onset is consistent with the speculation by earlier authors (3,4,51) that the regulatory change consists of the loss of what has been referred to as the wakefulness stimulus and that the loss of this component affects drive to both upper airway and respiratory pump muscles. Protective reflexes are also lost suddenly at sleep onset with the loss of alpha activity. However, studies over the sleep onset period have also indicated that the temporal changes in ventilation and airway resistance are different, as are the changes in different muscles. Different temporal patterns over sleep onset raise the possibility that changes in respiration during sleep may not be explainable by a single concept, such as the wakefulness stimulus.

Two further observations should be made about the changes in respiration during sleep onset. The first is that although the magnitude of the changes reported above vary widely over individuals, the changes occur in virtually all

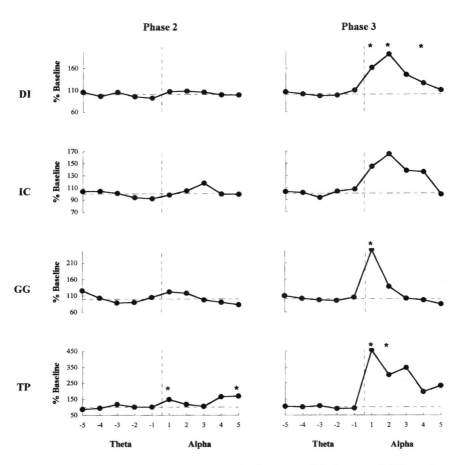

Figure 5   Average breath-by-breath changes in diaphragm (DI), intercostal (IC), genioglossus (GG), and tensor palatini (TP) EMG activity over transitions from theta to alpha
EEG activity. Muscle EMG activity for each data point has been represented as a percentage of the mean of the five pretransition alpha breaths. *Indicates posttransition values
that exceed the 95% confidence intervals derived from the five pretransition theta breaths.
The data illustrate the effect of arousals from sleep on respiratory muscle activity. (From
Ref. 36.)

individuals. Thus, the influence of sleep on the pattern of respiratory activity appears intrinsic to the normal sleep process. The second is that the association between state and respiratory instability during sleep onset in normal, healthy individuals closely matches the pattern of state-related changes in respiratory activity found in patients suffering from sleep apnea. Studies of the normal changes at alpha to theta transitions indicate that, for a brief period of time, perhaps 15 sec or so, there is a reduction in the activity of the diaphragm, both tonic and phasic upper airway muscles, including the protective activity of the genioglossus, and protective reflexes, such as the reflex response to inspiratory load. It is during this period that occlusion in the patient with obstructive sleep apnea occurs. Thus, the pattern of change in normal individuals at sleep onset is entirely consistent with the hypothesis that normal sleep-related changes in respiratory activity are one component in the development of sleep apnea, with the disorder developing either because the changes become exaggerated, or because normal changes interact with additional factors, such as a narrow airway. Indeed, it is not unreasonable to argue that sleep apnea, and in particular obstructive sleep apnea, is a disorder of sleep onset, as the attainment of a stable state (either sleep or wakefulness) in patients is typically associated with a stabilization of respiratory activity.

B. Cardiac Changes During Sleep Onset

There have been only a small number of studies of cardiac activity addressed specifically at the sleep onset process. Those studies that have been conducted indicate two effects in humans. Heart rate (HR) (52,53) and sympathetic neural activity (23) have been shown to fall in a progressive manner over the sleep onset period from presleep wakefulness to the initial period of stage 2 sleep. These changes are consistent with changes reported for established NREM sleep (see above). However, other measures of sympathetic activity, PEP, and T-wave amplitude (TWA) have not shown changes over the sleep onset period (18,52). Further, the one study to measure parasympathetic (RSA) activity between immediate presleep wakefulness and the first occurrence of stage 2 NREM sleep did not observe a sleep onset effect (52), a finding inconsistent with a number studies reporting an elevation of parasympathetic activity during sleep. However, in this experiment sleep onset was sampled on a number of occasions at different phases of subject's normal sleep period. Under these circumstances, the failure to observe an effect is consistent with the view that daily changes in parasympathetic activity are related to the circadian and not the sleep system, although such a conclusion leaves unexplained the fall in HR over the sleep onset period.

Only one preliminary study has evaluated cardiac activity as a function of the rapid alterations in sleep-wake state that occur during sleep onset (52). It reported a small and only marginally significant reduction in HR at alpha-to-theta transitions and an increase in TWA (reduction in sympathetic activity), but not changes in PEP or RSA. Sympathetic neural activity has not been assessed as a function of transitions between alpha and theta during sleep onset.

In summary, initial studies of cardiac activity over sleep onset have been consistent with studies comparing wakefulness with NREM sleep in showing a reduction in HR and efferent sympathetic activity. Whether BP falls over sleep onset has yet to be determined. In contrast to these effects, although consistent with stable NREM sleep, measurements reflecting central autonomic control have not shown consistent changes at sleep onset. There are several possible reasons for this. First, it is possible that changes in central autonomic control are relatively weak, and the current studies have insufficient power to observe effects. Second, it may indicate that sleep onset does not a affect central autonomic control. Third, the changes that occur in HR, sympathetic neural activity, and possibly BP may reflect secondary changes consequent upon metabolic and thermoregulatory effects of sleep. Thus, sleep onset is associated with marked changes in both metabolic rate (11) and thermoregulatory set point (12), either of which might mediate the observed changes in cardiac activity without changes in central autonomic tone. Finally, the failure to observe changes in RSA may reflect the possible circadian control of this variable, such that it is not specifically influenced by the sleep onset process itself.

IV.   Effect of Arousals from Sleep on Cardiac Activity

Although the fall in HR is quite small at wake to sleep or alpha-to-theta transitions, the change in both HR and BP is marked in transitions from sleep to wakefulness (54–56). Further, arousal from sleep is associated with transient increases in sympathetic neural activity (25,55,57). Indeed, the arousal effect appears to be primarily due to sympathetic activity, with an increase in HR and peripheral vasoconstriction and thus BP but not an increase in cardiac output (55). In disorders such as obstructive sleep apnea, the response of the cardiac system to arousals induced by the need to reestablish airway patency can be substantial (58). However, significant increases in HR, peaking at approximately five to seven heartbeats postarousal, occur at spontaneous arousals during sleep onset in normal young, healthy individuals (52). Consistent with the relative absence of wake-sleep differences in cardiac activity, HR rapidly returns to prearousal levels, indicating that the change at arousals is specifically associated with the arousal and not the resumption of a waking level of activity.

Current evidence suggests that the abrupt increase in both cardiac and respiratory activity at arousals from sleep is due to two components (56). One is the effect of respiratory stimuli, which accumulate during sleep but which stimulate both respiratory and cardiac activity once the awake state and thus waking regulatory control, is resumed. The second component is a reflex activation response that is engaged by the arousal process (56,59). This response is assumed to have adaptive significance and can be considered to be analogous with reflexes such as the orienting or startle reflexes.

V. Conclusion

Although the evidence with respect to the cardiac system is preliminary, the data suggest marked differences in the effect of sleep on regulatory control in the respiratory as opposed to cardiac systems at the time of sleep onset. In the respiratory system, there are large, abrupt, and pervasive changes in the nature of regulatory control that leave the system poorly controlled. In contrast, in the cardiovascular system, central control of the heart seems little effected during sleep onset, with the most dramatic changes being restricted to sympathetic outflow to motor neuron and small effects on overall cardiac activity. The functional significance of this fundamental difference between the influence of sleep over the respiratory and cardiac systems remains unclear.

References

1. Phillipson EA, Bowes G. Control of breathing during sleep. In: Handbook of Physiology: The Respiratory System. Vol. II, Sec. 3, pt. 2. Bethesda, MD: American Physiological Society, 1986, pp. 649–690.
2. Dempsey JA, Smith CA, Harms CA, Chow C, Saupe KW. Sleep-induced breathing instability. Sleep 1996; 19:236–247.
3. Phillipson EA. Control of breathing during sleep. Am Rev Respir Dis 1978; 118: 909–939.
4. Orem J, Osorio I, Brooks E, Dick T. Activity of respiratory neurones during NREM sleep. J Neurophysiol 1985; 54:1144–1156.
5. Henke KG, Badr MS, Skatrud JB, Dempsey JA. Load compensation and respiratory muscle function during sleep. J Appl Physiol 1992; 72:1221–1234.
6. Morrell MJ, Harty HR, Adams L, Guz A. Breathing during wakefulness and NREM sleep in humans without an upper airway. J Appl Physiol 1996; 81:274–281.
7. Morrell MJ, Harty HR, Adams L, Guz A. Changes in total pulmonary resistance and PC_{O_2} between wakefulness and sleep in normal human subjects. J Appl Physiol 1995; 78:1339–1349.
8. Simon PM, Dempsey JA, Landry DM, Skatrud, JB. Effect of sleep on respiratory muscle activity during mechanical ventilation. Am Rev Respir Dis 1993; 147:32–37.
9. Mancia G. Autonomic modulation of the cardiovascular system during sleep. N Engl J Med 1993; 328:347–349.
10. Parmeggiani PL. The autonomic nervous system in sleep. In: Kryger MH, Roth T,

Dement WC, eds. Principles and Practice of Sleep Medicine, 2d ed. Philadelphia: Saunders, 1994:194–203.

11. Fraser G, Trinder J, Colrain I, Montgomery I. The effect of sleep and circadian cycle on sleep period energy expenditure. J Appl Physiol 1989; 63:2067–2074.

12. Glotzbach SF, Heller HC. Temperature regulation. In: Kryger MH, Roth T, Dement WC. eds. Principles and Practice of Sleep Medicine, 2d ed. Philadelphia: Saunders, 1994:260–276.

13. Baust W, Bohnert B. The regulation of heart rate during sleep. Exp Brain Res 1969; 7:169–180.

14. Berlad I, Shlitner S, Ben-Haim S, Lavie P. Power spectrum analysis and heart rate variability in stage 4 and REM sleep: evidence for state-specific changes in autonomic dominance. J Sleep Res 1993; 2:88–90.

15. Burgess HJ, Trinder J. Cardiac parasympathetic nervous system activity does not increase in anticipation of sleep. J Sleep Res 1996; 5:83–89.

16. Orr W, Lin B, Adamson P, Vanoli E. Autonomic control of heart rate variability during sleep. Sleep Res 1993; 22:26.

17. Vanoli E, Adamson PB, Lin B, Pinna GD, Lazzara R, Orr WC. Heart rate variability during specific sleep stages: a comparison of healthy subjects with patients after myocardial infarction. Circulation 1995; 91:1918–1822.

18. Burgess HJ, Trinder J, Kim Y, Luke D. Sleep and circadian influences on cardiac autonomic nervous system activity. Am J Physiol 1997; 273:H1761–H1768.

19. Baust W, Weidinger H, Kirchner F. Sympathetic activity during natural sleep and arousal. Arch Ital Biol 1968; 106:379–390.

20. Iwamura Y, Uchino Y, Ozawa S. Torii S. Spontaneous and reflex discharge of sympathetic nerve during "para-sleep" in decerebrate cat. Brain Res 1969; 16:359–367.

21. Reiner P. Correlational analysis of central noradrenergic neuronal activity and sympathetic tone in behaving cats. Brain Res 1986; 378:86–96.

22. Baccelli G, Guazzi M, Mancia G, Zanchetti A. Neural and non-neural mechanisms influencing circulation during sleep. Nature 1969; 223:184–185.

23. Hornyak M, Cejnar M, Elam M, Matousek M, Wallin BG. Sympathetic muscle nerve activity during sleep in man. Brain 1991; 114:1281–1295.

24. Okada H, Iwase S, Mano T, Sugiyama Y, Watanabe T. Changes in muscle sympathetic nerve activity during sleep in humans. Neurology 1991; 41:1961–1966.

25. Somers VK, Dyken ME, Mark AL, Abboud FM. Sympathetic-nerve activity during sleep in normal subjects. N Engl J Med 1993; 328:303–307.

26. Van de Bourne P, Nguyen H, Biston P, Linkowski P, Degaute JP. Effects of wake and sleep stages on the 24-hr autonomic control of blood pressure and heart rate in recumbent men. Am J Physiol 1994; 266(2 pt 2):H548–H554.

27. Varoneckas G. Cardiac abnormalities in relation to autonomic heart rate control and hemodynamics during individual sleep stages in ischemic heart disease patients. Sleep Res 1995; 24A:8.

28. Vaughn BV, Quint SR, Messenheimer JA, Robertson KR. Heart period variability in sleep. Electroencephalog Clin Neurophysiol 1995; 94:155–162.

29. Berntson GG, Bigger JT, Eckberg DL, Grossman P, Kaufman PG, Malik M, Nagaraja HN, Porges SW, Saul JP, Stone PH, Van der Molen MW. Heart rate variability: origins, methods, and interpretive caveats. Psychophysiology 1997; 34:623–648.

30. Burgess HJ, Trinder J, Kim Y. Cardiac autonomic nervous system activity during presleep wakefulness and stage 2 NREM sleep. J Sleep Res 1999; 8(2):113–122.

31. Cajochen C, Pischke J, Aeschbach D, Borbely AA. Heart rate dynamics during human sleep. Physiol Behav 1994; 55:769–774.

32. Kay A, Trinder J, Bowes G, Kim Y. Changes in airway resistance during sleep onset. J Appl Physiol 1994; 76:1600–1607.

33. Henke KG, Dempsey JA, Badr MS, Kowitz JM, Skatrud JB. Effect of sleep-induced increases in upper airway resistance on respiratory muscle activity. J Appl Physiol 1991; 70:158–168.

34. Skatrud JB, Dempsey JA, Badr S, Begle RL. Effect of airway impedance on CO_2 retention and respiratory muscle activity during NREM sleep. J Appl Physiol 1988; 65:1676–1685.

35. Tabachnik E, Muller NL, Bryan AC, Levison H. Changes in ventilation and chest wall mechanics during sleep in normal adolescents. J Appl Physiol 1981; 51:557–564.

36. Worsnop C, Kay A, Pierce AJ, Kim Y, Trinder J. The activity of respiratory pump and upper airway muscles during sleep onset. J Appl Physiol 1998; 85(3):908–920.

37. Colrain IM, Trinder J, Fraser G, Wilson GV. Ventilation during sleep onset. J Appl Physiol 1987; 63:2067–2074.

38. Trinder J, Whitworth F, Kay A, Wilkin P. Respiratory instability during sleep onset. J Appl Physiol 1992; 73:2462–2469.

39. Bulow K. Respiration and wakefulness in man. Acta Physiol Scand Suppl 1963; 209:5–110.

40. Trinder J, Van Beveren J, Smith P, Kleiman J, Kay A. Correlation between ventilation and EEG defined arousal during sleep onset in young subjects. J Appl Physiol 1997; 83:2005–2011.

41. Dunai J, Kleiman J, Trinder J. Individual differences in peripheral chemosensitivity and state related ventilatory instability. J Appl Physiol 1999; 87(2):661–672.

42. Dunai J, Trinder J, Wilkinson M. Peripheral chemoreceptor contribution to ventilatory instability during sleep onset. J Appl Physiol 1996; 81:2235–2243.

43. Kay A, Trinder J, Kim Y. Individual differences in the relationship between upper-airway resistance and ventilation during sleep onset. J Appl Physiol 1995; 79:411–419.

44. Gora J, Trinder J, Kay A, Colrain IM, Kleiman J. Load compensation as a function of state during sleep onset. J Appl Physiol 1998; 84(6):2123–2131.

45. Mezzanotti WS, Tangel DJ, White DP. Influence of sleep onset on upper-airway muscle activity in apnea patients versus normal controls. Am J Respir Crit Care Med 1996; 153:1880–1887.

46. Kay A, Trinder J, Kim Y. Progressive changes in airway resistance as a function of slow wave EEG activity. J Appl Physiol 1996; 81:282–292.

47. Trinder J, Kay A, Kleiman J, Dunai J. Gender differences in airway resistance during sleep. J Appl Physiol 1997; 83:1986–1997.

48. Tangel DJ, Mezzanotte WS, White DP. The influence of sleep on the activity of tonic vs. inspiratory phasic muscles in normal men. J Appl Physiol 1992; 73:1058–1068.

49. White DP. Pathophysiology of obstructive sleep apnea. Thorax 1995; 50:797–804.

50. Mezzanotti WS, Tangel DJ, White DP. Waking genioglossal EMG in sleep apnea patients versus normal controls (a neuromuscular compensatory mechanism). J Clin Invest 1992; 89:1571–1579.
51. Fink BR. Influence of cerebral activity in wakefulness on regulation of breathing. J Appl Physiol 1961; 16:15–20.
52. Burgess HJ, Trinder J, Kleiman J. Cardiac activity during sleep onset. Psychophysiology 1999; 36(3):298–306.
53. Pivik RT, Busby K. Heart rate associated with sleep onset in preadolescents. J Sleep Res 1996; 5:33–36.
54. Davies RJO, Belt PJ, Roberts SJ, Ali NJ, Stradling JR. Arterial blood pressure responses to graded transient arousal from sleep in normal humans. J Appl Physiol 1993; 74:1123–1130.
55. Morgan BJ, Crabtree DC, Puleo DS, Badr MS, Toiber F, Skatrud JB. Neurocirculatory consequences of abrupt change in sleep state in humans. J Appl Physiol 1996; 80:1627–1636.
56. Horner RL. Auronomic consequences of arousal from sleep: mechanisms and implications. Sleep 1996; 19:S193–S195.
57. Takeuchi S, Iwase S, Mano T, Okada H, Sugiyama Y, Watanabe T. Sleep-related changes in human muscle and skin sympathetic nerve activities. J Auton Nerv Syst 1994; 47:121–129.
58. Tilkian AG, Guilleminault C, Schroeder JS, Lehrman KL, Simmons FB, Dement WC. Hemodynamics in sleep-induced apnea: studies during wakefulness and sleep. Ann Intern Med 1976; 85:714–719.
59. Horner RL, Sanford LD, Pack AI, Morrison AR. Activation of a distinct arousal state immediately after spontaneous awakening from sleep. Brain Res 1997; 778:127–134.

16

Theoretical Models of Periodic Breathing

MICHAEL C. K. KHOO

University of Southern California
Los Angeles, California

I. Introduction

The detailed reports of Cheyne (1) and Stokes (2) in the late nineteenth century on periodic breathing were also the first to link congestive heart failure to the exaggerated form of ventilatory pattern that now bears both physicians' names. However, autopsy of the patient described by Cheyne also revealed neurological lesions. Thus, Traube (3) later suggested that there were two kinds of Cheyne-Stokes respiration (CSR), one caused by heart disease and the other resulting from the medullary damage produced by decreased cerebral blood supply. This spawned the long-running controversy on whether the pathogenetic mechanisms underlying CSR are primarily neurological or cardiovascular in origin. This controversy has persisted until relatively recent times, since there is experimental or clinical evidence to support both hypotheses. For instance, Guyton et al. (4) induced CSR in anesthestized dogs by artificially lengthening the carotid arteries, thereby prolonging lung-to-brain circulation time. Since it was known that patients with congestive heart failure commonly have prolonged circulation times (5), these workers concluded that their results supported a cardiovascular mechanism for CSR. On the other hand, careful analysis of their results shows that only one-third of the experimental preparations developed CSR in spite of extremely long circulation times that ranged from 2 to 5 min. Furthermore, with such drastic interventions, one cannot rule out neurological damage in some of the animals. In support of the neurological mechanism, Brown and Plum (6) found that 5 of the 28 patients with CSR that they studied were free of heart disease, although all had some kind of neurological lesion. The debate over cardiovascular versus neurological theories of CSR became even more muddled upon the appearance of numerous reports showing that periodic breathing can also appear in healthy subjects under a variety of circumstances. It is now well known that periodic breathing is a common occurrence in normal sojourners to high altitude, particularly when these subjects are asleep (7–11). This condition disappears when the subjects return to sea level. Douglas and Haldane (12) found that periodic breathing could be induced transiently following forced hyperventilation for about 2 min or during administration of a hypoxic gas mixture. Normals also commonly exhibit periodic breathing during sleep onset and in the light stages of sleep (13,14). Furthermore, periodic breathing frequently occurs in apparently healthy infants in the first few months of life but becomes uncommon thereafter (15,16).

The appearance of periodic breathing under relatively physiological circumstances as well as in highly pathological conditions suggests that there might be some commonality to these apparently disparate entities. Since respiration is regulated by a highly complex and dynamic control system with multiple feedback pathways, it is highly likely that these periodicities in ventilation may simply reflect the dynamics of an automatic control system that is constantly attempting to restore itself toward equilibrium as it responds to perturbations from the external environment or as the properties of certain of its components are altered by disease. This "instability hypothesis" forms the basis of most theoretical models of periodic breathing that have been proposed (17,18).

Since periodic breathing has been the subject of several review articles published over the past decade or so (19–26), our intent here is not to present yet another comprehensive survey of work done in this area. Instead, in this chapter, we examine various important aspects of periodic breathing from a modeling perspective, paying particular attention to the factors most likely to precipitate CSR in congestive heart failure (CHF). We also provide an in-depth discussion of some key modeling details that are often misunderstood or misinterpreted. Although much attention has been paid in recent years to the mechanisms underlying upper airway obstruction during sleep, the present work focuses primarily on central apnea.

II. Respiratory Control Instability: Theoretical Considerations

A. Basic Notions

The homeostatic control of most physiological processes, from basic cellular interactions up to the level of integrated multiorgan systems, is achieved through the use of negative feedback. In respiratory control, alterations in arterial blood gas tensions stimulate the chemoreflexes to produce ventilatory adjustments that act to restore Pa_{CO_2} and Pa_{O_2} toward their equilibrium levels. It is important to note that the feedback is "negative" because the corrective action taken by the respiratory controller is always opposite in sign to the original change in ventilation. Thus, a transient bout of hyperpnea would produce lower Pa_{CO_2} and higher PA_{O_2}, which, acting through the chemoreflexes, would subsequently elicit a decrease in ventilation. Homeostatic regulation would work perfectly if the corrective change in ventilation (i.e., the decrease) were instantaneously produced, thereby cancelling the effects of the original bout of hyperpnea. However, in reality, there are delays in the feedback process, and it is this physical and temporal separation of chemoreception from the lungs that constitutes the fundamental reason for respiratory instability. This notion, that periodic breathing is the manifestation of feedback instability in respiratory control, is not new and was proposed in the early part of this century by Douglas and Haldane (12). Performing a number of experiments on themselves, these researchers found that periodic breathing could easily be induced by forced hyperventilation or by rebreathing hypoxic gas that had been scrubbed of CO_2 content. They likened the periodic breathing to the "hunting" of a governor as it regulates the pressure in a steam engine.

Figure 1 illustrates more clearly how this kind of instability can come about. For the sake of simplicity, we consider a very rudimentary model of the chemical control of respiration in which there is only one chemoreflex pathway and the effects of any hypoxia can be ignored (Fig. 1A). We assume that the system is operating at some equilibrium level when it is perturbed by a disturbance (X) that transiently lowers ventilation: this disturbance may be a spontaneous occlusion of the upper airways, for instance. As shown in Figures 1B, 1C, and 1D, the drop in ventilation produces an increase in PA_{CO_2} in the lungs. If the chemosensors were located in the lungs, the increase in PA_{CO_2} (ΔPA_{CO_2}) would translate rapidly into a compensatory increase in ventilation ($\Delta \dot{V}e$), which would partially or completely offset the effect of the rest of the original hypopnea. However, the chemosensors are not located in the lungs, and time is needed for the blood with higher Pa_{CO_2} to reach these receptors. As a consequence, the respiratory controller does not respond to the original disturbance until most of it has already entered the system. Since there is now nothing to offset this mistimed corrective action, the net result is an overcompensation of the original disturbance, which produces an undershoot in PA_{CO_2} and subsequently a decrease in ventilation. This cascade of events leads to an oscillatory ventilatory response, which Haldane had referred to as "hunting." A crucial ingredient of this oscillatory response is the totality of delays and lags inherent in the entire chemical control loop: if the corrective action by the controller is delayed to the extent that it becomes out of phase ($\phi = 180°$) with the preceding disturbance, there will be a tendency for the oscillation to propagate. This antisynchronous timing is crucial, since otherwise there will

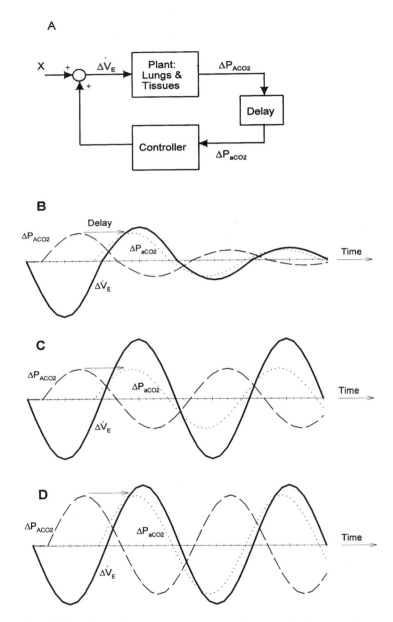

Figure 1 (A) Simplified schematic representation of the chemical control of respiration. (B–D) Illustration of how a sustained oscillation can come about (see accompanying text for details).

be cancellative interference between the propagated disturbance and subsequent corrective changes.

Whether the closed-loop response to the initial hypopneic disturbance will be a brief oscillation that is quickly damped out (as in Fig. 1B) or a more sustained oscillation (as in Figs. 1C and 1D) depends on factors other than the circulatory delay. In Fig. 1C, the initial hypopnea produces an increase in $P_{A_{CO_2}}$ that is of the same magnitude as in Fig. 1B. However, the increase in $P_{a_{CO_2}}$ subsequently produces an overshoot in ventilation that is twice as large as that in Figure 1B. In this case, a doubling in "controller gain" or ventilatory response to CO_2 is the factor responsible for propagating the oscillation, which otherwise would have been damped out.

Figure 1D illustrates another way in which the initial hypopneic disturbance can produce a sustained oscillation. In this case, the controller gain is assumed to be the same as that in Figure 1B. Thus, the only way in which an oscillatory response can be sustained is for changes in ventilation to produce larger changes in $P_{A_{CO_2}}$ compared to those in Figure 1B. The ratio of the magnitude of $P_{A_{CO_2}}$ to the magnitude of $\Delta \dot{V}_E$ is known as the "plant gain." In Figure 1D, the plant gain is doubled, leading to a sustained oscillatory response similar to that displayed in Figure 1C. The plant gain is inversely related to the amount of "damping" in the gas exchanger portion of the system. In a system that has large CO_2 and O_2 stores, there will be a large amount of damping in the system, since a given change in ventilation will lead to a smaller fluctuation in $P_{A_{CO_2}}$ or $P_{A_{O_2}}$. This is equivalent to saying that the system in this case has a low plant gain.

In the situations depicted in Figures 1C and 1D, either controller gain or plant gain was doubled while the other was assumed constant. These cases reflect only two out of an infinite number of possible combinations that would produce a sustained oscillatory response. For instance, a 50% increase in both controller and plant gains can also lead to a self-sustained oscillation. Thus, the stability of the closed-loop response depends on the *combined* gains of the plant and controller, as well as the total lag inherent in the forward and feedback portions of the respiratory control system. In the parlance of control engineering, stability is dependent on the system property known as "loop gain" (LG). To take into account both magnitude and phase considerations, LG can be represented in the form of a complex variable:

$$LG = |LG|e^{-j\phi} \tag{1a}$$

where

$$|LG| = G_{cont}\, G_{plant} \tag{1b}$$

and

$$\phi = \phi_{cont} + \phi_{plant} + \phi_{delay} \tag{1c}$$

In the above set of equations, j is the square root of -1, and G_{cont} and G_{plant} are the magnitudes of controller and plant gains, respectively, while ϕ represents the sum of the phase lags of all components that make up the plant (ϕ_{plant}) and controller (ϕ_{cont}) as well as the phase lag contribution (ϕ_{delay}) from the circulatory delay. An oscillation becomes self-sustaining when ϕ equals 180° and the product $G_{cont}G_{plant}$ attains the value of unity (27–29). These conditions constitute the Nyquist stability criterion (30), a fundamental theorem in classic control theory. Other previous models of respiratory control have employed different stability criteria (31,32). A common limitation of all these analyses is the assumption of small perturbations, so that the nonlinear equations characterizing the system can be linearized around some equilibrium point. As such, the quantitative predictions that arise from these analyses must be interpreted as estimates of those system parameters in the period immediately following the initiation of oscillatory behavior.

When the magnitude of LG is larger than unity, the system becomes unstable, so that any small perturbations due to noise entering the chemoreflex loop will be amplified, spawning an oscillation of rapidly increasing magnitude. Eventually, this growth will be limited by saturating nonlinearities in the controller and plant as these become progressively more dominant with increasing oscillation amplitude. However, the conversion of an initially low amplitude ventilatory oscillation into a stable limit cycle with repetitive episodes of central apnea can occur very rapidly, in the time course of only a few breaths (33). In a sense, the term *respiratory instability* is a misnomer, since fully developed CSR patterns generally represent highly stable oscillations.

B. Analysis of Loop Gain

Although the preceding discussion is useful for describing in a general way how respiratory instability can come about, there are a number of important details that need to be highlighted. These details strongly affect the predictions that can be made, which, in turn, provide the means for validating or improving the model. The first important point is that controller gain and plant gain, as shown in Eq. (1b), are not constant values but are complex functions of frequency. Consider, for instance, plant gain. Plant gain encompasses all the influences that would affect the translation of a given change in ventilation into a change in Pa_{CO_2} or PA_{O_2}. For simplicity, we limit the present discussion here to only CO_2, although similar considerations apply also to O_2. Lung and tissue gas stores of CO_2 affect the rapidity of the CO_2 exchange process and thus have a direct influence on system damping or, conversely, plant gain. When CO_2 stores are large, fluctuations in ventilation exert a smaller effect on alveolar and arterial P_{CO_2} changes. Thus, these stores act like a low-pass filter, attenuating the effects of rapid ventilatory fluctuations more than those of slow changes in ventilation. Further insight can be obtained by considering some of the mathematics behind this assertion. Assuming the simplest flow-through model of CO_2 exchange in the lungs, we have:

$$V_L \frac{dP_{A_{CO_2}}}{dt} = (\dot{V}_E - \dot{V}_D)(P_{I_{CO_2}} - P_{A_{CO_2}}) + MR_{CO_2} \qquad (2)$$

where V_L represents the effective volume of CO_2 stored in the lungs, pulmonary blood, and lung tissue; $P_{I_{CO_2}}$ is the inspired CO_2 gas tension, and MR_{CO_2} is the metabolic production rate of CO_2. To deduce the plant gain magnitude, G_{plant} (defined as $\Delta P_{A_{CO_2}}/\Delta \dot{V}_E$), from this simplified gas exchange model, we assume small sinusoidal fluctuations in $\dot{V}_E$ ($\Delta \dot{V}_E$) and solve Eq. (2) to deduce how these translate into sinusoidal fluctuations in $P_{A_{CO_2}}$ ($\Delta P_{A_{CO_2}}$). This can be done with the application of some calculus and the use of Laplace transforms (27–29). The resulting expression shows that G_{plant} depends strongly on the frequency f of the oscillations in $\dot{V}_E$ and $P_{A_{CO_2}}$:

$$G_{plant}(f) = \frac{P_{A_{CO_2}} - P_{I_{CO_2}}}{\sqrt{4\pi^2 f^2 V_L^2 + \frac{MR_{CO_2}^2}{(P_{A_{CO_2}} - P_{I_{CO_2}})^2}}} \qquad (3)$$

In the above equation, it can be seen that G_{plant} is largest when $f = 0$—i.e., plant gain magnitude is maximized in the steady state. However, as f increases, the expression on the right-hand side of Eq. (3) decreases, since its denominator becomes progressively larger. The inherent response time of the gas exchange process also produces a lag in the phase of the resulting sinusoidal fluctuations in $P_{A_{CO_2}}$ relative to those in $\dot{V}_E$. This lag, ϕ_{plant}, contributes to the overall lag ϕ associated with loop gain. For the simple gas exchange model represented by Eq. (2), ϕ_{plant} takes the form:

$$\phi_{plant}(f) = \tan^{-1}\left(\frac{2\pi f V_L}{\dot{V}_E - \dot{V}_D}\right) \qquad (4)$$

From the expression for G_{plant} in Eq. (3), it can be seen that administration of inhaled CO_2 raises $P_{I_{CO_2}}$ as well as $P_{A_{CO_2}}$. But since $P_{A_{CO_2}}$ does not increase as much as $P_{I_{CO_2}}$, this reduces G_{plant} at all frequencies. Therefore, hypercapnia induced by exogenous means enhances system stability. On the other hand, Eq. (3) also predicts that endogenously induced hypercapnia (increasing $P_{A_{CO_2}}$ without changing $P_{I_{CO_2}}$), such as what occurs during sleep onset, raises G_{plant} over the whole range of frequencies and makes respiratory control less stable. A somewhat unexpected prediction is that G_{plant} is also increased when the metabolic rate is reduced. As discussed below, this is another factor that promotes instability during sleep.

Equations (3) and (4) provide the simplest possible mathematical descriptions of plant gain. Much more complicated expressions arise when other important components, such as the influences of body CO_2 stores and mixing in the vasculature are taken into account. Detailed consideration of these factors may be found in Khoo et al. (27). However, the key point is that all these components contribute to the frequency dependence of plant gain magnitude and phase. Moreover, the respiratory controller is also frequency dependent, since both central and peripheral chemoreflexes have response times that span a range from 10–200 sec (34–36). The net result is that loop gain magnitude and phase also vary with frequency. Figure 2 illustrates these considerations. Using the model of Khoo et al. (37), we have computed how LG would change with frequency under conditions simulating a normal subject during wakefulness. Only the range of frequencies from 0.01–0.05 Hz is shown, since this covers the range of periodicites (20–100 sec) generally observed in periodic breathing. While LG magnitude falls with increasing frequency, the phase lag rises. To determine whether spontaneous oscillations can occur, we apply the criteria for stability that were outlined earlier. We begin by searching for the frequency at which φ becomes

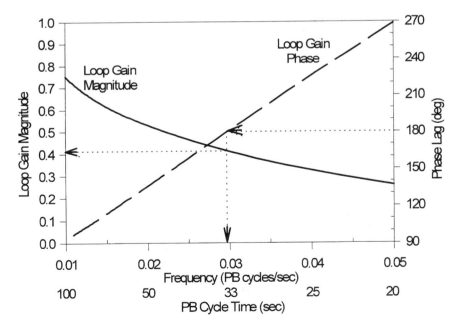

Figure 2 Loop gain magnitude and phase as functions of frequency (or equivalently, periodic breathing cycle time) in a simulated ''normal'' subject during wakefulness.

180°. In this case (as indicated by the dotted arrows), the corresponding oscillation cycle time is 34 sec. Next, we determine the loop gain magnitude at this
periodicity, which turns out to be slightly above 0.4. Thus, under the conditions
simulated by the model, the system will tend to "resonate" with a frequency of
~0.03 Hz (corresponding to the 34-sec periodicity) when perturbed by noise or
other extraneous influences. However, these oscillations will be rapidly damped
out since the LG magnitude is substantially lower than unity.

The second important detail that is often not discussed is the multifactorial
nature of LG. This arises because ventilatory fluctuations produce simultaneous
changes in both Pa_{CO_2} and Pa_{O_2}. At the level of the controller, changes in both
Pa_{CO_2} and Pa_{O_2} produce responses in ventilatory output. This may be further decomposed into contributions arising from the central and peripheral chemoreceptors. Thus, from a functional viewpoint, there is more than one feedback loop.
Consider the following steady state description of the ventilatory response to
hypercapnia and hypoxia:

$$\dot{V}_E = G_C(P_{a_{CO_2}} - I_C) + G_P(\lambda + e^{-0.05Pa_{O_2}})(P_{a_{CO_2}} - I_P) \tag{5}$$

where G_C and G_P are the central and peripheral gain factors, and I_C and I_P are
the corresponding apneic thresholds. The above controller model assumes that
central chemoreflex drive is not affected by hypoxia and that all hypercapnic-
hypoxic interaction exists at the peripheral chemoreflex level. It should be noted
that Eq. (5) is essentially the same as the controller equation of Khoo et al. (27),
with a small modification added to ensure that a residual peripheral chemoreflex
drive λ exists during hyperoxia [see review by Cunningham et al. (38)]. Using
perturbation analysis, it can be shown that the response of the above controller
($\Delta\dot{V}_E$) to small changes in both Pa_{CO_2} (ΔPa_{CO_2}) and Pa_{O_2} (ΔPa_{O_2}) can be decomposed
into 3 ventilatory drive contributions:

$$\Delta\dot{V}_E = \Delta\dot{V}_C + \Delta\dot{V}_{P^{CO_2}} + \Delta\dot{V}_{P^{O_2}} \tag{6}$$

where

$$\Delta\dot{V}_C = G_C\Delta Pa_{CO_2} \tag{7}$$

$$\Delta\dot{V}_{P^{CO_2}} = G_P(\lambda + e^{-0.05Pa_{O_2}})\Delta Pa_{CO_2} \tag{8}$$

and

$$\Delta\dot{V}_{P^{O_2}} = -0.05G_P(Pa_{CO_2} - I_P)e^{-0.05Pa_{O_2}}\Delta Pa_{O_2} \tag{9}$$

$\Delta\dot{V}_c$ represents the contribution from the central chemoreflex, which depends only
on ΔPa_{CO_2}. $\Delta\dot{V}_{P^{CO_2}}$ and $\Delta\dot{V}_{P^{CO_2}}$ represent the responses of the peripheral chemoreflexes to ΔPa_{CO_2} and ΔPa_{O_2}, respectively. This delineation is important since it
highlights the fact that stability considerations now must be extended to incorpo-

rate the effects of at least three feedback loops, as depicted schematically in Figure 3A.

In order to determine LG for this multiloop model, we define the individual components that correspond to each of the feedback loops: LGc for the central chemoreflex loop, LGP_{CO_2} for the peripheral CO_2 loop, and LGP_{O_2} for the peripheral O_2 loop. Since each of these loops has its own dynamic characteristics, at any given frequency of stimulation the responses from these different contribution sources will differ in both magnitude and phase. Thus, although $\dot{V}E$ is assumed to be the sum of $\dot{V}_c$, $\dot{V}P^{CO_2}$ and $\dot{V}P^{O_2}$, computation of the overall loop gain involves the vectorial addition of LGc, LGP_{CO2} and LGP_{O2}, so that the differences in magnitude and phase can be accounted for—i.e.:

$$|LG(f)| = \sqrt{|LG_C(f)|^2 + |LGP^{CO_2}(f)|^2 + |LGP^{O_2}(f)|^2} \tag{10}$$

$$\phi(f) = \phi_C(f) + \phi P^{CO_2}(f) + \phi P^{O_2}(f) \tag{11}$$

To illustrate how these three components affect overall loop gain, we present the results of this kind of computation performed for the example of the awake normal subject discussed earlier (see Fig. 2). The gain factors representing the central (Gc) and peripheral (GP) chemoreflexes were assigned values so that, under normoxic conditions, peripheral CO_2 chemosensitivity would constitute roughly 28% of the combined steady state hypercapnic response slope. Figure 3B shows a vector diagram in which the overall LG is decomposed into its three components: LGc, LGP^{CO_2} and LGP^{O_2}. Using the right horizontal axis to represent $\phi = 0°$, we adopt the convention that depicts an increase in ϕ as a clockwise rotation of any given vector. Consistent with our earlier results in Fig. 2, at the frequency corresponding to a 34-sec cycle time, LG is represented as a vector of length 0.4 that points horizontally to the left ($\phi = 180°$). Because of vectorial summation, both magnitude and phase of each individual component play important roles in determining the magnitude of overall LG. For example, the central chemoreflex component contribution is only about 2%, due to the fact that the magnitude of LGc is small and ϕc is 262° (almost perpendicular to the horizontal axis) at this oscillation frequency; this may be attributed to the sluggishness of the medullary chemoreflex response. At this periodicity, the peripheral CO_2 component contributes most ($\sim$77%) to overall LG. However, it is interesting to note that the peripheral O_2 component, even under these relatively normoxic circumstances, remains significant, contributing substantially more ($\sim$21%) to overall LG than the central component.

C. Nonlinear Models

It is important to recognize that a key assumption implicit in all that has been discussed thus far is linearity. This assumption is approximately valid when the

A

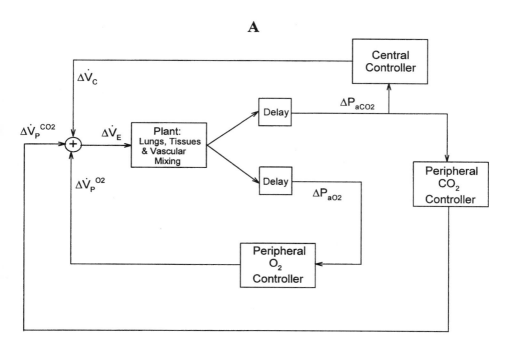

B

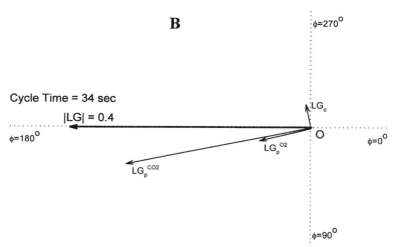

Figure 3 (A) Functional decomposition of chemoreflex control into multiple feedback pathways. (B) Vectorial decomposition of loop gain into its central, peripheral CO_2, and peripheral O_2 components.

fluctuations in $\dot{V}_E$, Pa_{CO_2} and Pa_{O_2} do not exceed certain limits. When larger changes occur, these computations of local stability must be repeated at new system "set points." For example, the expression for G_{plant} in Eq. (3) assumes that we are considering small changes in $\dot{V}_E$ and PA_{CO_2} around a fixed average level of PA_{CO_2}-PI_{CO_2}. Changes in the operating levels of PI_{CO_2}, PA_{CO_2}, metabolic rate, and lung CO_2 stores will lead to changes in G_{plant} and ϕ_{plant} at all frequencies—i.e., the curves shown in Fig. 2 will shift with changes in these model parameters.

In the analysis summarized by Eqs. (6) to (9), we underestimated the controller response to simultaneous changes in Pa_{CO_2} and Pa_{O_2}, since the calculations did not include the nonlinear term that reflects multiplicative interaction between hypercapnia and hypoxia. We have estimated that the linearity assumption would produce an error no higher than 25% in model predictions as long as the swings in blood gases do not exceed 10 torr. However, the errors increase dramatically when the changes in blood gases or ventilation become larger or when the effects of a "hard nonlinearity," such as the occurrence of apnea, begin to dominate the dynamics of the system.

To overcome these limitations, it is necessary to resort to the use of computer simulation models. The general procedure here is to model respiratory control as a system of coupled differential equations which are solved numerically by finite difference methods. Numerical solution allows stability characteristics to be explored over a wide range of parameter variations. Over the past few decades, several of these computer models have been proposed (37,39–43), each differing from the others in the level of complexity being represented and in the assumptions made about the physiological processes underlying various system components. The advantage of these models is that they allow the complexity of physiological reality to be better represented. This can lead to improved quantitative predictions. On the other hand, the increased complexity often leaves one with little physical insight into which factors are most responsible in initiating and propagating the ventilatory periodicities. We believe a prudent approach would be to employ linear analysis to gain insight into the problem and then to turn to computer simulation to fill in the details.

D. Empirical Evidence of Respiratory Control Instability

A considerable body of evidence from human and animal studies has accumulated over the years to support the notion that, in most cases, periodic breathing is the result of unstable respiratory control. We have seen from the example illustrated in Figure 3B that, under normal physiological conditions, loop gain is derived predominantly from peripheral CO_2 and O_2 contributions, with the central chemoreflex contribution playing a minimal role. It follows that since hypoxia increases peripheral chemoreflex gain, periodic breathing should also become more preva-

lent. Indeed, various studies have demonstrated significant increases in the incidence and strength of ventilatory oscillations with growing severity of hypoxia
(7–12,44,45). Taking into account the rise in cardiac output and the lowering of
the lung washout time constant for O_2 (due to steeper slope of the blood O_2
dissociation curve in hypoxia), our model also predicts a decrease in cycle time
with increasing hypoxia (27). This prediction has been validated with the empirical finding that the intensity of ventilatory oscillations increases and cycle time
decreases with ascent to high altitude (9). On the other hand, at more extreme
altitudes, the decrease in cycle time appears to level off at $\sim$20 sec (8,10). This
is predicted by the model if the assumption is made that there is no further increase in cardiac output and shortening of circulatory delay at these extremely
hypoxic levels. In several studies involving animal preparations, interventions
that enhance the relative importance of peripheral drive have also been found to
increase the incidence of periodic breathing. Examples of such interventions are
the administration of hypoxic inhalation mixtures (46), central drive depression
by focal cooling of the medulla (47), and augmentation of carotid chemoreceptor
sensitivity by blocking dopamine receptors (48).

The instability hypothesis predicts that inhalation of hypercapnic or hyperoxic mixtures depress plant gain, and therefore should eliminate or attenuate periodic breathing. This is consistent with most experimental and clinical studies of
PB (47–49), although some researchers have reported the persistence of PB despite O_2 administration (13,50,51). One possible explanation for this discrepancy
is that O_2 inhalation tends to increase oscillation cycle time and thus lengthen
the duration of apnea; this, in turn, could act to offset the reduction in plant gain.

As one can deduce from Eq. (3), a decrease in lung stores for CO_2 and O_2
increases plant gain since smaller volumes would lead to reduced damping of
fluctuations in alveolar and arterial blood gases. This explains the increased incidence of periodic breathing in subjects that are in the supine position relative to
those that are seated, since the horizontal posture leads to a reduction in functional
residual capacity (52). Several models have also predicted the transient appearance of periodic breathing following passive hyperventilation and the ensuing
apnea (27,39,41). These predictions have been validated in anesthetized dogs
(46) and humans during sleep (53).

Substantial differences in hypercapnic and hypoxic chemosensitivities exist
between individuals. It follows from the instability hypothesis that the incidence
of periodic breathing should be higher in subjects with larger chemosensitivities.
A number of studies on humans have demonstrated strong statistical correlations
between incidence of periodic breathing and hypoxic or hypercapnic gains
(8,11,54,55). Xie et al. (54) found that the central and peripheral chemosensitivities of patients with periodic breathing and idiopathic central sleep apnea are
roughly twice as large as the corresponding measures of controller gain in normal
controls. Data from the study of Chapman et al. (55) also suggest that a stronger

degree of hypercapnic-hypoxic interaction may promote greater susceptibility to the development of periodic respiration.

According to the instability hypothesis, repetitive episodes of apnea are produced when an oscillation has grown to a sufficiently large amplitude that its hypoventilatory portions attain zero ventilation. With further growth in amplitude, the apneic fraction of the oscillatory cycle duration would increase. Support for this mechanism of apnea production is evident in the study of Waggener et al. (56), who demonstrated, using a comb-filtering technique, that the vast majority of periodic apneas seen in premature infants coincide with the minimum phase of the dominant ventilatory oscillation.

III. Respiratory Control Instability in Congestive Heart Failure

Several mathematical models of periodic breathing have shown that the prolongation of circulatory delay destabilizes chemoreflex control (27,31,32,40,41). However, close analysis of the behavior of these models indicates that the relationship between stability and circulatory delay is highly dependent on other key model parameters. Consequently, in some cases, CSR could only be produced under highly unrealistic conditions. For example, in Milhorn's study (40), the circulatory delay had to be increased to 3 $\frac{1}{2}$ min before the model was able to oscillate spontaneously. We believe that this was probably due to the exclusion of the peripheral chemoreflex from their controller. The model of Longobardo et al. (41), assuming a more reasonable circulatory delay of 30 sec for CHF and normal chemoreflex gain, was able to simulate CSR with a periodicity of about 2 min. However, the model did not oscillate spontaneously and CSR occurred only after posthyperventilation apnea. This "inertia" may have resulted from the considerable amount of damping that was assumed by the inclusion of the entire volume of arterial blood (2.4 L) as a component of lung CO_2 and O_2 storage.

Applying the kind of analysis that was presented in Section II.B, we have computed the loop gain for a hypothetical subject with CHF. The results of these calculations are displayed in Figures 4A and 4B. All model parameters were assigned the same values as those employed for the normal subject (see Figs. 2 and 3B), except that cardiac output was halved and the lung-to-ear circulation delay was doubled to 18 sec. As Figure 4B clearly demonstrates, the longer delay is reflected in the much steeper rate of increase in phase lag ϕ with frequency relative to the normal case. LG magnitude is also increased over the whole range of frequencies displayed. The frequency at which ϕ becomes 180° now corresponds to a cycle time of 70 sec. However, loop gain magnitude at this periodicity is 0.8, a value large enough to permit the occurrence of underdamped oscillations in ventilation but insufficient for engendering self-sustained periodic behavior. The vector diagram in Figure 4A shows the breakdown of LG into its three com-

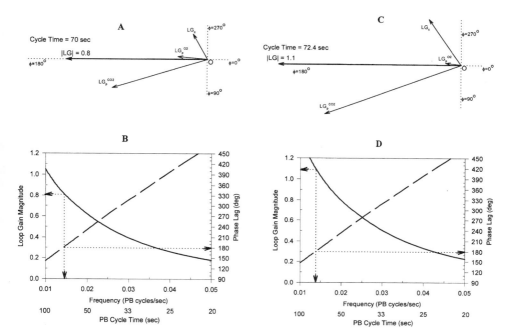

Figure 4 Dependence of loop gain on frequency and component contributions. (A,B) A simulated subject with prolonged circulatory delay and reduced cardiac output. (C, D) A simulated subject with prolonged circulatory delay, reduced cardiac output, and increased hypercapnic ventilatory response.

ponents at the periodicity of 70 sec. The peripheral CO_2 component continues to dominate, accounting for ~68% of the overall LG. However, the central contribution now plays a significantly larger role (>10%) in determining overall LG, compared to 2% in the case for the normal subject. This example shows that a doubling of circulatory delay by itself promotes instability but may not be sufficient for the generation of self-sustained oscillation. Figures 4C and 4D illustrate the results of another simulation of CSR in CHF. Here, in addition to the assumption of a doubling in circulatory delay, we have also assumed a doubling of the hypercapnic sensitivities of both central and peripheral chemoreceptors; the hypoxic sensitivity in normocapnia was left unchanged (see 61). The computations indicate that these alterations in model parameters elevate the loop gain magnitude (at $\phi = 180°$) to a value exceeding unity, thus allowing self-sustained oscillation to occur at a periodicity of approximately 72 sec.

The model calculations displayed in Figure 4 suggest that an increased controller gain or some other supplemental factor may be the distinguishing parameter that differentiates subjects with CSR from those without CSR in the population of patients with CHF. Indeed, while CSR is a common occurrence, it does not occur in all subjects with CHF (57). Both groups of CHF patients have been found to have similar left ventricular ejection fraction (58–60) and similar lung-to-ear circulatory delay (60). Recently, Wilcox et al. (61) found, in 34 CHF patients with CSR, hypercapnic ventilatory response slopes that were, on average, approximately twice the levels found in normals and patients with obstructive sleep apnea. Hypoxic sensitivities were not different. In an earlier study, Andreas et al. (62) found a significant relationship between amount of periodic breathing in sleep and the hypercapnic ventilatory response slope. However, in the group of subjects studied, the hypercapnic sensitivities measured fell within the normal range.

We have also performed model computations using other circulatory delay times, ranging from 8 to 20 sec. In each case, we determined the cycle duration of the sustained oscillation that would occur when the hypercapnic controller gains were increased to sufficiently high levels. We found a linear relationship between lung-to-ear delay (T_D) and circulation time (CT) that followed the regression equation:

$$CT = -2.91 + 4.14 \ T_D \tag{12}$$

This result is remarkably consistent with experimental studies that have also examined the relationship between circulatory delay and cycle time (63,64).

Patients with CHF and CSR have also been reported to be more hypocapnic than CHF controls without periodic breathing (60,64). In the light of Wilcox's recent report (61), it may well be that the hypocapnia and hyperventilation stem from the higher controller gain in these subjects. Comparison of subjects from these two groups with similar left ventricular ejection fractions and cardiac output have led to the finding that left ventricular diastolic volume is larger in the subjects with both CHF and CSR (65). Increased filling pressures can lead to pulmonary vascular congestion and consequently a decrease in pulmonary gas volume. The reduction in gas stores [V_L in Eq. (3)] would certainly promote instability by elevating plant gain. Although the mechanisms remain unclear, pulmonary congestion could also be partly responsible for the hyperventilation and hypocapnia generally found in this type of patient (65). The hypocapnia itself could be a destabilizing factor if it acts to silence the medullary chemoreceptors, leaving the regulation of breathing to the sole custody of the peripheral chemoreflex, which would subject the system to considerably greater volatility.

IV. Periodic Breathing During Sleep

A. Effect of Sleep on Loop Gain

While CSR can occur during wakefulness in CHF, the periodicities that are generally observed are patterns that include episodes of hypopneas or ventilatory oscillations that are barely visible unless analyzed by spectral analysis or comb-filtering techniques (66,67). Ventilatory periodicities that include apnea and the accompanying large fluctuations in blood gases generally occur during sleep. Reduction of Pa_{CO_2} by a few torrance through passive hyperventilation can easily induce apnea in sleeping subjects, whereas the same intervention rarely leads to the cessation of breathing in wakefulness (53). These observations are due to some extent to the changeover in the behavioral control mode that so dominates wakefulness to the automatic chemoreflex-based control of ventilation that occurs during sleep. Thus, the removal of voluntary and nonspecific environmental influences may simply unmask the underlying oscillatory dynamics of a marginally stable system (68).

Fink suggested the existence of an input to the respiratory centers, a "wakefulness stimulus," that is dependent on the level of vigilance (69). The withdrawal of this supplemental drive to breathe during sleep onset is equivalent to a rightward shift of the CO_2 ventilatory response line or increase in the CO_2 apneic threshold. This produces an increase in the operating level of Pa_{CO_2}. As one can deduce from Eq. (3), this endogenous increase in Pa_{CO_2} raises plant gain which, in turn, increases loop gain, thereby making the chemoreflex control of ventilation less stable. This prediction is consistent with Bulow's observation that individuals with the largest increases in apneic threshold are also most likely to exhibit periodic breathing during sleep (13).

We have also demonstrated in model simulations that for a given magnitude of wakefulness drive, the increase in Pa_{CO_2} that accompanies sleep onset is dependent on controller gain (37). For subjects with normal hypercapnic ventilatory response slopes, the model predicts the sleep-induced increase in Pa_{CO2} to be on the order of 4 torr. However, a doubling of controller gain can reduce this Pa_{CO_2} increase to <2 torr. The form of this predicted dependence of Pa_{CO_2} increase on controller gain is consistent with experimental data (70). The explanation for this result becomes self-evident when the effect of sleep is conceptualized as a downward shift (by an amount equal to the wakefulness drive) of the CO_2 response line. This produces an increase in the apneic threshold. More importantly, for the same wakefulness drive magnitude, this downward shift produces a larger increase in apneic threshold for CO_2 responses with low gain compared to hypercapnic responses with high gain. In the extreme case where CO_2 gain is infinite (i.e., the CO_2 response line becomes vertical), the downward shift would lead to zero change in Pa_{aCO_2}. At the other extreme, where hypercapnic sensitivity is zero, the downward shift would yield an infinite increase in Pa_{CO_2}.

As alluded to earlier, Eq. (3) (see Section II.B) predicts that changes in two other factors that normally accompany sleep also predispose the system to elevated plant gain and consequently increased LG. First, as we have noted in the previous section, the change in posture from standing or sitting to the supine position leads to a decrease in functional residual capacity and lung CO_2 stores, which reduces system damping. Second, the reduction in metabolic rate that accompanies sleep can also lead to an increase in plant gain. Furthermore, low metabolic rates tend to produce longer apneas, since Pa_{CO_2} takes a longer time to recover to levels necessary to reinitiate breathing during apnea (43). This is consistent with the greater amounts of periodic breathing observed in patients with hypothyroidism (71) as well as in diabetics during hemodialysis using acetate-buffered dialysate (72).

On the other hand, it is known that the ventilatory responses to hypercapnia and hypoxia are depressed with increasing depth of sleep (73,74). This decreased controller gain would act to promote stability in respiratory control. However, we have demonstrated in a computer model that the elevation in plant gain that accompanies sleep onset is likely to more than offset any depression in controller gain during the light stages of quiet sleep, thus leading to a greater propensity for instability (75). As sleep depth increases, the progressive depression of chemoresponsiveness eventually becomes the more dominant factor, leading to decreased loop gain and greater stability during slow-wave sleep. This explanation is compatible with the well-known finding that periodic breathing occurs mostly in the light stages of quiet sleep and only rarely in stage 4 sleep (13,14,73,74). In a recent study, Modarreszadeh et al. (76) found that the closed-loop ventilatory response to dynamic changes in inhaled CO_2 (under hyperoxic conditions) was preserved during stage 2 sleep, while central controller gain decreased significantly. This suggested that plant gain was increased with sleep. In another study also employing pseudorandom-binary forcing of inhaled CO_2, Khoo et al. (77) found no significant decrease in dynamic controller (central + peripheral) gain in normal subjects during normoxic sleep. This again highlights the importance of recognizing the dynamic properties of respiratory control: decreased steady state hypercapnic or hypoxic sensitivities do not necessarily imply similarly decreased dynamic sensitivities.

B. Respiratory Effects of Transient State Changes

The process of the wakefulness stimulus withdrawal in itself constitutes a large disturbance to the respiratory chemoreflexes. For individuals with normal levels of hypercapnic sensitivity, model calculations predict that the magnitude of the wakefulness drive has to be on the order of 6 to 7 L min^{-1} to achieve the increases in Pa_{CO_2} of 4–5 torr that have been reported frequently in sleep studies (13,74). This implies that if Pa_{CO_2} could be maintained at waking levels during sleep onset [e.g., through passive hyperventilation (53)], most subjects would be apneic. Colrain and co-workers (78) have demonstrated that the reduction in ventilatory drive at sleep onset is not only substantial, but that much of this loss can take effect in the course of a few breaths. Withdrawal of a large wakefulness drive with such a rapid time course could lead to a period of apnea, since there would not be sufficient time for the respiratory chemostat to compensate for the imposed disturbance. The large changes in arterial blood gases accompanying this initial period of apnea could subsequently push the system into oscillation if LG were sufficiently high. There have indeed been a number reports of a greater tendency for periodic breathing to occur in subjects who fall asleep abruptly (13,74).

In cases where LG is greatly depressed due to substantial reduction in controller gain during sleep—e.g., in patients with primary alveolar hypoventilation syndrome—a different kind of "instability" may appear. Rapid withdrawal of wakefulness drive would lead to apnea. Since there is little or no controller gain, there is insufficient drive to terminate the apnea. Consequently, blood gases deteriorate to the point where an arousal is triggered, restoring the wakefulness drive to some extent. Breathing is reinitiated with large inspiratory drives in the initial breaths because of the poor blood gas levels. As blood gases return to normal, drowsiness may set in again and the next transition to sleep occur. Recent model simulations show that this type of instability can lead to repetitive large fluctuations in ventilation and arterial blood gases with periodicities that are roughly double those reported in normals under high-LG conditions (37,75). In a situation of low LG, the respiratory control system is also more susceptible to being affected by external influences. Therefore, respiratory oscillations secondary to oscillations in other organ systems, such as primary fluctuations in arterial blood pressure (79), may appear.

It is most likely, however, that the CSR that occurs in patients with CHF involves both chemoreflex- and arousal-mediated instabilities, since hypercapnic chemosensitivity in this group of subjects is either normal or higher-than-normal (61,62). In our previous modeling study (37), we have shown that conditions of moderate-to-high controller gain can give rise to a variety of patterns in which the chemoreflex-mediated instability interacts with the arousal-driven instability. In some situations, arousal may accompany every hyperpneic episode in the periodic breathing cycle. In other situations, arousal may occur on every other cycle. Another simulation study has shown a similar wealth of complex oscillatory patterns under conditions of hypoxic sleep (80). Figure 5 shows two examples of model-generated CSR, simulated under conditions of prolonged circulatory delay and increased hypercapnic sensitivity (as in Figs. 4C and 4D). In Figure 5A, sleep onset rapidly leads to the generation of sustained cycles of CSR, with arousal occurring a few breaths following the termination of each apneic episode. This kind of pattern is reminiscent of the relationship between arousal and CSR that has been observed in CHF during sleep (63). A study by Hanly and Zuberi-Khokar (81) has shown the frequency of arousals in CHF patients with CSR to be significantly higher than that in normals as well as CHF patients without CSR. The result of simulating the administration of a hyperoxic mixture (starting at time = 0 sec) is displayed in Figure 5B. Oxygen administration leads to a clear dampening of the periodic breathing cycles as well as the supression of respiratory-related arousals after a few minutes. This beneficial effect of oxygen therapy in reducing CSR and frequency of arousals has been demonstrated in clinical studies (82,83). One other feature in the simulation result of Fig. 5B is noteworthy. Prior to eliminating the periodic breathing, the initial effect of hyperoxia was to produce longer central apneas (35 sec versus 22 sec without O_2) and longer cycle times ($\sim$120 sec versus 90 sec without O_2). Again, this is consistent with what has been reported in the literature (51).

From the simulation examples presented in Figure 5, it can be seen that the arousal which occurs during the hyperpneic phase of each CSR cycle contributes to the amplification of the hyperpnea that is already present, thereby promoting an even more potent level of hypocapnia that acts subsequently to prolong the apnea that follows. In an analysis of breathing patterns at extreme altitude (33), we found that ventilation was significantly higher in those hyperpneic phases of the periodic breathing cycle that were accompanied by arousal than in cycles not associated with arousal. Xie et al. (84) showed in patients with idiopathic central sleep apnea that apnea duration lengthened as the degree of hyperventilation in the preceding hyperpneic phase increased.

Recent work in our laboratory suggests that the time course of the transient bout of increased ventilatory drive that accompanies arousal may be as important as the magnitude of this hyperpnea in affecting subsequent respiratory stability (85,86). Using acoustic stimulation to provoke transient arousal, we measured the time course of the ventilatory increase accompanying the arousals. These experiments were conducted on normal subjects and patients with obstructive sleep apnea breathing under continuous positive airway pressure to minimize the influence of changes in upper airway resistance. The measurements allowed us to incorporate into our original model (37) the time course of the wakefulness drive during arousal, which, until then, took on a highly unrealistic form (see Fig. 5) since this empirical information was not available previously. The results obtained from computer simulations performed with the modified model are displayed in Fig. 6. Stability of the model was assessed by determining the lowest value of the wakefulness drive accompanying arousal that would predict sustained oscillatory activity: values above this "stability boundary" produced periodic breathing with apnea, while values below the boundary produced an inherently stable response to arousal. Figure 6A shows the two types of arousal-induced ventilatory profiles found in our subjects that were employed in the simulations: one depicting a very abrupt bout of hyperpnea lasting about 20 sec (OSA subjects), and the other representing a somewhat more gradual time-course lasting over 40 sec (normals). The effects of the different arousal time courses on model stability are displayed in Figure 6B for a range of controller gains. Both cases show stability boundaries that are tilted to the right—i.e., it is easier for an arousal to lead to subsequent sustained periodic breathing when the controller gain is high. However, the "fast" arousal time course was substantially more destabilizing at low-to-moderate values of controller gain.

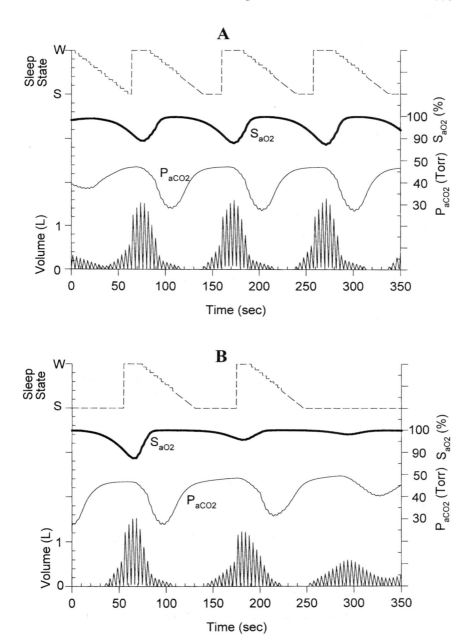

Figure 5 Model simulations of Cheyne-Stokes respiration in congestive heart failure during air breathing (A) and during oxygen administration (B). Sleep state (top tracings) fluctuate in phase with respiratory pattern and arterial blood gases.

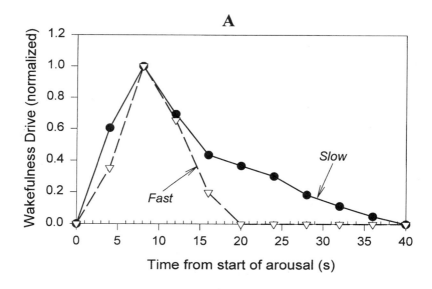

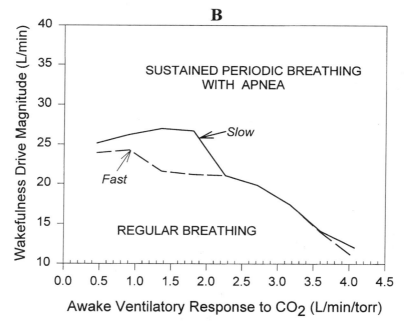

Figure 6   Effect of the magnitude and time course of the ventilatory increase induced by transient arousal on respiratory stability. (A) Time-courses of the "fast" and "slow" types of arousal patterns. (B) Stability boundaries corresponding to the "fast" and "slow" arousals (see accompanying text for details). (Modified from Ref. 85.)

V. Other Mechanisms Affecting Ventilatory Stability

A. Upper Airway Resistance

The loss of wakefulness stimulus that accompanies sleep also leads to a general reduction in tonic activity of the upper airway muscles (73). Thus, airway resistance is generally higher during sleep than in wakefulness. This may account for part of the apparent decrease in chemoresponsiveness that accompanies sleep (87). Although apneas are generally not of the obstructive variety in the periodic breathing of patients with CHF, it is likely that less dramatic fluctuations in upper airway resistance do occur. These can play a significant role in precipitating and amplifying periodic ventilation in the following way (19): if upper airway resistance were to increase with increasing ventilatory motor output, the resulting changes in inspiratory airflow would be attenuated. Conversely, negative synchronization between upper airway resistance and ventilatory motor output would lead to an amplification of fluctuations in airflow, thereby exerting a destabilizing influence on respiratory control. The consequent fluctuations in blood gases, ventilatory pump activity and upper airway muscle activity could eventually lead to events that include complete upper airway closure (88,89).

During hypoxia-induced periodic breathing in sleeping normals, Hudgel et al. (90) found in 6 of the 9 subjects that upper airway resistance fluctuated between low values at the most hyperpneic breath and high values at the most hypopneic breath; in the remaining 3 subjects, there were no significant fluctuations. It is noteworthy that, in the first group of subjects, upper airway resistance increased substantially during the periodic breathing cycle only when the ratio of upper airway to chest wall inspiratory electromyographic activity decreased below 0.8; on the other hand, in the second group of subjects who did not show significant fluctuations in resistance, this ratio did not fall below 0.8. This finding suggests one of two possibilities for the development of obstructed breaths during periodic breathing. The first is that the electrical activities of the upper airways and chest may be related to the respective pressures in a highly nonlinear fashion, while the second is that the recruitment of the upper airway muscles may be slower than that of the inspiratory pump muscles. Warner et al. (91), who studied a group of snorers, showed that the tendency for resistance to fluctuate during hypoxia-induced periodic breathing was higher in those subjects who already had a high baseline airway resistance during sleep, whereas the subjects with close to normal baseline resistance exhibited little change.

B. Short-Term Potentiation

It has been demonstrated in anesthetized animals (92) and awake humans (93) that the abrupt removal of any drive that produces active hyperventilation leads not to apnea but to a more gradual decay in ventilation. Although this phenomenon was previously referred to as the *ventilatory afterdischarge*, it is now generally known as *short-term potentiation*, since it is believed to be the respiratory manifestation of a general form of central nervous system memory. The presence of a short-term potentiation would improve the stability of respiratory control by providing additional damping to the system, in effect low-pass filtering the neural output from the respiratory controller.

Following a period of ventilatory excitation, short-term potentiation exerts an counterbalancing influence to the hypopnea or apnea that might be expected to follow the loss of chemical drive. It has been suggested that the impairment of short-term potentiation, either structural or functional, may be necessary for a given individual to develop PB with apnea (19). Some recent evidence suggests that this might be the case in CHF patients who have CSR. Ahmed et al. (94) measured the ventilatory responses to hyperoxia immediately following a brief exposure to hypoxia in awake CHF patients who exhibited CSR during sleep and age-matched normals. In the CHF-CSR group, posthypoxic-hyperoxic ventilation fell much more rapidly than in the normals, who showed the expected gradual decline characteristic of short-term potentiation.

Apart from the possible loss of this stabilizing mechanism through disease, several studies have demonstrated that short-term potentiation appears to highly sensitive to various factors that may be present under nonpathological conditions. Short-term potentiation has been shown to be attenuated by hypocapnia (95) and sustained hypoxia (96). Since CSR is generally associated with some hypoxia and repetitive phases of hypocapnia, it is conceivable that these conditions may interact to override the stabilizing mechanism after each period of hyperpnea, allowing the subsequent apnea to occur. Although it has been reasonably well established that the short-term potentiation mechanism remains intact during NREM sleep in normals (95), a recent study by Gleeson and Sweer (97) suggests that its damping effects on ventilatory changes are reduced in sleep relative to wakefulness. This, along with several other factors, may help to account for the greater prevalence of CSR during sleep. However, the connection between sleep state and short-term potentiation remains unclear and provides fertile ground for future research. Although the general consensus is that short-term potentiation increases ventilatory stability, very recent modeling work (25,26) in our laboratory suggests that this is true only when the general level of neural drive is operating above threshold; in contrast, when part of this process operates at subthreshold levels, its influence on respiratory motor output can be destabilizing. However, this result is purely theoretical and remains speculative at the present time.

VI. Concluding Remarks

While we now know much more about the mechanisms that give rise to Cheyne-Stokes respiration, there remain many unresolved issues, particularly those that pertain to the neural control of breathing and the interaction between the respiratory and cardiovascular control systems. As new empirical findings come to light, it is likely that our current models will become inadequate and newer models will have to be developed to assimilate and ''explain'' the expanded array of observations. Clinical researchers can play an important role in enhancing this process of model advancement by applying more quantitative approaches during data collection. For instance, recent techniques for estimating loop gain would be useful in quantifying the level of ventilatory stability (29,76,98,99). More informative measures of the pattern of periodic breathing can also be had by applying quantitative descriptors, such as the ''strength index'' of Waggener et al. (9) or the ''relative stability'' index of Carley and Shannon (29).

In this chapter, we have attempted to closely weave together knowledge derived from modeling with what has been derived from observation, for it is this continual interplay between theory and experiment—between deduction and induction—that drives the scientific endeavor forward. It is therefore appropriate to bring our discussion to a close with the following indelible remarks by Fred Grodins (100), who championed this approach:

> The process of modeling is slow, careful work. If it is to be more than a meaningless mathematical game, its deliberate aim must always be to explore observable implications in order to test the ability of particular physiological hypotheses to ''explain'' old observations and to support new experiments to challenge them. Since some scientists are by nature theoreticians and others are by nature experimentalists, model prediction and experimental testing may not be carried out by the same persons. This may cause emotional strains among scientists, but clearly both are necessary for the progress of science.

Acknowledgment

The author's original work described herein and the preparation of this chapter were supported by NIH grants RR-01861, HL-02536, and the American Lung Association.

References

1. Cheyne J. A case of apoplexy in which the fleshy part of the heart was converted into fat. Dublin Hosp Rep II; 1818;216–223.
2. Stokes W. The Diseases of the Heart and the Aorta. Dublin, Ireland: Hodge and Smith, 1854:302–340.
3. Traube L. Zur Theorie des Cheyne-Stokes 'schen Atsmungsphanomen. Berl Klin Wochenschr 1874; 11:185–209.
4. Guyton AC, Crowell JW, Moore JW. Basic oscillating mechanism of Cheyne-Stokes breathing. Am J Physiol 1956; 187:395–398.

5. Pryor WW. Cheyne-Stokes respiration in patients with cardiac enlargement and prolonged circulation time. Circulation 1951; 4:233–238.
6. Brown HW, Plum F. The neurological basis of Cheyne-Stokes respiration. Am J Med 1961; 30:849–861.
7. Mosso A. Life of Man on the High Alps. London: T Fisher-Unwin, 1898.
8. Lahiri S, Maret K, Sherpa MG. Dependence of high altitude sleep apnea on ventilatory sensitivity to hypoxia. Respir Physiol 1983; 52:281–301.
9. Waggener TB, Brusil PJ, Kronauer RE, Gabel RA, Inbar GF. Strength and cycle time of high-altitude ventilatory patterns in unacclimatized humans. J Appl Physiol 1984; 56:576–581.
10. West JB, Peters RM Jr, Aksnes G, Maret KH, Milledge JS, Schoene RB. Nocturnal periodic breathing at altitudes of 6,300 and 8,050 m. J Appl Physiol 1986; 61:280–287.
11. White DP, Gleeson K, Pickett C, Rannels AM, Cymerman A, Weil JV. Altitude acclimatization: influence on periodic breathing and chemoresponsiveness during sleep. J Appl Physiol 1987; 63:401–412.
12. Douglas CG, Haldane JS. The causes of periodic or Cheyne-Stokes breathing. J Physiol (Lond) 1909; 38:401–419.
13. Bulow K. Respiration and wakefulness in man. Acta Physiol Scand 1963; 59(suppl 209):1–110.
14. Webb P. Periodic breathing during sleep. J Appl Physiol 1974; 37:899–903.
15. Shannon DC, Carley DW, Kelly DH. Periodic breathing: quantitative analysis and clinical description. Pediatr Pulmonol 1988; 4:98–102.
16. Waggener TB. The relationship between abnormalities in respiratory control and apnea in infants. Respir Care 1986; 31:622–627.
17. Cherniack NS, Longobardo GS. Abnormalities in respiratory rhythm. In: Handbook of Physiology. The Respiratory System II. Bethesda, MD: American Physiological Society, 1986:729–749.
18. Khoo MCK, Yamashiro SM. Models of control of breathing. In: Chang HK, Paiva M, eds. Respiratory Physiology: An Analytical Approach. New York: Marcel Dekker, 1989:799–829.
19. Younes M. The physiologic basis of central apnea and periodic breathing. Curr Pulmonol 1989; 10:265–326.
20. Bradley TD, Phillipson EA. Central sleep apnea. Clin Chest Med 1992; 13:493–507.
21. Cherniack NS, Longobardo GS. Periodic breathing during sleep. In: Saunders NA, Sullivan CE, eds. Sleep and Breathing, 2d ed. New York: Marcel Dekker, 1994:157–190.
22. Bruce EN, Daubenspeck JA. Mechanisms and analysis of ventilatory stability. In: Dempsey JA, Pack AI, eds. Regulation of Breathing, 2d ed. New York: Marcel Dekker, 1995:285–314.
23. Khoo MCK. Periodic breathing. In: Crystal RG, West JB, Barnes PJ, Cherniack NS, Weibel ER, eds. The Lung: Scientific Foundations, 2d ed. New York: Raven Press, 1996:1851–1863.
24. Dempsey JA, Smith CA, Harms CA, Chow C, Saupe KW. Sleep-induced breathing instability. Sleep 1996; 19:236–247.

25. Khoo MCK. Periodic breathing and central apnea. In: Altose M, Kawakami Y, eds. Control of Breathing in Health and Disease. New York: Marcel Dekker, 1998.

26. Dempsey JA, Smith CA, Khoo MCK. Sleep-induced respiratory instabilities. In: Pack AI, ed. Pathogenesis, Diagnosis and Treatment of Sleep Apnea. New York: Marcel Dekker. In press.

27. Khoo MCK, Kronauer RE, Strohl KP, Slutsky AS. Factors inducing periodic breathing in humans: a general model. J Appl Physiol 1982; 53:644–659.

28. Nugent ST, Finley JP. Periodic breathing in infants: a model study. IEEE Trans Biomed Eng 1987; 34:482–485.

29. Carley DW, Shannon DC. A minimal mathematical model of human periodic breathing. J Appl Physiol 1988; 65:1400–1409.

30. Milsum JH. Biological Control Systems Analysis. New York: McGraw-Hill, 1966.

31. Glass L, Mackey MC. Pathological conditions resulting from instabilities in physiological control systems. Ann NY Acad Sci 1979; 316:214–235.

32. ElHefnawy A, Saidel GM, Bruce EN. CO_2 control of the respiratory system: plant dynamics and stability analysis. Ann Biomed Eng 1988; 16:445–461.

33. Khoo MCK, Anholm JD, Ko SW, Downey R, Powles ACP, Sutton JR, Houston CS. Dynamics of periodic breathing and arousal during sleep at extreme altitude. Respir Physiol 1996; 103:33–43.

34. Bellville JW, Whipp BJ, Kaufmann RD, Swanson GD, Aqleh KA, Wiberg DM. Central and peripheral chemoreflex loop gain in normal and carotid body-resected subjects. J Appl Physiol 1979; 46:843–853.

35. Robbins PA. The ventilatory response of the human respiratory system to sine waves of alveolar carbon dioxide and hypoxia. J Physiol (Lond) 1984; 350:461–474.

36. Berkenbosch A, Ward DS, Olievier CN, DeGoede J, Hartevelt. Dynamics of ventilatory response to step changes in P_{CO_2} of blood perfusing the brain stem. J Appl Physiol 1989; 66:2168–2173.

37. Khoo MCK, Gottschalk A, Pack AI. Sleep-induced periodic breathing and apnea: a theoretical study. J Appl Physiol 1991; 70:2014–2024.

38. Cunningham DJC, Robbins PA, Wolff CB. Integration of respiratory responses to changes in alveolar partial pressures of CO_2 and O_2 and in arterial pH. In: Fishman AP, ed. Handbook of Physiology: The Respiratory System. Bethesda, MD: American Physiological Society 1987:475–528.

39. Horgan JD, Lange DL. Analog computer studies of periodic breathing. IRE Trans Biomed Eng 1962; 9:221–228.

40. Milhorn HT Jr, Guyton AC. An analog computer analysis of Cheyne-Stokes breathing. J Appl Physiol 1965; 20:328–333.

41. Longobardo GS, Cherniack NS, Fishman AP. Cheyne-Stokes breathing produced by a model of the human respiratory system. J Appl Physiol 1966; 21:1839–1846.

42. Nugent ST, Tan GA, Finley JP. An analytical study of the infant respiratory control system. Biomed Meas Inform Contr 1988; 2:212–221.

43. Longobardo GS, Cherniack NS, Gothe B. Factors affecting respiratory system stability. Ann Biomed Eng 1989; 17:377–396.

44. Carley DW, Shannon DC. Relative stability of human respiration during progressive hypoxia. J Appl Physiol 1988; 65:1389–1399.

45. Anholm JD, Powles ACP, Downey R, Houston CS, Sutton JR, Bonnett MH, Cymerman A. Operation Everest II: arterial oxygen saturation and sleep at extreme simulated altitude. Am Rev Respir Dis 1992; 145:817–826.

46. Cherniack NS, Longobardo GS, Levine OR, Mellins R, Fishman AP. Periodic breathing in dogs. J Appl Physiol 1966; 21:1847–1854.

47. Cherniack NS, von Euler C, Homma I, Kao FF. Experimentally induced Cheyne-Stokes breathing. Respir Physiol 1979; 37:185–200.

48. Lahiri S, Hsiao C, Zhang R, Mokashi A, Nishino T. Peripheral chemoreceptors in respiratory oscillations. J Appl Physiol 1985; 58:1901–1908.

49. Dowell AR, Buckley CE III, Cohen R, Whalen RE, Sieker HO. Cheyne-Stokes respiration: a review of clinical manifestations and critique of physiological mechanisms. Arch Intern Med 1971; 127:712–726.

50. Greene AJ. Clinical studies of respiration IV: some observations on Cheyne-Stokes respiration. Arch Intern Med 1933; 52:454–463.

51. Motta J, Guilleminault C. Effects of oxygen administration on sleep-induced apneas. In: Guilleminault C, Dement WC, eds. Sleep Apnea Syndromes. New York: Alan R Liss, 1978.

52. Anthony AJ, Cohn AE, Steele JM. Studies on Cheyne-Stokes respiration. J Clin Invest 1932; 11:1321–1341.

53. Dempsey JA, Skatrud JB. A sleep-induced apneic threshold and its consequences. Am Rev Respir Dis 1986; 133:1163–1170.

54. Xie A, Rutherford R, Rankin F, Wong B, Bradley TD. Hypocapnia and increased ventilatory responsiveness in patients with idiopathic sleep apnea. Am J Respir Crit Care 1995; 152:1950–1955.

55. Chapman KR, Bruce EN, Gothe B, Cherniack NS. Possible mechanisms of periodic breathing during sleep. J Appl Physiol 1988; 64:1000–1008.

56. Waggener TB, Stark AR, Cohlan BA, Frantz ID III. Apnea duration is related to ventilatory oscillation characteristics in newborn infants. J Appl Physiol 1984; 57:536–544.

57. Quaranta AJ, D'Alonzo GE, Krachman SL. Cheyne-Stokes respiration during sleep in congestive heart failure. Chest 1997; 111:467–473.

58. Findley LJ, Zwillich CW, Ancoli-Israel S, Kripke D, Tisi G, Moser KM. Cheyne-Stokes breathing during sleep in patients with congestive heart failure. South Med J 1985; 78:11–15.

59. Hanly PJ, Zuberi-Zhokhar NS. Increased mortality associated with Cheyne-Stokes respiration in patients with congestive heart failure. Am J Respir Crit Care Med 1996; 153:272–276.

60. Naughton MT, Benard D, Tam A, Rutherford R, Bradley TD. Role of hyperventilation in the pathogenesis of central apneas in patients with congestive heart failure. Am Rev Respir Dis 1993; 148:330–338.

61. Wilcox I, McNamara SG, Dodd MJ, Sullivan CE. Ventilatory control in patients with sleep apnoea and left ventricular dysfunction: comparison of obstructive and central sleep apnoea. Eur Respir J 1998; 11:7–13.

62. Andreas S, von Breska B, Kopp E, Figulla HR, Kreuzer H. Periodic respiration in patients with heart failure. Clin Invest 1993; 71:281–285.

63. Millar TW, Hanly PJ, Hunt B, Frais M, Kryger MH. The entrainment of low frequency breathing periodicity. Chest 1990; 98:1143–1148.

64. Hall MJ, Xie A, Rutherford R, Ando S, Floras JS, Bradley TD. Cycle length of periodic breathing in patients with and without heart failure. Am J Respir Crit Care Med 1996; 154: 376–381.

65. Tkacova R, Hall MJ, Liu PP, Fitzgerald FS, Bradley TD. Left ventricular volume in patients with heart failure and Cheyne-Stokes respiration during sleep. Am J Respir Crit Care Med 1997; 156:1549–1555.

66. Goodman L. Oscillatory behavior of ventilation in resting man. IEEE Trans Biomed Eng 1964; 11:81–93.

67. Brusil PJ, Waggener TB, Kronauer RE, Gulesian P. Methods for identifying respiratory oscillations disclose altitude effects. J Appl Physiol 1980; 48:545–556.

68. Cherniack NS. Sleep apnea and its causes. J Clin Invest 1984; 73:1501–1506.

69. Fink BR. Influence of cerebral activity in wakefulness on regulation of breathing. J Appl Physiol 1961; 16:15–20.

70. Gothe B, Altose MD, Goldman MD, Cherniack NS. Effect of quiet sleep on resting and CO_2-stimulated breathing in humans. J Appl Physiol 1981; 50:724–730.

71. Skatrud J, Iber C, Ewart R, Thomas G, Rasmussen H, Schultze B. Disordered breathing during sleep in hypothyroidism. Am Rev Respir Dis 1981; 124:325–329.

72. DeBacker WA, Heyrman RM, Wittesaele WM, van Waeleghem J, Vermeire PA, Broe ME. Ventilation and breathing patterns during hemodialysis-induced carbon dioxide unloading. Am Rev Respir Dis 1987; 136:406–410.

73. Douglas NJ. Control of breathing during sleep. Clin Sci 1984; 67:465–471.

74. Phillipson EA, Bowes G. Control of breathing during sleep. In: Handbook of Physiology: The Respiratory System II. Bethesda, MD: American Physiological Society, 1987:649–690.

75. Khoo MCK. Modeling the effect of sleep state on respiratory stability. In: Khoo MCK, ed. Modeling and Parameter Estimation in Respiratory Control. New York: Plenum Press, 1989:193–204.

76. Modarreszadeh M, Bruce EN, Hamilton H, Hudgel DW. Ventilatory stability to CO_2 disturbances in wakefulness and quiet sleep. J Appl Physiol 1995; 79:1071–1081.

77. Khoo MCK, Yang F, Shin JW, Westbrook PR. Estimation of dynamic chemoreflex gain in wakefulness and NREM sleep. J Appl Physiol 1995; 78:1052–1064.

78. Colrain IM, Trinder J, Fraser G. Ventilation during sleep onset. J Appl Physiol 1987; 50:2067–2074.

79. Preiss G, Iscoe S, Polosa C. Analysis of a periodic breathing pattern associated with Mayer waves. Am J Physiol 1975; 228:768–774.

80. Saunders KB, Stradling J. Chemoreceptor drives and short sleep-wake cycles during hypoxia: a simulation study. Ann Biomed Eng 1993; 21:465–474.

81. Hanly P, Zuberi-Khokhar N. Daytime sleepiness in patients with congestive heart failure and Cheyne-Stokes respiration. Chest 1995; 107:952–958.

82. Hanly PJ, Millar TW, Steljes DG, Baert R, Frais MA, Kryger MH. The effect of oxygen on respiration and sleep in congestive heart failure. Ann Intern Med 1989; 111:777–782.

83. Franklin KA, Eriksson P, Sahlin C, Lundgren R. Reversal of central sleep apnea with oxygen. Chest 1997; 111:163–169.

84. Xie A, Wong B, Phillipson EA, Slutsky AS, Bradley TD. Interaction of hyperventilation and arousal in the pathogenesis of idiopathic central sleep apnea. Am J Respir Crit Care Med 1994; 150:489–495.

85. Khoo MCK, Koh SSW, Shin JJW, Westbrook PR, Berry RB. Ventilatory dynamics during transient arousal from NREM sleep: implications for respiratory control stability. J Appl Physiol 1996; 80:1475–1484.

86. Khoo MCK, Berry RB. Modeling the interaction between arousal and chemical drive in sleep-disordered breathing. Sleep 1996; 19:S167–S169.

87. Dempsey JA, Skatrud JB. Fundamental effects of sleep state on breathing. Curr Pulmonol 1988; 9:267–304.

88. Onal E, Lopata M. Periodic breathing and the pathogenesis of occlusive sleep apneas. Am Rev Respir Dis 1982; 126:676–680.

89. Alex CG, Onal E, Lopata M. Upper airway occlusion during sleep in patients with Cheyne-Stokes respiration. Am Rev Respir Dis 1986; 133:42–45.

90. Hudgel DW, Chapman KR, Faulks C, Hendricks C. Changes in inspiratory muscle electrical activity and upper airway resistance during periodic breathing induced by hypoxia during sleep. Am Rev Respir Dis 1987; 135:899–906.

91. Warner G, Skatrud JB, Dempsey JA. Effect of hypoxia-induced periodic breathing on upper airway obstruction during sleep. J Appl Physiol 1987; 62:2201–2211.

92. Eldridge FL. Maintenance of respiration by central neural feedback mechanisms. Fed Proc 1977; 36:2400–2404.

93. Tawadrous FD, Eldridge FL. Posthyperventilation breathing patterns after active hyperventilation in man. J Appl Physiol 1974; 37:353–356.

94. Ahmed M, Serrette C, Kryger MH, Anthonisen NR. Ventilatory instability in patients with congestive heart failure and nocturnal Cheyne-Stokes breathing. Sleep 1994; 17:527–534.

95. Holtby SG, Berezanski DJ, Anthonisen NR. The effect of 100% oxygen on hypoxic eucapnic ventilation. J Appl Physiol 1988; 65:1157–1162.

96. Badr MS, Skatrud JB, Dempsey JA. Determinants of poststimulus potentiation in humans during NREM sleep. J Appl Physiol 1992; 73:1958–1971.

97. Gleeson K, Sweer LW. Ventilatory pattern after hypoxic stimulation during wakefulness and NREM sleep. J Appl Physiol 1993; 75:397–404.

98. Ghazanshahi SD, Khoo MCK. Estimation of chemoreflex loop gain using pseudo-random binary CO_2 stimulation. IEEE Trans Biomed Eng 1997; 44:357–366.

99. Oku Y. The application of ARX modeling to ventilatory control. In: Khoo MCK, ed. Bioengineering Approaches to Pulmonary Physiology and Medicine. New York: Plenum Press, 1996:51–63.

100. Grodins FS. Models. In: Hornbein TF, ed. Regulation of Breathing Part II. New York: Marcel Dekker, 1981:1313–1351.

17

Pathophysiological Interactions Between Sleep Apnea and Congestive Heart Failure

T. DOUGLAS BRADLEY

The Toronto General Hospital
University Health Network
The Toronto Rehabilitation Institute
The Mount Sinai Hospital
University of Toronto
Toronto, Ontario, Canada

JOHN S. FLORAS

The Mount Sinai Hospital
The Toronto General Hospital
University Health Network
University of Toronto
Toronto, Ontario, Canada

I. Introduction

There is increasing recognition of the importance of sleep-related breathing disorders in the pathophysiology, evaluation, and treatment of congestive heart failure (CHF). Augmented sympathetic nervous system activity, loss of nocturnal hypotension, and increased left ventricular wall stress, which accompany these disorders, have important adverse implications for cardiac function. Obstructive and central sleep apnea (OSA and CSA, respectively) are very common in patients with CHF (1–4) and reduce life expectancy in this condition independently of other known risk factors (5,6). Their treatment by nasal continuous positive airway pressure (CPAP) can lead to remarkable improvements in objective measures of cardiac function and in patient well-being (1,7–10). Findings such as these emphasize the importance of including OSA and CSA in the differential diagnosis of conditions which could contribute to the development or progression of CHF. These observations also indicate that treatments targeted specifically at these co-existing sleep-related breathing disorders, such as CPAP or supplemental oxygen (1,7,11,12), have promise as nonpharmacological adjunctive therapy for patients with CHF. In spite of the rapidly growing body of evidence in support of these concepts, sleep apnea disorders have been given scant attention in the heart failure literature. For example, in two current review articles on the pathophysiology, investigation and therapy of CHF, sleep apnea was only briefly alluded to as a pathological entity that could contribute to disease progression in one of these (13) and was not mentioned in the other (14). Moreover, the demonstrated benefits and potential role of therapy for sleep apnea, independent of and in addition to conventional or novel pharmacological approaches, were not considered.

Why is this an important question? CHF affects approximately 5 million Americans and is the largest source of inpatient hospital costs for any single disease in the United States for patients over 65 years of age (13). Over the last 25 years, the prevalence of CHF has more than doubled, and it continues to grow as the population ages and more patients survive myocardial infarction (15). Mortality remains high despite advances in medical therapy (16): in the SOLVD treatment study, for example, mortality at 41 months was still 35% in those patients allocated to angiotensin-converting enzyme inhibition (17). Clearly, if the prognosis of this condition is to improve, new diagnostic and therapeutic approaches to CHF must be developed.

At the outset it is important to recognize that the diagnosis and appropriate treatment of sleep-related breathing disorders in the setting of CHF necessitates a novel and collaborative approach to the management of these patients, guided by specialized knowledge of sleep disorders medicine and access to specialized laboratory facilities and expertise in the use of respiratory devices. The diagnosis of OSA and CSA rests on the demonstration of recurrent apneas and hypopneas during polysomnography. When these sleep-related breathing disorders persist despite optimal medical therapy for CHF, they may require treatment through nonpharmacological means, such as CPAP, that require care and expertise for their successful delivery (1,7,8,18).

In this chapter we present evidence in support of the concept that coexistent sleep-related breathing disorders affect adversely the cardiovascular and autonomic nervous systems of patients with CHF. Evidence that therapy targeted at these breathing disorders can alleviate such dysfunction is presented elsewhere in this text. Our specific goals are 1) to present the epidemiological evidence for a link between sleep-related breathing disorders and CHF and 2) to describe the pathophysiological consequences of OSA and CSA and their impact on the cardiovascular system, with particular reference to the failing heart. We confine our discussion of CHF to patients with systolic as opposed to diastolic left ventricular (LV) dysfunction. Right heart failure is not considered. This subject has been reviewed in depth in previous publications (19–21).

II. Epidemiology of Sleep-Related Breathing Disorders in Congestive Heart Failure

Although the epidemiology of sleep-related breathing disorders is discussed in detail elsewhere in this volume, a brief overview of this subject is necessary here to put the problem of these breathing disorders in patients with CHF in perspective. Few studies report specifically on the epidemiology of sleep apnea in patients with CHF. In the course of a randomized trial of CPAP to treat CSA in patients with CHF, Naughton and colleagues (1) found that 56% of 74 functional class 2 and 3 male outpatients with CHF referred to this study had either OSA (7%) or CSA (49%). Javaheri et al. (2) reported a comparably high prevalence of OSA and CSA in a study involving a similar group of male outpatients with CHF. In a subsequent publication, these investigators reported on 81 male subjects with CHF and LV ejection fraction <45% (4). Using a definition for a sleep apnea disorder of at least 15 apneas and hypopneas per hour of sleep (apnea-hypopnea index, or AHI) 40% had CSA and 11% had OSA. When patients with CSA and OSA were grouped together, they had worse LV systolic function (ejection fraction 22% versus 27%), and were more likely to have atrial fibrillation and ventricular ectopy. Those with OSA were more obese, had higher diastolic blood pressure, and were more likely to snore than those with CSA (4). Other features specific to these disorders could not be identified with certainty owing to the small number of men studied. Furthermore, since these studies were confined to men, their findings may not apply to women with CHF. More recently, Sin and colleagues (3) reported that sleep apnea was common in women with CHF as well: 47% referred to our sleep laboratory had an AHI $\geq$ 10 per hour of sleep.

Because the means of patient referral for the above studies are not clear, the prevalences of CSA and OSA that were reported may not be representative of the heart failure population in general. However, it is important to note that the prevalence of OSA in both studies was similar to that reported in an otherwise healthy population aged between 30 and 60 years, namely 9% among males and 4% among females. CSA was rare in that cohort (22). Sleep-related breathing disorders as a whole are therefore almost certainly more common in patients with CHF than in the general population because of their high prevalence of CSA.

III. Effects of Sleep on Cardiovascular Function in Healthy Subjects

Normally, metabolic rate, sympathetic nervous system activity (SNA), heart rate, stroke volume, cardiac output, and systemic blood pressure all fall progressively from wakefulness through stages 1 to 4 of non–rapid-eye-movement (NREM) sleep (23–26), whereas vagal tone increases (24,27). The net effect of these changes is to reduce myocardial workload. Although the deeper stages of NREM sleep are characterized by relative stability of the autonomic and circulatory systems, from time to time NREM sleep is punctuated by spontaneous K complexes and arousals from sleep followed by transient increases in muscle sympathetic nerve activity (MSNA), heart rate, and blood pressure (26,28). These observations emphasize the important influence of subtle changes in sleep state on the autonomic and circulatory systems.

Sleep-related alterations in respiratory patterns parallel those of the autonomic and circulatory systems: as subjects proceed from stage 1 to stage 4 sleep, there are progressive reductions in central respiratory drive and minute ventilation and an increase in Pa_{CO_2} (29). Respiratory rhythm and ventilatory output are also very stable in the deeper stages of NREM sleep. It is presumed that this is because ventilation is under purely chemical-metabolic control (29,30). Brief arousals into wakefulness are associated with transient increases in respiratory drive and ventilation (29,31) paralleled by increases in MSNA during NREM sleep (24,26). These observations should not be surprising. Hypercapnia and hypoxia stimulate both the respiratory chemoreceptors and central sympathetic neurons, and the neural connections between the respiratory control and the central cardiovascular sympathetic centers in the nucleus tractus solitarius permit the modulation of central sympathetic outflow by respiratory drive and rhythm (32).

During rapid eye movement (REM) sleep, breathing becomes less dependent on metabolic drive and more so on behavioral factors, such as dream content (29,33). Patterns of breathing and SNA become irregular and begin to diverge: there is a further depression of respiratory drive with reductions in ventilation (29), but SNA and blood pressure increase (24,26). The cause of this dissociation between central respiratory drive and central sympathetic outflow during REM sleep is not yet clear. One possibility is that the sympathetic nervous system is not subject to any functional equivalent of the postsynaptic REM-related inhibition of skeletal muscle activity that affects the respiratory system. In any case, since adults spend approximately 80–85% of their total sleep time in NREM sleep, in general sleep relaxes the cardiovascular system. However, if recurrent apneas occur during sleep, this tranquil state is disrupted. This can have disturbing effects on the heart and circulation.

IV. Pathophysiological Effects of Obstructive Sleep Apnea in Subjects with Normal Ventricular Function

Upper airway occlusion during sleep is caused by a sleep-related withdrawal of upper airway inspiratory muscle tone superimposed upon a narrow, highly compliant pharynx (34–36). As a result, the pharynx collapses during sleep, leading to obstructive apnea. Several key pathophysiological features of OSA can adversely affect the cardiovascular system: generation of exaggerated negative intrathoracic pressure (Pit) against the occluded airway, development of hypoxia during apnea, arousal from sleep at termination of apnea, and marked surges in systolic blood pressure.

During obstructive apnea, Pa_{O_2} falls and Pa_{CO_2} rises, causing an increase in respiratory drive. Exaggerated negative Pit is generated during vigorous but ineffectual inspiratory efforts against the occluded upper airway (Fig. 1). These persist until apnea is terminated by an arousal (37). This exaggerated negative Pit disturbs the loading conditions of the heart in several ways. First, the pressure gradient between intracavitary (LV) and extracavitary (i.e., intrathoracic or pericardial) pressure is augmented, thus increasing end-systolic LV transmural pressure (LVPtm) (38–41), a principal determinant of LV afterload. In some OSA patients with normal ventricular function, these increases in afterload can trigger ischemic changes in the electrocardiogram (42). Second, the exaggerated negative intrathoracic pressure increases venous return to the right atrium. The resultant right ventricular (RV) distention can shift the intraventricular septum leftwards during diastole, thereby impeding LV filling (43–46). The higher LV afterload caused by this negative intrathoracic pressure can also reduce the rate of LV

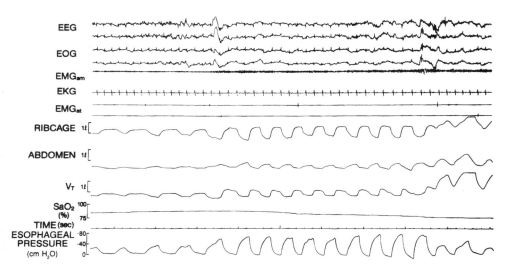

Figure 1 Polysomnographic recording of an obstructive hypopnea in a patient with idiopathic dilated cardiomyopathy during stage 2 non–rapid-eye-movement (NREM) sleep. Note the pronounced negative intrathoracic (i.e., esophageal) pressure swings during the hypopnea, which would increase left ventricular afterload by increasing transmural pressure during systole. In addition, hypoxia during the hypopnea, as indicated by the falling oxyhemoglobin saturation (Sa_{O2}), and an arousal from sleep at its termination, would increase sympathetic nervous system activity. EEG, electroencephalogram; EOG, electrooculogram; EMG_{sm}, submental electromyogram; ECG, electrocardiogram; EMG_{at}; anterior tibial EMG; V_T, tidal volume. (From Ref. 7.)

relaxation thereby increasing the impedance to LV filling and increasing LV filling pressures (39,47). By one or more of these mechanisms, generation of exaggerated negative Pit during Mueller maneuvers or obstructive apneas can induce marked reductions in stroke volume and cardiac output that are proportional to the degree of negative Pit (41,46–48). This could explain the occurrence of nocturnal ischemia and acute pulmonary edema in some patients with OSA (49–52). The extent to which each of these factors contributes to reductions in cardiac output probably varies over the course of each apnea and may be further influenced by the underlying contractile state of the myocardium.

Intermittent hypoxia during obstructive apneas can adversely affect cardiac performance through several mechanisms. Hypoxia is a systemic arterial vasodilator but causes pulmonary vasoconstriction and increases pulmonary artery pressures (19,48,53). The resultant increase in RV afterload may reduce right-sided cardiac output or cause RV distension and a leftward intraventricular septal shift during diastole (43–46,54). Hypoxia can also reduce cardiac output by depressing cardiac contractility directly (55) and by impairing the relaxation of both ventricles (56). It is also a potent stimulator of the sympathetic nervous system. The effect of increasing Pa_{CO_2} during apnea on MSNA is additive to that of hypoxia (57).

Obstructive apnea is almost invariably terminated by a brief arousal in response to hypoxia, hypercapnia, and ineffectual inspiratory efforts. In this setting, arousal from sleep is a critical defense mechanism that provokes stimulation of the pharyngeal dilator muscles permitting restoration of upper airway patency and airflow (29,37). However, arousals from sleep also have pathological effects. They disrupt sleep and play a key role in the development of symptoms of sleep apnea, such as excessive daytime sleepiness and fatigue. Arousals from sleep are also a form of startle response and, either alone or in concert with other stimuli discussed below, provoke increases in SNA and blood pressure (26,28,37).

Activation of the sympathetic nervous system is an important consequence of obstructive apnea triggered by the synergistic interactions between at least five factors: hypoxia, hypercapnia, apnea, reduced cardiac output, and arousal from sleep (24,26,57–61) (Fig. 2). During normal breathing, lung inflation stimulates pulmonary vagal afferents, which tonically suppress sympathetic outflow (60–62). When lung inflation ceases during apnea, this sympathoinhibitory reflex is disengaged, permitting augmented central sympathetic outflow. During Mueller maneuvers and obstructive apneas, there are initial increases in LV transmural pressure, decreases in blood pressure (40,41), and a concomitant reduction in MSNA, probably due to stimulation of cardiac and aortic arch baroreceptors (58,63). Later in these events, however, there are marked increases in MSNA. These could be due to chemical stimuli (58) or to reductions in cardiac output and blood pressure (41,46,53,63). At the termination of airway occlusion, blood pressure rises to or above the baseline level just after the peak MSNA is reached

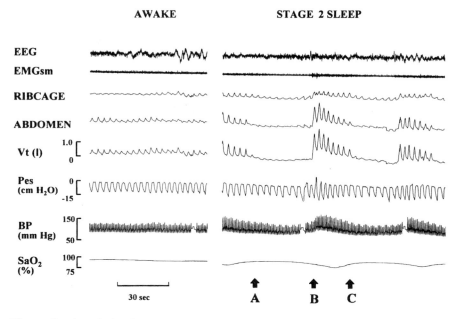

Figure 2 A typical polysomnographic recording from a patient with congestive heart failure and obstructive sleep apnea while awake and during stage 2 sleep: (A-B) obstructive apnea, (B-C) ventilatory period, and (A-C) entire apnea-ventilatory cycle. Inspiratory Pes swings during apnea indicate their obstructive nature. BP increases from wakefulness to stage 2 sleep and is higher during the ventilatory period than during apnea. These increases in blood pressure occur even though the patient was normotensive while awake and was on blood pressure lowering drugs. Pes, esophageal pressure; BP, blood pressure. Otherwise as for Figure 1. (From Ref. 69.)

(58,59,63–65). However, in two studies of healthy humans, there was no difference in the degree of increase in MSNA at the end of breath-holds with and without negative intrathoracic pressure indicating an important effect of chemical stimuli at this point (58,63). Whether this is also true in patients with CHF remains to be determined.

One possible hemodynamic consequence of this increase in sympathetic nerve traffic is a surge in blood pressure (Fig. 3). MSNA and systemic blood pressure tend to peak just after the onset of ventilation rather than at the exact termination of apnea (59,63–69). This apparent delay may be due to the time lag required for changes in arterial blood gas tension in the lung to be detected by the carotid body, owing to circulatory delay, to the time between the onset of arousal and its maximum influence on sympathetic nerve traffic, or to the

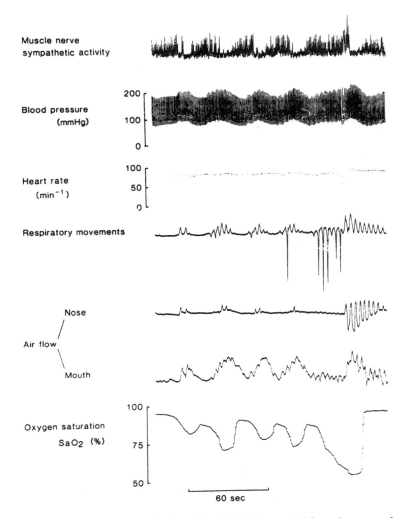

Figure 3 Muscle-nerve sympathetic activity (MSNA) recorded from the peroneal nerve of a patient with obstructive sleep apnea during NREM sleep. Note that MSNA increases throughout the apneas as Sa_{O2} falls and abruptly drops upon termination of the apneas. Conversely, blood pressure falls during apneas and rises to a peak just after their terminations corresponding to arousals from sleep. This suggests that MSNA increases in response to hypoxia and reductions in blood pressure during apnea and is acutely inhibited by sudden increases in lung inflation and blood pressure, and increases in Sa_{O2} following termination of apneas. Thus, while it is clear that recurrent obstructive apneas stimulate increased MSNA, it is not clear whether MSNA is changing in response to blood pressure or vice versa. (From Ref. 59.)

entrainment of blood pressure by the increasing depth and frequency of breathing at this time (69,70). Moreover, maximum blood pressure peaks after the peak in MSNA, suggesting either that there is a time lag between changes in MSNA and changes in blood pressure or that sudden rises in blood pressure actually inhibit MSNA reflexively through activation of peripheral baroreceptors. Thus it is not clear whether MSNA is changing in response to blood pressure or vice versa. These surges in MSNA and systemic blood pressure, in conjunction with reductions in Pit increase LVPtm not only during but also just after the termination of apnea, rendering such patients susceptible to the development of myocardial ischemia, cardiac arrhythmias, and reduced cardiac output tens or hundreds of times each night (42,47–49,51,71–74). Patients with underlying coronary artery disease or CHF would be particularly susceptible to these adverse effects (51,75,76).

Even when studied while awake, patients with OSA have greater MSNA and blood pressure variability but lower heart rate variability than matched healthy subjects (77,78). Systemic hypertension during wakefulness occurs in approximately 50–60% of patients with OSA (37,79–81). The degree to and mechanism by which acute apnea-induced decreases in Pa_{O_2} and elevations in Pa_{CO_2}, MSNA, and blood pressure might mediate long-term increases in blood pressure in OSA remain to be determined. The evidence for a role of intermittent apnea-related hypoxia in causing hypertension in OSA is conflicting. In a recent study, Brooks et al. (82) demonstrated that exposure of dogs to experimentally induced OSA for several months caused marked elevations in nocturnal blood pressure that persisted into the daytime. Nocturnal and daytime blood pressure fell to baseline levels within a few weeks following reversal of OSA. This was the first demonstration in an animal model that OSA could cause nocturnal as well as diurnal hypertension. However, exposure of the same dogs to acoustic stimuli during sleep that provoked arousals and elevations in blood pressure equal to those observed during OSA did not lead to diurnal hypertension. These findings indicated that arousals from sleep were insufficient to induce diurnal hypertension but that additional stimuli, likely intermittent hypoxia during obstructive apneas, were essential to its development. Further evidence favoring hypoxia as an instigator of sustained hypertension comes from experiments in rats. In these animals, chronic intermittent exposure to hypoxia induced sustained arterial hypertension that was mediated by the carotid chemoreceptors and the sympathetic nervous system (83–85). However, the potential role of hypoxia in provoking sustained hypertension in humans with OSA is not as clear cut.

Evidence in favor of this proposition includes the observations that chemoreceptor reflex deactivation by the application of 100% O_2 suppresses MSNA in OSA patients but not in healthy control subjects (77) and that patients with OSA and hypertension have greater pressor responses to hypoxia than those without hypertension (86). However, against this proposition are the observations that acute administration of O_2 to patients with OSA does not prevent increases in blood pressure at the termination of apnea (64), and no relationship between the degree of nocturnal hypoxia and daytime systemic blood pressure has been detected thus far in patients with OSA (79,80). Therefore, the relative contribution of hypoxia to acute and chronic blood pressure elevations in OSA remains to be elucidated.

In patients with OSA but without CHF sympathetic nervous activity decreases abruptly just after the onset of ventilation following apneas (59,65,66) owing to the sympathoinhibitory effects of abrupt lung inflation, elevated blood pressure, and correction of blood gas derangements (62,65,67). Blood pressure decreases shortly thereafter. Even so, these nocturnal events appear to have aftereffects that persist into wakefulness: daytime MSNA and plasma norepinephrine (PNE) concentrations are higher in such patients than in appropriately matched controls (59,65,87). The mechanism for this sustained sympathetic activation is uncertain but could involve an upward resetting of baseline central sympathetic outflow during the awake state. Should the same hold true for CHF, this might explain some of the variability in SNA that seems excessive or inappropriate in that it cannot be explained by the extent of hemodynamic impairment (88). Because survival in CHF is inversely proportional to cardiac noradrenergic drive (89) and to awake PNE concentration, (90), excessive sympathetic activation, in turn, may have implications for prognosis.

Finally, OSA has a number of adverse effects on cardiac rhythm that are related to the severity of hypoxia. These include sinus bradycardia, second-degree heart block, and supraventricular and ventricular ectopy and tachycardia (25,91–93).

V. Implications for Patients with Congestive Heart Failure

How might these five adverse consequences of OSA particularly disadvantage patients with CHF? Sympathoadrenal activation is a major risk factor for premature death in patients with CHF (89,90). Neurally released and circulating catecholamines have detrimental effects on cardiovascular homeostasis, symptoms, and disease progression, whether at the level of the myocyte (direct catecholamine toxicity or induction of apoptosis), the myocardial beta-receptor complex (number, affinity, or responsiveness to endogenous and exogenous agonists), organ function (altered loading conditions, development of arrhythmias), or functional status of the afflicted patient (60,94). Because sympathetic activation during sleep arises as a result of apneas and arousals from sleep and not necessarily as a compensatory response to defend tissue perfusion, it may be particularly noxious to the diseased myocardium.

The contractile function of the failing heart is highly sensitive to changes in afterload (95,96). Thus, it is of particular concern to note that the normal fall in blood pressure during sleep is reversed in patients with CHF and OSA (69). Some patients with treated CHF may be normotensive during daytime clinic visits but hypertensive at night. In eight pharmacologically treated patients, studied during overnight polysomnography, average systolic blood pressure increased from 120 mmHg during wakefulness to 132 mmHg during stage 2 sleep ($p < 0.05$) (Fig. 2) (69). The highest systolic blood pressure was observed during the ventilatory period of stage 2 sleep (Table 1). However, systolic arterial blood pressure is not the only source of increased LV afterload in these patients. During paroxysms of apnea, patients abruptly generate levels of negative Pit reaching as much as −90 cmH_2O, (−65 mmHg) (Fig. 1). The effects of this increase in LV transmural pressure on afterload are functionally equivalent to those caused by sudden surges in systemic arterial blood pressure of the same magnitude. It should therefore not be surprising that we (and others) have observed profound reductions in stroke volume and cardiac output, right from the onset of simulated

Table 1 The effects of obstructive sleep apnea on cardiovascular and respiratory variables

		Stage 2 Sleep		
Variable	Awake	Mean Stage 2 Sleep	Apnea	Ventilatory Period
BP_{dias} (mmHg)	74.7 ± 4.1	79.3 ± 6.1	77.1 ± 5.6	80.6 ± 6.5[b]
BP_{sys} (mmHg)	120.4 ± 7.8	131.8 ± 10.6[a]	129.4 ± 10.6	133.9 ± 10.9[a,c]
Pes_{sys} (mmHg)	−4.2 ± 0.6	−5.4 ± 1.0	−4.6 ± 1.2	−6.1 ± 1.0[a,c]
$LVPtm_{sys}$ (mmHg)	124.4 ± 7.7	137.2 ± 10.8[a]	133.9 ± 10.0	140.2 ± 10.6[b,d]
HR (beats per minute)	83.3 ± 5.8	82.1 ± 5.8	80.1 ± 5.9[a]	83.9 ± 5.6[d]
Pes_{amp} (mmHg)	9.3 ± 1.4	12.2 ± 1.4	9.1 ± 1.3	15.2 ± 2.0[a,c]
RR (breaths per minute)	19.9 ± 2.6	20.5 ± 1.7	19.1 ± 1.7	20.8 ± 1.8

These data demonstrate that, in patients with congestive heart failure, obstructive sleep apnea increases BP, negative Pes_{sys} swings, $LVPtm_{sys}$, HR, and inspiratory Pes_{amp} during stage 2 NREM sleep compared to wakefulness. These increasd loads to the cardiovascular and respiratory systems, however, occur mainly during the ventilatory period between apneas.

Abbreviations: BP_{dias}, diastolic blood pressure; BP_{sys}, systolic blood pressure; Pes_{sys}, systolic esophageal pressure; $LVPtm_{sys}$, systolic left ventricular transmural pressure; HR, heart rate; Pes_{amp}, amplitude of esophageal pressure swings; RR, respiratory rate.

[a]$p < 0.05$,

[b]$p < 0.01$ versus wakefulness;

[c]$p < 0.05$,

[d]$p < 0.01$ versus apnea.

Source: From Ref. 69.

obstructive apneas, at more modest levels of negative Pit (38,41,97). These changes are greater in magnitude than those evoked by the same stimulus in matched control subjects with normal ventricular function (97,98). Moreover, recent observations in our laboratory suggest that these adverse effects on hemo-dynamics persist well into the recovery period, after the termination of simulated obstructive apnea (98). These findings suggest that the contractile function of the myocardium is impaired by this extra load, to the extent that there may be a sustained impairment of contractility lasting beyond the stimulus exposure.

When one considers that the typical patient with OSA experiences between 20 and 60 obstructive events per hour of sleep, each lasting between 15 to 60 sec, the implications of these repetitive and profound nocturnal changes in loading conditions become particularly significant for the patient with compro-mised ventricular function, regardless of etiology. But if flow-limiting coronary artery lesions are also present, these exaggerated negative Pit swings could precipitate myocardial ischemia even in the absence of hypoxia (44). Hypoxia can also directly impair myocardial contractility (55). These effects may be more pronounced in patients with associated coronary artery disease than in those without. Indeed, increased systolic LVPtm causes greater reductions in LV ejection fraction in patients with ischemic heart disease than in healthy subjects (97).

Brady- and tachyarrhythmias are frequent causes of death in CHF (75,76). The combination of increases in LV afterload, hypoxia, and increased SNA dur-ing OSA could all facilitate development of myocardial ischemia and arrhythmias during sleep, especially in patients with CHF due to coronary artery disease (25,92,93). However, the role that OSA might play in provoking arrhythmias in patients with CHF has not been formally studied.

In patients with preexisting ventricular dysfunction, these abrupt and recur-rent reductions in Pit, in conjunction with elevations in systemic arterial pressure and hypoxia, could trigger acute contractile impairment and nocturnal pulmonary edema, as has been reported in some patients with OSA (49,50,52,74). Over time, these repetitive increases in LV afterload (due to negative Pit alone) may be sufficient to stimulate ventricular hypertrophy or exacerbate preexisting heart fail-ure (7,99). Apnea-associated hypertension and hypoxia-induced myocardial con-tractile impairment would further aggravate these processes. It is noteworthy that 6 of the 8 subjects with CHF and OSA in whom we measured blood pressure during wakefulness and stage 2 sleep had idiopathic dilated cardiomyopathy (69). This raises the question of whether OSA might have played a role in the pathogen-esis of their heart failure. The marked improvement in daytime ejection fraction observed in such patients after treatment of apnea with nocturnal CPAP provides further evidence that OSA could stimulate progressive deterioration in the LV function of susceptible individuals with otherwise unexplained dilated cardiomy-opathy (7).

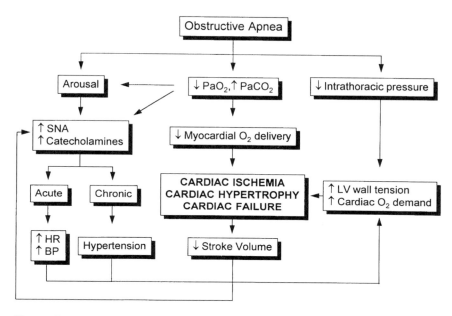

Figure 4 Pathophysiological effects of obstructive sleep apnea (OSA) on the cardiovascular system. OSA exposes the myocardium to increased afterload, hypoxia and increased sympathetic nervous system activity (SNA), all of which could contribute to the progression of myocardial failure. LV, left ventricular; HR, heart rate. Otherwise as for Figure 3. (Modified from Ref. 127.)

As summarized in Figure 4, OSA has a number of pathophysiological effects that could worsen pump failure and possibly lead to increased morbidity and mortality in patients with CHF. Moreover, OSA may also be a hitherto unappreciated cause of sympathetic activation in this condition.

VI. Central Sleep Apnea (Cheyne-Stokes Respiration)

Central sleep apnea in association with Cheyne-Stokes respiration is a form of periodic breathing in which central apneas during sleep alternate regularly with hyperpneas that have a crescendo-decrescendo pattern of tidal volume (V_T) (20). In contrast to OSA, CSA appears to result from rather than to cause CHF. For similar degrees of LV dysfunction, patients with CSA hyperventilate more, and are more hypocapnic when awake and asleep than those without CSA (100,101). Low Pa_{CO_2}, close to the apneic threshold, is a key predisposing factor. Hyperventilation is probably caused mainly by vagally mediated pulmonary irritant receptors, stimulated by pulmonary congestion (102). In favor of this concept, Solin et al. (103) recently demonstrated that CHF patients with CSR-CSA have higher pulmonary capillary wedge pressures in association with lower Pa_{CO_2} than do CHF patients without CSR-CSA. Tkacova and associates (104) have shown that CHF patients with CSA have greater LV volumes that those without CSA, which is consistent with higher LV filling pressures. Abrupt increases in ventilation quickly drive their Pa_{CO_2} below this threshold, precipitating central apneas (100). In addition, mild hypoxia during apneas, arousals from sleep at the end of apneas, and increased ventilatory responsiveness to chemical respiratory stimuli could also contribute to augmented ventilation and hypocapnia following termination of apneas. Older CHF patients (3) may be at higher risk for nocturnal hyperventilation because of less compliant left ventricles with higher end-diastolic pressures than are found in younger patients. The higher risk for CSA associated with the presence of atrial fibrillation in CHF patients (3) may also be due to higher left atrial pressures resulting from the loss of atrial contraction.

Central apneas are triggered by reductions in Pa_{CO_2}, and their length is proportional to the preceding ventilation and the magnitude of fall on Pa_{CO_2} (31,100,105). Moreover, the time from the nadir of end-tidal P_{CO_2}, which occurs at the height of ventilation in the middle of the ventilatory period, until the onset of central apnea is the same as the circulatory delay from the lung to the carotid body (105). These data demonstrate that central apneas are triggered by a reduction in Pa_{CO_2} detected at the level of the carotid chemoreceptors.

Based on the above pathophysiological schema, Lorenzi-Filho et al. (105) were able to demonstrate that inhalation of a CO_2-enriched gas mixture abolishes central apneas and hypopneas in CHF patients with CSA (Fig. 5). Although dips in Sa_{O_2} during central apneas could augment ventilatory drive during hyperpnea and facilitate subsequent reductions in Pa_{CO_2} below the apnea threshold, short-term inhalation of O_2 alone in these same patients did not cause any reduction in the frequency of central events. These observations indicate that whereas hypocapnia and dips in Pa_{CO_2} below the apnea threshold are the cause of central apneas, dips in Pa_{O_2} appear to be their result.

The length of the hyperpneic portion of the periodic breathing cycle is directly proportional to lung-to–carotid body circulatory delay and inversely proportional to cardiac output (106). Nevertheless, lung-to–carotid body circulatory delay in CHF patients with CSA is no different than that in those without CSA (100). Compared to patients with CSA but without CHF, those with CHF experience a slower apnea-related decline in Sa_{O_2} detected at the carotid body. Accordingly, the rate of rise of V_T is slower and the length of hyperpnea is longer than in patients without CHF, giving their hyperpneas their characteristic crescendo-decrescendo appearance (106). However, the length of central apnea is similar in patients with and without CHF (31,100,106). Taken together, these data indicate that prolonged circulatory delay does not play an important role in the causa-

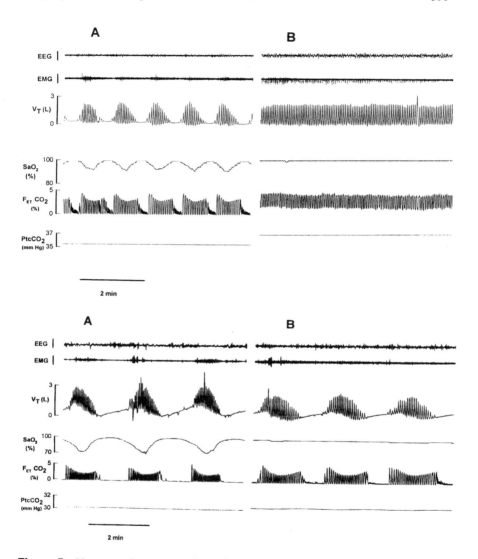

Figure 5 Upper panel: representative polysomnographic recordings from a patient during stage 2 sleep while breathing air (A) and CO_2 (B). Central apneas are abolished by CO_2 inhalation in association with an increase in the fraction of end-tidal CO_2 (FET_{CO_2}) above the level during hyperpneas preceding apneas, and a 1.6-mmHg increase in transcutaneous P_{CO_2} (Ptc_{CO_2}). Abolition of Cheyne-Stokes respiration with central sleep apneas was also associated with elimination of dips in Sa_{O_2}. Lower panel: recordings from a different patient than shown in the upper panel while breathing air (A) and O_2 (B). Although O_2 inhalation abolishes dips in Sa_{O_2}, Cheyne-Stokes respiration with central sleep apneas persists. There were no significant effects of O_2 inhalation on either FET_{CO_2} or Ptc_{CO_2}. Abbreviations as for Figure 1 unless otherwise indicated. (From Ref. 105.)

tion of central apneas in patients with CHF but that it sculpts the ventilatory pattern and prolongs its duration.

The breathing patterns of patients with CHF entrain oscillations in heart rate and blood pressure and exert an important modulatory influence on central sympathetic outflow (107,109). These effects are complex and differ between normal rhythmic breathing and periodic breathing. For example, oscillations in heart rate and blood pressure during normal breathing are entrained by respiration, such that the spectral power of these oscillations is concentrated in the high-frequency range (0.15–0.5 Hz) at the respiratory frequency—the so-called respiratory sinus arrhythmia (70). The very low frequency (0.0049–0.05 Hz) heart rate and blood pressure oscillations normally observed during rhythmic breathing, however, are not related to respiration. The major effect of periodic breathing and CSA is to shift the majority of power in the heart rate variability and blood pressure spectra from the high- and low-frequency (0.05–0.15 Hz) ranges into the very low frequency band at precisely the periodic breathing-cycle frequency (70,109), even though respiratory sinus arrhythmia is still present. This shift of spectral power is a marker for poor prognosis in CHF patients.

Cardiovascular entrainment appears to be modulated by the respiratory pattern itself. By applying spectral analysis and time-domain methods in subjects trained to perform simulated periodic breathing, Lorenzi-Filho et al. (70) demonstrated that the periodic ventilatory pattern can amplify oscillations in blood pressure and heart rate and entrain them at precisely the same very low frequency as the periodic breathing cycle (Fig. 6). This duplicates the pattern of cardiovascular oscillations observed during CSA in CHF patients (109,110). Those changes were observed in awake subjects with normal ventricular function in the absence of hypoxia and were not affected by inhalation of CO_2. They also occurred in the absence of arousals from sleep. The implication of these data are that surges in blood pressure and heart rate just after the termination of central and possibly obstructive apneas in patients with CHF are related in part to increases in V_T and respiratory frequency (70). The fact that heart rate increases as blood pressure rises indicates that these effects are not modulated predominantly by the baroreceptors but may be due to an increase in sympathetic outflow or to synchronization of central respiratory and sympathetic neuronal output to the respiratory and cardiovascular systems, respectively. Further research will be required to determine the mechanisms involved in these cardiorespiratory interactions. During sleep, CHF patients with CSA would be expected to manifest even greater surges in blood pressure, heart rate, and MSNA in response to oscillations in ventilation as a result of additional exacerbating mechanisms, including hypoxia and arousals from sleep.

We have recently described a significant independent and previously unrecognized correlation between spontaneous breathing pattern and MSNA in patients with CHF during wakefulness. Patients with rapid shallow breathing exhibit the

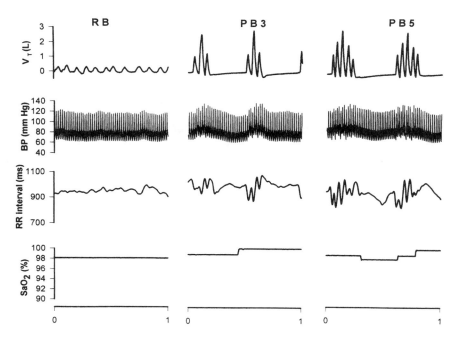

Figure 6 Recording of tidal volume (V_T), blood pressure (BP), interval from R wave to R wave (RR), and Sa_{O_2} in one subject during regular breathing (RB), and during voluntary periodic breathing with three (PB3) or five breaths between central apneas (PB5) while awake. Oscillations in BP and RR interval were present during RB, but they became more prominent and regular and were entrained at the periodic breathing cycle frequency during PB3 and PB5. Sa_{O_2} does not fall during PB3 and PB5 because overall the subjects hyperventilated. This figure also illustrates that oscillations in BP and RR interval can occur in the absence of hypoxia and arousals from sleep. (From Ref. 70.)

highest degree of sympathetic activation (107). This activation is related directly to respiratory frequency and inversely to V_T. The relationship to respiratory frequency is consistent with observations in experimental animals, where central sympathetic outflow is related to the frequency of stimulation of the respiratory centers, which is, in turn, a function of central respiratory drive (32). The inverse relationship of MSNA to V_T, on the other hand, is probably a function of suppression of the pulmonary vagally mediated sympathoinhibitory effects of lung inflation: the greater the inspiratory V_T, the lower the MSNA, and vice versa (62). These data indicate that even during normal rhythmic breathing, sympathetic outflow to muscle is related to or may even be modulated by respiratory pattern.

Periodic breathing disrupts this pattern of sympathetic activity. MSNA tends to parallel oscillations in ventilation, heart rate, and blood pressure such that it declines over the course of central apnea and gradually rises to a peak in concert with ventilation as it increases just after termination of apnea (111,112). This pattern is probably due to prolonged circulatory delay, such that reductions in Pa_{CO_2} and increases in Pa_{O_2} during hyperventilation are not detected at the chemoreceptors until the onset of apnea, while the rise in Pa_{CO_2} and fall in Pa_{O_2} during apnea is not detected until after the onset of ventilation (106). Not surprisingly, however, overnight urinary norepinephrine (UNE) concentrations are markedly higher in CHF patients with CSA than in CHF patients of similar age, sex, and LV ejection fraction but without CSA and are directly related to the frequency of arousals from sleep and degree of apnea-related hypoxia but not to LV ejection fraction (9). These data strongly suggest, first, that CSA can trigger sympathetic activation in certain patients with CHF, and, second, that the increased SNA in these patients is not simply a compensatory response to low cardiac output but is directly related to the sleep apnea disorder. It may therefore represent excessive and pathological sympathoexcitation. These changes transcend the sleeping state: in the same study we were somewhat surprised by the observation that daytime PNE concentration was also higher in those with than those without CSA and was also directly related to the frequency of arousals from sleep and the degree of apnea-related hypoxia but not to LV ejection fraction. Indeed, our preliminary observations (111) and those of others (112) also suggest that CSA patients with CHF have higher daytime MSNA than corresponding CHF patients without CSA. The mechanism for this effect remains to be elucidated.

In contrast to obstructive apneas, no inspiratory efforts are made during central apneas (Fig. 7)(8). Consequently, any changes in LV afterload during the apneic phase would be mediated primarily by changes in systemic arterial pressure. In sedated animals, prolonged central apneas lower heart rate because of hypoxia but have no effect on stroke volume (113), whereas in conscious humans with CHF, central apneas do not seem to cause significant alterations in heart rate, stroke volume, or cardiac output, probably because afterload is not increased and hypoxia is too mild to reduce heart rate or impair cardiac contractility (41,114).

By contrast, a substantial degree of negative intrathoracic pressure can be generated during hyperpnea. Thus, in some respects, the hyperpneic phase of these cycles replicates some of the adverse loading conditions of OSA. In addition, this inspiratory effort is probably one factor provoking arousal from sleep (115–117). It has been reported that paroxysmal nocturnal dyspnea in patients with CHF can be related to the hyperpneic phase of CSA, probably through this mechanism (8,118,119).

Although hypoxia during central apneas is usually mild, it also appears to trigger arousal from sleep. As with OSA, sleep fragmentation due to arousal at

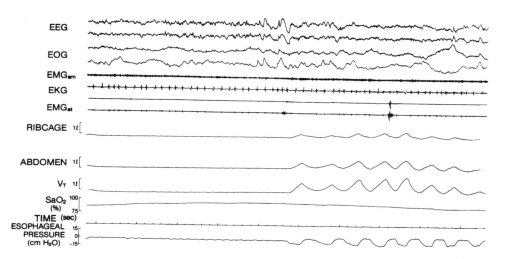

Figure 7 Central apnea during stage 2 NREM sleep in a patient with CHF. It illustrates the absence of negative intrathoracic (i.e., esophageal) pressure swings and the development of hypoxia during the apnea. The apnea is terminated by an arousal, as indicated by the increase in EEG and EMG$_{at}$ activity. Abbreviations as for Figure 1. (From Ref. 8.)

the termination of apnea is probably an important cause of excessive daytime sleepiness and fatigue in patients with CHF and CSA (1,8,37). Hypoxia and arousals from sleep also stimulate the sympathetic nervous system, as discussed above (59,65,66).

Surges in blood pressure, heart rate, and central sympathetic outflow place marked metabolic demands upon the already failing heart that may eventually exceed its capacity to meet. Hypoxia and high nocturnal and daytime catecholamine release could aggravate myocardial dysfunction. These mechanisms may contribute to the progression of myocardial failure and underlie part of the increased mortality reported in patients with CHF and CSA as compared to those without CSA (5,6). Thus, CSA could participate in a vicious pathophysiological cycle involving the cardiovascular, respiratory and autonomic nervous systems, as illustrated in Figure 8.

One other pathological consideration that warrants further investigation is the impact of sleep deprivation or disruption on the progression of heart failure. Sleep apnea, whether obstructive or central, is characterized by fragmented sleep architecture as well as sleep deprivation; the total amount of sleep in such patients has been consistently reported to average only 4.5 hr per night (1,4). Indeed, these patients experience such frequent arousals and spend such little time in

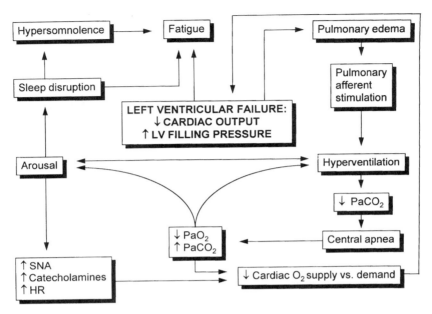

Figure 8 Pathophysiological scheme of central sleep apnea (CSA) in CHF. Note that CHF itself contributes to the development of CSA, which, in turn, has adverse effects on the myocardium including hypoxia and increased SNA. In addition, arousals disrupt sleep and contribute to symptoms of hypersomnolence and fatigue. Abbreviations as for Figures 3 and 4. (Modified from Ref. 127.)

stages III–IV of NREM sleep (1,2,7,8,100) that the cardiovascular system may not enjoy the restorative effects of uninterrupted sleep.

VII. Treatment of Sleep Apnea in Patients with Congestive Heart Failure

Conventional drug management of CHF is unlikely to affect OSA and therefore would not be expected to attenuate or abolish its hemodynamic or sympathoneural consequences. Therefore, the maximum benefits to be derived from identifying OSA in CHF patients would most likely accrue from its elimination by specific therapy. Indeed, as discussed in more detail elsewhere in this volume, the approach to OSA in the setting of CHF should be similar to that for OSA in the absence of CHF. The specific therapy of choice in most cases of OSA is CPAP.

A number of approaches to the therapy of CSA in patients with CHF can be taken, depending on the weight one places on the pathophysiological significance of this breathing disorder. If one takes the view that CSA itself is simply a reflection of the severity of cardiac failure, then pharmacological therapy of CHF might alleviate this breathing disturbance. If, on the other hand, CSA is accompanied by symptoms of sleep disruption or sleep apnea such as restless sleep, insomnia, paroxysmal nocturnal dyspnea, or excessive daytime sleepiness, then specific treatment of CSA should be of additional and independent benefit. Finally, if one takes the approach that CSA plays a role in the progression of CHF, then considerable attention should be directed toward the specific abolition of this condition. The most thoroughly tested treatment for CSA in the setting of CHF—and the one so far shown to have the greatest clinical benefit in terms of respiratory, cardiovascular, and symptomatic outcomes—is also CPAP. Although trials from our center have consistently shown improvements in CSA, cardiovascular function, and neurohumoral activity and symptoms of CHF (1,8,9), studies by other groups have not shown such benefits (120–122). The reasons for this are discussed in detail elsewhere in this volume. Nocturnal supplemental O_2 has also been shown to alleviate CSA (11), and causes modest short-term (1 to 4 weeks) reductions in nocturnal UNE concentrations (123) and daytime exercise capacity (12). However, no direct benefits of O_2 therapy to the cardiovascular system have been demonstrated.

VIII. Conclusions and Future Directions

In the course of this chapter we have reviewed recent evidence that sleep apnea, whether primarily obstructive or central in nature, can have pathological effects on the failing heart and may be associated with a worse prognosis in patients with CHF. Furthermore, sleep apnea may elicit symptoms of paroxysmal nocturnal dyspnea, restless sleep, daytime hypersomnolence, and fatigue. These effects are by and large not amenable to pharmacological therapy but may be specifically attenuated or eliminated by CPAP in the case of OSA and by CPAP or possibly O_2 in the case of CSA. These findings highlight the need to consider OSA and CSA in the differential diagnosis of conditions that could contribute to the development and progression of LV dysfunction in patients with CHF. Indeed, consideration of sleep apnea and polysomnography may become an important aspect of cardiac transplant evaluation. Recent epidemiological studies suggest that clinical markers and a few simple laboratory tests may direct physicians toward the diagnosis of a sleep-related breathing disorder in a patient with CHF. These studies also raise the question of whether sleep apnea is a primary cause of death during sleep in many patients with CHF (124).

There are few well-controlled clinical trials of treatment of CSA and OSA in such patients, but those studies in which CPAP was used have reported favorable medium-term outcomes with respect to sleep apnea and sleep quality, LV function, SNA, respiratory muscle strength, and quality of life. These studies also demonstrate reductions in PNE concentration and atrial natriuretic peptide concentration, which are important markers of increased mortality in patients with CHF (125,126). These observations provide a strong rationale for undertaking larger, longer-term clinical trials of CPAP to assess its effects on cardiovascular clinical outcomes, including mortality, in patients with CHF and sleep-related breathing disorders.

Acknowledgments

Work described in this chapter was supported by Operating Grants from the Medical Research Council of Canada (MT 11607 and MA 12422) and the Heart and Stroke Foundation of Ontario. J.S. Floras is a Career Investigator of the Heart and Stroke Foundation of Ontario.

References

1. Naughton MT, Liu PP, Benard DC, Goldstein RS, Bradley TD. Treatment of congestive heart failure and Cheyne-Stokes respiration during sleep by continuous positive airway pressure. Am J Respir Crit Care Med 1995; 151:92–97.
2. Javaheri S, Parker TJ, Wexler L, Michaels SE, Stanberry E, Nishyama H, Roselle GA. Occult sleep-disordered breathing in stable congestive heart failure. Ann Intern Med 1995; 122:487–492.
3. Sin D, Fitzgerald F, Bradley TD. Risk factors for sleep apnea in heart failure. Am J Respir Crit Care Med 1998; 157:A62.
4. Javaheri S, Parker TJ, Liming JD, Corbett WS, Nishiyma H, Wexler L, Roselle GA. Sleep apnea in 81 ambulatory male patients with stable heart failure: types and their prevalence, consequences, and presentations. Circulation 1998; 97:2154–2159.
5. Findley LJ, Zwillich CW, Ancoli-Israel S, Kripke D, Tisi G, Moser KM. Cheyne-Stokes breathing during sleep in patients with left ventricular heart failure. South Med J 1985; 78:11–15.
6. Hanly PJ, Zuberi-Khokhar. Increased mortality associated with Cheyne-Stokes respiration in patients with congestive heart failure. Am J Respir Crit Care Med 1996; 153:272–276.
7. Malone S, Liu PP, Holloway R, Rutherford R, Xie A, Bradley TD. Obstructive sleep apnea in patients with dilated cardiomyopathy: Effects of continuous positive airway pressure. Lancet 1991; 338:1480–1484.
8. Takasaki Y, Orr D, Popkin J, Rutherford R, Liu P, Bradley TD. Effect of nasal

continuous positive airway pressure on sleep apnea in congestive heart failure. Am Rev Respir Dis 1989; 140:1578–1584.

9. Naughton MT, Benard DC, Liu PP, Rutherford R, Rankin F, Bradley TD. Effects of nasal CPAP on sympathetic activity in patients with heart failure and central sleep apnea. Am J Respir Crit Care Med 1995; 152:473–479.

10. Granton JT, Benard DC, Naughton MT, Goldstein RS, Liu PP, Bradley TD. CPAP improves inspiratory muscle strength in patients with heart failure and central sleep apnea. Am J Respir Crit Care Med 1996; 153:277–282.

11. Hanly PJ, Millar TW, Steljes DG, Baert R, Frais MA, Kryger MH. The effect of oxygen on respiration and sleep in patients with congestive heart failure. Ann Intern Med 1989; 111:777–782.

12. Andreas S, Clemens C, Sandholzer H, Figulla HR, Kreuzer H. Improvements in exercise capacity with treatment of Cheyne-Stokes respiration in patients with congestive heart failure. J Am Coll Cardiol 1996; 27:1486–1490.

13. American College of Cardiology/American Heart Association Task Force Report. Guidelines for the evaluation and management of heart failure. J Am Coll Cardiol 1995; 26:1376–1398.

14. Dec GW, Fuster V. Medical Progress: idiopathic dilated cardiomyopathy. N Engl J Med 1994; 331:1564–1575.

15. Yusuf S, Thom T, Abbot RD. Changes in hypertension treatment and congestive heart failure mortality in the United States. Hypertension 1989; 13(supp I):I174–I179.

16. Center For Disease Control. Changes in moratality for heart faiure—United States, 1980–1995. MMWR 1998; 47:633–637.

17. The SOLVD Investigators. Effect of enalapril on survival in patients with reduced left ventricular ejection fraction and congestive heart failure. N Engl J Med 1991; 325:293–302.

18. Benard DC, Naughton MT, Bradley TD. Administration of continuous positive airway pressure to patients with congestive heart failure and Cheyne-Stokes respiration. J Polysomnogr 1992; Dec:9–11.

19. Bradley TD, Rutherford R, Grossman RF, Lue F, Zamel N, Moldofsky H, Phillipson EA. Role of daytime hypoxemia in the pathogenesis of right heart failure in the obstructive sleep apnea syndrome. Am Rev Respir Dis 1985; 131:835–839.

20. Bradley TD. Right and left ventricular functional impairment and sleep apnea. Clin Chest Med 1992; 13:459–479.

21. Bradley TD. Breathing during sleep in cardiac disease. In: Saunders NA and Sullivan CE, eds. Sleep and Breathing. 2d ed. (Lung Biology in Health and Disease, vol. 17) New York, Marcel Dekker, 1994:787–821.

22. Young TB, Palta M, Dempsey JA, Skatrud JB, Weber S, Badr S. The occurrence of sleep-disordered breathing among middle-aged adults. N Engl J Med 1993; 328:1230–1235.

23. White DP, Weil JV, Zwillich CW. Metabolic rate and breathing during sleep. J Appl Physiol 1985; 59:384–391.

24. Somers VK, Dyken ME, Mark AL, Abboud FM. Sympathetic-nerve activity during sleep in normal subjects. N Engl J Med 1993; 328:303–307.

25. Shepard JW Jr. Gas exchange and hemodynamics during sleep. Med Clin North Am 1985; 69:1243–1264.

26. Hornyak M, Cejnar M, Elam M, Matousek M, Wallin BG. Sympathetic muscle nerve activity during sleep in man. Brain 1991; 114:1281–1295.

27. Furlan R, Guzzetti S, Crivellaro W, Dossi S, Tinelli M, Baselli G, Cerutti S, Lombardi F, Pagani M, Milliani A. Continuous 24-hour assessment of neural regulation of systemic arterial pressure and RR variabilities in ambulant subjects. Circulation 1990; 81:537–547.

28. Davies RJ, Belt PJ, Roberts SJ, Ali NJ, Stradling JR. Arterial blood pressure responses to graded transient arousal from sleep in normal humans. J Appl Physiol 1993; 74:1123–1130.

29. Phillipson EA, Bowes G. Control of breathing during sleep. In: Cherniack NS, Widdicombe JG, eds. Handbook of Physiology. Vol. 2: Control of Breathing Bethesda MD: American Physiological Society, Williams & Wilkins, 1986:649–849.

30. Orem J, Osario I, Brooks E, Dick T. Activity of respiratory neurons during NREM sleep. J Neurophysiol 1985; 54:1144–1156.

31. Xie A, Wong B, Phillipson EA, Slutsky AS, Bradley TD. Interaction of hyperventilation and arousal in the pathogenesis of idiopathic central sleep apnea. Am J Respir Crit Care Med 1994; 150:489–495.

32. Guyenet PG, Koshiya N, Huangfu D, Verberne AJ, Riley TA. Central respiratory control of A5 and A6 pontine noradrenergic neurons. Am J Physiol 1993; 264: R1035–R1044.

33. Orem J. Neuronal mechanisms of respiration in REM sleep. Sleep 1980; 3:251–267.

34. Remmers JE, Degroot WJ, Sauerland EK. Pathogenesis of upper airway occlusion during sleep. J Appl Physiol 1978; 44:931–938.

35. Brown IG, Bradley TD, Phillipson EA, Zamel N, Hoffstein V. Pharyngeal compliance in snoring subjects with and without obstructive sleep apnea. Am Rev Respir Dis 1985; 132:211–215.

36. Bradley TD, Brown IG, Grossman RF, Zamel N, Martinez D, Phillipson EA, Hoffstein V. Pharyngeal size in snorers, non-snorers, and patients with obstructive sleep apnea. N Engl J Med 1986; 315:1327–1331.

37. Bradley TD, Phillipson EA. The pathophysiology of obstructive sleep apnea. Med Clin North Am 1985; 69:1169–1185.

38. Buda AJ, Pinsky MR, Ingels NB Jr, Daughters GT, Stinson EB, Alderman EL. Effect of intrathoracic pressure on left ventricular performance. N Engl J Med 1979; 301:453–459.

39. Virolainen J, Ventila M, Turto H, Kupari M. Effect of negative intrathoracic pressure on left ventricular pressure dynamics and relaxation. J Appl Physiol 1995; 79: 455–460.

40. Magder SA, Lichtenstein S, Adelman AG. Effects of negative pleural pressure on left ventricular hemodynamics. Am J Cardiol 1983; 52:588–593.

41. Hall MJ, Ando SI, Floras JS, Bradley TD. Magnitude and time course of hemodynamic responses to Mueller maneuvers in patients with congestive heart failure. J Appl Physiol 1998; 85:1476–1484.

42. Hanly P, Sasson Z, Zuberi N, Lunn K. ST-segment depression during sleep in obstructive sleep apnea. Am J Cardiol 1993; 71:1341–1345.

43. Robotham JL, Rabson J, Permutt S, Bromberger-Barnea B. Left ventricular hemodynamics during respiration. J Appl Physiol 1979; 47:1295–1303.

44. Scharf SM, Graver LM, Balaban K. Cardiovascular effects of periodic occlusions of the upper airways in dogs. Am Rev Respir Dis 1992; 146:321–329.

45. Peters J, Fraser C, Stuart RS, Baumgartner W, Robotham JL. Negative intrathoracic pressure decreases independently left ventricular filling and emptying. Am J Physiol 1989; 257:H120–H131.

46. Tolle FA, Judy WV, Yu PL, Markand ON. Reduced stroke volume related to pleural pressure in obstructive sleep apnea. J Appl Physiol 1983; 55:1718–1724.

47. Buda AJ, Schroeder JS, Guilleminault C. Abnormalities of pulmonary artery wedge pressures in sleep-induced apnea. Int J Cardiol 1981; 1:67.

48. Tilkian AG, Guilleminault C, Schroeder JS, Lehrman KL, Simmons FB, Dement WC. Hemodynamics in sleep-induced apnea: studies during wakefulness and sleep. Ann Intern Med 1976; 85:714–719.

49. Chan HS, Chiu HF, Tse LK, Woo KS. Obstructive sleep apnea presenting with nocturnal angina, heart failure and near-miss sudden death. Chest 1991; 99:1023–1025.

50. Chaudhary BA, Nadimi M, Chaudhary TK, Speir WA. Pulmonary edema due to obstructive sleep apnea. South Med J 1984; 77:499–501.

51. Franklin KA, Nilsson JB, Sahlin C. Sleep apnoea and nocturnal angina. Lancet 1995; 345:1085–1087.

52. Chaudhary, BA, Ferguson DS, Speir WA Jr. Pulmonary edema as a presenting feature of sleep apnea syndrome. Chest 1982; 82:122–124.

53. Schroeder JS, Motta J, Guilleminault C. Hemodynamic studies in sleep apnea. In: Guilleminault C, Dement WC, eds. Sleep Apnea Syndromes. Kroc Foundation Series Vol. II. New York, Liss, 1978:177.

54. Stoohs R, Guilleminault C. Cardiovascular changes associated with obstructive sleep apnea syndrome. J Appl Physiol 1992; 72:583–589.

55. Kusuoka H, Weisfeldt ML, Zweier JL, Jacobus WE, Marban E. Mechanism of early contractile failure during hypoxia in intact ferret heart: evidence for modulation of maximal Ca^{2+}-activated force by inorganic phosphate. Circ Res 1986; 59: 270–282.

56. Cargill RI, Kiely DG, Lipworth BJ. Adverse effects of hypoxaemia on diastolic filling in humans. Clin Sci 1995; 89:165–169.

57. Somers VK, Mark AL, Zavala DC, Abboud FM. Contrasting effects of hypoxia and hypercapnia on ventilation and sympathetic activity in humans. J Appl Physiol 1989; 67:2101–2106.

58. Morgan BJ, Denahan T, Ebert TJ. Neurocirculatory consequences of negative intrathoracic pressure vs. asphyxia during voluntary apnea. J Appl Physiol 1993; 74: 2969–2975.

59. Hedner J, Ejnell H, Sellgren J, Hedner T, Wallin G. Is high and fluctuating muscle nerve sympathetic activity in the sleep apnoea syndrome of pathogenetic importance for the development of hypertension? J Hypertens 1988; 6(suppl):S529–S531.

60. Floras JS. Clinical aspects of sympathetic activation and parasympathetic withdrawal in heart failure. J Am Coll Cardiol 1993; 22:(suppl A):72A–84A.

61. Somers VK, Mark AL, Zavala DC, Abbound FM. Influence of ventilation and hypocapnia on sympathetic nerve responses to hypoxia in normal humans. J Appl Physiol 1989; 67:2095–2100.

62. Seals DR, Suwarno NO, Dempsey JA. Influence of lung volume on sympathetic nerve discharge. Circ Res 1990; 67:130–140.

63. Somers VK, Dyken ME, Skinner JL. Autonomic and hemodynamic responses and interactions during the Mueller maneuver in humans. J Auton Nerv Syst 1993; 44: 253–259.

64. Ringler J, Basner RC, Shannon R, Schwartzstein R, Manning H, Weinberger SE, Weiss JW. Hypoxemia alone does not explain blood pressure elevations after obstructive apneas. J Appl Physiol 1990; 69:2143–2148.

65. Somers VK, Dyken ME, Clary MP, Abbound FM. Sympathetic neural mechanisms in obstructive sleep apnea. J Clin Invest 1995; 96:1897–1904.

66. Shimizu T, Takahashi Y, Kogawa S, Takahashi K, Kanbayashi T, Saito Y, Hishikawa Y. Muscle sympathetic nerve activity during apneic episodes in patients with obstructive sleep apnea syndrome. Electroencephalogr Clin Neurophysiol 1994; 93: 345–352.

67. O'Donnell CP, King ED, Schwartz AR, Robotham JL, Smith PL. Relationship between blood pressure and airway obstruction during sleep in the dog. J Appl Physiol 1994; 77:1819–1828.

68. Ringler J, Garpestad E, Basner RC, Weiss JW. Systemic blood pressure elevation after airway occlusion during NREM sleep. Am J Respir Crit Care Med 1994; 150: 1062–1066.

69. Tkacova R, Rankin F, Fitzgerald FS, Floras JS, Bradley TD. Effects of continuous positive airway pressure on obstructive sleep apnea and left ventricular afterload in patients with heart failure. Circulation 1998; 98:2269–2275.

70. Lorenzi-Filho G, Dajani HR, Leung RST, Floras JS, Bradley TD. Entrainment of blood pressure and heart rate oscillations by periodic breathing. Am J Respir Crit Care Med 1999; 159:1147–1154.

71. Hung J, Whitford EG, Parsons RW, Hillman DR. Association of sleep apnoea with myocardial infarction in men. Lancet 1990; 336:261–264.

72. Galatius-Jensen S, Hansen J, Rasmussen V, Bildsoe J, Therboe M, Rosenberg J. Nocturnal hypoxaemia after myocardial infarction: association with nocturnal myocardial ischaemia and arrhythmias. Br Heart J 1994; 72:23–30.

73. Garpestad E, Parker JA, Katayama H, Lilly J, Yasuda T, Ringler J, Strauss HW, Weiss JW. Decrease in ventricular stroke volume at apnea termination is independent of oxygen desaturation. J Appl Physiol 1994; 77:1602–1608.

74. Loui WS, Blackshear JL, Fredrickson PA, Kaplan J. Obstructive sleep apnea manifesting as suspected angina: report of three cases. Mayo Clin Proc 1994; 69:244–248.

75. Francis GS. Development of arrhythmias in the patient with congestive heart failure: pathophysiology, prevalence and prognosis. Am J Cardiol 1986; 57:3B–7B.

76. Middlekauff HR, Stevenson WG, Stevenson LW, Saxon LA. Syncope in advanced

heart failure: high risk of sudden death regardless of origin of syncope. J Am Coll Cardiol 1993; 21:110–116.

77. Narkiewicz K, van de Borne PJH, Montano N, Dyken ME, Phillips BG, Somers VK. Contribution of tonic chemoreflex activation to sympathetic activity and blood pressure in patients with obstructive sleep apnea. Circulation 1998; 97:943–945.

78. Narkiewicz K, Montano N, Cogliata C, van de Borne PHJ, Dyken ME, Somers VK. Altered cardiovascular variability in obstructive sleep apnea. Circulation 1998; 98:1071–1077.

79. Carlson JT, Hedner JA, Ejnell H, Peterson LE. High prevalence of hypertension in sleep apnea patients independent of obesity. Am J Respir Crit Care Med 1994; 150:72–77.

80. Hoffstein V. Blood pressure, snoring, obesity, and nocturnal hypoxaemia. Lancet 1994; 344:643–645.

81. Hla KM, Young TB, Bidwell T, Palta M, Skatrud JB, Dempsey J. Sleep apnea and hypertension. A population-based study. Ann Intern Med 1994; 120:382–388.

82. Brooks D, Horner RL, Kozar LF, Render-Teixeira CL, Phillipson EA. Obstructive sleep apnea as a cause of systemic hypertension: evidence from a canine model. J Clin Invest 1997; 99:106–109.

83. Fletcher EC, Lesske J, Qian W, Miller CC III, Unger T. Repetitive, episodic hypoxia causes diurnal elevation of blood pressure in rats. Hypertension 1992; 19:555–561.

84. Fletcher EC, Lesske J, Behm R, Miller CC III, Stauss H, Unger T. Carotid chemoreceptors, systemic blood pressure, and chronic episodic hypoxia mimicking sleep apnea. J Appl Physiol 1992; 72:1978–1984.

85. Fletcher EC, Lesske J, Culman J, Miller CC III, Unger T. Sympathetic denervation blocks blood pressure elevation in episodic hypoxia. Hypertension 1992; 20:612–619.

86. Hedner JA, Wilcox I, Laks L, Grunstein RR, Sullivan CE. A specific and potent pressor effect of hypoxia in patients with sleep apnea. Am Rev Respir Dis 1992; 146:1240–1245.

87. Carlson JT, Hedner J, Elam M, Ejnell H, Sellgran J, Wallin BJ. Augmented resting sympathetic activity in awake patients with obstructive sleep apnea. Chest 1993; 103:1763–1768.

88. Ferguson DW, Berg WJ, Sanders S. Clinical and hemodynamic correlates of sympathetic nerve activity in normal humans and patients with heart failure: evidence from direct microneurographic recordings. J Am Coll Cardiol 1990; 16:1125–1134.

89. Kaye DM, Lambert GM, Lefkovits J, Morris M, Jennings G, Esler MD. Neurochemical evidence of cardiac sympathetic activation and increased central nervous system norepinephrine turnover in severe congestive heart failure. J Am Coll Cardiol 1994; 23:570–578.

90. Cohn JN, Levine TB, Olivari MT, Garberg V, Lura D, Francis GS, Simon AB, Rector T. Plasma norepinephrine as a guide to prognosis in patients with congestive heart failure. N Engl J Med 1984; 311:819–823.

91. Shepard JW Jr, Garrison MW, Grither DA, Dolan GF. Relationship of ventricular ectopy and oxyhemoglobin desaturation in patients with obstructive sleep apnea. Chest 1985; 88:335.

92. Shepard JW Jr. Hypertension, cardiac arrhythmias, myocardial infarction, and stroke in relation to obstructive sleep apnea. Clin Chest Med 1992; 13:437.

93. Millar WP. Cardiac arrhythmias and conduction disturbances in the sleep apnea syndrome. Am J Med 1982; 73:317–321.

94. Daly PA, Sole MJ. Moycardial catecholamines and the pathophysiology of heart failure. Circulation 1990; 82 (suppl I):I-35–I-43.

95. Ross J Jr. Afterload mismatch and preload reserve: a conceptual framework for the analysis of ventricular function. Progr Cardiovasc Dis 1976; 18:254–264.

96. Ross J Jr, Covell JW, Mahler F. Contractile responses of the left ventricle to acute and chronic stress. Eur J Cardiol 1974; 1:325–332.

97. Scharf SM, Bianco JA, Tow DE, Brown R. The effects of large negative intrathoracic pressure on left ventricular function in patients with coronary artery disease. Circulation 1981; 63:871–875.

98. Hall MJ, Ando S, Senn B, Wong A, Fitzgerald FS, Floras JS, Bradley TD. Sustained hemodynamic impairment after simulated obstructive apneas in congestive heart failure. Am J Respir Crit Care Med 1996; 153(part 2):A125.

99. Hedner J, Ejnell K, Caidahl K. Left ventricular hypertrophy independent of hypertension in patients with obstructive sleep apnea. J Hypertens 1990; 8:941–946.

100. Naughton M, Benard D, Tam A, Rutherford R, Bradley TD. Role of hyperventilation in the pathogenesis of central sleep apnea in patients with congestive heart failure. Am Rev Respir Dis 1993; 148:330–338.

101. Hanly P, Zuberi N, Gray R. Pathogenesis of Cheyne-Stokes respiration in patients with congestive heart failure: relationship to arterial P_{CO_2}. Chest 1993; 104:1079–1084.

102. Churchill ED, Cope E. The rapid shallow breathing resulting from pulmonary congestion and edema. J Exp Med 1929; 49:531–537.

103. Solin P, Bergin P, Richardson M, Kaye DM, Walters HE, Naughton MT. Influence of pulmonary capillary wedge pressure on central sleep apnea in heart failure. Circulation. 1999; 99:1574–1579.

104. Tkacova R, Hall MJ, Liu PP, Fitzgerald FS, Bradley TD. Left ventricular volume in patients with heart failure and Cheyne-Stokes respiration during sleep. Am J Respir Crit Care Med 1997; 156:1549–1555.

105. Lorenzi-Filho G, Rankin F, Bies I, Bradley TD. Effects of inhaled CO_2 and O_2 on Cheyne-Stokes respiration in patients with heart failure. Am J Respir Crit Care Med 1999; 159:1490–1498.

106. Hall MJ, Xie A, Rutherford R, Ando SI, Floras JS, Bradley TD. Cycle length of periodic breathing in patients with and without heart failure. Am J Respir Crit Care Med 1996; 154:376–381.

107. Naughton MT, Floras JS, Rahman MA, Jamal M, Bradley TD. Respiratory correlates of muscle sympathetic nerve activity in heart failure. Clin Sci 1998; 95:277–285.

108. Ando S, Dajani HR, Floras JS. Frequency domain characteristics of muscle sympa-

thetic nerve activity in heart failure and healthy humans. Am J Physiol 1997; 273: R205–R212.

109. Mortara A, Sleight P, Pinna GD, Maestri R, Prpa A, La Rovere MT, Cobelli F, Tavazzi L. Abnormal awake respiratory patterns are common in chronic heart failure and may prevent evaluation of autonomic tone by measures of heart rate variability. Circulation 1997; 96:246–252.

110. Franklin KA, Sandstrom E, Johansson G, Balfors EM. Hemodynamics, cerebral circulation, and oxygen saturation in Cheyne-Stokes respiration. J Appl Physiol 1997; 83:1184–1191.

111. Yu E, Ando S, Senn B, Fitzgerald F, Hall M, Bradley TD, Floras JS. Sleep-related breathing disorders and daytime sympathetic activity in heart failure. Can J Cardiol 1997; 13:97C.

112. van de Borne P, Oren R, Abouassaly C, Anderson E, Somers VK. Effect of Cheyne-Stokes respiration on muscle sympathetic nerve activity in severe congestive heart failure secondary to ischemic or idiopathic dilated cardiomyopathy. Am J Cardiol 1998; 81:432–436.

113. Tarasiuk A, Scharf SM. Cardiovascular effects of periodic obstructive and central apneas in dogs. Am J Respir Crit Care Med 1994; 150:83–89.

114. Faber J, Lorimier P, Sergysels R. Cyclic haemodynamic and arterial blood gas changes during Cheyne-Stokes breathing. Intens Care Med 1990; 16:208–209.

115. Yasuma F, Kozar LF, Kimoff RJ, Bradley TD, Phillipson EA. Interaction of chemical and mechanical respiratory stimuli in the arousal response to hypoxia in sleeping dogs. Am Rev Respir Dis 1991; 143:1274–1277.

116. Gleeson K, Zwillich CW, White DP. The influence of increasing ventilatory effort on arousal from sleep. Am Rev Respir Dis 1992; 72:985–992.

117. Vincken W, Guilleminault C, Silvestri L, Cosio M, Grassino A. Inspiratory muscle activity as a trigger causing the airways to open in obstructive sleep apnea. Am Rev Respir Dis 1987; 1356:372–377.

118. Bradley TD, Chartrand DC, Fitting JW, Killian KJ, Grassino A. The relation of inspiratory effort sensation to fatiguing patterns of the diaphragm. Am Rev Respir Dis 1986; 134:1119–1124.

119. Harrison TR, King CE, Calhoun JA, Harrison WG Jr. Congestive heart failure: Cheyne-Stokes respiration as the cause of dyspnea at the onset of sleep. Arch Intern Med 1934; 53:891–910.

120. Guilleminault CE, Clerk A, Labonowski M, Simmons J, Stoohs R. Cardiac failure and benzodiazepines. Sleep 1993; 16:524–528.

121. Buckle P, Millar T, Kryger M. The effect of short-term nasal CPAP on Cheyne-Stokes respiration in congestive heart failure. Chest 1992; 102:31–35.

122. Davies RJ, Harrington KJ, Ormerod OJ, Stradling JR. Nasal continuous positive airway pressure in chronic heart failure with sleep-disordered breathing. Am Rev Respir Dis 1993; 147:630–634.

123. Staniforth AD, Kinnear WJM, Starling R, Hetmanski DJ, Cowley AJ: Effect of oxygen on sleep quality, cognitive function and sympathetic activity in patients with chronic heart failure and Cheyne-Stokes respiration. Eur Heart J 1998; 19: 922–928.

124. Pratt CM, Greenway PS, Schoenfeld MH, Hibben ML, Reiffel JA. Exploration of

the precision of classifying cardiac sudden death: implications of the interpretation of clinical trials. Circulation 1996; 93:519–524.

125. Gottlieb SS, Kukin ML, Ahern D, Packer M. Prognostic importance of atrial natri-uretic peptide in patients with chronic heart failure. J Am Coll Cardiol 1989; 13: 1534–1539.

126. Swedberg K, Eneroth P, Kjekshus J, Wilhelmsen L. Hormones regulating cardio-vascular function in patients with severe congestive heart failure and their relation to mortality. Circulation 1990; 82:1730–1736.

127. Hall MJ, Bradley TD. Cardiovascular disease and sleep apnea. Curr Opin Pulm Med 1995; 1:512–518.

18

Prevalence and Prognostic Significance of Sleep Apnea in Heart Failure

SHAHROKH JAVAHERI

Department of Veterans Affairs Medical Center
and University of Cincinnati College of Medicine
Cincinnati, Ohio

I. Introduction

Despite recent advances in the treatment of heart failure, it is still a highly prevalent syndrome associated with excess morbidity and mortality (1). While multiple factors may contribute to the progressive downhill course of heart failure, the pathophysiological consequences of sleep apnea, such as nocturnal arterial oxyhemoglobin desaturation and neurohormonal activation, may play an important role.

Although Hippocrates (2) and George Cheyne (3) may have noticed periodic breathing and John Hunter (4) described it in a patient with heart failure and intracerebral bleeding in 1781, John Cheyne (5) and William Stokes (6) have been credited for their visual description of periodic breathing in heart failure (Cheyne-Stokes respiration, or CSR). In 1818, John Cheyne described an obese patient with probable alcohol-related cardiomyopathy (fatty heart):

> A.B. sixty years of age, of a sanguine temperament, circular chest, and full habit of body, for years had lived a very sedentary life, while he indulged habitually in the luxuries of the table....For several days his breathing was irregular; it would entirely cease for a quarter of a minute, then it would become perceptible, though very low, then by degrees it became heaving and quick, and then it would gradually cease again.

On postmortem exam, there was "anasarcous swelling of the inferior extremities," and the heart was about three times the normal size, with an enlarged left ventricle.

Referring to periodic breathing, William Stokes wrote (6):

> ... it consists in the occurrence of a series of inspirations, increasing to a maximum, and then declining in force and length, until a state of apparent apnea is established. In this condition the patient may remain for such a length of time as to make his attendants believe that he is dead, when a low inspiration, followed by one more decided, marks the commencement of a new ascending and then descending series of inspirations.

In their description of CSR, neither Cheyne nor Stokes spoke of these events occurring during sleep. The description of CSR during sleep in patients with heart failure dates back to 1925, when Sir James Mackenzie first noted it (7). In addition, he also indicated that there may be either an apnea or hypopnea with CSR, and that arousal may occur with hyperpnea. Mackenzie wrote:

> Another form of distressed breathing is Cheyne-Stokes respiration. Many elderly people exhibit Cheyne-Stokes respiration without being conscious of it. But in certain forms of heart failure it may occur and become so marked that the patient's rest is disturbed during the period of increased breathing. This is preceded by a period when the breathing almost ceases, or completely ceases, it may be for a period of a half a minute to a minute, during which the patient may fall asleep, to be wakened up, it may be, by a sense of suffocation; on its resumption the breathing is often exaggerated.

However, it appears that there was some confusion between apnea and what Mackenzie referred to as "cardiac asthma," which may have been paroxysmal nocturnal dyspnea. Regarding cardiac asthma, he wrote, "Occasionally the periods of apnea are so complete and prolonged that the patient wakes up with a sense of great distress, sometimes so severe that he may spring out of bed in his extremity, and may then have to breathe heavily and in labored fashion for many minutes."

About 10 years later, in 1934, Harrison and associates (8) systematically described the effects of sleep on breathing in patients with heart failure. Using a pneumograph and a kymograph, these investigators recorded breathing patterns of patients with heart failure while awake and asleep (visually determined). The studies were conducted in the evening and morphine was administered to facilitate sleep if necessary. They reported 1) the presence of periodic breathing while awake in some patients with acute decompensated heart failure, which diminished or disappeared when heart failure improved; 2) in some patients, periodic breathing appeared with the onset of sleep, and 3) apnea occurred during sleep and hyperpnea with arousal. These authors, therefore, confirmed the observations made by Mackenzie, emphasizing the destablizing effects of sleep on breathing. Furthermore, they noted that improvement in heart failure may result in disappearance of Cheyne-Stokes respiration (CSR). Harrison et al. (8) also distinguished CSR from orthopnea or paroxysmal nocturnal dyspnea, which are all different causes of shortness of breath (during sleep) in patients with heart failure.

In 1979, Rees and Clark (9) studied four patients with acute decompensated heart failure while asleep and not sedated. Three of the four patients were studied throughout the night. Thoracoabdominal excursions were monitored by a pair of magnetometers, and naso-oral airflow was monitored by thermistors. Rees and Clark (9) confirmed the observations of Harrison and associates (8). Interestingly, they described that one of the patients was admitted to the hospital ''for a study of his respiration during sleep because of daytime sleepiness and his wife's report of apneic periods at night.''

Although occurrence of CSR in heart failure was first reported in 1818 (5), the ability to conduct polysomnographic studies (10–15) had to await development of electrophysiological techniques that allowed the electroencephalographic definition of sleep and the systematic recording of respiratory parameters. Figure 1 shows a recording of CSR during sleep in a patient with severe left ventricular

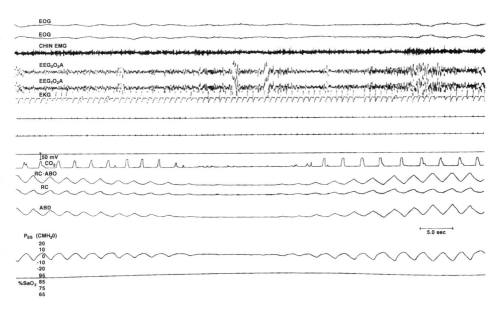

Figure 1 Polysomnographic depiction of classic Cheyne-Stokes respiration in stage 2 sleep. Note the smooth and gradual changes in the thoracoabdominal excursions and esophageal pressure of the crescendo and decrescendo arms of the cycle, with an intervening central apnea. EOG, electro-oculogram; EEG, electroencephalogram; EMG, electromyogram; CO_2 signal represents naso-oral airflow; RC, rib cage; ABD, abdomen; P_{ES}, esophageal pressure; Sa_{O_2}, arterial oxyhemoglobin saturation.

dysfunction. Changes in the chest wall (the rib cage and abdominal) excursions, esophageal pressure, and naso-oral airflow are characterized by gradually decreasing amplitude (reflecting tidal volume) ending in an apnea, followed by a gradually increasing tidal volume.

However, there are no quantitative criteria to define CSR; rather, it is a visual description of changes in the amplitudes of the thoracoabdominal excursions, esophageal pressure (if available), and naso-oral airflow. In this chapter, periodic breathing is used to refer to a pattern of breathing consisting of periodically recurring cycles of apnea or hypopnea followed by hyperpnea (irrespective of the obstructive or central nature of the events). Classic CSR is a form of periodic breathing with smooth and gradual changes (both decreases and increases) in breathing occurring over several breaths with an intervening central apnea. The crescendo and decrescendo arms of the respiratory cycle should be mirror images of each other (Fig. 1).

When the term *central apnea* is used, it includes all episodes of central apnea, irrespective of whether they occur in the context of CSR. Since there are no quantitative criteria for defining CSR (in contrast to what constitutes an apnea or hypopnea) and because what one observer may call CSR another may not, I

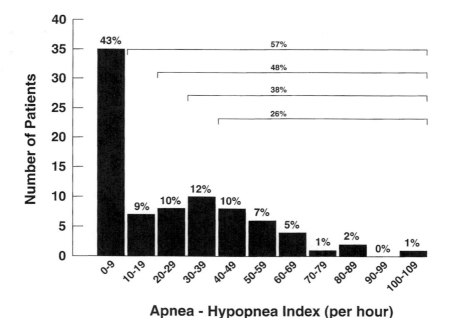

Figure 2 Frequency distribution of apnea-hypopnea index in 10-unit intervals in 81 patients with stable, compensated heart failure. (Modified from Ref. 17.)

prefer to use the term *central sleep apnea*, appreciating that in some patients with heart failure central apnea occurs in the context of CSR. However, in heart failure, periodic breathing consists of both obstructive and central disordered breathing events (13,15,17).

II. Prevalence and Consequences of Periodic Breathing in Heart Failure with Systolic Dysfunction

Although the presence of periodic breathing during sleep in patients with heart failure has been well known, its prevalence, predictors, and impact on the natural history of heart failure have been examined recently. The first polysomnographic study was reported by Findley and associates (10). They studied 15 patients with left ventricular systolic dysfunction, of whom 7 had polysomnography and 8 had portable sleep recordings that did not include electroencephalographic monitoring. Of the 15 patients, 6 (40%) had periodic breathing. It is unclear, however, how many of these were in acute phase of exacerbated heart failure. Dark and colleagues (11) studied six patients with decompensated heart failure (mean left ventricular ejection fraction of 28%) before and after medical therapy. All patients suffered from central sleep apnea, which improved after medical or surgical (transplantation) therapy of heart failure. Yasuma and associates (12) studied 11 patients with stable heart failure secondary to valvular disease on therapy (digoxin and diuretics) and found that 4 (36%) had central sleep apnea.

Takasaki and colleagues (13) studied five patients with stable NYHA class III and IV heart failure (left ventricular ejection fraction varied from 23 to 53%), all of whom demonstrated disordered breathing during sleep. All were loud snorers, two were massively obese, and one had predominantly obstructive sleep apnea. The mean apnea-hypopnea index was 69 per hour and the mean lowest arterial oxyhemoglobin saturation was 84%.

Hanly and associates (14) studied 10 stable, ambulatory patients with class III and IV heart failure, all but 1 of whom had a body-mass index below 30 kg/m^2. All had severe left ventricular dysfunction, with mean left ventricular ejection fraction of 22%. Polysomnography showed that all 10 patients had CSR, with an apnea-hypopnea index of about 37 per hour. The mean minimum arterial oxyhemoglobin saturation was 79%, and saturation was below 90% for 23% of total sleep time.

The prevalence, severity, and nature of periodic breathing in heart failure and systolic dysfunction are probably related to a number of factors, including severity of heart failure, stability of heart failure (presence of acute decompensation), level of arterial P_{CO_2}, left ventricular size, body weight [which may have impact on the presence of obstructive sleep apnea (OSA)], comorbid disorders, medications, and patient recruitment (e.g., patients referred to sleep laboratory versus random recruitment from outpatient clinics).

We have prospectively studied (16,17) 81 ambulatory male patients with stable heart failure due to systolic dysfunction (left ventricular ejection fraction < 45%), with details reported elsewhere (16,17). Clinical stability was defined as no change in symptoms or cardiac medications within the preceding 4 weeks. Seventy-eight patients were on a vasodilator (an angiotensin-converting enzyme inhibitor or hydralazine), 61 on digoxin, 34 on isosorbide dinitrate, and 69 on diuretics. Ambulatory patients were asked by their physicians (primary care physicians or cardiologists) to take part in the study. At the time of recruitment, no information was sought about symptoms or risk factors for sleep apnea. Of the 92 eligible patients, 81 (88% recruitment) agreed to participate. Therefore we believe that the results of this sample can be generalized to the represented male population (we studied only male patients, since female patients are seldom referred to our center).

The etiologies of heart failure were ischemic cardiomyopathy (30 patients without sleep apnea, group I, and 31 patients with sleep apnea, group II), dilated cardiomyopathy (7 patients in group I and 9 in group II) and presumed alcoholic cardiomyopathy (3 patients in group I and 1 in group II).

Exclusion criteria have been detailed previously (16,17). Briefly, they included instability in heart failure and a number of comorbid disorders (such as intrinsic pulmonary, renal, or liver diseases) and use of certain medications such as morphine derivatives, benzodiazepines, acetazolamide, or theophylline.

The frequency distribution of the apnea-hypopnea index in 10-unit intervals for 81 heart failure patients is depicted in Figure 2. Fifty-seven percent of all patients had an apnea-hypopnea index $\geq$ 10 per hour, and about a quarter of patients had suffered severe periodic breathing, with an apnea-hypopnea index $\geq$ 40 per hour. The apnea-hypopnea index includes both obstructive and central disordered-breathing events.

Using an apnea-hypopnea index of 15 per hour as the threshold, there were 40 patients (group I, 49% of all patients) who did not have "sleep apnea," with the mean ($\pm$SD) of the apnea-hypopnea index of 4 $\pm$ 3 per hour (Table 1). In the remaining 41 patients (group II, 51% of all patients), the mean apnea-hypopnea index was 44 $\pm$ 19 per hour. As noted above, the index consisted of both obstructive and central disordered-breathing events (Table 1). On average, however, episodes of central apnea accounted for more than 50% of all sleep-related breathing disorders, an observation that is quite different from that noted in OSA-hypopnea syndrome. In contrast to common belief, one-third of the episodes of central apnea occurred in rapid-eye-movement (REM) sleep, and two-thirds in non-REM (NREM) sleep (though in some patients, periodic breathing virtually occurred in NREM sleep).

There are several adverse pathophysiological consequences of periodic breathing, including sleep disruption, hypoxemia, both hypercapnia and hypocapnia, and changes in intrathoracic pressure (18–20). Because of periodic breathing,

Table 1 Sleep Disordered Breathing Episodes, Arterial Oxyhemoglobin Saturation, and Daytime Arterial Blood Gases and [H⁺] in 81 Heart Failure Patients Without (Group I) or With (Group II) Periodic Breathing[a]

Variable	Group I (n = 40, 49%)	Group II (n = 41, 51%)
Apnea-hypopnea index, number per hour		
Total	4 ± 3	44 ± 19[b]
NREM sleep	5 ± 5	50 ± 25[b]
REM sleep	3 ± 4	27 ± 24[b]
Central apnea index, number per hour		
Total	2 ± 2	24 ± 21[b]
NREM sleep	2 ± 3	28 ± 25[b]
REM sleep	0.4 ± 0.1	10 ± 14[b]
Baseline Sa_{O_2}, percent	95 ± 2	95 ± 2
Lowest Sa_{O_2}, percent		
Any sleep stage	89 ± 4	76 ± 12[b]
NREM sleep	89 ± 4	79 ± 11[b]
REM sleep	91 ± 3	80 ± 10[b]
$Sa_{O_2} < 90\%$, minutes	4 ± 10	49 ± 53[b]
$Sa_{O_2} < 90\%$, percent (%TST), percent	1 ± 3	19 ± 21[b]
Pa_{O_2}, mmHg	79 ± 11	85 ± 10[b]
Pa_{CO_2}, mmHg	39 ± 4	37 ± 5[b]
[H⁺], nmol/L	37 ± 2	36 ± 3

[a] Values are mean ± SD.
[b] $p < 0.05$ when compared to respective mean values in group I.
Abbreviations: NREM, non–rapid-eye-movement; REM, rapid-eye-movement; Sa_{O_2}, arterial oxyhemoglobin saturation (measured by pulse oximetry); TST, total sleep time.
Source: Data from Ref. 17.

heart failure patients (group II) had a poor sleep efficiency, owing to an inability to maintain sleep (interruption insomnia) (Table 2). On average, heart failure patients with periodic breathing spent approximately 2 hr awake in bed. Furthermore, heart failure patients with sleep apnea had more stage 1 sleep (light sleep), less stage 2 and REM sleep, and an excessive number of arousals (21). Periodic breathing also resulted in a moderate degree of arterial oxyhemoglobin desaturation (Table 1); the mean lowest saturation was 76% and saturation was below 90% for about 50 min, equivalent to 20% of total sleep time (Table 1). Arterial oxyhemoglobin desaturation during sleep occurred in spite of normal arterial P_{O2} while awake (Table 1).

In spite of marked differences in periodic breathing between group I and group II, there were no statistically significant differences in demographics, cardiac symptoms and signs, reports of habitual snoring, or subjective daytime sleepiness (Table 3). This observation is particularly unique to patients with CSA and

Table 2 Sleep Characteristics in 81 Heart Failure Patients Without (Group I) or With (Group II) Sleep-Disordered Breathing[a]

Variable	Group I	Group II
Total time in bed, minutes	392 ± 25	393 ± 19
Total sleep time, minutes	288 ± 64	264 ± 49[b]
Sleep efficiency (sleep time/time in bed), percent	73 ± 15	67 ± 13[b]
Sleep onset, minutes	18 ± 21	16 ± 16
Wakefulness after sleep onset, minutes	85 ± 46	111 ± 51[b]
Sleep stage 1, minutes	79 ± 64	111 ± 69[b]
Sleep stage 1/total sleep time, percent	28 ± 21	43 ± 26[b]
Sleep stage 2, minutes	143 ± 68	108 ± 80[b]
Sleep stage 2/total sleep time, percent	50 ± 20	40 ± 26
Sleep stages 3 and 4, minutes	4 ± 10	0.4 ± 1.4
Sleep stages 3 and 4/total sleep time, percent	1 ± 3	0.2 ± 0.5
REM sleep, minutes	62 ± 29	45 ± 35[b]
REM sleep/total sleep time percent	21 ± 8	17 ± 12[b]
NREM sleep, minutes	266 ± 51	219 ± 50
NREM sleep/total sleep time, percent	79 ± 8	83 ± 12[b]
Arousals, number per hour	20 ± 12	33 ± 21[b]
Arousals due to periodic breathing, number per hour	3 ± 3	20 ± 13[b]

[a] Values are means ± SD.
[b] $p < 0.05$ when compared to respective mean values in Group I. Periodic breathing resulted in considerable sleep disruption in patients with heart failure.
Abbreviations: REM, rapid-eye-movement; NREM, non–rapid-eye-movement.
Source: Data from Ref. 17.

heart failure (see further on) and is in marked contrast to the daytime symptomatology of the usual patients with OSA-hypopnea syndrome.

The lack of statistically significant differences in subjective daytime symptoms between the two groups is not necessarily surprising, since patients with heart failure and no periodic breathing may have daytime symptoms related to heart failure and sleep disruption. Fifteen percent of such patients (group I) reported excessive daytime sleepiness (Table 3), compared to 24% of heart failure patients with periodic breathing (the difference was not statistically significant). When excessive daytime sleepiness was measured objectively by multiple sleep latency tests, heart failure patients with sleep apnea had a significantly shorter sleep onset than those without sleep apnea (22).

Some important observations in our data were differences in left ventricular systolic function and atrioventricular irritability between groups I and II. Left ventricular ejection fraction was significantly lower (22 ± 8 versus 27 ± 9%, $p = 0.01$), and the prevalence of atrial fibrillation (22 versus 5%, $p = 0.026$) and

Table 3 Demographics, Historical Data, and Physical Examination Findings in 81 Heart Failure Patients Without (Group I) or With (Group II) Sleep Disordered Breathing[a]

Variable	Group I	Group II
Age, years	62 ± 12	66 ± 9
Weight, kilograms	85 ± 16	83 ± 25
Height, centimeters	174 ± 6	173 ± 6
Body-mass index, kilograms per square meter	28.0 ± 4.9	27.7 ± 7.3
Patients with habitual snoring, percent	50	44
Patients with excess daytime sleepiness, percent	15	24
Witnessed apnea, percent	15	22
Orthopnea, percent	25	24
Paroxysmal nocturnal dyspnea, percent	20	15
Crackles, percent	20	12
Systolic blood pressure, mmHg	124 ± 24	120 ± 18
Diastolic blood pressure, mmHg	73 ± 9	72 ± 11
New York Heart Association classification		
Classes I and II, percent	78	63
Class III, percent	23	37

[a] Values are means ± SD; there were no statistical differences between respective variables of the two groups.
Source: Data from Ref. 17.

nocturnal ventricular tachycardia (46 versus 25%, $p = 0.045$) were significantly higher in heart failure patients with sleep apnea than those without it. Similarly, during sleep the mean values for premature ventricular depolarizations (178 ± 272 vs 34 ± 58 per hour, $p = 0.0002$), couplets (15 ± 43 versus 0.4 ± 1 per hour, $p = 0.0001$) and ventricular tachycardias (1.3 ± 4 versus 0.1 ± 0.2 per hour, $p = 0.07$) were higher in patients with sleep apnea than those without it. There were significant correlations between the apnea-hypopnea index and left ventricular ejection fraction ($r = -0.35$), premature ventricular depolarization ($r = 0.42$), couplet ($r = 0.58$), and ventricular tachycardia ($r = 0.26$).

These data do not permit us to determine whether sleep-disordered breathing exacerbated left ventricular dysfunction or, alternatively, whether patients with more impaired cardiac function were more likely to have excessive sleep-disordered breathing. However, we speculate that the interaction between sleep-disordered breathing and left ventricular dysfunction could result in a vicious cycle (20), further increasing morbidity and mortality of patients with heart failure. Meanwhile, severe left ventricular systolic dysfunction and abnormalities in cardiac rhythm should serve as potential markers for the presence of significant periodic breathing during sleep in patients with heart failure.

III. Periodic Breathing and Central and Obstructive Sleep Apnea in Heart Failure with Systolic Dysfunction

We found that there was a surprisingly high prevalence (51% of the patients) of sleep-disordered breathing, which was not clinically suspected in our population (Table 3). Using arbitrary polysomnographic criteria (17), we classified the heart failure patients with sleep apnea (group II) into those with CSA (central apnea-hypopnea index ≥ 50% of overall apnea-hypopnea index) and OSA (obstructive apnea-hypopnea index > 50% of overall apnea-hypopnea index). In patients with CSA, the obstructive apnea-hypopnea index was less than 10 per hour; in patients with OSA, the obstructive apnea-hypopnea index was ≥ 15 per hour. This polysomnographic classification was done blindly without the knowledge of patients' demographic data. We found that 40% of all heart failure patients (32 out of 81 patients) had CSA and 11% had OSA (9 out of 81 patients) (Fig. 3). Only 9 (28%) of the 32 patients with CSA had habitual snoring, which was significantly less than the 78% of patients with heart failure and obstructive sleep apnea (Fig. 3). Furthermore, the body weight, body-mass index, and the diastolic blood pressure of the patients with OSA were significantly greater than in those with CSA

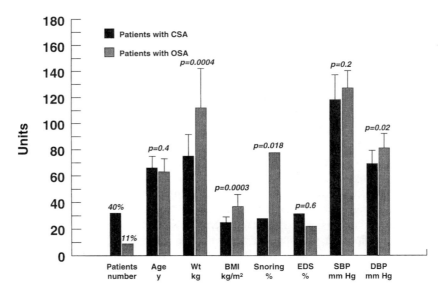

Figure 3   Demographic, historical data and physical examination findings in heart failure patients with either central sleep apnea (CSA) or obstructive sleep apnea (OSA). Wt, weight; BMI, body-mass index; EDS, excessive daytime sleepiness; SBP, systolic blood pressure; DBP, diastolic blood pressure. (From Ref. 17.)

(Fig. 3). Therefore, another reason why sleep-disordered breathing in heart failure remains relatively occult (Table 3) has to do with the predominance (40% of the patients) of CSA. Our data (Fig. 3) show that this disorder is less frequently associated with loud snoring and excessive body weight, which are the hallmarks of OSA-hypopnea syndrome. However, both CSA and OSA resulted in arterial oxyhemoglobin desaturation and arousals (Fig. 4).

In summary, 51% of patients with stable heart failure due to systolic dysfunction suffer from a moderate to severe degree of sleep-disordered breathing. Patients with heart failure and sleep apnea have a higher prevalence of atrial fibrillation, ventricular tachycardia, and lower left ventricular ejection fraction than heart failure patients without sleep apnea. CSA accounted for 40% and OSA for 11%. Heart failure patients with OSA are typically obese and have a history of habitual snoring, features that were relatively scarce in patients with CSA. Both CSA and OSA may result in recurrent episodes of arousal and arterial oxyhemoglobin desaturation.

In a recent abstract, Sin and associates (23) reported 422 heart failure patients who had been referred to a sleep laboratory for possible sleep apnea. Using an apnea-hypopnea index ≥ 10 per hour, 71% of patients were identified to have ''sleep apnea.'' In our study, 57% of the patients fell into this category (Fig. 1). We had the opportunity to study only male patients (17); however, the study of

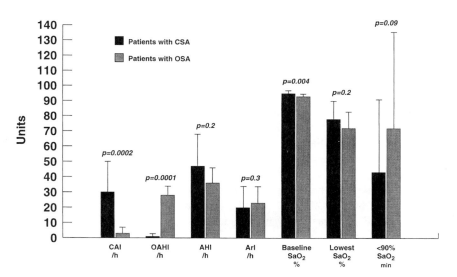

Figure 4 Polysomnographic findings in heart failure patients with either central sleep apnea (CSA) or obstructive sleep apnea (OSA). CAI, central apnea index; OAHI, obstructive apnea-hypopnea index; AHI, apnea-hypopnea index; ArI, arousal index; Sa_{O2}, arterial oxyhemoglobin saturation. (From Ref. 17.)

Sin and associates (23) included 53 women (13% of the patients). Interestingly, the male/female ratio was higher in central (3:1) than in obstructive (1:1) sleep apnea. Patients with CSA had a higher prevalence of atrial fibrillation, and they also had more pacemakers placed. Patients with OSA had a higher body-mass index than those without periodic breathing or those with CSA. The left ventricular ejection fraction in patients with CSA was lower than in those with OSA as well as in patients without sleep apnea. Given the different patterns of patient recruitment in the studies of Sin and associates (23) and our own (17), the similarities in the results are most impressive. Taken together, these two studies show the high prevalence of various forms of sleep apnea and the risk factors associated with periodic breathing in patients with heart failure and left ventricular systolic dysfunction.

IV. Periodic Breathing in Diastolic Heart Failure

Depending on their age, a considerable number of patients with symptoms of congestive heart failure may suffer from diastolic heart failure. In contrast to heart failure with systolic dysfunction, left ventricular ejection fraction is generally preserved in diastolic heart failure. In diastolic heart failure, the pathophysiological process is related to a stiff, noncompliant left ventricle that cannot fill adequately at normal diastolic pressure. As left ventricular end–diastolic pressure increases, however, symptoms of pulmonary congestion and edema prevail. Several factors may contribute to the development of a noncompliant left ventricle. For example, hypertension, a highly prevalent disorder, increases left ventricular afterload and results in ventricular hypertrophy.

Therefore, left ventricular diastolic dysfunction may be associated with both central and obstructive sleep apnea. Because of pulmonary congestion and the ensuing hyperventilation, Pa_{CO_2} could be close to the apneic point, predisposing the subject with diastolic heart failure to CSA (24–27). On the other hand, if left ventricular hypertrophy is due to hypertension and associated obesity, OSA may occur.

Only one study has been reported on periodic breathing in isolated diastolic heart failure; Chan et al. (28) studied 20 patients (13 female and 7 male), mean age 65 ± 6 (SD) years, body-mass index 28 ± 3.2 kg/m², 85% of whom had hypertension. Polysomnography showed that 55% (11 of 20) of the patients had an apnea-hypopnea index more than 10 per hour; 7 had predominantly obstructive and 4 central sleep apnea, with 2 of the latter demonstrating CSR. Comparing the two groups, the mean values for apnea-hypopnea index (20 ± 11 versus 4 ± 4 per hour) and the lowest arterial oxyhemoglobin saturation (76 ± 11% versus 82 ± 6%) were significantly different, but the mean body-mass index, although higher in patients with sleep apnea (29.1 ± 4.2 kg/m²), did not differ significantly from that in patients without sleep apnea (27.6 ± 1.3 kg/m²). As noted, however, 4 patients had CSA, and the body-mass indexes of the two subgroups (CSA and OSA patients) were not reported separately.

Research on periodic breathing in diastolic heart failure has not progressed as far as that in systolic dysfunction, with much work yet to be done.

V. Prognostic Significance of Periodic Breathing in Heart Failure

Long-term controlled studies of an adequate number of patients are necessary to determine the effects of sleep apnea on the natural history of heart failure. Heart failure is a major and growing public health problem. Its incidence and prevalence have been increasing because of increased survival from coronary heart disease and expansion of the aging population. At least 1–2% of the population suffer from heart failure, with an estimated annual incidence of 500,000. (If our data are generalizable to this population, the incidence of sleep apnea in heart failure patients is about 250,000 annually.) According to data compiled by National Heart, Lung, and Blood Institute (29), in 1993, heart failure was the first listed discharge diagnosis of 875,000 hospitalizations and the leading discharge diagnosis of hospitalized patients over 64 years of age. The average length of stay was 7.5 days. During the same year, heart failure accounted for 2,844,000 physicians' office visits. Economically, heart failure has a major impact, with an estimated health cost of $9 billion in 1989 (30), of which $6.4 billion was related to hospital care. Mortality from heart failure remains high in spite of vasodilator therapy. The annual mortality for patients with heart failure and systolic dysfunction is about 5% for asymptomatic patients [New York Heart Association (NYHA) class 1], 10–20% from mild to moderate heart failure (classes II and III), and 40% from patients with severe heart failure. Death rate during hospitalization from heart failure is estimated at 7–10% (29,30).

It is probably reasonable to speculate (20) that pathophysiological consequences of recurrent episodes of gas-exchange abnormalities (hypoxemia, hypercapnia, and hypocapnia), excessive arousals, and large negative swings in pleural pressure (occurring during OSA and the hyperventilation phase of CSA) may have adverse effects on myocardial cells and the function of an already failed left ventricle. The adverse effects of hypoxemia may be further augmented if myocardial blood supply is also limited because of coronary artery disease.

Large-scale studies, however, are needed to determine whether the natural history of heart failure is affected by sleep apnea and, furthermore, whether treatment of sleep apnea (obstructive and central) improves morbidity and mortality. In regard to OSA, studies (31) have suggested that this disorder per se may be associated with increased mortality. Adverse consequences of OSA could be further augmented in the presence of heart failure, as indicated above.

In regard to CSA in heart failure, few studies have been reported; these are summarized in Table 4. Although these studies may be criticized for various reasons, such as an inadequate number of patients and differences in ejection fraction among various groups, they all show a trend toward increased mortality of heart failure patients with sleep apnea than without. In the most recent study, Andreas and associates (32) followed 36 patients with heart failure for an average of 32 (range 11–53) months (Table 4). Cumulative survival between the two groups stratified by the amount of Cheyne-Stokes respiration (less than or equal to or greater than 20% of total sleep time) did not differ significantly. However, reviewing the data, it appears that the group with less than 20% CSR had mild sleep apnea. Furthermore, when survival analysis was performed after 3 months, 4 of 20 (20%) versus 1 of 16 (6%) of patients, respectively, with CSR $\geq$ 20 and CSR $<$ 20% died ($p = 0.24$). If we assume that the difference in survival (20 versus 6%) is clinically significant, then to have been statistically significant (alpha = 0.05, two sided, beta = 0.2), the number of patients in each arm should have been 109.

Trends toward a lower survival rate in patients with heart failure and sleep apnea were reported by Findley and associates (10) and Ancoli-Israel and colleagues (33) (Table 4). In another study by Hanly and Zuberi-Khokhar (34), when 16 heart failure patients were classified according to apnea-hypopnea index, there was a significant difference in the survival of patients with CSA (apnea-hypopnea index = 41 per hour) when compared to heart failure patients without sleep apnea (apnea-hypopnea index of 6 per hour) (Table 4).

In the study of Hanly and Zuberi-Khokhar (34) as well as the study by Ancoli-Israel and associates (33), the patients with excess mortality suffered from severe CSA. This may in part account for differences in mortality between those two studies (33, 34) and that of Andreas and colleagues (32), whose patients may have had less severe sleep apnea.

In the study of Hanly and Zuberi-Khokhar (34), all patients who died were hypocapnic (as determined by transcutaneous P_{CO_2}). Hypocapnia may be an important predictor of mortality in heart failure patients with CSA. In a recent study, we observed a strong association between hypocapnia and ventricular tachycardia in patients with heart failure (27). Of the 59 patients with heart failure, 18 were hypocapnic (awake $Pa_{CO_2} \leq 35$ mmHg). Although the mean left ventricular ejection fraction did not differ significantly, 78% of the hypocapnic (versus 39% of the eucapnic patients) patients had CSA. Hypocapnic patients with heart failure had more severe periodic breathing (and its associated consequences) than eucapnic patients. Hypocapnia was associated with excess ventricular irritability (premature ventricular contractions, couplets, and ventricular tachycardia). The number of ventricular tachycardias per hour of sleep was 20 times higher in the

Table 4 Survival in Heart Failure Patients With (Group I) and Without (Group II) Sleep Apnea

Author	Number of Patients		Age (Years)		LVEF (percent)		AHI/hr, CSR %TST		Death (percent)		F/U (months)
	Group I	Group II	Group I	Group II	Group I	Group II	Group I	Group II	Group I	Group II	
Findley et al.,[10]	6	9	68 ±11	56 ±11	28 ± 5	34 ± 9	30[a] ±29	1 ± 1	100[a]	33	6
Ancoli-Israel[33,b]	15	31	74* ±12	64 ± 4	NR (n = 3)	NR (n = 6)	52[a] ±15	3 ± 5	87[a]	45	NR
Hanly et al.[34]	9	7	61 ± 8	63 ± 4	22 ± 5	24 ± 5	41[a] ± 7	6 ± 5	78	14	36–54
Andreas[32]	20	16	59* ± 7	48 ± 7	20 ± 6	22 ± 9	CSR ≥ 20%	CSR < 20%	20	6	11–53

[a] $p \leq 0.05$

[b] In this study 66 and 13% of group I patients, and 27 and 39% of group II patients had, respectively, heart failure and chronic obstructive pulmonary disease.

Abbreviations: LVEF, left ventricular ejection fraction; AHI, apnea-hypopnea index; CSR, Cheyne-stokes respiration; F/U, follow-up; NR, not reported.

hypocapnic than the eucapnic patients. Ventricular tachycardia may be the mediator of sudden death in heart failure, as up to 40% of deaths in patients with heart failure may be sudden (35,36).

It is highly plausible that long-term treatment of sleep apnea in heart failure will significantly change the progressive downhill course of heart failure. Short-term therapeutic trials support this notion. First, application of nasal continuous positive airway pressure to patients with heart failure and sleep apnea has resulted in an increase in left ventricular ejection fraction (37) and reduced neurohormonal activation (decreased sympathoadrenal activation and atrial natriuretic peptide) (38,39). Since a low ejection fraction and activation of neurohormonal systems are important determinants of prognosis (36,40), the changes induced by continuous positive airway pressure may improve long-term survival of heart failure patients. Second, short-term treatment with low-flow nasal O_2 has been shown

Table 5 Comparison of Certain Variables Between Eucapnic and Hypocapnic Patients with Stable Heart Failure[a]

Variable	Eucapnic	Hypocapnic
Number	41	18
Patients with central sleep apnea, percent	39	78[b]
Age, years	63 ± 11	64 ± 9
Body mass index, kilograms per square meter	27 ± 5	26 ± 5
New York Heart Association classification		
Classes I and II, percent	80	44[b]
Class III, percent	20	56[b]
Pa_{O_2}, mmHg	83 ± 10	86 ± 10
Pa_{CO_2}, mmHg	39 ± 2	32 ± 3[b]
Left ventricular ejection fraction, percent	25 ± 8	21 ± 9
Total dark time, minutes	396 ± 23	393 ± 21
Total sleep time, minutes	287 ± 61	251 ± 52[b]
Apnea-hypopnea index, number per hour	20 ± 27	36 ± 25[b]
Central apnea index, number per hour	12 ± 19	26 ± 21[b]
Baseline Sa_{O_2}, percent	95 ± 2	95 ± 1
Lowest Sa_{O_2}, percent	84 ± 9	81 ± 14
Arousals due to periodic breathing, number per hour	9 ± 4	16 ± 3
Premature ventricular contractions, number per hour	68 ± 185	229 ± 262[b]
Couplets, number per hour	1 ± 2	13 ± 18[b]
Ventricular tachycardias, number per hour	0.1 ± 0.1	2 ± 3[b]

[a] Values are means ± SD.
[b] $p < 0.05$ when respective mean values were compared.
Abbreviations: Sa_{O_2}, arterial oxyhemoglobin saturation measured by pulse oximetry.
Source: Data from Ref. 27.

to improve periodic breathing, which could potentially improve sleep quality, cognitive function, and exercise capacity (41,42) and decrease urinary excretion of catecholamines (43).

We hope the results of well-designed studies with adequate numbers of heart failure patients with survival as an endpoint will become available in the next few years.

Acknowledgments

Supported by Merit Review Grants from the Department of Veterans Affairs. The author thanks C. Brown and F. Jones for their assistance.

References

1. Cohn JN. The management of chronic heart failure. N Engl J Med 1996; 335:490–498.
2. Major RH. Classic Descriptions of Disease. Springfield, IL: Charles C Thomas, 1932:508.
3. Tenney SM. Cheyne, Cheyne and Stokes. News Physiol Sci 1994; 9:96–97.
4. Ward M. Periodic respiration: A short historical note. Ann R Coll Surg Engl 1973; 52:330–334.
5. Cheyne J. A case of apoplexy, in which the fleshy part of the heart was converted into fat. Dublin Hosp Rep Commun 1818; 2:216–223.
6. Stokes W. The Diseases of the Heart and the Aorta. Dublin: Hodges and Smith, 1854.
7. Mackenzie J, Sir. Diseases of the Heart, 4th ed. London: Humphrey Milford, Oxford University Press, 1925:30–35.
8. Harrison TR, King CE, Calhoun JA, Harrison WG. Congestive heart failure: Cheyne-Stokes respiration as the cause of paroxysmal dyspnea at the onset of sleep. Arch Intern Med 1934; 53:891–910.
9. Rees PJ, Clark TJH. Paroxysmal nocturnal dyspnea and periodic respiration. Lancet 1979; 2:1315–1317.
10. Findley LJ, Zwillich CW, Ancoli-Israel S, Kripke D, Tisi G, Moser KM. Cheyne-Stokes breathing during sleep in patients with left ventricular heart failure. South Med J 1985; 78:11–15.
11. Dark DS, Pingleton SK, Kerby GR, Crabb JE, Gollub SB, Glatter TR, Dunn MI. Breathing pattern abnormalitites and arterial oxygen desaturation during sleep in the congestive heart failure syndrome. Chest 1987; 91:833–836.
12. Yasuma F, Nomura H, Hayashi H, Okada T, Tsuzuki M. Breathing abnormalities during sleep in patients with chronic heart failure. Jpn Circ J 1989; 53:1506–1510.
13. Takasaki Y, Orr D, Popkin J, Rutherford R, Liu P, Bradley TD. Effect of nasal continuous positive airway pressure on sleep apnea in congestive heart failure. Am Rev Respir Dis 1989; 140:1578–1584.

14. Hanly PJ, Millar TW, Steljes DG, Baert R, Frais MA, Kryger MH. Respiration and abnormal sleep in patients with congestive heart failure. Chest 1989; 96:480–488.

15. Dowdell WT, Javaheri S, McGinnis W. Cheyne-Stokes respiration presenting as sleep apnea syndrome: clinical and polysomnographic features. Am Rev Respir Dis 1990; 141:871–879.

16. Javaheri S, Parker TJ, Wexler L, Michaels SE, Stanberry E, Nishiyama H, Rosell GA. Occult sleep-disordered breathing in stable congestive heart failure. Ann Intern Med 1995; 122:487–492. [Erratum, Ann Intern Med 1995; 123:77.]

17. Javaheri S, Parker TJ, Liming JD, Corbett BS, Nishiyama H, Wexler L, Roselle GA. Sleep apnea in 81 ambulatory male patients with stable heart failure: types and their prevalences, consequences, and presentations. Circulation 1998; 97:2154–2159.

18. Yamashiro Y, Kryger MH. Sleep in heart failure. Sleep 1993; 16:513–523.

19. Bradley TD, Floras JS. Pathophysiologic and therapeutic implications of sleep apnea in congestive heart failure. J Cardiac Failure 1996; 2:223–240.

20. Javaheri S. Central sleep apnea-hypopnea syndrome in heart failure: prevalence, impact and treatment. Sleep 1996; 19:S229–S231.

21. ASDA Report: EEG arousals: scoring rules and examples. Sleep 1992; 15:174–184.

22. Hanly P, Zuberi-Khokhar N. Daytime sleepiness in patients with congestive heart failure and Cheyne-Stokes respiration. Chest 1995; 107:952–958.

23. Sin D, Fitzgerald F, Bradley TD. Risk factors for sleep apnea in heart failure. Am J Respir Crit Care Med 1998; 157:A62.

24. Skatrud JB, Dempsey JA. Interaction of sleep state and chemical stimuli in sustaining rhythmic ventilation. J Appl Physiol 1983; 55:813–822.

25. Naughton M, Benard D, Tam A, Rutherford R, Bradley TD. Role of hyperventilation in the pathogenesis of central sleep apnea in patients with congestive heart failure. Am Rev Respir Dis 1993; 148:330–338.

26. Hanly P, Zuberi N, Gray R. Pathogenesis of Cheyne-Stokes respiration in patients with congestive heart failure: relationship to arterial P_{CO2}. Chest 1993; 104:1079–1084.

27. Javaheri S, Corbett WS. Association of low $PaCO_2$ with central sleep apnea and ventricular arrhythmias in ambulatory patients with stable heart failure. Ann Intern Med 1998; 3:204–207.

28. Chan J, Sanderson J, Chan W, Lai C, Choy D, Ho A, Leung R. Prevalence of sleep-disordered breathing in diastolic heart failure. Chest 1997; 111:1488–1493.

29. National Institute of Health, National Heart Lung and Blood Institute. Factbook—Disease Statistics. Washington, DC: NIH/NHLBI, 1995:27–42.

30. National Institute of Health. Morbidity and Mortality: Chartbook on Cardiovascular Lung and Blood Diseases. Cardiovascular Diseases. Washington, DC: NIH, May 1996:15–47.

31. He J, Kryger MH, Zorick FJ, Conway W, Roth T. Mortality and apnea index in obstructive sleep apnea. Chest 1988; 94:9–14.

32. Andreas S, Hagenah G, Möller C, Werner GS, Kreuzer H. Cheyne-Stokes respiration and prognosis in congestive heart failure. Am J Cardiol 1996; 78:1260–1264.

33. Ancoli-Israel S, Engler RL, Friedman PJ, Klauber MR, Ross PA, Kripke DF. Comparison of patients with central sleep apnea with and without Cheyne-Stokes respiration. Chest 1994; 106:780–786.

34. Hanly P, Zuberi-Khokhar N. Increased mortality associated with Cheyne-Stokes respiration in patients with congestive heart failure. Am J Respir Crit Care Med 1996; 153:272–276.

35. Narang R, Cleland JGF, Erhardt L, Ball SG, Coats AJS, Cowley AJ, Dargie HJ, Hall AS, Hampton JR, Poole-Wilson PA. Mode of death in chronic heart failure: a request and proposition for more accurate classification. Eur Heart J 1996; 17:1390–1403.

36. Cohn JN. Prognosis in congestive heart failure. J Cardiac Failure 1996; 2:S225–S229.

37. Naughton MT, Liu PP, Benard DC, Goldstein RS, Bradley TD. Treatment of congestive heart failure and Cheyne-Stokes respiration during sleep by continuous positive airway pressure. Am J Respir Crit Care Med 1995; 151:92–97.

38. Naughton MT, Benard DC, Liu PP, Rutherford R, Rankin F, Bradley TD. Effects of nasal CPAP on sympathetic activity in patients with heart failure and central sleep apnea. Am J Respir Crit Care Med 1995; 152:473–479.

39. Tkacova R, Liu PP, Naughton MT, Bradley TD. Effect of continuous positive airway pressure on mitral regurgitant fraction and atrial natriuretic peptide in patients with heart failure. J Am Coll Cardiol 1997; 30:739–745.

40. Francis GS. Determinants of prognosis in patients with heart failure. J Heart Lung Transplant 1994; 12:S113–S116.

41. Hanly PJ, Millar TW, Steljes DG, Baert R, Frais MA, Kryger MH. The effect of oxygen on respiration and sleep in patients with congestive heart failure. Ann Intern Med 1989; 111:777–782.

42. Andreas S, Clemen C, Sandholzer H, Figulla HR, Kreuzer H. Improvement of exercise capacity with treatment of Cheyne-Stokes respiration in patients with congestive heart failure. J Am Coll Cardiol 1996; 27:1486–1490.

43. Staniforth AD, Kinneart WJM, Starling R, Hetmanski DJ, Cowley AJ. Effects of oxygen on sleep quality, cognitive function and sympathetic activity in patients with chronic heart failure and Cheyne-Stokes respiration. Eur Heart J 1998; 19:922–928.

19

Effects of Continuous Positive Airway Pressure in Animal Models of Congestive Heart Failure

STEVEN M. SCHARF

Long Island Jewish Medical Center
and Albert Einstein College of Medicine
New Hyde Park, New York

I. Introduction

The respiratory and cardiovascular systems are both concerned with delivery of oxygen to peripheral tissues. As such, it is not surprising that they interact on many levels: mechanical, humoral, and neuroreflex. Failure of one system is often associated with dysfunction or failure of the other. While various forms of positive-pressure ventilatory therapy have been known to improve gas exchange and work of breathing in patients with congestive heart failure (CHF), it has become clear in recent years that, under the right circumstances, this type of therapy can lead to improved function of the failing heart. Specifically, clinical studies indicate that continuous positive airway pressure (CPAP), delivered by face mask, may lead to dramatic improvements in cardiac function in patients with CHF both acutely (1,2) and chronically (3). However, the clinical literature does not uniformly demonstrate improved cardiac function and outcome in CHF with CPAP (4–6). Some of the differences in reported efficacy of CPAP in CHF no doubt relate to the presence of numerous comorbid conditions, different therapeutic and clinical environments, and nonuniformity of diagnoses in small clinical studies. In addition, the necessary limitations of clinical studies may make elucidation of responsible mechanisms difficult. Animal studies offer some advantages

435

in this regard, especially uniformity of and control over experimental conditions. Principles learned from animal studies may then be coupled with human disease states to better explain the role of CPAP therapy in treatment of patients. This chapter is written in five major sections. First, we discuss the theoretical background concerning possible effects of CPAP on cardiocirculatory function. Second, we review some of the relevant previous animal studies on the effects of increasing airway pressure on cardiac function in normal and failing hearts during positive-pressure ventilation. Third, we describe animal studies performed in our laboratory on the effects of CPAP on cardiac function in normal and failing hearts. Fourth, we discuss different models to explain the experimental findings. We hope to convince the reader that the theoretical background predicting improvement in cardiac function under some circumstances is incomplete, and we suggest some alternative factors that might be at work. Finally, we try to draw some conclusions and point out some directions for future studies.

II. The Control of Cardiac Output with Positive Airway Pressure—Theory

The determination of cardiac output (CO) with increasing airway pressure may be understood in terms of the interaction between venous return and cardiac function according to the classic theory of Guyton et al. (7), the basic principles of which remain valid today, in spite of numerous modifications to the theory. Venous return is determined by the gradient between the pressure in the common peripheral circulatory reservoir, called the mean circulatory pressure, and right atrial pressure, which acts as the back pressure to venous return as well as an index of the diastolic filling (preload) of the heart. As such, the following equation applies:

$$VR = \frac{MCP - RAP}{Rv} \tag{1}$$

where VR = venous return; MCP = mean circulatory pressure, the upstream pressure for venous return; RAP = right atrial pressure, and Rv is the resistance to venous return. This model has proven to be a powerful tool for understanding many aspects of circulatory physiology. The reader is referred elsewhere for a more complete discussion of newer modifications of the venous return model (8). Figure 1 demonstrates a venous return curve along with some cardiac function curves to be discussed shortly. If RAP is raised to the level of MCP, then the pressure gradient driving VR is zero and VR is zero. As RAP is lowered, VR increases linearly, with a slope equal to 1/Rv. At some point, further decreases in RAP fail to elicit increases in VR and VR becomes flow-limited. This point is represented by the flow-limiting (FL) point in the VR curve. Flow limitation occurs because of collapse of the great veins at or close to the entrance to the

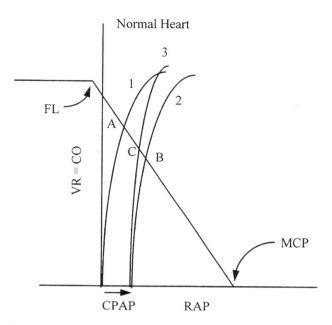

Figure 1   Venous return (VR)–cardiac function interactions that determine cardiac output (CO). Cardiac function curve 1 is normal. Cardiac function curve 2 is shifted to the right on the *x* axis by the amount by which continuous positive airway pressure (CPAP) increases intrathoracic pressure (ITP), but there is no effect on cardiac function. Cardiac function curve 3 shows a beneficial effect of increased ITP. See text for discussion. MCP, mean circulatory pressure; RAP, right atrial pressure; FL, point of flow limitation in VR curve.

thorax as RAP falls below their surrounding pressure. A Frank-Starling type of cardiac function curve may be superimposed on the VR curve. Three cardiac function curves, labeled 1, 2, and 3, are shown in Figure 1. The curves plot CO as a function of RAP, which is an index of diastolic cardiac filling. For now, we concentrate on curve 1, a "normal" cardiac function curve. At equilibrium, VR must equal CO; therefore, under steady-state conditions, the system exists at the point of intersection of the VR and cardiac function curves, indicated as point A in Figure 1.

A.   Effects of Increased Intrathoracic Pressure

If airway pressure increases, lung volume increases. This leads to an increase in intrathoracic pressure (ITP), the degree of which is determined by lung and chest wall compliance in addition to the increase in airway pressure. If there were no effect on cardiac function, then the cardiac function curve would shift to the right along the *x* axis by an amount equal to the increase in ITP. This is shown in Figure 1 as curve 2. The point of steady-state intersection of the VR and cardiac function curves moves to point B. Essentially, because of rightward shift in the cardiac function curve with increased ITP, the point of intersection between VR and cardiac function curves "slides" down the VR curve. This is because increases in ITP are transmitted through to the right atrium, raising RAP and reducing the gradient for VR (MCP − RAP). Thus, with increased airway pressure, VR would decrease. It should be noted that the situation is actually more complicated than this. As airway pressure increases and CO decreases, there are compensatory increases in MCP, which tend to buffer the decreases in VR, and there are probably shifts in the FL point as well. However, the importance of these changes at the relatively low levels of airway pressure used to deliver CPAP is not great; the reader is referred elsewhere for complete discussion of changes in the VR curve with high levels of airway pressure (8,9). Even if, as discussed below, cardiac function is improved by the increase in ITP, this has little effect on the changes in CO in normal hearts. In Figure 1, the theoretical possibility of improved cardiac function with increased ITP is demonstrated by curve 3, which is steeper than curves 1 and 2. In this case, the intersection of VR and cardiac function curves is found at C, with CO only slightly higher than at point B but still lower than at point A. This is because the theoretical "best" cardiac function curve would be a vertical line. Since normal cardiac function curves are not far off the vertical, there is really little room for improvement. Thus, with normal hearts, when ITP is increased with CPAP, VR effects predominate over the cardiac function effects and CO decreases.

The somewhat scary Figure 2 shows the effects of increased ITP when there is a failing heart. In this case the cardiac function curve (curve 1) is depressed, shifted down to the right. That is, CO is lower and RAP is greater than normal. The intersection of VR and cardiac function curves (point A) is at a lower CO and greater RAP than the normal curves. With application of increased airway pressure, if there were no change in the cardiac function curve, then there would be a shift from curve 1 to curve 2 and VR/CO would decrease (point B). However, if increased ITP improved cardiac function, then the point of intersection of VR and cardiac function curves would move back up the VR curve and CO could even increase with ITP (point C). This is because, with a severely depressed cardiac function curve, there is a great deal of room for improvement in cardiac function, and ITP-induced changes in cardiac function could predominate over changes in VR. Curve 4 shows that if ITP pressure continued to increase, eventually VR effects would lead to a decrease in CO (point D). Thus, theory predicts that if increased ITP with increasing airway pressure improves cardiac function, this effect could be sufficient with failing hearts to allow CO to actually increase. However, there would be an "optimal" increase in ITP beyond which further increases would again lead to decreased CO.

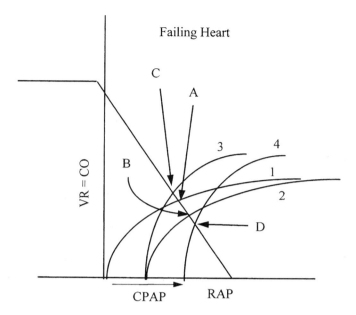

Figure 2 VR–cardiac function curves with failing hearts. Cardiac function curves 1– 3 are as for Figure 1. Cardiac function curve 4 shows what happens if higher levels of CPAP are applied, thus continuing to increase ITP. See text for discussion. Abbreviations as in Figure 1.

B. Effects of Increased ITP on Cardiac Function

Since the middle of the nineteenth century (10), it has been recognized that just as decreasing ITP during inspiration can aid the entrance of blood into the chest from the periphery, it will impede the egress of blood from the chest to the periphery. There are a number of ways of looking at this. This is because the heart and great vessels are exposed to ITP. Normally, ITP changes are small and respiration has a small effect on blood flow. However, with abnormal ventilatory maneuvers, the situation can change. Figure 3 presents a simplified scheme of the left ventricle (LV) (apparently hanging by its own aorta) within the chest. At "baseline" during systole, we have shown the LV pressure as 100 units and intrathoracic pressure as −3 units. From the point of view of the LV, it "sees" a pressure not of 100 units across its wall but of 103 units. Thus the stress across the LV wall may be expressed as the pressure gradient, called the transmural pressure, across its wall. If a Mueller maneuver (sustained decrease in ITP) is performed, decreasing ITP to −40 units in this example, then at systole, for the same intracavitary LV pressure of 100 units, the LV actually is contracting against a pres-

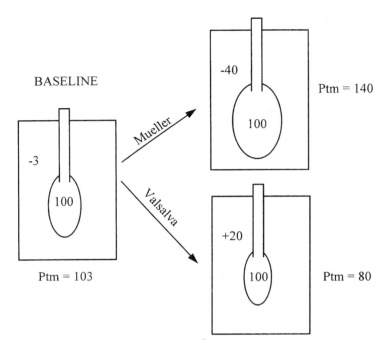

Figure 3 Model for mechanical effects of Mueller and Valsalva maneuver on left ventricular (LV) function. Ptm, end-systolic transmural LV pressure (difference between LV intracavitary and intrathoracic pressure). See text for discussion.

sure 140 units across its wall. Thus, although arterial pressure (equal to LV systolic pressure) need not be different between baseline and the Mueller maneuver, the LV is actually contracting against an increased LV systolic transmural pressure. This is sensed by the LV as an increase in LV afterload, and the ventricle dilates. During the performance of a Valsalva maneuver, ITP increases to, in this example, +20. Hence, for the same LV intracavitary pressure of 100 units, LV transmural systolic pressure decreases to 80 units, and the LV senses this as a decrease in afterload with improved ventricular ejection. Thus, under the right circumstances, increasing ITP could aid in ventricular ejection. Numerous studies in humans and animals have confirmed these basic principles of the effects of changes in ITP on ventricular function (11–18).

From what has been said above, there are theoretical reasons to believe that purely on a mechanical basis, increasing ITP would be harmful to CO in normal hearts but would be of potential benefit in patients with abnormal or failing hearts. We next consider the experimental findings addressing this issue in animal studies.

III. Effects of Increasing Airway Pressure on Cardiac Output Hearts During Mechanical Ventilation

In reviewing experimental data, one must be careful about extrapolating results between studies. This is because conditions may vary greatly between studies. Also, mechanical ventilation with positive end-expiratory pressure (PEEP) is often considered to be equivalent to CPAP. However, with mechanical ventilation and PEEP, increases in ITP occur throughout all phases of the respiratory cycle, while with CPAP, ITP is increased at end-expiration but ITP decreases during inspiration. Thus, VR effects of PEEP are far greater than those of CPAP. In addition, experimental studies with PEEP are usually performed on anesthetized, often paralyzed animals. Anesthetic effects on baseline cardiovascular function are profound. It is known that there are sympathetic homeostatic reflexes that buffer the adverse hemodynamic effects of PEEP (19,20). These are likely to be depressed more with general anesthesia, used for studying PEEP, than with sedation, used in some studies of CPAP. Even more caution is urged in extrapolating to clinical situations.

A. Effects of Increased ITP in Heart Failure—Anesthetized Animals

Following up on clinical studies suggesting improved CO with positive-pressure ventilation in heart failure, Pinsky et al. produced heart failure (21) by injecting large doses of propanalol in anesthetized dogs. The animals were ventilated using large-tidal-volume (30 mL/kg) ventilation and, to further increase ITP, the chest and abdomen were bound with elastic bandages. With binding, inspiratory ITP increased by 12.1 mmHg. With the mechanical ventilation under the bound condition, there was a upward-leftward shift in the Starling function curve of the LV, indicating improved cardiac function. In a similar study on anesthetized humans with heart failure, Pinsky and Summer demonstrated improved cardiac output (22) when ITP was increased during mechanical ventilation by binding the chest and abdomen. The term *ventilator-assisted myocardial performance* (VAMP) was suggested by Robotham to describe the use of the ventilator to improve the function of failing hearts (23).

Theoretically, increased ITP during cardiac diastole would exert its maximum adverse effect on ventricular filling and its minimal beneficial effect on cardiac ejection. To minimize adverse effects of increased ITP on VR and to maximize the beneficial effects on LV function, increased ITP could be gated to cardiac systole. Pinsky et al. (24) studied the use of phasic increases in ITP produced by a jet ventilator in dogs with propanalol-induced cardiac failure. With normal cardiac function, LV stroke volume decreased with phasic pulsed increased ITP. However, when cardiac function was abnormal, LV stroke volume increased with this form of ventilatory assist. As predicted, effects were maximum when the pulsed increases in ITP were gated to cardiac systole (25). Similar findings were later observed in anesthetized humans with heart failure (26). Using a mathematical model, Beyer et al. (27) predicted that maximum flow augmentation would occur when the onset of the pulsed increase in ITP was simultaneous with onset of LV isovolumic contraction. Thus, by proper timing of the pulsed increase in ITP, ventricular assist may be obtained with minimal adverse effect on VR.

Peters and Ihle (28) used chronically instrumented unanesthetized dogs before and after coronary occlusion to study the effects of timed pulsed increases in ITP. They produced these pulses by electrocardiographic gated inflations of a vest. Although single inflations coupled to late systole augmented stroke volume, repetitive inflations coupled to any cardiac cycle phase led to nonspecific increases in flow. This was not observed after β-adrenergic blockade. Thus, the effects of vest inflation were related to changes in sympathoadrenal tone rather than increased ITP. They felt that direct compression of the heart, not increased ITP, was responsible for increased stroke volume in this model. The demonstration of the importance of sympathoadrenal function in determining the effects of phasic increases in ITP suggests a dimension that is not considered by purely mechanical models of the circulation and studies in animals in which sympathetic blockade is used to produce heart failure.

B. CHF and Sympathoadrenal Function

Patients with chronic CHF experience substantial changes in sympathoadrenal function. These include elevation in tonic sympathetic tone resulting in chronic elevations in baseline plasma norepinephrine levels (29–31), downregulation of cardiac β-receptors (32), decreased myocardial norepinephrine levels (33), and increased myocardial norepinephrine turnover (34,35). While enhancement of sympathoadrenal function acutely acts to maintain blood pressure and cardiac function, the chronic effects of CHF on sympathoadrenal function could actually worsen cardiac function by leading to increased LV afterload (vasoconstriction), myocardial necrosis (chronic sympathetic stimulation), and depletion of myocardial catechols and inotropic receptors. By further increasing sympathetic tone, the recurrent hypoxemia seen in sleep apnea patients could even worsen this situation in patients with combined disease. Reversal of CHF-induced changes in sympathetic tone—whether by downregulation of the whole system, selective vasodilation, or restoration of myocardial adrenergic responsiveness—could lead to increased CO and clinical improvement. Thus, in addition to mechanical effects, CPAP-induced changes in heart function could be related to changes in neurohumoral function. With this in mind, we now consider the effects of CPAP some recent experimental studies.

IV. Studies of CPAP in Preinstrumented Sedated Animals

In our laboratory, we have developed a previously instrumented preparation in pigs that allows for study under sedation rather than anesthesia. In stage 1, animals are instrumented using sterile technique under general anesthesia for study of LV function. This includes placement of a catheter into the left atrium, sonomicrometer crystals across the orthogonal axes of the LV for later measurement of LV volume, and an electromagnetic flow probe around the ascending aorta. Catheters and leads are brought out into a subcutaneous pocket. Following recovery of several days, animals are sedated with either fentanyl-droperidol or alphaloxone-alphadolone, a steroidal analgesic-anesthetic. Animals remain tranquil but still responsive to pain and loud noises. Under local anesthesia, femoral arterial and venous catheters are placed for administration of fluids and recording of blood pressure; the subcutaneous pocket is then opened and a high-fidelity catheter-tipped manometer is passed into the LV via the left atrial catheter. Thus, LV end-diastolic pressure (LVEDP), end-systolic pressure (LVESP), and LV volumes may be measured.

A. Effects of CPAP on CO

In sedated pigs, the effects of increasing CPAP in 5-cmH_2O increments were studied in the normal condition and then following infusion of hetastarch 35 mL/kg (36). This infusion was enough to increase LVEDP from the normal value of 10.6 ± 5.9 to 19.1 ± 6.4 mmHg ($p < 0.001$). Thus, the hypervolemic condition represents at state of volume expansion and central circulatory conditions similar to that seen with CHF. Cardiac index (CI) changes are illustrated in Figure 4 (37). In the figure, values are shown normalized to baseline, which was set at 1. Note that with normovolemic animals (NV), increasing CPAP to 15 cmH_2O led to decreased CI. When the animals were made hypervolemic, however, CI increased at low-level CPAP before decreasing with continued increases in CPAP. The maximum increase in CI was seen at the lowest level of CPAP, 5 cmH_2O. In another series of experiments, CHF was produced in the animals using rapid ventricular pacing for 7–10 days before studying the hemodynamics (38). In this case, LVEDP at baseline was even higher than with hypervolemia, 21.6 ± 5.3 mmHg. Changes in CI with CHF are also shown in Figure 4. Note that the increase in CI was also maximal at the lowest level of CPAP, as in the hypervolemia studies. However, even though CI decreased as CPAP was increased, it did not reach baseline even at the greatest level of CPAP. Finally, an extremely interesting phenomenon was observed following removal of CPAP. In the normovolemic

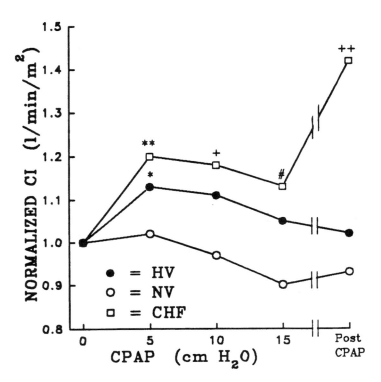

Figure 4 Changes in cardiac index (CI) normalized to baseline in two sets of experiments: Studies of normal animals while normovolemic (NV) and after being made hypervolemic (HV) and studies of animals following induction of congestive heart failure (CHF). See text for discussion. (From Ref. 37.)

and hypervolemic studies (36), CI returned to baseline following removal of CPAP. However, with CHF, there was a secondary increase in CI following CPAP removal that lasted from 30–60 min before returning to baseline. The implications of this finding for the mechanism of action of CPAP are important, as discussed below.

B. Effects of CPAP on Ventricular Afterload

In the studies of Genovese et al. cited above (36,38), LV end-systolic volume was used as one indicator of changes in LV afterload. Decreased LV end-systolic volume was taken as prima facie evidence of a decrease in LV afterload, since changes in contractility were assumed not to have occurred. Figure 5 shows raw-

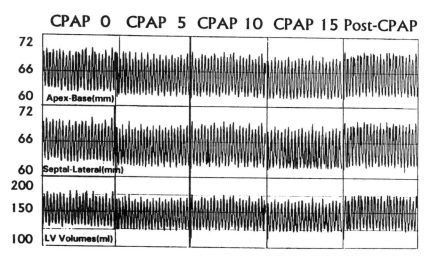

Figure 5 Changes in two of the three LV orthagonal LV dimensions and calculated LV volume during CPAP in pigs with pacing induced CHF. (From Ref. 38.)

data traces and calculated LV volumes from the CHF studies (38). Note that there was a decrease in end-systolic (minimal) LV volume with increasing CPAP. Figure 6 shows mean changes in LV volumes from the normal animals. LV ejection fraction was also found to increase with CPAP in both the hypervolemic animals (36) and animals with CHF (38).

In the studies of Pinsky et al. (22,24–26), LV afterload was measured as LV end-systolic transmural pressure. This was calculated as LV end-systolic cavitary pressure minus esophageal pressure—a reasonable assumption for many studies. However, when the pericardium is intact, changes in cardiac volume may complicate matters. When the heart is small, changes in ITP are transmitted to the cardiac surface, and the effect of pericardial elasticity on cardiac surface pressure is small. On the other hand, with cardiac dilation, the elasticity of the pericardium becomes greater and may have greater effects on calculations of LV transmural pressure. This is because cardiac surface pressure is the arithmetic sum of intrathoracic pressure and pericardial elastic pressure. As the heart becomes larger, pericardial elastic pressure becomes an increasingly important component of cardiac surface pressure during positive-pressure maneuvers (39,40). This means that change in esophageal pressure during a respiratory maneuver may be a poor indicator of pressure on the cardiac surface when the heart is dilated, as in CHF or hypervolemia (40). It follows, then, that using esophageal pressure to estimate LV transmural pressure may lead to inaccurate overestimations of LV transmural pressure.

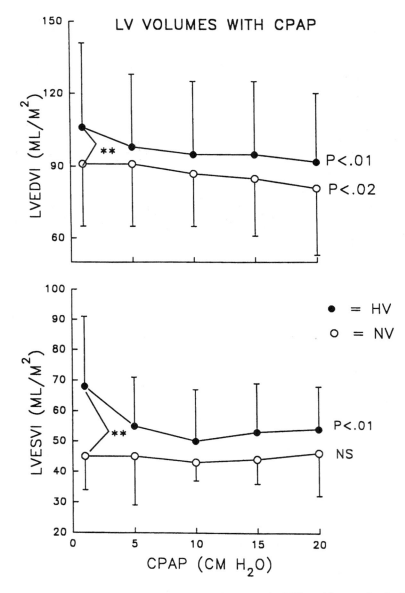

Figure 6   Cardiac volumes with CPAP in normovolemic (NV) and hypervolemic (HV) animals. **statistical significant difference between NV and HV. The *p* values are for change with CPAP (analysis of variance). Open symbols, normovolemia; closed symbols, hypervolemia. (Modified from Ref. 36.)

In the initial studies in CHF (38), cardiac surface pressure was not measured. Therefore, change in airway pressure was used as a maximal estimate of change in cardiac surface pressure. In other words, it was assumed that there was complete transmission of CPAP to the pleural space. Hence, the degree to which LV transmural pressure would decrease during CPAP would have been overestimated using airway pressure to calculate LV transmural pressure. Figure 7 illustrates the values of LV end-systolic transmural pressure from these calculations in CHF. There was no decrease in LV end-systolic transmural pressure with CPAP using airway pressure to estimate cardiac surface pressure. Similar results were found in human studies by Liston et al. (41). On the other hand, using esophageal pressure as an estimate of cardiac surface pressure, Naughton et al. (42) demonstrated decreased LV transmural pressure with increased CPAP in patients with CHF. This occurred because CPAP decreased the work of breathing of their patients and reduced the magnitude of inspiratory swings in esophageal

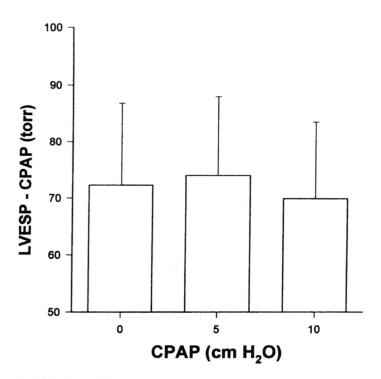

Figure 7 LV end-systolic (LVESP) transmural pressure calculated as the difference between intracavitary LVESP and CPAP level in CHF studies.

pressure. Since mean esophageal pressure increased, mean LV transmural pressure was calculated to have decreased.

In sedated pigs, Huberfeld et al. (43) measured both esophageal and cardiac surface (pericardial) pressure during the application of CPAP in normal and hypervolemic animals. They confirmed increased CO with CPAP in the hypervolemic animals. Figure 8 shows the changes in esophageal and pericardial pressure with CPAP in their studies. With increasing CPAP in normovolemia, there were parallel increases in pericardial and esophageal pressure. Thus estimates of LV transmural pressure made from esophageal pressure would reflect those made using pericardial pressure. However, in hypervolemia, the situation was different. There was an increase in baseline pericardial pressure with hypervolemia, reflecting cardiac dilation, which led to an increase in pericardial pressure. However, as CPAP increased, esophageal pressure rose but pericardial pressure actually fell. In fact calculated LV end-systolic transmural pressure actually increased slightly with CPAP. Thus, with hypervolemia, decreasing LV end-systolic transmural pressure could not account for increased CO with CPAP. These studies demonstrated that simple transmission of increased ITP to the cardiac surface

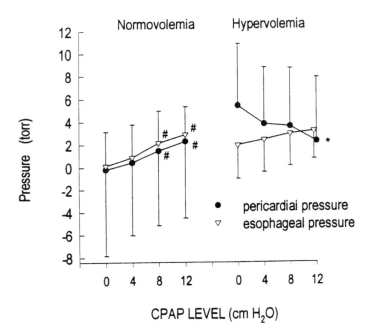

Figure 8 Pericardial and esophageal pressure in normovolemic and hypervolemic animals during the application of CPAP.

did not lead to decreased LV afterload as measured by decreased LV end-systolic transmural pressure.

Although the finding that cardiac surface pressure decreased with increasing CPAP in hypervolemia seems surprising, it is not unprecedented. In studies on the effect of PEEP on pericardial pressure Cabrera et al. (44) found that, after volume loading, there were no changes in pericardial pressure with application of PEEP even though ITP increased. They concluded that the "changes in pericardial pressure in response to PEEP reflect both the transmission of airway pressure to the pericardial surface and, presumably, PEEP related changes in cardiac volume and ventricular compliance" (44). The explanation can be understood in terms of a model in which cardiac surface pressure can be understood as the sum of two pressures, as follows:

$$PCs = ITP + Pperi \qquad (2)$$

where PCs = cardiac surface pressure and Pperi = pericardial elastic or transpericardial pressure. Transpericardial pressure is determined by the pericardial pressure-volume curve and the volume of heart within the pericardial sac, as illustrated in Figure 9. The pericardial pressure-volume curve is shown curvilinear. At relatively high pericardial volumes, there are large decreases in pressure (ΔP) associated with decreases in heart volume (ΔV). This is because with increased cardiac volume the pericardium begins to approach its elastic limit and becomes stiff. For relatively low cardiac volumes, decreases in cardiac volume are associated with relatively small changes in transpericardial pressure. Thus, if CPAP is associated with decreased cardiac volume by any mechanism whatsoever, then the decrease in transpericardial pressure (Pperi) will be greater (more negative) if initial heart volume is increased (distended heart). Thus, for a given increase in ITP, PCs could decrease (large enough decrease in Pperi) with CPAP if cardiac volume were large enough to put the pericardium close to the limits of diastolic distention. Under these conditions, the decrease in Pperi would be larger than the increase in ITP with CPAP and PCs would decrease [Eq. (2)]. The question then remains: If cardiac volume did not decrease because of increased cardiac surface pressure, then how does CPAP decrease cardiac volume? This is considered in the last section of this chapter.

C. Effects of CPAP on Coronary Blood Flow and Myocardial Energetics

An increase in cardiac surface pressure can lead to a decrease in coronary blood flow because of increased epicardial surface pressure and/or increased right atrial pressure. Indeed, in 1973, Tucker and Murray (45) observed decreases in coronary blood flow with application of PEEP that were out of proportion to decreases in cardiac work. Subsequently, other studies in animals (46–48) and humans (49)

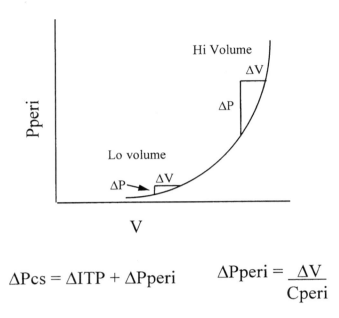

$$\Delta Pcs = \Delta ITP + \Delta Pperi \qquad \Delta Pperi = \frac{\Delta V}{Cperi}$$

Figure 9 Theoretical effects of decreased heart volume on transpericaridial pressure beginning from high and low initial cardiac volumes. For a given decrease in heart volume ΔV, the decrease in transpericardial pressure ΔP is greater when initial cardiac volume is close to the limits of pericardial distention. PCs, cardiac surface pressure; ITP, intrathoracic pressure; Pperi, transpericardial pressure; Cperi, pericardial compliance, much less at high than at low cardiac volumes. We assume that ITP increases with CPAP, but heart volume decreases. If initial heart volume is great enough, pericardial pressure could decrease more than ITP increases. Thus, PCs could decrease. See text for explanation.

demonstrated that positive-pressure maneuvers could be associated with decreased coronary blood flow and even signs of cardiac ischemia. This could be of special concern in patients with coronary artery disease. Huberfeld et al. (50), in fact, observed a small decrease in coronary blood flow with CPAP in hypervolemic animals (Fig. 10). However, no changes in several indices of myocardial O_2 consumption, O_2 extraction, or regional or global myocardial function were observed. The authors felt that decreased coronary flow was associated with systemic vasodilation and slightly decreased coronary perfusion pressure with CPAP and did not constitute a threat for the development of ischemia. Possibly the animals were protected from decreased coronary flow because cardiac surface pressure does not decrease with CPAP in hypervolemic animals when CO increases.

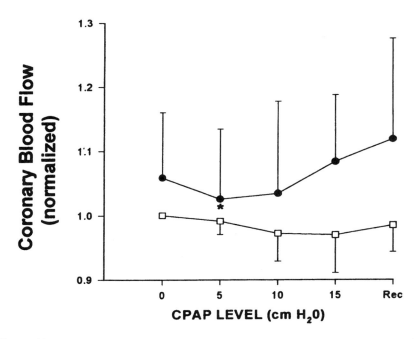

Figure 10 Effects of CPAP on coronary blood flow in normal and hypervolemic sedated pigs. Data are normalized to normovolemic baseline. Open circles, normovolemia; Closed circles, hypervolemia; * = significant compared to baseline. (Adapted from Ref. 50.)

D. CPAP and Sympathoadrenal Function in Sedated Pigs

As noted above, CHF is associated with an upregulation of baseline sympatho-adrenal tone, which could itself be a source of cardiac dysfunction. In humans, Naughton et al. (51) observed evidence of decreased sympathoadrenal tone in patients with CHF undergoing chronic CPAP treatment. Using plasma norepi-nephrine (PNE) as an index of overall sympathoadrenal tone, Scharf et al. (52) studied the effects of CPAP on sympathoadrenal tone in normovolemia, hyper-volemia, and CHF in sedated pigs. Figure 11 illustrates the results. Both hy-pervolemia and CHF were associated with increased PNE at baseline relative to normovolemia. However with hypervolemia there was a decrease in PNE with low-level CPAP, whereas with CHF there was a small increase. However, low-level CPAP led to increased CO with both hypervolemia and CHF. This showed that in this model, increased CO with low-level CPAP could not be associated with a specific change in PNE. Thus, changes in total-body integrated sympatho-adrenal activity, as measured by PNE, were not responsible for increased CO with

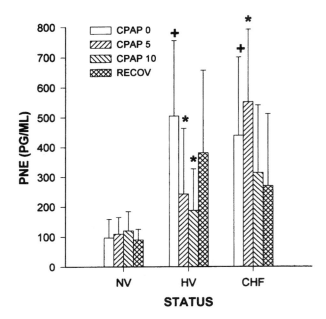

Figure 11   Plasma norepinephrine levels (PNE) with CPAP in sedated pigs. NV, normo-volemia; HV, hypervolemia; CHF, congestive heart failure. * = statistically different from baseline for each condition. (From Ref. 52.)

CPAP. Differences between the pig study and the human study were explained by differences in species, degree and chronicity of CHF, concomitant cardiac medications in patients, and other variables that might have been present in chronic patient studies but not in the pig studies. These results illustrate the difficulty of interpreting studies of this type in a simple fashion and suggest that the explanation may be far more complicated.

V.   Models for Explaining Decreased Cardiac Volumes and Increased CO with CPAP

It would appear that increased CO with low-level CPAP observed in the animal studies cannot be easily explained either by a decrease in LV afterload due to increased cardiac surface pressure (decreased LV transmural pressure) or by a decrease or increase in overall sympathetic activity (as measured by PNE). It also appears that increased CO is associated with a decrease in cardiac volume. Thus, decreased cardiac volume and increased CO appear to be linked with

CPAP. There are two explanations for this that we have presented in previous studies and will be reviewed here.

A. CPAP-Induced Systemic Vasodilation

In the studies of the sedated pig presented so far as well as in acute studies of humans with CPAP (1), systemic vascular resistance has been observed to decrease with CPAP under conditions where CO increases (hypervolemia and CHF). This is illustrated in Figure 12. As noted above, CO increases with hypervolemia and CHF at low-level (5 cmH$_2$O) CPAP. In CHF, there was a secondary increase in CO during the recovery period (Fig. 4). These changes in CO correspond to decreases in systemic vascular resistance with CPAP. Thus, changes in CO may be explained by systemic vasodilation during CPAP, possibly on a reflex basis, which leads to a decrease in the impedance to LV ejection and increases stroke volume and cardiac output. This would result in decreases in cardiac volume secondary to decreased LV afterload. The reflex basis for vasodilation with

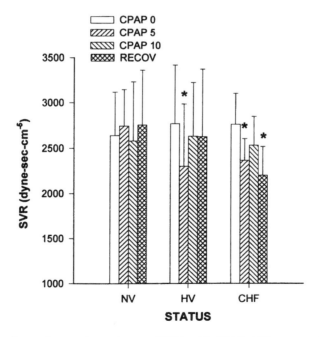

Figure 12 Systemic vascular resistance (SVR) with CPAP. NV, normovolemia; HV, hypervolemia; CHF, congestive heart failure. * = statistically different from baseline for any condition. Note that when CO was observed to increase (CPAP 5 cmH$_2$O for HV and CHF, and recovery period for CHF), SVR was observed to decrease. (From Ref. 52.)

CPAP is poorly understood. As noted, with CHF and with hypervolemia, there are changes in baseline sympathoadrenal tone. These changes in baseline autonomic function may predispose to different types of reflex vascular response to CPAP between normal and hypervolemic (including CHF) conditions. Whatever the basis for vasodilation, decreased impedance to LV emptying on this basis could explain both increased CO and decreased cardiac volumes with CPAP. Another explanation, that cardiac contractility may increase, is considered unlikely, since changes in indices of contractility do not change with hypervolemia (36,50). Changes in contractility may act synergistically to vasodilation to increase CO with CPAP in CHF, since small increases in indices of cardiac contractility were observed with CPAP during CHF (38,52). However, whether reflex vasodilation with CPAP is a prime cause or a secondary finding, possibly due to activation of baroreceptors, is not known; further work will need to be done to clarify the role and mechanisms of vasodilation with CPAP in hypervolemic states.

B. Transfer of Blood Volume from Intrathoracic to Extrathoracic Compartments

Increasing ITP with increased airway pressure can transfer blood volume from intrathoracic to extrathoracic volume compartments (53). Figure 13 illustrates the coupling of peripheral and central (intrathoracic) reservoirs. For simplicity, the normal gradient of pressure for venous return is not shown. P_1 and P_3 represent the initial pressures in intra- and extrathoracic compartments, respectively. P_2 and P_4 represent pressure in the reservoirs after an increase in ITP. For a given increase in intrathoracic or pleural pressure (Ppl), the following must be true:

$$\Delta Ppl = (P_1 - P_2) + (P_4 - P_3) \tag{3}$$

The volume transferred from intrathoracic to extrathoracic compartments, ΔV, is:

$$\Delta V = (P_1 - P_2){*}C_c = (P_4 - P_3){*}C_p \tag{4}$$

where C_c and C_p are the compliances of the central and peripheral compartments, respectively. Rearranging:

$$\frac{(P_1 - P_2)}{(P_4 - P_3)} = \frac{C_p}{C_c} \tag{5}$$

Thus, it follows that the amount by which the level in the central reservoir decreases $(P_1 - P_2)$ is less than the increase in Ppl, and the transmural pressure in the central reservoir (the level in the reservoir minus Ppl) decreases.

The principles of coupling between heart and peripheral circulation have been mathematically modeled by Permutt and Wise (54). Depending on whether heart volume is high or low, the consequences for CO of a decrease in transmural pressure can be quite different. This is illustrated in Figure 14. In the figure are

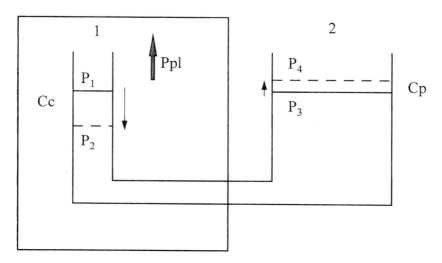

Figure 13 Model of coupling between central and peripheral vascular reservoirs. Cc, central compliant reservoir (heart and lungs); Cp, peripheral vascular reservoir. When pleural pressure (Ppl) increases, there is transfer of volume from intrathoracic to extrathoracic reservoirs. P_1 and P_2, pressure in central reservoir before and after increase in Ppl respectively, P_3 and P_4, pressure in peripheral reservoir before and after increase in Ppl respectively. See text for discussion.

shown diastolic and systolic pressure-volume curves for cardiac contractions. For the purposes of this analysis, the pericardium may be thought of as part of the ventricular wall, adding its constraint to filling to that of the myocardium. The pressure-volume history of single beats is shown stylistically at baseline and following equal decreases in cardiac transmural pressures at end-systole and end-diastole. The horizontal distance between end-diastolic and end-systolic volumes represents stroke volume. When initial cardiac volume is low (normal situation), because of the shape of the pressure-volume curves, the heart is stiffer (steeper volume-pressure curve) during systole than during diastole. Thus, for equal decreases in transmural pressure due to increased ITP, volume decreases more at end-diastole than at end-systole. In this case stroke volume decreases.

However, when initial cardiac volume is increased enough to push the heart up toward the limits of diastolic distention (hypervolemia, CHF) an interesting phenomenon occurs. The heart is actually stiffer in diastole (steeper volume-pressure curve) than in systole. Thus, for equal decreases in transmural pressure, there is actually a greater decrease in end-systolic than end-diastolic volume. This leads to an *increase* in stroke volume. According to this concept, anytime the heart is pushed toward the limit of its diastolic distention, transfer of volume

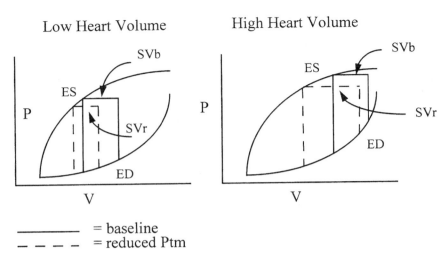

Low Heart Volume   High Heart Volume

————— = baseline
— — — — = reduced Ptm

Figure 14 Effects of increased pleural pressure and decreased cardiac transmural pressure on end-diastolic (ED) and end-systolic (ES) volume, as well as stroke volume (SV). ED and ES pressure-volume curves are shown when initial cardiac volume is low and when initial cardiac volume is high. The cardiac pressure-volume histories are shown stylized. The effects of equal reductions in ED and ES transmural pressures (Ptm) with increased intrathoracic pressure on SV are shown for both volume ranges. SV is represented as the horizontal distance between ED and ES volume. SVb, baseline stroke volume; SVr, stroke volume when Ptm is decreased because of an increase in intrathoracic pressure.

out from central reservoirs can lead to an increase in stroke volume. Thus, on a purely mechanical basis, increased ITP could increase stroke volume when the heart is distended. This could explain the clinical and experimental observations cited above that, in normals, CPAP leads to decreased CO, whereas with cardiac distention, CPAP could lead to increased CO. Alterations in sympathoadrenal function could be secondary to improved cardiac function or could act additively to these mechanical effects. Actually, the observation that, with cardiac distention, removal of blood can lead to improved CO is not new. This was reported in the classic older clinical studies of Howarth et al. (55), who reported that phlebotomy in the presence of CHF led to an increase in CO.

VI. Conclusions and Questions

The experimental studies described here support clinical observations that, in the presence of CHF, low-level CPAP can lead to improved cardiac function and increased CO. Further, the presence of CHF per se is not sufficient to observe this effect; cardiac distention is required (56). What is less easy to understand is the mechanism whereby this occurs. Interactions between VR and cardiac function with increased ITP explain this finding, assuming that increased ITP leads to improved function. Experimental data do not support the concept that with low-level CPAP, increased ITP with CPAP decreases LV afterload by simple transmission of changes in ITP to the cardiac surface, thus decreasing LV end-systolic transmural pressure. However, based on considerations of peripheral-central circulatory coupling and transfer of volume from intrathoracic to extrathoracic compartments, a purely mechanical explanation may be adequate to explain the clinical and experimental observations. This does not rule out concomitant changes in autonomic function, which is altered with CHF, possibly leading to vasodilation and adding to the mechanical effects. Elucidation of the mechanisms involved could lead to a better understanding of why some patients appear to benefit from CPAP while others do not.

Additionally, there is the matter of the carryover effects of CPAP removal on CO (Figs. 4 and 9), where CO actually increased for a time following CPAP removal. The length of time that this effect is observed suggests an alteration in autonomic function. Possibly this carryover effect is related to the clinical observation that, following several months of CPAP therapy, patients with CHF and Cheyne-Stokes respiration demonstrated sustained improvements in cardiac function (3) when CPAP is not applied. Clearly more work is needed to explain this phenomenon more completely.

Thus, experimental observations support the clinical studies showing that CPAP can be an effective adjunct to cardiac function with CHF. Future work needs to be directed to specifying under what circumstances and for which patients this holds. Additional studies elucidating the mechanisms by which CPAP can have its beneficial effect will help in improving the clinical efficacy of this mode of therapy for failing hearts.

References

1. Bradley TD, Holloway RM, Mclaughlin PR, Ross, BL, Walters J, Liu PP. Cardiac output response to continuous positive airway pressure in congestive heart failure. Am Rev Respir Dis 1992; 145:377–382.
2. Lenique F, Habis M, Lofaso F, Dubois RJL, Harf A, Bochard L. Ventilatory and hemodynamic effects of continuous positive airway pressure in left heart failure. Am J Respir Crit Care Med 1997; 155:500–505.
3. Naughton MT, Liu PP, Benard DC, Goldstein RS, Bradley RD. Treatment of congestive heart failure and Cheyne-Stokes respiration during sleep by continuous positive airway pressure. Am J Respir Crit Care Med 1995; 151:92–97.
4. Baratz DM, Westbrook PRE, Shah PK, Mohsenifar Z. Effect of nasal continuous

positive airway pressure on cardiac output and oxygen delivery in patients with congestive heart failure. Chest 1992; 102:1397–1401.

5.   Buckle P, Millar T, Kryger M. The effect of short-term nasal CPAP on Cheyne-Stokes respiration in congestive heart failure. Chest 1992; 102:31–35.

6.   Calverley PM. Nasal CPAP in cardiac failure: case not proven. Sleep 1996; 10(suppl): S236–S239.

7.   Guyton AC, Jones CE, Coleman TB. Circulatory Physiology: Cardiac output and Its Regulation. Philadelphia: Saunders, 1973.

8.   Scharf SM. Mechanical Cardiopulmonary interactions in critical care. In: Dantzker DR, Scharf SM, eds. Cardiopulmonary Critical Care, 3d ed. Philadelphia: Saunders, 1997:75–92.

9.   Scharf SM. Cardiovascular effects of positive pressure ventilation. J Crit Care 1992; 7:168–279.

10. Donders FC. Contribution to the mechanism of respiration and circulation in health and disease [1853]. In: West JB, ed. Translations in Respiratory Physiology. Stoudsburg, PA, Dowden, Hutchinson and Ross, 1975: 298–318.

11. Buda AJ, Pinsky MR, Ingles NB, Daughters GT, Stenson EB, Alderman EL. Effect of intrathoracic pressure and LV performance. N Engl J Med 1979; 301:453–459.

12. Scharf SM, Brown R, Tow DE, Parisi AF. Cardiac effects of increased lung volume and decreased pleural pressure in man. J Appl Physiol 1979; 47:257–262.

13. Scharf SM, Bianco JA, Tow DE, Brown R. The effects of large negative intrathoracic pressure on left ventricular function in patients with coronary artery disease. Circulation 1981; 63:871–875.

14. Scharf SM, O'Beirne Woods B, Brown R, Parisi AF, Miller MM, Tow DE. Effects of Mueller maneuver on global and regional left ventricular function in angina pectoris with or without previous myocardial infarction. Am J Cardiol 1987; 59:1305–1309.

15. Robotham J, Scharf SM. The effects of positive and negative pressure ventilation on cardiac performance. In: Matthay RA, Matthay MA, Dantzker D, eds. Cardiovascular pulmonary interaction in normal and disease lung. Philadelphia: Saunders, 1983:161–187.

16. Charlier AA. Beat to Beat Hemodynamic Effects of Lung Inflation and Normal Respiration in Anesthetized and Conscious Dogs. Brussels, Editions Arscia, 1967.

17. Brinker JA, Weiss JL, Lappe DL, Rabson JL, Summer WR, Permutt S, Weisfeldt ML. Leftward septal displacement during right ventricular loading in man. Circulation 1980; 61:626–633.

18. Lichtenstein SV, Slutsky A, Salerno TA. Noninvasive right and left ventricular assist. Surg Forum 1985; 36:306–308.

19. Scharf SM, Ingram RH. Influence of abdominal pressure and sympathetic vasoconstriction on the cardiovascular response to PEEP. Am Rev Respir Dis 1977; 116: 661–670.

20. Fessler HE, Brower RG, Wise RA. Effects of positive end-expiratory pressure on the gradient for venous return. Am Rev Respir Dis 1990; 143:19–24.

21. Pinsky MR, Summer WR, Wise RA, Permutt S, Bromberger-Barnea B. Augmentation of cardiac function by elevation of intrathoracic pressure. J Appl Physiol 1983; 54:950–955.

22. Pinsky MR, Summer WR. Cardiac augmentation by phasic high intrathoracic pressure support in man. Chest 1983; 84:370–375.
23. Robotham JL, ventilatory-assisted myocardial performance (VAMP). Chest 1983; 84:366–367.
24. Pinsky MR, Matuschak GM, Klain M. Determinants of cardiac augmentation by elevations in intrathoracic pressure. J Appl Physiol 1985; 58:1189–1198.
25. Pinsky MR, Matuschak GM, Bernardi L, Klain M. Hemodynamic effects of cardiac cycle–specific increases in intrathoracic pressure. J Appl Physiol 1986; 60:604–612.
26. Pinsky MR, Marquez J, Martin D, Klain M. Ventricular assist by cardiac cycle-specific increases in intrathoracic pressure. Chest 1987; 91:709–715.
27. Beyar R, Halperin, HR, Tsitlik JE, Guerci AD, Kass D, Weisfeldt M, Chandra NC. Circulatory assistance by intrathoracic pressure variations: optimization and mechanisms studied by a mathematical model in relation to experimental data. Circ Res 1989; 64:703–720.
28. Peters J, Ihle P. ECG synchronized thoracic vest inflation during autonomic blockade, myocardial ischemia or cardiac arrest. J Appl Physiol 1992; 73:2263–2273.
29. Cohn JN, Levine TB, Oliveri MT, Garberg V, Lura D, Francis GS, Simon AB, Rector T. Plasma norepinephrine as a guide to prognosis in patients with chronic congestive heart failure. N Engl J Med 1984; 311:819–823.
30. Daly PA, Sole MJ. Myocardial catecholamines and the pathophysiology of heart failure. Circulation 1990; 82(suppl 1):134–138.
31. Swedberg K, Enroth P, Kjekshus J, Wilhelmsen L. Hormones regulating cardiovascular function in patients with severe CHF and their relation to mortality. Circulation 1990; 82:1730–1736.
32. Bristow MR, Ginsburg P, Minobe W, Cubicciotti RS, Sageman WS, Lurie K, Billingham ME, Harrison DC, Stinson EB. Decreased catecholamine sensitivity and β-adrenergic receptor density in failing human hearts. N Engl J Med 1982; 307:205–211.
33. Chidsey CA, Braunwald E, Morrow AG. Catecholamine excretion and cardiac stores of norepinephrine in congestive heart failure. Am J Med 1965; 39:442–451.
34. Kaye DM, Lambert GW, Lefkovits J, Morris M, Jennings G, Esler MD. Neurochemical evidence of cardiac sympathetic activation and increased central nervous system norepinephrine turnover in severe congestive heart failure. J Am Coll Cardiol 1994; 23:570–578.
35. Kendall MJ, Lynch KP, Hjalmarson A, Kjekshus J. β-blockers and sudden cardiac death. Ann Intern Med 1995; 123:358–367.
36. Genovese J, Moskowitz M, Tarasiuk A, Graver LM, Scharf SM. Effects of CPAP on cardiac output in normal and hypervolemic unanesthetized pigs. Am J Respir Crit Care Med 1994; 150:752–758.
37. Scharf SM. Ventilatory support in cardiac failure. Curr Opin Crit Care. 1997; 3:71–77.
38. Genovese J, Huberfeld S, Tarasiuk A, Moskowitz M, Scharf SM. Effects of CPAP on cardiac output in pigs with pacing induced congestive heart failure. Am J Respir Crit Care Med 1995; 152:1847–1853.
39. Takata M, Robotham JL. Ventricular external constraint by the lung and pericardium during positive end-expiratory pressure. Am Rev Respir Dis 1991; 143:872–875.

40. Scharf SM, Brown R, Warner KG, Khuri S. Esophageal and pericardial pressures and left ventricular configuration with respiratory maneuvers. J Appl Physiol 1989; 66:481–491.

41. Liston R, Deegan PC, McCreery C, Costello R, Maurer B, McNicholas WT. Haemodynamic effects of nasal continuous positive airway pressure in severe congestive heart failure. Eur Respir J 1995; 8:430–435.

42. Naughton MT, Rahman MA, Hara K, Floras JS, Bradley TD. Effect on continuous positive airway pressure on intrathoracic and left ventricular transmural pressures in patients with congestive heart failure. Circulation 1995; 91:1725–1731.

43. Huberfeld S, Genovese J, Tarasiuk A, Scharf SM. Effects of CPAP on pericardial pressure, transmural left ventricular pressures and respiratory mechanics in hypervolemic unanesthetized pigs. Am J Respir Crit Care Med 1995; 152:142–147.

44. Cabrera MR, Nakamura GE, Montague DA, Cole RA. Effect of airway pressure on pericardial pressure. Am Rev Respir Dis 1989; 140:659–667.

45. Tucker HJ, Murray JF. Effects of end-expiratory pressure on organ blood flow in normal and diseased dogs. J Appl Physiol 1973; 34:573–577.

46. Venus B, Jacobs HF. Alterations in regional myocardial blood flows during different levels of positive end-expiratory pressure. Crit Care Med 1984; 12:96–101.

47. Hassapoyannes C, Harper JF, Struck LM, Hornung CA, Abel FL. Effects of systole-specific pericardial pressure increases on coronary flow. J Appl Physiol 1991; 71:104–111.

48. Fessler HE, Brower RG, Wise R, Permutt S. Positive pleural pressure decreases coronary perfusion. Am J Physiol 1990; 258:H814–H820.

49. Tittley JG, Fremes SE, Weisel RD, Christakis GT, Evans PJ, Madonik M, Ivanov J, Teasdale SF, Mickle DAG, McLaughlin PR. Hemodynamic and myocardial metabolic consequences of PEEP. Chest 1985; 88:496–502.

50. Huberfeld SI, Genovese J, Patel U, Scharf SM. Myocardial mechanics and energetics during continuous positive end-expiratory pressure in sedated pigs. Crit Care Med 1996; 24:2027–2034.

51. Naughton MT, Bernard DC, Liu PP, Rutherford R, Rankin F, Bradley TD. Effects of nasal CPAP on sympathetic activity in patients with heart failure and central sleep apnea. Am J Respir Crit Care Med 1995; 152:473–479.

52. Scharf SM, Chen L, Slamowitz D, Rao PS. Effects of continuous positive airway pressure on cardiac output and plasma norepinephrine in sedated pigs. J Crit Care 1996; 11:57–64.

53. Braunwald E, Binion JT, Morgan WL, Sarnoff SF. Alterations in central blood volume and cardiac output induced by positive pressure breathing and counteracted by metarimal (Aramine). Circ Res 1957; 5:670–680.

54. Permutt S, Wise RA. The control of cardiac output through coupling of heart and blood vessels. In: Yin FCP, ed. Ventricular/Vascular Coupling, New York: Springer-Verlag, 1987:159–179.

55. Howarth SJ, McMichael J, Sharpey-Schaefer EP. Effects of venesection in low output heart failure. Clin Sci 1946; 6:41–50.

56. DeHoyos A, Liu PP, Benard DC, Bradley TD. Haemodynamic effects of continuous positive airway pressure in humans with normal and impaired left ventricular function. Clin Sci 1995; 88:173–178.

20

Therapy of Obstructive and Central Sleep Apnea in Patients with Congestive Heart Failure

RUZENA TKACOVA

The Toronto General Hospital
University Health Network
The Toronto Rehabilitation Institute
University of Toronto
Toronto, Onatrio, Canada

T. DOUGLAS BRADLEY

The Toronto General Hospital
University Health Network
The Toronto Rehabilitation Institute
The Mount Sinai Hospital
University of Toronto
Toronto, Onatrio, Canada

I. Introduction

Congestive heart failure (CHF) is a major clinical and public health problem (1). For example, in the United States, the prevalence of CHF among those aged 50–59 years is 1%, and it doubles with each 10-year increment in age thereafter (2). In addition, the prevalence of CHF has doubled in the past 20 years in association with improved survival from myocardial infarction (3). Despite remarkable advances in cardiovascular therapeutics over the past decade, only a modest impact has been made on the mortality rate of CHF. Therefore, given the increasing prevalence of CHF and the limited effectiveness of pharmacological therapies, novel approaches to its management must be developed if the dismal prognosis of this condition is to improve.

One such approach may be the diagnosis and specific treatment of coexisting sleep apnea disorders in patients with CHF. From the very beginning of clinical interest in sleep-disordered breathing, an association between sleep apnea and cardiovascular disease, especially hypertension, was recognized (4–6). Recent studies indicate that approximately 40–50% of stable symptomatic outpatients with CHF suffer from either obstructive sleep apnea (OSA) or Cheyne-Stokes respiration with central sleep apnea (CSR-CSA) (7,8). These sleep-related breathing disorders can generate profound mechanical and adrenergic stresses upon the failing myocardium that may not be reversed by standard pharmacological therapy (9). Consequently, sleep-related breathing disorders likely contribute to the progression of heart failure and may adversely affect its prognosis. Indeed, several studies have reported higher mortality rates in CHF patients with CSR during either wakefulness (10) or sleep (11,12) than in those without this breathing disorder. Conversely, successful treatment of either type of sleep apnea in patients with CHF can result in objective and subjective improvement in the severity of heart failure (8,13,14).

Thus, there is now emerging a body of evidence supporting the assessment of potentially treatable sleep-related breathing disorders in selected patients with CHF. Where recurrent hypoxia, sleep fragmentation, paroxysmal nocturnal dyspnea, or symptoms of sleep apnea are present in association with a sleep-related breathing disorder in patients with CHF, treatment of this breathing disorder should be considered. Therefore, the purpose of this chapter is to review the current knowledge on the types and efficacy of various treatments for sleep apnea in patients with CHF.

II. Treatment of Obstructive Sleep Apnea in Patients with Congestive Heart Failure

Patients with OSA are at increased risk for hypertension, myocardial ischemia, and stroke (15–18). Those who also suffer from CHF are particularly susceptible to the adverse effects of OSA, such as hypoxia, hypercapnia, arousals from sleep, increased sympathetic nervous system activity, and increased left ventricular (LV) afterload (19,20). Although the prevalence of OSA in patients with CHF is not certain, it has been reported to occur in approximately 10% (7,20) to 22% (19) compared to 2–9% in the otherwise healthy population (21,22). Treatment of OSA is therefore liable to be relevant to a significant proportion of the CHF population in whom abolition of OSA may provide clinical benefits over and above those due to pharmacological therapies.

The therapeutic approach to OSA in patients with CHF is generally similar to that in patients with normal heart function. Since upper airway instability is the final common mechanism resulting in recurrent episodes of partial or complete airway obstruction, therapy is aimed at stabilizing the upper airway in order to prevent obstructive apneas and hypopneas.

A. General Measures

There are three general measures modifying the function of the upper airway and thus potentially preventing its occlusion: 1) weight loss, 2) avoidance of muscle relaxants, and 3) changes in body position.

Patients with OSA are commonly overweight and have abnormal pharyngeal properties, such as pharyngeal narrowing due to fat depositions surrounding the collapsible segment of the pharynx (23) and increased pharyngeal collapsibility (24). These factors predispose them to upper airway occlusion during sleep (25). Weight loss in obese patients with OSA has been shown to reduce or, in some cases, to abolish obstructive apneas (26). This effect is likely due to an increase in upper airway caliber, owing to reduced pharyngeal fat deposition, and improved neuromuscular control of upper airway function. Unfortunately, the long-term success rates of weight-loss programs are rather disappointing in most patients.

Substances that are known to aggravate sleep apnea should be avoided. Alcohol and sedative medications increase the tendency for the upper airway to collapse by relaxing upper airway muscles (27,28). Exacerbation of OSA by alcohol and sedatives appears to be mediated through a selective reduction in respiratory motor activity to the pharyngeal dilator muscles without diminishing diaphragmatic activity. This effect tilts the balance of forces in favor of upper airway occlusion during inspiration. Consequently, by increasing upper airway resistance, alcohol and sedatives increase the frequency of obstructive apneas and hypopneas (29,30) and should therefore be avoided.

In the supine position, the gravitational force causes the tongue and soft palate to relapse passively against the posterior pharyngeal wall, predisposing to upper airway occlusion. Therefore, in some OSA patients whose apneas occur mainly while they are supine, the frequency of obstructive events can be markedly reduced by assuming the lateral decubitus rather than the supine position (31).

Although the effects on OSA of these general measures have not been addressed in patients who also suffer from CHF, there is no reason to believe that they would respond differently from OSA patients without CHF. Therefore, these general measures should be routinely advised to OSA patients with coexisting CHF. Nevertheless, most CHF patients will require more specific and definitive treatment for OSA.

There is some indirect evidence to suggest that increases in vascular pressure or interstitial edema in the neck might render the upper airway more collapsible (32). This evidence comes from measurements of upper airway caliber in OSA patients when their legs are raised to increase venous return and distend the neck veins as compared to when the legs are lowered. Although direct evidence is lacking, it is possible that increased neck vein distension and/or neck edema due to fluid overload in CHF could increase pharyngeal collapsibility and predispose to OSA. Consequently, to the extent that edema narrows the upper airway, diuresis induced by pharmacological agents could theoretically reduce upper airway edema and collapsibility. However, this hypothesis is highly speculative and remains to be tested.

B. Specific Therapy

Treatment of Obstructive Sleep Apnea by Continuous Positive Airway
Pressure (CPAP) in Patients with Congestive Heart Failure

Acute Respiratory Effects of CPAP

The most effective and best tolerated therapy for OSA, and the only therapy yet
tested in OSA patients with coexisting CHF, is continuous positive airway pressure (CPAP) applied via a nasal mask during sleep. CPAP functions as a pneu-
matic splint that increases the cross-sectional area of the entire upper airway
throughout the respiratory cycle (33). In so doing, it eliminates occlusion in all
upper airway segments rather than only in isolated segments, as is the case in
most upper airway surgical procedures. In CHF patients with OSA, CPAP causes
immediate and long-term abolition of obstructive apneas and hypopneas in association with improvements in oxyhemoglobin saturation (Sa_{O_2}), and sleep quality.

CPAP unloads inspiratory muscles in CHF patients both while they are
awake (34) and during sleep (19). Naughton et al. (34) found a 36% reduction
in intrathoracic pressure (Pit) amplitude in 15 CHF patients during the day while
on 10 cmH_2O of CPAP. Pit amplitude provides a good index of the degree of
inspiratory muscle force generation and energy expenditure per breath (35). Its
reduction by CPAP is likely due to redistribution of lung water induced by the
positive intrathoracic pressure (34,36), resulting in reductions in lung and airway
resistance and the elastic and resistive components of work of breathing as well
as increased lung compliance (37). In CHF patients also suffering from OSA,
Pit becomes more negative during sleep as the inspiratory muscles contract to
overcome the resistance of the occluded upper airway (13). Therefore, the inspiratory unloading effect of CPAP observed during wakefulness becomes amplified
during sleep owing to the relief of upper airway obstruction and elimination of
exaggerated negative Pit in such patients. In a recent study involving CHF patients with OSA, Tkacova et al. (19) documented both a 56% reduction in Pit
amplitude and a reduction in respiratory rate during sleep while on CPAP. The
product of Pit amplitude and respiratory rate, an index of inspiratory force generation over time (34,35), was profoundly reduced by 58%. Because CPAP also
alleviated OSA, inspiratory muscle unloading occurred in association with improved oxygenation at the same level of PC_{O_2} and alveolar ventilation (19). Accordingly, better gas exchange was achieved at a much lower energy expenditure
of the inspiratory muscles while on CPAP. Elimination of OSA by CPAP also
consolidates sleep by reducing the frequency of arousals and increasing the
amount of slow-wave sleep in patients with CHF (13).

Acute Effects of CPAP on Left Ventricular Afterload and Heart Rate

Despite their adherence to optimum pharmacological therapy and the presence
of normal daytime blood pressure (BP), CHF patients with OSA experience recur-

rent increases in left ventricular (LV) afterload in association with obstructive apneas during sleep that rise above levels during wakefulness (19). These result from surges in systolic BP and reductions in Pit, which together increase systolic LV transmural pressure (LVPtm), an important determinant of LV afterload. The presence of LV hypertrophy and dilated cardiomyopathy of unknown etiology in patients with OSA who are normotensive while awake (13,38) suggest that, over time, nocturnal increases in LV afterload related to obstructive apneas have detrimental effects on myocardial function. However, the relative contributions of negative Pit and surges in BP to increased LV afterload appear to vary considerably from one patient to another (13,19). We have therefore recently studied the effects of CPAP on the two components of LV afterload influenced by OSA: Pit and BP.

In patients with CHF, CPAP increases Pit even during wakefulness in the absence of OSA (Fig. 1). Naughton et al. (34) found that CPAP of 10 cmH$_2$O increased Pit during systole by approximately 6 mmHg and reduced heart rate by 10%, but it had no effect on BP. Consequently, CPAP induced a 6-mmHg reduction in systolic LVPtm due entirely to the increase in Pit. In contrast, when CPAP was applied during stage 2 sleep to eight patients with CHF who also had

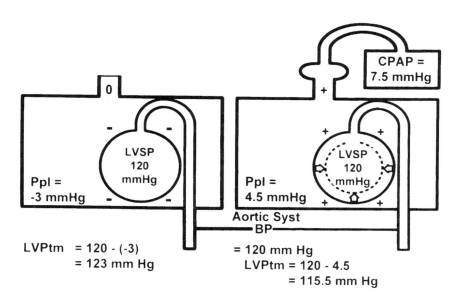

Figure 1 Schematic representation of the effects of continuous positive airway pressure (CPAP) on left ventricular transmural pressure (LVPtm). LVPtm is the difference between left ventricular systolic pressure (LVSP) and pleural pressure (Ppl) (left panel). During wakefulness and during sleep in patients without sleep apnea, CPAP reduces LVPtm by increasing Ppl (right panel).

OSA, the major component of the fall in systolic LVPtm was a 16 mmHg decrease in systolic BP due to the abolition of OSA (19) (Fig. 2). The increase in Pit in these patients was comparable (4–6 mmHg) to that reported by Naughton et al. (34) However, because these patients experienced both a 16-mmHg reduction in systolic BP and 4-mmHg increase in Pit, the net effect of the abolition of OSA in these patients was a highly significant 20 mmHg decrease in systolic LVPtm and therefore in LV afterload. These reductions in nocturnal BP occurred even though

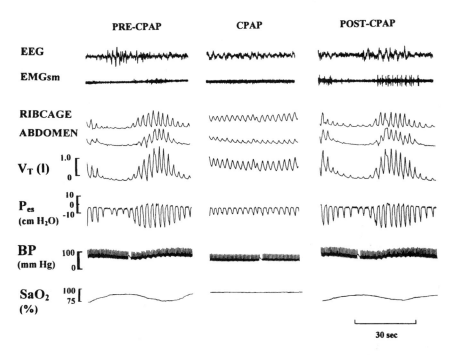

Figure 2 Polysomnographic recording during stage 2 sleep before, during, and after continuous positive airway pressure application (PRE-CPAP, CPAP, and POST-CPAP, respectively) in a patient with congestive heart failure and obstructive sleep apnea. The middle panel illustrates that by eliminating obstructive apnea, CPAP reduces systolic LVPtm (i.e., left ventricular afterload) both by reducing negative Pes swings and decreasing blood pressure (BP). In addition, reductions in Pes amplitude indicate unloading of the inspiratory muscles. The ventilatory period in this patient has a waxing and waning pattern of V_T typical of Cheyne-Stokes ventilation but obstructive apnea as indicated by the recurrent generation of negative Pes during apnea. Abolition of obstructive apnea also improves Sa_{O2} and eliminates apnea-related arousals. EEG, electroencephalogram; EMG_{sm}, submental electromyogram; V_T, tidal volume; Pes, esophageal pressure; BP, blood pressure; Sa_{O2}, oxyhemoglobin saturation. (From Ref. 19.)

these patients were receiving optimum pharmacological afterload-reducing therapy and were normotensive while awake. These findings indicate that OSA-induced surges in BP are relatively resistant to pharmacological afterload-reducing agents. Therefore, elimination of OSA by CPAP causes reductions in nocturnal BP and LV afterload over and above those due to vasodilators. It therefore has the potential to further improve long-term outcomes in such patients.

In addition to reducing BP and LV afterload, abolition of OSA by CPAP lowers heart rate in CHF patients while they are asleep (19). There are two possible mechanisms by which CPAP reduces heart rate in these patients: reduced sympathetic and/or increased parasympathetic nervous system activity. In patients with OSA but without CHF, CPAP has been shown to decrease sympathetic discharge to muscle and to reduce plasma and urinary norepinephrine concentrations (39,40). On the other hand, there is evidence that application of CPAP to awake patients with CHF increases cardiac parasympathetic activity. Butler et al. (41) demonstrated that, in CHF patients while awake, CPAP increases cardiac parasympathetic activity, as evidenced by an increase in the high-frequency component of heart rate variability (Fig. 3). This increase in cardiac parasympathetic activity while on CPAP was probably due to stimulation of pulmonary vagal stretch receptors by CPAP-induced lung inflation. Since low heart rate variability has been associated with increased mortality in general and with a greater risk of sudden death in particular (42), the main clinical implications of the reductions in heart rate and increases in heart rate variability in patients with CHF by CPAP are the potential to reduce myocardial O_2 consumption and to improve prognosis.

Acute Effect of CPAP on Cardiac Output

The effects of positive airway pressure on cardiac output depend on the underlying contractile state of the heart and its preload and on the balance between the preload- and afterload-reducing effects of positive airway pressure. Accordingly, the effects of CPAP on cardiac output differ between the failing and the normal heart. In the normal heart, cardiac output is more sensitive to changes in preload than in afterload, whereas in the failing heart, the converse is true (43–45). Based on these considerations, the effects of CPAP on cardiac output are predictable. In the normal heart, application of CPAP causes a reduction in cardiac output because it impedes venous return and LV filling (45,46). In addition, CPAP does not reduce LV afterload in humans with normal heart function because the increased Pit it causes is offset by a slight increase in systolic BP (34). As a result, there is no net change in systolic LVPtm. However, cardiac output in the failing heart is less responsive to changes in preload and more responsive to changes in afterload (43,44). Indeed, patients with decompensated CHF have increased preload (i.e., increased LV end-diastolic volume and pressure), which is the cause of pulmonary venous hypertension and congestion. In this setting, reductions in preload by diuretics relieve pulmonary edema, whereas increases in preload

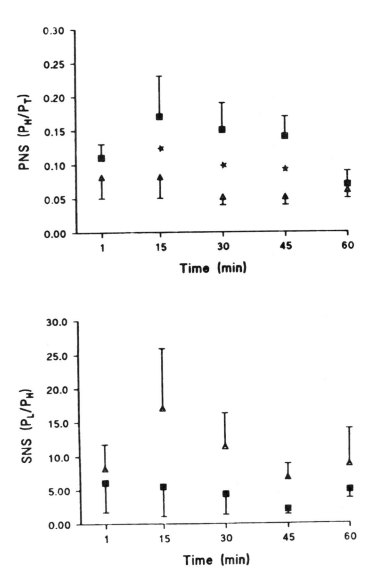

Figure 3 Effects of continuous positive airway pressure (CPAP) on the high-frequency/ total heart rate variability spectral power (P_H/P_T) and low-frequency/high-frequency heart rate variability spectral power (P_L/P_H), which are indicators of parasympathetic (PNS) and sympathetic nervous system (SNS) influence on heart rate variability, respectively, in patients with congestive heart failure. Data are shown at baseline (1 min) and after 15, 30, and 45 min with (■, $n = 14$) and without ($\triangle$, $n = 7$) CPAP of 10 cmH$_2$O, and after 15 min of recovery (60 min). Note that CPAP caused a significant increase in the PNS indicator but had no significant effect on the SNS indicator. *Significant between group difference ($p < 0.0036$). P_L, harmonic power in the low-frequency band (0.00–0.15 Hz); P_H, harmonic power in the high-frequency band (0.15–0.50 Hz); P_T, total harmonic and nonharmonic spectral power (0.00–0.50 Hz). (From Ref. 41.)

worsen it. Application of CPAP in this setting reduces LV afterload because Pit is increased, whereas BP is not affected (34). The net result is a reduction in LVPtm during systole. At the same time, because the failing heart with a high LV filling pressure is on the flat portion of the Starling curve, reductions in preload have little effect on cardiac output. Accordingly, the afterload-reducing effects of CPAP predominate, causing an augmentation in stroke volume and cardiac output (50). In a group of 11 CHF patients with high pulmonary capillary wedge pressure ($\geq$12 mmHg), Bradley et al. (47) found that application of 5 cmH_2O of CPAP increased cardiac index from 2.48 $\pm$ 0.26 to 2.82 $\pm$ 0.26 L/min/m^2. In contrast, among CHF patients with normal pulmonary capillary wedge pressure (<12 mmHg), stroke volume and cardiac output fell significantly. In another study, these investigators found that cardiac output and stroke volume increased in a dose-related fashion while on CPAP of 5 and 10 cmH_2O among those CHF patients with elevated LV filling pressures (48). Among healthy subjects and CHF patients with normal LV filling pressures, there were dose-related reductions in cardiac output and stroke volume. These findings suggest that the cardiac output response to CPAP in CHF patients with low LV filling pressures is similar to healthy subjects, probably because their cardiac output is to some extent preload-dependent as well. However, recent studies in hypervolemic pigs indicate that although low CPAP pressure of 5–10 cmH_2O can augment cardiac output, once CPAP increases to 15–20 cmH_2O, cardiac output falls (49). This implies that once CPAP increases above a certain level, its preload-reducing effect becomes predominant and more than offsets its afterload-reducing effect on cardiac output. A more detailed review of the effects of positive airway pressure in animal models of heart failure is provided in Chapter 19 in this volume.

Acute Effects of CPAP on Myocardial Ischemia and Cardiac Arrhythmias

A number of epidemiological studies have described an association between cardiac ischemic events and OSA. For example, Hung et al. (50) and Galatius-Jensen et al. (51) found a higher prevalence of OSA following myocardial infarction in men and women than among age- and sex-matched control subjects with no history of ischemic heart disease. In another study, Franklin et al. (18) found that 9 of 10 patients with documented coronary artery disease and frequent episodes of nocturnal angina pectoris had OSA with associated ischemic changes on the electrocardiogram. Abolition of OSA by CPAP in these patients markedly reduced the number of ischemic events on the electrocardiogram and virtually eliminated episodes of nocturnal angina over the next few weeks to months. It is very likely that these nocturnal ischemic events were precipitated by increased myocardial O_2 demand due to surges in sympathetic nervous system activity, BP, and heart rate in the face of reduced O_2 supply due to apnea-related hypoxia. Therefore, reversal of these processes by CPAP probably improved the balance between O_2 demand and supply and alleviated myocardial ischemia. In another report, ST-segment depressions during sleep were seen in 7 out of 23 OSA patients without a history of coronary artery disease (17). The frequency and duration of ST-segment depressions was significantly reduced when OSA was eliminated acutely by nasal CPAP.

Cardiac arrhythmias appear to occur frequently in patients with OSA. Among 400 OSA patients, sustained ventricular tachycardia was found in 8, sinus arrest in 43, second-degree atrioventricular conduction block in 31, and frequent premature ventricular contractions in 75 (52). Cardiac arrhythmias are a common cause of death in CHF (53). In 16 patients with OSA and nocturnal heart block, Koehler et al. (54) described a substantial reduction in the number of bradyarrhythmias in association with the abolition of OSA while on CPAP during sleep (from 651 to 72 per night). In another study (55), 7 out of 8 patients referred for pacemaker therapy with asymptomatic bradyarrhythmia consisting of severe sinus bradycardia, second-degree atrioventricular block, and complete heart block were diagnosed as having OSA by overnight polysomnography. When OSA was alleviated by either CPAP or tracheostomy, all 7 patients had an improvement in symptoms of sleep apnea and a reduction in the frequency of heart block without pacemaker therapy over an average follow-up period of 22 months. However, neither the prevalence of cardiac arrhythmias nor the potential for CPAP to alleviate such rhythm disturbances in CHF patients with OSA has been examined.

Effects of CPAP on Hemostasis

Increases in platelet activation and aggregability and in plasma fibrinogen concentrations and whole-blood viscosity have been reported in patients with OSA but without CHF (56,57). Such changes may contribute to an increased risk of cardiovascular and cerebrovascular ischemic events. Treatment of OSA by CPAP in these patients reduced their platelet activation and aggregability (56) as well as their plasma fibrinogen concentrations and whole-blood viscosity (57). It is possible that similar long-term reductions in platelet adhesiveness and blood coagulability could reduce the frequency of cardiovascular and cerebrovascular events in patients with OSA. Any such beneficial effects could be especially pronounced in patients at risk for these events, including those with CHF, coronary artery disease, or atrial fibrillation. However, the effects of CPAP on hemostasis has not been tested in OSA patients with these concurrent disorders.

Carryover effects of CPAP in OSA and CHF

Many of the beneficial effects of CPAP on cardiorespiratory function are not limited to the duration of its application but persist following its withdrawal. Genovese et al. (58) observed sustained increases in cardiac output during CPAP application and following its withdrawal in pigs with experimental CHF. However, the mechanism of that effect was not determined. In humans with CHF, CPAP-induced reductions in heart rate during wakefulness were sustained into the post-CPAP withdrawal period (34). When CPAP is applied during sleep to CHF patients with OSA, the carryover effects into the immediate post-CPAP withdrawal period include reductions in apnea-hypopnea index, heart rate, the product of systolic LVPtm and heart rate, Pit amplitude, respiratory rate, and the product of Pit amplitude and respiratory rate (19). More importantly, in the only study that systematically addressed the long-term effects of CPAP on cardiac function in patients with CHF and coexistent OSA, Malone et al. (13) observed that abolition of OSA by CPAP in eight such male patients led to a highly significant improvement in LV ejection fraction (LVEF) (from 37–49%, $p < 0.001$) over a 1-month period (Fig. 4). This improvement was more pronounced than previously described in OSA patients without CHF (from 59–63%) (59). Since the improvements in LVEF were observed during wakefulness at least 4 hr after CPAP had been removed, they indicated a prolonged beneficial carryover effect of CPAP on cardiac function. The most likely mechanisms responsible for this improvement in cardiac function are reductions in LV afterload due to the combined effects of reduced BP and increased Pit, improvements in Sa_{O_2}, and reductions in sympathetic nervous system activity (SNA) (19,39). In addition, symptoms of sleep apnea were alleviated and New York Heart Association (NYHA) functional class improved. Regardless of the mechanisms involved, beneficial carryover effects of CPAP have important clinical implications. They may explain, for example, sustained reductions in dyspnea lasting into the daytime in CHF patients with OSA treated with nocturnal CPAP (13). The improvement in LVEF suggests the potential for improvement in prognosis. Nevertheless, it seems that CPAP must be continued over the long term for such improvement

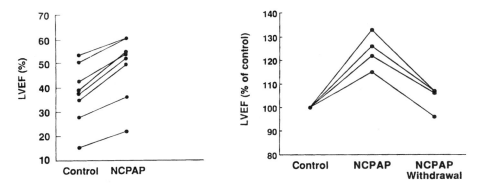

Figure 4 Individual left ventricular ejection fractions (LVEF) at baseline and after 4 weeks of nasal continuous positive airway pressure (NCPAP) therapy in patients with congestive heart failure and obstructive sleep apnea (left panel). Note that the improvement in LVEF by CPAP occurred in all studied subjects. In four patients, CPAP was withdrawn later for 1 week, which resulted in reduction in LVEF back to baseline (right panel). (From Ref. 13.)

to be maintained, since a 1-week withdrawal of CPAP led to a deterioration in LVEF and cardiac functional class back to the baseline level in a subset of four of the patients studied by Malone et al. (13). Most likely, recurrence of OSA led to this worsening of cardiac function. At the present time, CPAP should be considered the treatment of choice for most cases of OSA in patients with CHF.

Oral Appliances in the Treatment of OSA in Patients with CHF

Oral appliances modify the upper airway by changing the position of the mandible and tongue. There are two main types of oral appliances: mandibular advancement and tongue-retaining devices. Despite considerable variation in their design, their clinical effects are remarkably consistent. In his review, Schmidt-Nowara et al. (60) summarized the results of 21 papers analyzing the efficacy of oral appliances in 320 OSA patients with normal heart function. On average, the apnea-hypopnea index (AHI) was reduced from 47–19 events per hour of sleep. However, in only half of these patients was the AHI reduced to <10 while on oral appliances. In addition, application of these devices does not reliably abolish nocturnal hypoxemia, and does not reduce daytime sleepiness to the same extent as CPAP (61). Since oral appliances are less effective than CPAP in alleviating OSA and improving oxygenation and have not been specifically tested in patients with CHF, they should not be considered as first-line therapy for CHF patients with OSA. Studies demonstrating the efficacy of oral appliances in this patient population are required before their therapeutic role in this setting can be ascertained.

Surgery in the Treatment of OSA in Patients with CHF

Although several surgical approaches have been investigated for the treatment of OSA, none of them has been studied specifically in patients with CHF. In general, surgical procedures aim to improve upper airway patency either by eliminating a specific anatomic abnormality, such as hypertrophied tonsils, by widening the pharyngeal lumen at the presumed site of collapse during sleep or by bypassing the site of collapse (33,62,63). Clearly, where hypertrophied tonsils or adenoids impinge in the pharyngeal lumen, surgical removal could bring complete or partial relief of OSA (64). However, the risk of general anesthesia is higher in OSA patients with CHF than in those with normal cardiac function and must be taken into account in contemplating surgery for OSA in such patients.

The role of uvulopalatopharyngoplasty (UPPP), laser-assisted UPPP (LAUP), and more extensive maxillofacial surgeries is unclear (33,62,63,65). There are no randomized trials in which the effectiveness of UPPP, LAUP, and other surgical approaches to treat OSA have been tested, and results of case series have been inconsistent (62,66). For example, using meta-analysis on the effects of UPPP in OSA, Sher et al. (66) found an overall response rate defined as a

50% or greater reduction in AHI, of only 41%. Similarly, LAUP failed to reduce AHI below 15 obstructive events per hour of sleep in most patients (65). Although proper assessment of the upper airway by physical examination, cephalometric imaging, and pharyngoscopy is believed to predict the outcome of surgical procedures in treatment of OSA by some authors (67), others (33,68) consider upper airway narrowing to be diffuse rather than localized, such that no method is able to accurately predict the success of these types of surgery for any individual patient. Another drawback of these surgical approaches is the unpredictability of their long-term effects. Contrary to the results of treatment with CPAP, which are very stable over time, with UPPP or LAUP it is evident that the patient's condition may evolve and sleep apnea may reappear (62). Considering that surgical treatments of OSA in patients without CHF have a low success rate and are associated with anesthesia-related risks and surgical complications, they should be avoided in CHF patients suffering from OSA if at all possible.

In those patients who do not tolerate CPAP due to deviated nasal septum, surgical repair of this deformity should be considered, as it may improve compliance with CPAP (69). Tracheostomy is universally effective in eliminating OSA in patients without CHF because it completely bypasses the site of upper airway obstruction (63). In these patients it also improves Sa_{O_2}, reduces pulmonary and systemic BP, and alleviates cardiac arrhythmias (63,70). However, tracheostomy is unsightly and can cause local complications, such as wound infections and tissue breakdown, as well as lower respiratory tract infections (71). The effects of tracheostomy on OSA in patients with CHF have not been reported, but there is no reason why it should not work in this setting. Nevertheless, if there is a periodic breathing disorder underlying OSA in some patients with CHF, by-passing the upper airway with a tracheostomy could lead to periodic breathing with central apneas (72).

III. Treatment of Cheyne-Stokes Respiration with Central Sleep Apnea (CSR-CSA) in Patients with CHF

CSR-CSA is a form of periodic breathing during sleep characterized by central apneas alternating with prolonged hyperpnea with a characteristic crescendo-decrescendo pattern of tidal volume (73). Recent studies show that the key pathophysiological feature of CSR-CSA is a tendency to hyperventilate, resulting in dips in Pa_{CO_2} below an apneic threshold during sleep (74). In the setting of poor LV function, hyperventilation probably arises from pulmonary vagal afferent stimulation due to pulmonary venous congestion (75,76). Therefore, unlike OSA, CSR-CSA is likely a consequence rather than a cause of CHF.

Although CSR-CSA likely arises secondary to CHF, once present, it probably has adverse effects similar to those of OSA. Indeed, CSR-CSA is associated with increased mortality (7,11,12) in CHF patients, suggesting that therapy directed specifically at alleviating CSR-CSA might benefit this group of patients. Since CSR-CSA is common in the setting of CHF, with a prevalence of approximately 40% (7,20,24), its treatment has the potential to benefit a very significant proportion of the CHF population.

A. Pharmacological Treatment

Because CSA-CSR arises secondary to CHF, appropriate pharmacological therapy for CHF should be considered the first line of therapy for this breathing disorder. However, only a few studies have directly addressed this issue. Dark et al. (77) performed polysomnography on six patients with decompensated CHF before and then after vigorous medical treatment for CHF. The number of central apneas and hypopneas decreased from 153 ± 87 episodes per night before treatment to 72 ± 100 episodes per night after treatment. The one patient whose sleep study remained unchanged after medical therapy underwent cardiac transplantation, following which sleep apnea and severe apnea-related hypoxia were abolished. In one case-controlled open observational study, the addition of captopril to diuretics and digoxin in eight CHF patients with CSR-CSA was associated with a reduction in the central AHI from 35–20 events per hour over 4 weeks (78). Unfortunately, neither symptoms of CSR-CSA nor cardiac function was assessed in that study. There have been no randomized controlled trials examining the effects of drugs commonly used for the treatment of CHF on sleep-related breathing disorders. Murdock and associates also described a case report of the alleviation of CSR-CSA in a CHF patient after heart transplantation (79).

B. CPAP

Since CPAP has beneficial effects on cardiac loading conditions, heart rate, heart rate variability, and cardiac output in CHF patients while awake, it seems reasonable that it could also have longer-lasting beneficial effects even in the absence of recurrent upper airway obstruction. Indeed, CPAP is the most extensively studied therapy for CSR-CSA in patients with CHF and is the only treatment shown to alleviate this breathing disorder in association with substantial beneficial effects on cardiovascular and neurohumoral function as well as symptoms of CHF.

Effects of CPAP on CSR-CSA and Respiratory Muscles

Takasaki et al. (14) were the first to study the effects of CPAP in patients with CHF and CSR-CSA in a before-and-after case-controlled trial in 1989. These patients complained of paroxysmal nocturnal dyspnea, fatigue, and excessive daytime sleepiness. Application of CPAP of 8 to 12.5 cmH$_2$O at night to these five patients for 4–6 weeks was associated with a highly significant reduction in the AHI from 60 ± 12 to 9 ± 7/hr of sleep, an increase in nocturnal Sa_{O_2}, and improvements in sleep structure characterized by a significant increase in slow-wave sleep time and a reduction in movement arousals. At the 4- to 6-week follow-up assessment, nocturnal dyspnea was completely resolved, and fatigue and excessive daytime sleepiness were alleviated.

These initial observations of beneficial effects of CPAP on CSR-CSA were confirmed by Naughton et al. (80) in a controlled but unblinded trial of CPAP in patients with stable CHF and CSR-CSA. These patients were on optimal pharmacological treatment for CHF. Whereas in the control group there were no changes from baseline to the 1-month follow-up study in the frequency of central apneas and hypopneas, the group treated with CPAP experienced a significant decrease in the frequency of central events, associated with a significant reduction in minute ventilation and a significant increase in transcutaneous P_{CO_2} (Fig. 5). Since the key determinant of CSR-CSA in patients with CHF is hyperventilation with hypocapnia during sleep (74), these findings indicated that one mechanism through which CPAP attenuates CSR-CSA is by reducing minute ventilation and rising Pa_{CO_2} toward or above the apneic threshold (81). Indeed, CPAP was previously shown to reduce minute ventilation and increase Pa_{CO_2} in experimental animals (82). The means by which CPAP reduces minute ventilation in CHF patients with CSR-CSA in not clear. The most likely mechanism is attenuation of pulmonary edema by increasing Pit, reducing LV filling pressure, augmenting cardiac output, and shifting interstitial lung fluid to the extrathoracic vascular compartment (34,36,37,47).

In initiating CPAP therapy in CHF patients with CSR-CSA, two important points need to be kept in mind. First, CPAP is being used primarily to treat CHF,

Table 1 Respiratory Effects of Continuous Positive Airway Pressure in Congestive Heart Failure

Acute effects
   Unloading of inspiratory muscles
   Prevention of upper airway occlusion (OSA)
Chronic effects
   Elimination of upper airway occlusion and OSA
   Reduced minute volume of ventilation and increased Pa_{CO_2} above apnea threshold
     (CSR-CSA)
   Reduced frequency of central apneas
   Improvement in nocturnal oxygenation (OSA and CSR-CSA)
   Alleviation of symptoms of sleep apnea (OSA and CSR-CSA)
   Increased inspiratory muscle strength (CSR-CSA)

Abbreviations: OSA, obstructive sleep apnea; CSR, Cheyne-Stokes respiration; CSA, central sleep apnea.

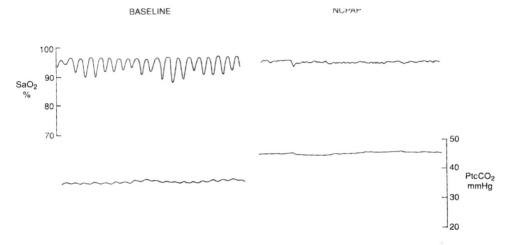

Figure 5 Tracings of oxyhemoglobin saturation (Sa_{O_2}) and transcutaneous P_{CO_2} (Ptc_{CO_2}) during stage 2 sleep in a patient with Cheyne-Stokes respiration with central sleep apnea (CSR-CSA) at baseline and on nasal continuous positive airway pressure (NCPAP). Note the typical pattern of dips in Sa_{O_2} at baseline in association with apneas during CSR-CSA associated with a low Ptc_{CO_2}. In contrast, there is an absence of dips in Sa_{O2}, indicating elimination of central apneas, associated with a markedly higher Ptc_{CO_2} in the same patient at the 1-month follow-up study while on CPAP. (From Ref. 80.)

not CSR-CSA per se. Second, in contrast to OSA, CSR-CSA generally does not respond rapidly to CPAP. Therefore, the most important goal in initiating CPAP in such patients is not the immediate relief of CSR-CSA but rather to get the patient comfortable wearing the CPAP appliance. To this end we allow patients to acclimatize to CPAP over 2–3 days. Initially, patients start off on a low pressure for a few hours while they are awake before attempting to use it during sleep. CPAP is then raised by 2- to 3-cmH₂O increments a day at a time until 10 to 12 cmH₂O is reached (83). During this time, sleep and respiration are not monitored. Once patients are used to CPAP, they are sent home with it. They then return for overnight polysomnography on CPAP 4–6 weeks later, by which time the frequency of central events is generally markedly reduced (80).

In those studies where this protocol has not been adhered to—either because there was no acclimatization period, CPAP was less than 10 cmH₂O or was rapidly titrated up over a single night, or was used for less than 1 month at the time of follow-up polysomnography—there were no reductions in the frequencies of central apneas and hypopneas while on CPAP (84–86). The slow titration of CPAP up into the therapeutic range that we advocate is similar to the approach taken when titrating angiotensin-converting enzyme (ACE) inhibitors or beta blockers into the therapeutic range in patients with CHF (87,88). In addition, it appears to take several weeks to months for the beneficial effects of CPAP on the respiratory and cardiovascular systems to accumulate. Again, this is analogous to the effects of ACE inhibitors and beta blockers on the cardiovascular system in patients with CHF (87,88).

Patients with CHF often suffer from respiratory muscle weakness (89), which may play a role in the pathogenesis of their dyspnea. Muscle weakness is likely due to structural and functional abnormalities of skeletal muscle related to insufficient energy supply (90). Inspiratory muscle weakness could be aggravated by the increased magnitude of pleural pressure swings during inspiration required to overcome reduced lung compliance and increased airway resistance resulting from pulmonary congestion (34,89,91). In response to angiotensin-converting enzyme inhibitor therapy, there is a partial reversal of abnormal ultrastructure and improvement in oxidative enzyme capacity of peripheral skeletal muscle in CHF patients. These effects are most likely due to improved hemodynamics, with increases in blood flow and oxygen delivery to skeletal muscles (92).

CPAP unloads inspiratory muscles by reducing the amplitude of inspiratory pleural pressure swings (19,34). Under conditions of low cardiac output and limited energy supply, unloading of inspiratory muscles by CPAP may improve the balance between respiratory muscle energy supply and demand. If part of respiratory muscle weakness in CHF patients is due to fatigue, then unloading of these muscles should increase their strength. In fact, Granton and associates observed a 14% improvement in maximum static inspiratory pressure after 3 months of CPAP in nine CHF patients suffering from CSR-CSA (93). It was concluded that inspiratory muscle weakness in CHF is at least partially reversible with CPAP therapy. Concurrent improvements in LVEF only accounted for about 25% of the variability in the improvement in maximum inspiratory pressure; therefore the beneficial effect of CPAP on inspiratory muscle strength was most likely due to unloading of these muscles by CPAP (93). The lack of significant improvement in expiratory muscle strength is consistent with this notion, because expiratory muscles are not unloaded by CPAP.

Effects of CPAP on Cardiac Function and Neurohumoral Activity

In the first uncontrolled trial of nightly CPAP for the treatment of chronic CHF patients with CSR-CSA, Takasaki et al. (14) demonstrated a significant increase in LVEF (from 31 ± 8 to $38 \pm 10\%$) measured during wakefulness, in association with alleviation of CSR-CSA. Following that study, Naughton et al. (8) conducted a randomized controlled clinical trial of nightly CPAP of 3 months duration in patients with stable CHF and CSR-CSA. All patients in the control and treatment groups were on optimal pharmacological treatment for their CHF. Patients ran-

Table 2 Effects of Continuous Positive Airway Pressure on Cardiac Function and Neurohumoral Activity in Congestive Heart Failure

Acute effects
   Increased intrathoracic pressure
   Reduced systolic blood pressure during sleep (OSA)
   Reduced systolic left ventricular transmural pressure (i.e., decreased afterload)
   Increased cardiac output in patients with elevated left ventricular filling pressure
   Reduced frequency of nocturnal cardiac arrhythmias (OSA)
Chronic effects
   Alleviation of symptoms of sleep apnea (OSA and CSR-CSA)
   Alleviation of symptoms of congestive heart failure (OSA and CSR-CSA)
   Increased left ventricular ejection fraction (OSA and CSR-CSA)
   Reduced mitral regurgitation (CSR-CSA)
   Reduced atrial natriuretic peptide concentration (CSR-CSA)
   Reduced awake plasma and overnight urinary norepinephrine concentrations (CSR-CSA)

Abbreviations: OSA, obstructive sleep apnea; CSR, Cheyne-Stokes respiration; CSA, central sleep apnea.

domized to CPAP used it for an average of 6 hr per day at an average pressure of 10 cmH$_2$O. In association with alleviation of CSR-CSA, they experienced a progressive improvement in LVEF, which reached 8% above baseline at the end of 3 months (Fig. 6). These findings emphasize the need for CPAP to be used for several weeks to months in order for its beneficial effects on LV function to occur. In contrast, the control group experienced no improvements in any of those factors. Such improvements in LVEF are greater than those described during treatment with vasodilators and ACE inhibitors but are similar to those observed during treatment with beta blockers (88,94,95). In addition to improved LV systolic function, CPAP-treated patients experienced a significant improvement in NYHA functional class and other symptoms of CHF (8).

In a subsequent study from our laboratory, Tkacova et al. (96) found that improvement in LVEF caused by nocturnal CPAP in patients with CHF and CSR-CSA was accompanied by a 41% reduction in functional mitral regurgitation and a 26% decrease in plasma atrial natriuretic peptide (ANP) concentration (Figs. 7 and 8). Mitral regurgitation is an integral part of the vicious cycle whereby cardiac dilation leads to functional mitral regurgitation, which, in turn, leads to further ventricular and atrial dilation, elevations in pulmonary venous pressure, and pulmonary congestion (97). Interruption of the vicious cycle by CPAP improves the forward pumping efficiency of the failing heart and may be particularly effective in retarding the progression of ventricular dilation that follows myocardial injury (96,98). The physiological significance of the reduction in mitral re-

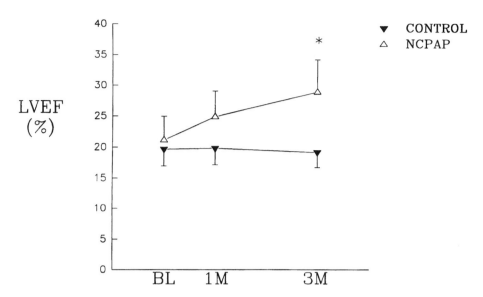

Figure 6 Left ventricular ejection fractions (LVEF) in patients with congestive heart failure and Cheyne-Stokes respiration with central sleep apnea at baseline (BL), 1 month (1M), and 3 months (3M). Filled triangles represent mean values in the control group and open triangles in the CPAP-treated group. Note the progressive increase in LVEF from baseline to 1 and 3 months in the CPAP-treated group. *Change from BL to 3M greater than in control group ($p = 0.019$). (From Ref. 8.)

gurgitation due to CPAP is further emphasized by the concomitant reduction in ANP. Since chronic regurgitant flow probably contributes to increased ANP in CHF by worsening atrial pressure and volume overload, its reduction by CPAP should relieve atrial overload and reduce ANP production and release. The significant correlation between baseline ANP and mitral regurgitation and the reduction in ANP in proportion to the decrease in mitral regurgitation at 3 months in the CPAP-treated patients are consistent with these concepts (96). Most importantly, reductions in the degree of mitral regurgitation and lowering of ANP concentrations together strongly suggest that cardiac size and filling pressures are reduced by CPAP. Also, elevated plasma ANP concentrations are predictors of increased mortality in severe CHF (99); therefore their reductions by CPAP may suggest improved prognosis.

The mechanisms by which CPAP leads to remarkable improvements in LVEF, reductions in mitral regurgitation, and decreases in ANP in patients with severe CHF and CSR-CSA could include reductions in cardiac filling pressures, diastolic volumes, and LV afterload (19,34,37,45,46). However, these improve-

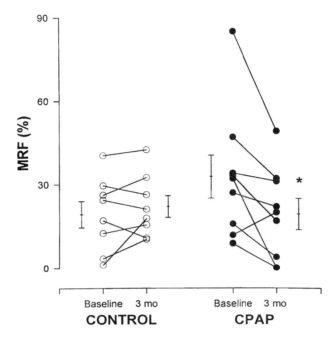

Figure 7   This figure illustrates significant reduction in mitral regurgitant fraction (MRF) from baseline to 3 months in patients with congestive heart failure and Cheyne-Stokes respiration with central sleep apnea treated with continuous positive airway pressure (CPAP). *$p < 0.02$ compared to baseline. (From Ref. 96.)

ments cannot be attributed solely to a temporary alteration in loading conditions, since these measurements were made after the patients had been off CPAP for several hours (8,96). The mechanism(s) responsible for these carryover effects remain to be determined but almost certainly involve favorable chronic alterations in the energetics and biological properties of the myocardium.

Although increased sympathoadrenal activity is an important acute compensatory response to maintain cardiac output in CHF, prolonged increases in sympathoadrenal activity may actually impair LV systolic and diastolic function and thus contribute to progression of the disease (100). High sympathetic nervous system activity and circulating catecholamine levels can stimulate cardiac myocyte hypertrophy and damage (101). In addition, high plasma norepinephrine (NE) concentration is an independent marker of higher mortality in CHF (102). Naughton et al. (103) demonstrated that CHF patients with CSR-CSA had higher overnight urinary and daytime plasma NE concentrations than CHF patients without CSR-CSA, despite similar LVEF. Among those CHF patients with CSR-CSA randomized to receive nightly CPAP for 1 month, there was a 40% reduction in

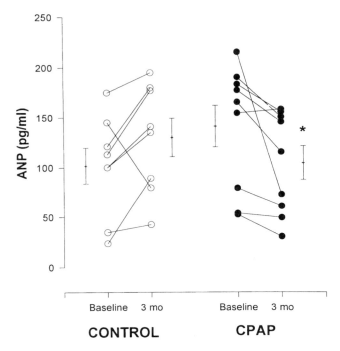

Figure 8 Individual atrial natriuretic peptide (ANP) concentrations at baseline and 3 months from the same patients shown in Figure 6. *$p < 0.05$ compared to baseline. (From Ref. 96.)

overnight urinary NE and a 24% reduction in daytime plasma NE (Fig. 9). These reductions in NE concentrations were associated with a significant decrease in heart rate. The mechanisms responsible for these reductions in NE concentrations likely include attenuation of CSR-CSA, with a reduction in the frequency of apneas and arousals, elimination of apnea-related hypoxic dips, as well as improvement in LV systolic function. Regardless of the mechanisms involved, these findings have significant clinical implications, because treatments for CHF that reduce SNA, heart rate, and LV afterload and increase LVEF cause greater improvements in survival than treatments that only reduce afterload (95,104,105).

C. Respiratory Stimulants

Respiratory stimulants, such as theophylline, acetazolamide, or medroxyprogesterone could theoretically alleviate CSR-CSA by providing a constant stimulus to breathe, thus overriding the lack of respiratory drive due to low Pa_{CO_2} and

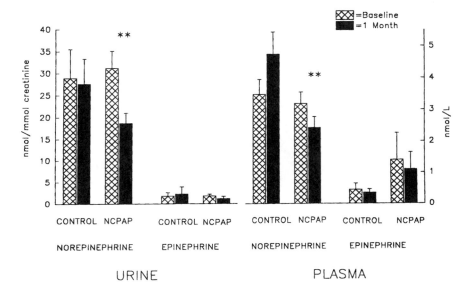

Figure 9   This figure illustrates that nasal continuous positive airway pressure (NCPAP) caused significant reductions in overnight urinary (UNE) and plasma norepinephrine (PNE) concentrations from baseline to 1 month in congestive heart failure patients with Cheyne-Stokes respiration and central sleep apnea. *Differences from baseline to 1 month in the NCPAP group versus the control group are significant ($p < 0.025$). (From Ref. 103.)

preventing the occurrence of central apneas (106,107). Raising Pa_{CO_2} by inhalation of CO_2 could potentially eliminate CSR-CSA by increasing Pa_{CO_2} above the apneic threshold (108–110).

Theophylline

In addition to its bronchodilating property, theophylline increases respiratory drive by a direct stimulatory effect on brainstem respiratory centers (111). However, only one study systematically addressed its effects on CSR-CSA in adults with CHF. Javaheri et al. (106) studied the effects of theophylline on CSR-CSA in 15 male patients with CHF for 5 days using a double-blind, randomized, placebo-controlled crossover design. Use of theophylline was associated with a significant reduction in the AHI (from 47 ± 21 to 18 ± 17 events per hour), but no increase in Sa_{O_2}, reduction in the frequency of arousals, or improvements in sleep structure. However, the interpretation of their findings was confounded by the unusual design of their study: nocturnal supplemental O_2 was started at the same time as theophylline and placebo and was discontinued at the time of the follow-up sleep study.

The rationale for this design was that, since recurrent dips in Sa_{O_2} during CSR-CSA might trigger cardiac arrhythmias, supplemental O_2 had to be administered to counteract this potential effect on ethical grounds. This rationale, however, is questionable, because there is no evidence as yet that mild hypoxic dips, typical of CSR-CSA, cause serious cardiac arrhythmias, or that supplemental O_2 eliminates them or has any beneficial effects on prognosis. On the other hand, one cannot be certain that supplemental O_2 did not play a role beyond that due to theophylline in reducing the severity of CSR-CSA, since it had previously been shown that O_2 administration reduces the severity of CSR-CSA in stable CHF patients (112). Most importantly, theophylline did not lead to any improvement in cardiac function but resulted in a tendency (although not statistically significant) toward increased rates of ventricular premature beats. In addition, one patient developed supraventricular tachycardia while on theophylline. The tendency to increased cardiac arrhythmias is consistent with the known arrhythmogenicity of theophylline, which is related to its phosphodiesterase inhibitory, sympathoexcitatory, and positive inotropic effects (113). Other phosphodiesterase inhibitors, such as milrinone, have similar arrhythmogenic effects and invariably have been shown to increase mortality in patients with CHF (114). The same is true of other positive inotropic drugs, such as dobutamine (115). Another potential problem with theophylline is that it could increase minute ventilation in CHF patients with CSR-CSA whose minute ventilation is already higher and whose Pa_{CO_2} is reduced. In so doing, it would increase the load on already weakened inspiratory muscles and increase their metabolic demands in the face of low cardiac output. Therefore more data are required before a convincing case can be made that theophylline is a practical, effective, and safe treatment for CSR-CSA in patients with CHF.

Acetazolamide

Acetazolamide is a carbonic anhydrase inhibitor that stimulates central respiratory drive by causing a metabolic acidosis (116–118). General studies have shown that acetazolamide can reduce the frequency of central apneas and hypopneas in patients with CSA but without CHF (107,116,117). In the most recent of these studies, DeBacker et al. (107) administered acetazolamide to 14 patients with CSA but without CHF over 1 month. In association with a decrease in pH, they observed significant reductions in the frequencies of central respiratory events and arousals, an increase in Sa_{O_2}, and an improvement in symptoms of sleep apnea. In contrast, Sakamoto et al. (119) found that acetazolamide did not consistently reduce the frequency of respiratory events in patients with CSA. There are no published reports describing the effects of acetazolamide on CSR-

CSA in patients with CHF. Since patients with CHF and CSR-CSA hyperventilate, are hypocapnic (74), and have weak respiratory muscles (89), there is no strong rationale to use a drug that further increases ventilation and loads inspiratory muscles. Moreover, the creation of a metabolic acidosis by acetazolamide in such patients could precipitate malignant cardiac arrhythmias.

Carbon Dioxide

Hypocapnia caused by hyperventilation triggers central apneas in patients with or without CHF when Pa_{CO_2} is driven below the threshold for apnea (74,120–122). Lorenzi-Filho et al. (108) recently reported that raising P_{CO_2} in CHF patients with CSR-CSA by just 1–2 mmHg, through inhalation of a CO_2-enriched gas mixture, completely eliminated central apneas and hypopneas. Xie et al. (122) made similar observations in patients with idiopathic CSA using either CO_2 inhalation or rebreathing in a mask with increased dead space. Although Steens et al. (115) also found that inhalation of a gas mixture containing 3% CO_2 markedly reduced the frequency of central respiratory events in CHF patients with CSR-CSA, their definition of apnea and hypopnea did not conform to standard criteria, and they did not systematically evaluate P_{CO_2} during their experiments. Nevertheless, taken together, these findings indicate that raising P_{CO_2} above the apnea threshold eliminates CSR-CSA in patients with CHF. Although inhaled CO_2 or provision of a mask with increased dead space might alleviate CSR-CSA in patients with CHF, neither is liable to be clinically useful because, as with theophylline and acetazolamide, these increase minute ventilation and thereby increase the energy expenditure of the weakened inspiratory muscles. Raising P_{CO2} could also create a potentially dangerous respiratory acidosis.

There are no published reports on the use of medroxyprogesterone for the treatment of hypocapnic central sleep apnea, in patients either with or without CHF.

D. Respiratory Depressants

Another potential approach to the treatment of CSR-CSA would be to suppress arousals from sleep and blunt respiratory drive by administering sedative medications (123). In theory, this should reduce ventilation and allow Pa_{CO_2} to increase above the apneic threshold (124).

Sedative Medications

In patients with CHF and CSR-CSA, Biberdorf et al. (125) found that although temazepam reduced the number of arousals from sleep, it neither reduced the severity of CSR-CSA nor improved Sa_{O_2}. Guilleminault et al. (84) made similar observations when they administered three different benzodiazepines to nine CHF patients. Thus, the available evidence does not support the use of sedatives as a treatment for CSR-CSA in patients with CHF.

Oxygen

The rationale for using O_2 to treat CSR-CSA in patients with CHF is that correction of apnea-related dips in Sa_{O_2} may suppress peripheral chemoreceptor drive, thereby preventing subsequent ventilatory overshoot. If this were the case, then alleviation of CSR-CSA by supplemental O_2 should be accompanied by an increase in Pa_{CO_2} toward or above the apnea threshold (126). Hanly et al. (112) observed a modest but significant decrease in the central AHI (from 30 to 19 events per hour) with a single night of intranasal O_2 (2–3 L/min) in a randomized, single-blinded study in patients with CHF. However, because of the acute nature of this study, clinical outcomes were not assessed. Franklin et al. performed two trials of supplemental O_2 in patients with CSR-CSA related to either CHF or cerebrovascular accidents (127,128). In the first (127), they demonstrated that 50% O_2 administered via a venturi mask caused a marked reduction in central AHI in association with an increase in Pa_{CO_2}. In the second (128), low-flow O_2 was given via nasal cannula but caused only a slight decrease in central AHI. However, Pa_{CO_2} did not increase. These data are consistent with the concept that inhalation of supplemental O_2 can alleviate CSR-CSA when it blunts peripheral chemoreceptor activity sufficiently to permit Pa_{CO_2} to rise above the apnea threshold. Both of the studies were performed over a single night and neither cardiac function nor symptoms were assessed.

In a subsequent randomized double-blind crossover study of intranasal O_2 given at 4 L/min for 7 days to 22 patients with CHF, Andreas et al. (129) also documented a modest decrease in central AHI (from 26–10 events per hour) in patients with CSR-CSA. In addition, these patients experienced a slight but significant increase in peak O_2 consumption during exercise but no change in the duration of exercise, peak heart rate, or quality of life while on O_2. Cardiac function was not assessed. The clinical significance of these findings therefore remains unclear. More recently, Staniforth et al. (130) documented significant reductions in AHI and in overnight urinary NE excretion in 11 patients with stable CHF and CSR-CSA while they were on nocturnal O_2 over 4 weeks during a double-blind crossover study. However, supplemental O_2 did not reduce daytime plasma NE concentration and did not improve symptoms of heart failure or cognitive performance. Again, cardiac function was not assessed.

To summarize, although treatment of CSR-CSA by supplemental O_2 may be promising for some patients, it is unlikely to be of benefit where hypoxic dips are minimal. Moreover, trials conducted to date have been small and of short duration, and they have not demonstrated improvements in cardiac function or symptoms of CHF. Nevertheless, O_2-induced reductions in overnight urinary catecholamine excretion suggest the potential for benefits to the cardiovascular system. Balanced against the potential benefits of supplemental O_2, however, are potential detrimental effects demonstrated in patients with CHF by other investigators. These include increases in systemic vascular resistance, BP, and LV filling pressure and reductions in cardiac output (131). The mechanism(s) for these adverse effects have not been demonstrated but may involve elaboration of oxygen free radicals. Thus, it is not clear that long-term supplemental O_2 would be a safe and effective therapy for CSR-CSA in CHF patients. This issue can be resolved only by longer trials with larger numbers of patients in which the effects of nocturnal O_2 on heart function and prognosis in patients with CHF and CSR-CSA are assessed.

IV. Conclusions

Sleep-related breathing disorders are common in patients with CHF and are associated with acute pathological effects on the cardiovascular system. Such effects, over time, have the potential to cause progression of CHF and to worsen its prognosis. As this review indicates, specific treatment of these disorders, especially with CPAP, can have beneficial short- and medium-term effects on cardiovascular and respiratory function. In the case of treatment with CPAP, the benefits to LVEF, mitral regurgitation, ANP, and NE imply the potential to improve survival. To date, however, studies of various interventions for OSA and CSR-CSA in CHF patients have involved too few subjects over too short a duration to provide definitive evidence of long-term benefits. Nevertheless, these studies have provided sufficient evidence of medium-term benefit to warrant larger, longer-term trials of CPAP or supplemental O_2 in order to evaluate their effects on prognosis in CHF patients with either OSA or CSR-CSA.

Acknowledgments

This work was partially supported by operating grants MT-11607 and MA-12422 from the Medical Research Council of Canada. R. Tkacova is supported by a Research Fellowship from Respironics Inc.

References

1. McAlister FA, Teo KK. The management of congestive heart failure. Postgrad Med J 1997; 73:194–200.
2. Kannel WB, Belanger AJ. Epidemiology in heart failure (abstr). Am Heart J 1991; 121:951–957.

3. Yusuf S, Thom T, Abbot RD. Changes in hypertension treatment and congestive heart failure mortality in the Unites States. Hypertension 1989; 13(suppl 1):1174–1179.
4. Guilleminault C, Tilkian A, Dement WC. The sleep apnea syndromes. Annu Rev Med 1976; 27:465–484.
5. Hla KM, Young TB, Bidwell T, Palta M, Skatrud JB, Dempsey J. Sleep apnea and hypertension: a population-based study. Ann Intern Med 1994; 120:382–388.
6. Carlson JT, Hedner JA, Ejnell H, Peterson LE. High prevalence of hypertension in sleep apnea patients independent of obesity. Am J Respir Crit Care Med 1994; 150:72–77.
7. Javaheri S, Parker TJ, Wexler L, Michaels SE, Stanberry E, Nishyama H, Roselle GA. Occult sleep-disordered breathing in stable congestive heart failure. Ann Intern Med 1995; 122:487–492.
8. Naughton MT, Liu PP, Bernard DC, Goldstein RS, Bradley TD. Treatment of congestive heart failure and Cheyne-Stokes respiration during sleep by continuous positive airway pressure. Am J Respir Crit Care Med 1995; 151:92–97.
9. Bradley TD, Floras JS. Pathophysiologic and therapeutic implications of sleep apnea in congestive heart failure. J Cardiac Failure 1996; 2:223–240.
10. Andreas, S, Hagenah G, Moller C, Werner GS, Kreuzer H. Cheyne-Stokes respiration and prognosis in congestive heart failure. Am J Cardiol 1996; 78:1260–1264.
11. Findley LJ, Zwillich CW, Ancoli-Israel S, Kripke D, Tisi G, Moser KM. Cheyne-Stokes breathing during sleep in patients with left ventricular heart failure. South Med J 1985; 78:11–15.
12. Hanly PJ, Zuberi-Khokhar NS. Increased mortality associated with Cheyne-Stokes respiration in patients with congestive heart failure. Am J Respir Crit Care Med 1996; 153:272–276.
13. Malone S, Liu PP, Holloway R, Rutherford R, Xie A, Bradley TD. Obstructive sleep apnoea in patients with dilated cardiomyopathy: effects of continuous positive airway pressure. Lancet 1991; 338:1480–1484.
14. Takasaki Y, Orr D, Popkin J, Rutherford R, Liu P, Bradley TD. Effect of nasal continuous positive airway pressure on sleep apnea in congestive heart failure. Am Rev Respir Dis 1989; 140:1578–1584.
15. Young T, Peppard P, Palta M, Hla KM, Finn L, Morgan B, Skatrud J. Population-based study of sleep-disordered breathing as a risk factor for hypertension. Arch Intern Med 1997; 157:1746–1752.
16. Palomaki H, Partinin M, Juvela S, Kaste M. Snoring as a risk factor for sleep-related brain infarction. Stroke 1989; 10:1311–1315.
17. Hanly P, Sasson Z, Zuberi N, Lunn K. ST-segment depression during sleep in obstructive sleep apnea. Am J Cardiol 1993; 71:1341–1345.
18. Franklin KA, Nilsson JB, Sahlin C. Sleep apnoea and nocturnal angina. Lancet 1995; 345:1085–1087.
19. Tkacova R, Rankin F, Fitzgerald F, Floras JS, Bradley TD. Effects of continuous positive airway pressure on obstructive sleep apnea and left ventricular afterload in patients with heart failure. Circulation 1998; 98:2269–2275.
20. Javaheri S, Parker TJ, Liming JD, Corbett WS, Nishiyama H, Wexler L, Roselle GA. Sleep apnea in 81 ambulatory male patients with stable heart failure: types

and their prevalences, consequences, and presentations. Circulation 1998; 97:2154–2159.

21. Young TB, Palta M, Dempsey JA, Skatrud JB, Weber S, Badr S. The occurrence of sleep-disordered breathing among middle-aged adults. N Engl J Med 1993; 328: 1230–1235.

22. Stradling JR, Crosby JH. Predictors and prevalence of obstructive sleep apnoea and snoring in 1001 middle aged men. Thorax 1991; 46:85–89.

23. Horner RL, Mohiaddin RH, Lowell DG, Shea SA, Burman ED, Longmore DB, Guz A. Sites and sizes of fat deposits around the pharynx in obese patients with obstructive sleep apnoea and weight matched controls. Eur Respir J 1989; 2:613–622.

24. Brown IG, Bradley TD, Phillipson EA, Zamel N, Hoffstein V. Pharyngeal compliance in snoring subjects with and without sleep apnea. Am Rev Respir Dis 1985; 132:211–215.

25. Issa FG, Sullivan CE. Upper airway closing pressures in obstructive sleep apnea. J Appl Physiol 1984; 57:520–527.

26. Rubinstein I, Colapinto N, Rotstein LE, Brown IG, Hoffstein V. Improvement in pharyngeal properties after weight loss in patients with obstructive sleep apnea. Am Rev Respir Dis 1988; 138:1192–1195.

27. Bonora M, Shields GI, Knuth SL, Bartlett D Jr, St John WM. Selective depression by ethanol of upper airway respiratory motor activity in cats. Am Rev Respir Dis 1984; 130:156–161.

28. Bonora M, St John WM, Bledsoe TA. Differential elevation by protryptyline and depression by diazepam of upper airway respiratory motor activity. Am Rev Respir Dis 1985; 131:41–45.

29. Issa FG, Sullivan CE. Alchohol, snoring, and sleep apnea. J Neurol Neurosurg Psychiatry 1982; 45:353–359.

30. Mendelson WB, Garnett D, Gillin JC. Flurazepam-induced sleep apnea syndrome in a patient with insomnia and mild sleep-related respiratory changes. J Neurol Ment Dis 1981; 169:261–264.

31. George CF, Millar TW, Kryger MH. Sleep apnea and body position during sleep. Sleep 1988; 11:90–99.

32. Shepard JW Jr, Pevernagie DA, Stanson AW, Daniels BK, Sheedy PF. Effects of changes in central venous pressure on upper airway size in patients with obstructive sleep apnea. Am J Respir Crit Care Med 1996; 153:250–254.

33. Hoffstein V. How and why should we stabilize the upper airway? Sleep 1996; 19: S57–S60.

34. Naughton MT, Rahman MA, Hara K, Floras JS, Bradley TD. Effect of continuous positive airway pressure on intrathoracic and left ventricular transmural pressures in patients with congestive heart failure. Circulation 1995; 91:1725–1731.

35. McGregor M, Becklake MR. The relationship of oxygen cost of breathing to respiratory mechanical work and respiratory force. J Clin Invest 1961; 40:971–980.

36. Manyari DE, Wang Z, Cohen J, Tyberg JV. Assessment of human splanchnic volume-pressure relation using radionuclide plethysmography: effect of nitroglycerine. Circulation 1993; 87:1142–1151.

37. Lenique F, Habis M, Lofaso F, Dubois-Rnade JL, Harf A, Brochard L. Ventilatory

and hemodynamic effects of continuous positive airway pressure in left heart failure. Am J Respir Crit Care Med 1997; 155:500–505.

38. Hedner J, Ejnell H, Caidahl K. Left ventricular hypertrophy independent of hypertension in patients with obstructive sleep apnoea. J Hypertens 1990; 8:941–946.

39. Somers VK, Dyken ME, Clary MP, Abbound FM. Sympathetic neural mechanisms in obstructive sleep apnea. J Clin Invest 1995; 96:1897–1904.

40. Barruzzi A, Riva R, Cirignotta F, Zucconi M, Cappelli M, Lugaresi E. Atrial natriuretic peptide and catecholamines in obstructive sleep apnea syndrome. Sleep 1991; 14:83–86.

41. Butler GC, Naughton MT, Rahman MA, Bradley TD, Floras JS. Continuous positive airway pressure increases heart rate variability in congestive heart failure (see comments). J Am Coll Cardiol 1995; 25:672–679.

42. Bigger JT, Fleiss JL, Rolnitzky LM, Steinman RC. Frequency domain measures of heart rate variability to assess risk late after myocardial infarction. J Am Coll Cardiol 1993; 21:729–736.

43. Pinsky MR, Matuschak GM, Klain M. Determinants of cardiac augmentation by elevations in intrathoracic pressure. J Appl Physiol 1985; 58:1189–1198.

44. Pinsky MR, Summer WR, Wise RA, Permutt S, Brobmerger-Barnea B. Augmentation of cardiac function by elevation of intrathoracic pressure. J Appl Physiol 1983; 54:950–955.

45. Fewell JE, Abendschein DR, Carlson CJ, Murray JF, Rapaport E. Continuous positive-pressure ventilation decreases right and left ventricular end-diastolic volumes in the dog. Circ Res 1980; 46:125–132.

46. Johnston WE, Vinten-Johansen J, Santamore WP, Case LD, Little WC. Mechanisms of reduced cardiac output during positive end expiratory pressure in the dog. Am Rev Respir Dis 1919; 140:1257–1264.

47. Bradley TD, Holloway RM, McLaughlin PR, Ross BL, Walters J, Liu PP. Cardiac output response to continuous positive airway pressure in congestive heart failure. Am Rev Respir Dis 1992; 145:377–382.

48. De Hoyos A, Liu PP, Benard DC, Bradley TD. Haemodynamic effects of continuous positive airway pressure in humans with normal and impaired left ventricular function. Clin Sci (Colch) 1995; 88:173–178.

49. Genovese J, Moskowitz M, Tarasiuk A, Graver LM, Scharf SM. Effects of continuous positive airway pressure on cardiac output in normal and hypervolemic unanesthetized pigs. Am J Respir Crit Care Med 1994; 150:752–758.

50. Hung J, Whitford EG, Parsons RW, Hillman DR. Association of sleep apnoea with myocardial infarction in men. Lancet 1990; 336:261–264.

51. Galatius-Jensen S, Hansen J, Rasmussen V, Bildsoe J, Therboe M, Rosenberg J. Nocturnal hypoxaemia after myocardial infarction: association with nocturnal myocardial ischaemia and arrhythmias. Br Heart J 1994; 72:23–30.

52. Guilleminault C, Connolly SJ, Winkle RA. Cardiac arrhythmia and conduction disturbances during sleep in 400 patients with sleep apnea syndrome. Am J Cardiol 1983; 52:490–494.

53. Francis GS. Development of arrhythmias in the patient with congestive heart failure: pathophysiology, prevalence and prognosis. Am J Cardiol 1986; 57:3B–7B.

54. Koehler U, Fus E, Grimm W, Pankow W, Schafer H, Stammintz A, Peter JH. Heart

block in patients with obstructive sleep apnoea: pathogenetic factors and effects of treatment. Eur Respir J 1998; 11:434–439.

55. Stegman SS, Burroughs JM, Henthorn RW. Asymptomatic bradyarrhythmias as a marker for sleep apnea: appropriate recognition and treatment may reduce the need for pacemaker therapy. Pacing Clin Electrophysiol 1996; 19:899–904.

56. Bokinsky G, Miller M, Ault K, Husband P, Mitchell J. Spontaneous platelet activation and aggregation during obstructive sleep apnea and its response to therapy with nasal continuous positive airway pressure: a preliminary investigation. Chest 1995; 108:625–630.

57. Chin K, Ohi M, Kita H, Noguchi T, Otsuka N, Tsuboi T, Mishima M, Kuno K. Effects of NCPAP therapy on fibrinogen levels in obstructive sleep apnea syndrome. Am J Respir Crit Care Med 1996; 153:1972–1976.

58. Genovese J, Huberfeld S, Tarasiuk A, Moskowitz M, Scharf SM. Effects of CPAP on cardiac output in pigs with pacing-induced congestive heart failure. Am J Respir Crit Care Med 1995; 152:1847–1853.

59. Krieger J, Grucker D, Sforza E. Left ventricular ejection fraction in obstructive sleep apnea: effects of long-term treatment with nasal continuous positive airway pressure. Chest 1991; 100:917–921.

60. Schmidt-Nowara W, Lowe A, Wiegand L, Cartwright R, Perez-Guerra F, Menn S. Oral appliances for the treatment of snoring and obstructive sleep apnea: a review. Sleep 1995; 18:501–510.

61. Ferguson KA, Ono T, Lowe AA, Keenan SP, Fleetham JA. A randomized crossover study of an oral appliance vs nasal-continuous positive airway pressure in the treatment of mild-moderate obstructive sleep apnea. Chest 1996; 109:1269–1275.

62. Pepin JL, Veale D, Mayer P, Bettega G, Wuyam B, Levy P. Critical analysis of the results of surgery in the treatment of snoring, upper airway resistance syndrome (UARS), and obstructive sleep apnea (OSA). Sleep 1996; 19:S90–S100.

63. Guilleminault C, Simmons FB, Motta J, Cummiskey J, Rosekind M, Schroeder JS, Dement WC. Obstructive sleep apnea syndrome and tracheostomy: long-term follow-up experience. Arch Intern Med 1981; 141:985–988.

64. Moser RJ, Rajagopal KR. Obstructive sleep apnea in adults with tonsillar hypertrophy. Arch Intern Med 1987; 147:1265–1267.

65. Walker RP, Grigg-Damberger MM, Gopalsami C. Uvulopalatopharyngoplasty versus laser-assisted uvulopalatoplasty for the treatment of obstructive sleep apnea. Laryngoscope 1997; 107:76–82.

66. Sher AE, Schechtman KB, Piccirillo JF. The efficacy of surgical modifications of the upper airway in adults with obstructive sleep apnea syndrome. Sleep 1996; 19: 156–177.

67. Launois SH, Feroah TR, Campbell WN, Issa FG, Morrison D, Whitelaw WA, Isono S, Remmers JE. Site of pharyngeal narrowing predicts outcome of surgery for obstructive sleep apnea. Am Rev Respir Dis 1993; 147:182–189.

68. Rubinstein I, Bradley TD, Zamel N, Hoffstein V. Glottic and cervical tracheal narrowing in patients with obstructive sleep apnea. J Appl Physiol 1989; 67:2427–2431.

69. Heimer D, Scharf SM, Lieberman A, Lavie P. Sleep apnea syndrome treated by repair of deviated nasal septum. Chest 1983; 84:184–185.

70. Motta J, Guilleminault C, Schroeder JS, Dement WC. Tracheostomy and hemodynamic changes in sleep-inducing apnea. Ann Intern Med 1978; 89:454–458.

71. Harlid R, Andersson G, Frostell CG, Jorbeck HJ, Ortquist AB. Respiratory tract colonization and infection in patients with chronic tracheostomy: a one-year study in patients living at home. Am J Respir Crit Care Med 1996; 154:124–129.

72. Badr MS, Grossman JE, Weber SA. Treatment of refractory sleep apnea with supplemental carbon dioxide. Am J Respir Crit Care Med 1994; 150:561–564.

73. Hall MJ, Xie A, Rutherford R, Ando S, Floras JS, Bradley TD. Cycle length of periodic breathing in patients with and without heart failure. Am J Respir Crit Care Med 1996; 154:376–381.

74. Naughton M, Benard D, Tam A, Rutherford R, Bradley TD. Role of hyperventilation in the pathogenesis of central sleep apneas in patients with congestive heart failure. Am Rev Respir Dis 1993; 148:330–338.

75. Paintal AS. Mechanisms of stimulation of type J pulmonary receptors. J Physiol 1969; 203:511–532.

76. Sackner MA, Krieger BP. Noninvasive respiratory monitoring in Scharf SM, Cassidy SS, eds. Heart and Lung Interactions in Health and Disease. New York: Marcel Dekker, 1991: 663–805.

77. Dark DS, Pingleton SK, Kerby GR, Crabb JE, Gollub SB, Glatter TR, Dunn MI. Breathing pattern abnormalities and arterial oxygen desaturation during sleep in the congestive heart failure syndrome: improvement following medical therapy. Chest 1987; 91:833–836.

78. Walsh JT, Andrews R, Starling R, Cowley AJ, Johnston ID, Kinnear WJ. Effects of captopril and oxygen on sleep apnoea in patients with mild to moderate congestive heart failure. Heart 1995; 73:237–241.

79. Murdock DK, Lawless CE, Loeb HS, Scanlon PJ, Pifarre R. The effect of heart transplantation on Cheyne-Stokes respiration associated with congestive heart failure. J Heart Transplant 1986; 5:336–337.

80. Naughton MT, Benard DC, Rutherford R, Bradley TD. Effect of continuous positive airway pressure on central sleep apnea and nocturnal P_{CO_2} in heart failure. Am J Respir Crit Care Med 1994; 150:1598–1604.

81. Skatrud JB, Dempsey JA. Interaction of sleep state and chemical stimuli in sustaining rhythmic ventilation. J Appl Physiol 1983; 55:813–822.

82. Torres A, Kamarek RM, Kimball WR, Qvist J, Stanek K, Whyte R, Zapol WM. Regional diaphragmatic length and EMG activity during inspiratory pressure support and CPAP in awake sheep. J Appl Physiol 1993; 74:695–703.

83. Benard DC, Naughton MT, Bradley TD. Administration of continuous positive airway pressure to patients with congestive heart failure and Cheyne-Stokes respiration. J Polysomnogr 1992; 9–11.

84. Guilleminault C, Clerk A, Labanowski M, Simmons J, Stoohs R. Cardiac failure and benzodiazepines. Sleep 1993; 16:524–528.

85. Davies RJO, Harrington KJ, Ormerod OJM, Stradling JR. Nasal continuous positive airway pressure in chronic heart failure with sleep-disordered breathing. Am Rev Respir Dis 1993; 147:630–634.

86. Buckle P, Millar T, Kryger M. The effect of short-term nasal CPAP on Cheyne-Stokes respiration in congestive heart failure. Chest 1992; 102:31–35.

87. The SOLVD Investigators. Effect of enalapril on survival in patients with reduced left ventricular ejection fraction and congestive heart failure. N Engl J Med 1991; 325:293–302.

88. Cohn JN, Fowler MB, Bristow MR, Colucci WS, Gilbert EM, Kinhal V, Krueger SK, Lejemtel T, Narahara KA, Packer M, Young ST, Holcslaw TL, Lukas MA. Safety and efficacy of carvedilol in severe heart failure: the U.S. carvedilol heart failure study group. J Cardiac Failure 1997; 3:173–179.

89. McParand C, Krishnan B, Wang Y, Gallagher C. Inspiratory muscle weakness and dyspnea in chronic heart failure. Am Rev Respir Dis 1992; 146:467–472.

90. Sullivan MJ, Green HJ, Cobb FK. Skeletal muscle biochemistry and histology in ambulatory patients with long-term heart failure. Circulation 1990; 81:518–528.

91. Rasanen J, Heikkila J, Downs J, Nikki P, Vaisanen I, Vitanen A. Continuous positive airway pressure by face mask in acute cardiogenic pulmonary edema. Am J Cardiol 1985; 55:296–300.

92. Drexler H, Banhardt U, Meinertz T, Wollschlager H, Lehmann M, Just H. Contrasting peripheral short-term and long-term effects of converting enzyme inhibition in patients with congestive heart failure: a double-blind, placebo controlled trial. Circulation 1989; 79:491–502.

93. Granton JT, Naughton MT, Benard DC, Liu PP, Goldstein RS, Bradley TD. CPAP improves inspiratory muscle strength in patients with heart failure and central sleep apnea. Am J Respir Crit Care Med 1996; 153:277–282.

94. Veterans Administration Cooperative Study Group. Effect of vasodilator therapy on mortality in chronic congestive heart failure: results of a Veterans Administration Cooperative Study. N Engl J Med 1986; 314:1547–1552.

95. Veterans Administration Cooperative Study Group. A comparison of enalapril with hydralazine-isosorbide dinitrate in the treatment of chronic congestive heart failure. N Engl J Med 1991; 325:303–310.

96. Tkacova R, Liu PP, Naughton MT, Bradley TD. Effect of continuous positive airway pressure on mitral regurgitant fraction and atrial natriuretic peptide in patients with heart failure. J Am Coll Cardiol 1997; 30:739–745.

97. Vanoverschelde JLJ, Raphael DA, Robert DA, Cosyns JR. Left ventricular filling in dilated cardiomyopathy: relation to functional class and hemodynamics. J Am Coll Cardiol 1990; 15:1288–1295.

98. Weiland DS, Konstam MA, Salem DN, Martin TT, Cohen SR, Zile MR, Das D. Contribution of reduced mitral regurgitant volume to vasodilator effect in severe left ventricular failure secondary to coronary artery disease or idiopathic dilated cardiomyopathy: Am J Cardiol 1986; 58:1046–1050.

99. Gottlieb SS, Kukin ML, Ahern D, Packer M. Prognostic importance of atrial natriuretic peptide in patients with chronic heart failure. J Am Coll Cardiol 1989; 13: 1534–1539.

100. Daly PA, Sole MJ. Myocardial catecholamines and the pathophysiology of heart failure. Circulation 1990; 82:I35–I43.

101. Francis GS, McDonald KM, Cohn JN. Neurohumoral activation in preclinical heart failure: remodeling and the potential for intervention. Circulation 1993; 87:IV90–IV96.

102. Cohn JN, Levine TB, Olivari MT. Plasma norepinephrine as a guide to prognosis

in patients with chronic congestive heart failure. N Engl J Med 1984; 311:819–823.

103. Naughton MT, Benard DC, Liu PP, Rutherford R, Rankin F, Bradley TD. Effects of nasal CPAP on sympathetic activity in patients with heart failure and central sleep apnea. Am J Respir Crit Care Med 1995; 152:473–479.

104. Swedberg K, Eneroth P, Kjekshus J, Wilhelmsen L. Hormones regulating cardiovascular function in patients with severe congestive heart failure and their relation to mortality. Circulation 1990; 82:1730–1736.

105. Francis GS, Cohn JN, Johnson G, Rector TS, Goldman S, Simon A and the V-HeFT VA Cooperative Studies Group. Plasma norepinephrine, plasma renin activity, and congestive heart failure. Circulation 1993; 87(suppl VI):40–48.

106. Javaheri S, Parker TJ, Wexler L, Liming JD, Lindower P, Roselle GA. Effect of theophylline on sleep-disordered breathing in heart failure. N Engl J Med 1996; 335:562–567.

107. DeBacker WA, Verbraecken J, Willemen M, Wittesaele W, DeCock W, Van de-Heyning P. Central apnea index decreases after prolonged treatment with acetazolamide. Am J Respir Crit Care Med 1995; 151:87–91.

108. Lorenzi-Filho G, Rankin F, Bies I, Merson R, Rosenberg J, Bradley TD. Effects of inhaled CO_2 and O_2 on Cheyne-Stokes respiration in patients with heart failure. Am J Respir Crit Care Med 1999; 159:1490–1498.

109. Andreas S, Hagenah G, Moller C, Heindl S. Treatment of Cheyne-Stokes respiration with nasal oxygen and carbon dioxide. Am J Respir Crit Care Med 1998; 157: A776.

110. Steens RD, Millar TW, Su X, Biberdorf D, Buckle P, Ahmed M, Kryger MH. Effect of inhaled 3% CO_2 on Cheyne-Stokes respiration in congestive heart failure. Sleep 1994; 17:61–68.

111. Eldridge FL, Millhorn DE, Waldrop TG. Mechanism of respiratory effects of methylxanthines. Respir Physiol 1983; 53:239–261.

112. Hanly PJ, Millar TW, Steljes DG, Baert R, Frais MA, Kryger MH. The effect of oxygen on respiration and sleep in patients with congestive heart failure. Ann Intern Med 1989; 111:777–782.

113. Bittar G, Friedman HS. The arrhythmogenicity of theophylline: a multivariate analysis of clinical determinants. Chest 1991; 99:1415–1420.

114. Packer M, Carver JR, Rodeheffer RJ, Ivanhoe RJ, DiBianco R, Zeldis SM, Hendrix GH, Bommer WJ, Elkayam U, Kukin ML, Mallis GI, Sollano JA, Shannon J, Tandon PK, DeMets DL. Effect of oral milrinone on mortality in severe chronic heart failure. N Engl J Med 1991; 325:1468–1475.

115. Dies F, Krell MJ, Whitlow P. Intermittent dobutamine in ambulatory outpatients with chronic cardiac failure. Circulation 1986; 74(suppl II):II–39.

116. White DP, Zwillich CW, Pickett CK, Douglas NJ, Findley LJ, Weil JV. Central sleep apnea: improvement with acetazolamide therapy. Arch Intern Med 1982; 142: 1816–1819.

117. Tojima H, Kunitomo F, Kimura H, Tatsumi K, Kuriyama T, Honda Y. Effects of acetazolamide in patients with sleep apnoea syndrome. Thorax 1988; 43:113–119.

118. Bickler PE, Litt L, Banville D, Severinghaus JW. Effects of acetazolamide on cerebral acid-base balance. J Appl Physiol 1988; 65:422–427.

119. Sakamoto T, Nakazawa Y, Hashizume Y, Tsutsumi Y, Mizuma H, Hirano T, Mukai M, Kotorii T. Effects of acetazolamide on the sleep apnea syndrome and its therapeutic mechanism. Psychiatry Clin Neurosci 1995; 49:59–64.

120. Xie A, Rutherford R, Rankin F, Wong B, Bradley TD. Hypocapnia and increased ventilatory responsiveness in patients with idiopathic central sleep apnea. Am J Respir Crit Care Med 1995; 152:1950–1955.

121. Xie A, Wong B, Phillipson EA, Slutsky AS, Bradley TD. Interaction of hyperventilation and arousal in the pathogenesis of idiopathic central sleep apnea. Am J Respir Crit Care Med 1994; 150:489–495.

122. Xie A, Rankin F, Rutherford R, Bradley TD. Effects of inhaled CO_2 and added deadspace on idiopathic central sleep apnea. J Appl Physiol 1997; 82:918–926.

123. Bonnet MH, Dexter JR, Arand DL. The effect of triazolam on arousal and respiration in central sleep apnea. Sleep 1990; 13:31–41.

124. Dalen JE, Evans GL, Banas JS. The hemodynamic and respiratory effects of diazepam (Valium). Anesthesiology 1969; 30:259–263.

125. Biberdorf DJ, Steens R, Millar TW, Kryger MH. Benzodiazepines in congestive heart failure: effect of temazepam on arousabillity and Cheyne-Stokes respiration. Sleep 1993; 16:529–538.

126. Berssenbrugge A, Dempsey J, Iber C, Skatrud J, Wilson P. Mechanisms of hypoxia-induced periodic breathing during sleep in humans. J Physiol 1983; 343:507–524.

127. Franklin KA, Eriksson P, Sahlin C, Lundgren R. Reversal of central sleep apnea with oxygen. Chest 1997; 111:163–169.

128. Franklin KA, Sandstrom E, Johansson G, Balfors EM. Hemodynamics, cerebral circulation, and oxygen saturation in Cheyne-Stokes respiration. J Appl Physiol 1997; 83:1184–1191.

129. Andreas S, Clemens C, Sandholzer H, Figulla HR, Kreuzer H. Improvement of exercise capacity with treatment of Cheyne-Stokes respiration in patients with congestive heart failure. J Am Coll Cardiol 1996; 27:1486–1490.

130. Staniforth AD, Kinnear WJM, Starling R, Hetmanski DJ, Cowley AJ. Effect of oxygen on sleep quality, cognitive function and sympathetic activity in patients with chronic heart failure and Cheyne-Stokes respiration. Eur Heart J 1998; 19: 922–928.

131. Haque WA, Boehmer J, Clemson BS, Leuenberger UA, Silber DH, Sinoway LI. Hemodynamic effects of supplemental oxygen administration in congestive heart failure. J Am Coll Cardiol 1996; 27:353–357.

AUTHOR INDEX

Numbers in italics give the page on which the complete reference is listed.

Stricker EM, 197, *210*
Strohl KP, 220, *225*, 243, *258*, 274,
  282, 360, 361, 362, 363, *381*
Struck LM, 449, *460*
Stuart RS, 389, 393, *409*
Su X, 482, *493*
Suadicani P, 273, 275, *281*, 282
Suda T, 323, *335*
Sugita Y, 291, *303*
Sugiyama Y, 118, 120, 122, 124, 125,
  129, 139, 141, 143, *154*, *155*, 339,
  350, *352*, *354*
Sulkava R, 286, *301*
Sullivan CE, 153, *158*, 215, 221, *224*,
  275, *282*, 296, *306*, 370, 373, *382*,
  393, *411*, 463, *488*
Sullivan MJ, 477, 484, *492*
Sullivan PJ, 218, 222, *225*
Summer WR, 17, *30*, 440, 441, 445,
  458, *459*, 467, *489*
Sun MK, 64, 68, 71, 73, 76, 82, 85, 87,
  89, *91*, *92*, *93*, *94*, 97, *98*
Sun QJ, 76, 82, 86, *95*, 97, *98*
Sundaram K, 63, 66, 83, *88*, 90
Sundlof G, 139, *154*
Surawicz B, 256, *259*
Sutton JR, 360, 367, 374, *381*, *382*
Sutton TW, 309, 315, 320, *324*, *328*
Suwarno NO, 10, 14, 15, 16, 17, 22, *28*,
  119, 123, *130*, 391, 394, 401, *410*
Suzuki K, 319, 321, *331*
Suzuki M, 153, *158*, 275, *282*
Suzuki S, 86, *98*
Suzuki T, 144, *155*
Svardsudd K, 275, *282*
Sved AF, 72, 73, *93*
Svensson TH, 128, *133*
Swan HJC, 101, *111*
Swan JW, 52, *59*
Swanson GD, 34, *56*, 362, *381*
Swedberg K, 406, *414*, 442, *459*, 481,
  493
Sweer L, 220, *225*
Sweer LW, 378, *384*
Switzer DA, 286, 292, *301*
Swoyer J, 321, 322, *333*

Syper KM, 12, 13, *28*
Szulczyk A, 21, *30*
Szulczyk P, 21, *30*

T

Tabachnik E, 342, *353*
Tafil M, 145, *156*
Taguchi K, 74, *94*
Taguchi O, 165, 166, 168, 174, *178*
Taha BH, 1, 3, 4, 5, 6, 7, 8, 9, 10, *24*,
  25
Taichman GC, 101, *110*
Takahashi K, 391, 403, *410*
Takahashi Y, 391, 403, *410*
Takakura K, 321, *332*
Takasaki Y, 99, *109*, 385, 386, 402,
  403, 404, 405, *406*, 418, 419, *431*,
  462, 474, 477, *487*
Takata M, 445, *459*
Takayama K, 76, *95*
Take H, 320, *332*
Takeuchi S, 141, 143, *155*, 350, *354*
Takita K, 319, 321, *331*
Talajic M, 316, *328*
Tam A, 370, *382*, 397, 398, 404, *412*,
  426, *432*, 473, 475, 484, *491*
Tamminen M, 319, *331*
Tamura K, 320, *332*
Tan GA, 366, *381*
Tan TL, 153, *158*
Tanaka K, 243, *258*, 278, *283*
Tandon PK, 483, *493*
Tang PC, 17, *30*
Tangel DJ, 343, 347, *353*, *354*
Tanne D, 319, *331*
Tarasiuk A, 108, *112*, 162, 164, 165,
  169, *177*, 402, *413*, 443, 444, 445,
  446, 447, 448, 454, *459*, *460*, 469,
  470, *489*, *490*
Tarazi RC, 208, *212*
Tardy B, 311, *326*
Tateishi O, 323, *335*
Tatsumi K, 483, *493*
Tatu L, 319, 321, *330*
Taube A, 272, *281*, 286, 288, 289, *301*

SUBJECT INDEX

f refers to figures, t *to tables.*

A

α_1-adrenergic agonists, glycinergic PSPs and, 66

Acetazolamide, effect on CSR-CSA in congestive heart failure, 483–484

Acetylcholinesterase (AChE), 74–75
RVLM neurons, 73–74

Acute myocardial infarction, baroflex sensitivity, 37

Airway obstruction and coronary blood flow, 235–237

Airway pressure and cardiac output, mechanical ventilation in, 441–443

Airway resistance, sleep onset and, 342f, 343, 346f

Alcohol, OSA and, in congestive heart failure, 463

Anger and myocardial infarction, 312–313

Angina, ST-segment change in, 251, 251f

Angiotensin, baroflex sensitivity and, 37

Angiotensin II, central respiratory effects and, 38

Aortic arch baroreceptors, 13, 117

Aortic body chemoreceptors, hypoxia and, 34

Apnea, 4–5
vs. cardiac asthma, 416
central sleep. *See* Central sleep apnea
mixed sleep, 286–287
obstructive sleep. *See* Obstructive sleep apnea

Apnea-hypopnea index
frequency distribution, 418, 418f
heart failure, 419
left ventricular ejection fraction, 420

Apnea-recovery cycle, 214, 214f
heart rate changes, 215–216
systemic arterial pressure, 216–217

Arousal and obstructive apnea
acute response, 220–221
animal models, 170–173

Arrhythmias
circadian rhythm, 310
CPAP, 469–470
OSA, 396

Arrhythmogenesis, sleep and, 237–238

Arterial baroreceptors, 76
arterial blood pressure, 36

Arterial baroreflex sensitivity, 144

Arterial blood bases, heart failure and, 420–421, 421f